EXTRA CALORIES = EXTRA POUNDS

The most successful diet in the United States today is what people call "my own diet." Forget fads. With the sound advice and calorie information found in *The Calorie Counter*, 4th Edition, you can design your own diet that will help you achieve optimum health.

- **Understand calories**
- **Understand portions**
- **Determine the calories needed daily**
- **Calculate the calories used daily through exercise**
- **Find out the truth about dieting myths**
- **Manage "mindless eating"**
- **Lose weight**

Reading a book by Natow and Heslin is like having lunch with an old friend—you'll feel supported and encouraged to make the changes needed to eat right, lose weight, and keep it off.

THE CALORIE COUNTER

Books by Annette B. Natow and Jo-Ann Heslin

The Calorie Counter (Fourth Edition)

The Cholesterol Counter (Sixth Edition)

The Complete Food Counter (Second Edition)

The Diabetes Carbohydrate and Calorie Counter
(Third Edition)

Eating Out Food Counter

The Fat Counter (Sixth Edition)

The Healthy Heart Food Counter

The Most Complete Food Counter (Second Edition)

The Protein Counter (Second Edition)

The Ultimate Carbohydrate Counter

The Vitamin and Mineral Food Counter

Published by POCKET BOOKS

THE
CALORIE COUNTER

Fourth Edition

Annette B. Natow, Ph.D., R.D.

Jo-Ann Heslin, M.A., R.D.

With the assistance of Karen J. Nolan, Ph.D.

POCKET BOOKS

New York   London   Toronto   Sydney

POCKET BOOKS, a division of Simon & Schuster, Inc.
1230 Avenue of the Americas, New York, NY 10020

Copyright © 2003, 2007 by Annette B. Natow and Jo-Ann Heslin

ISBN-13: 978-1-4165-0982-0
ISBN-10:   1-4165-0982-8

This Pocket Books paperback edition January 2007

10   9   8   7   6   5

POCKET and colophon are registered trademarks of Simon & Schuster, Inc.

Cover photo by FoodPix

Manufactured in the United States of America

For information regarding special discounts for bulk purchases, please contact Simon & Schuster Special Sales at 1-800-456-6798 or business@simonandschuster.com.

To our families, who support us through every project:
Harry, Allen, Irene, Sarah, Meryl, Laura, Marty,
George, Emily, Steven, Rebecca, Joseph, Kristen,
Brian, Karen, and John.

ACKNOWLEDGMENTS

For graciously sharing her knowledge: Karen J. Nolan, Ph.D.

For all her continuous support and help, our agent, Nancy Trichter.

For her suggestions and editing skills, Sara Clemence.

Without the tireless cooperation of Stephen Llano and the production department at Pocket Books, *The Calorie Counter, 4th Edition* would never have been completed.

A special thank you to our editor, Micki Nuding.

And, we'd like to thank all our readers for their suggestions and questions. Your input helps us to provide you with the most useful information.

CONTENTS

"Man is to be compared to a clock, going all the time, rather than to an automobile engine, working only at intervals. . . .
"In order to have energy to spend . . . we must first acquire it . . . protein, fat and carbohydrate . . . are the fuels which supply energy for the human machine."

Mary Swartz Rose, Ph.D.
Feeding the Family
The Macmillan Company, 1919

INTRODUCTION

If losing weight were easy, no one would weigh too much.

If you're looking at this book, you are probably looking for help losing weight. You aren't alone; *losing weight has become one of the most important health concerns in America.*

Everyone is scrambling to solve the problem of America's expanding waistlines. The federal government, public health organizations, professional organizations, educators, pharmaceutical companies, food manufacturers, and even restaurant chains are all banding together to slow down the nation's weight gain epidemic. But new policies, programs, food formulations, and drug approvals occur slowly. Like most people we talk to every day, you are not willing to wait. *You want to lose weight now!*

So let's get started—

Weight gain results from a combination of your genes and your environment. There isn't much you can do about your genetic profile, which was fixed before you were born. But you *can* control your environment, especially your eating environment. And that's what we hope *The Calorie Counter* will help you do.

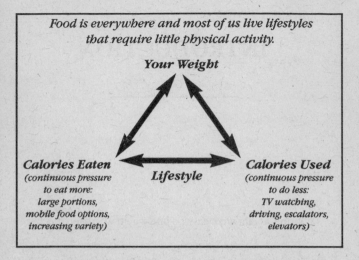

Food is everywhere and most of us live lifestyles that require little physical activity.

Your Weight

Calories Eaten
(continuous pressure to eat more: large portions, mobile food options, increasing variety)

Lifestyle

Calories Used
(continuous pressure to do less: TV watching, driving, escalators, elevators)

Two important things you should know:

The most successful diet in the U.S. today is what people call "my own diet." Forget fads. With the sound advice and the calorie information found in this book, you can design your own diet—one that works.

Consistent small changes will add up to big results. When it comes to losing weight and *maintaining* your weight loss, making many small changes in the way you relate to food will result in more success than making a few big changes, which usually don't last.

Skeptical?

If you eat 100 fewer calories each day for a year, and change nothing else in your life, you will lose 10 pounds. All you'd have to do is give up 1 slice of bread or 1 cookie or 1 small soda. A small change for a big result. Make a few more of those small changes and the end result could be very impressive.

Our best eating advice, in a nutshell:

- Eat less, but enjoy what you eat
- Eat lots of fruits and vegetables
- Eat whole grains instead of refined carbs (like white bread)
- Eat less sugar (but you don't have to give it up)
- Eat more good fats like olive oil, fish, and nuts
- Eat lean proteins
- Enjoy a glass of wine—but not the whole bottle
- Move more and move often—find ways to be active throughout the day

---

Aim for 10%

Losing 10% of your body weight—15 pounds for someone who weighs 150 pounds, 20 pounds for a person weighing 200 pounds, or 30 pounds if the scale tips in at 300 pounds—is all that is needed to significantly improve your health.

Lose 10% of your current body weight and you'll have:

> *Lower blood pressure*
> *Improved cholesterol levels*
> *Decreased risk for diabetes*
> *Better sex*

Reaching your ideal weight is great, but even just a 10% drop in body weight improves both your health and appearance.

UNDERSTANDING CALORIES

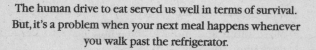

The human drive to eat served us well in terms of survival. But, it's a problem when your next meal happens whenever you walk past the refrigerator.

Calories are calories, whether they come from apples or chocolate fudge. Every time you eat, you take in calories. All foods, except water, have some. Your body is a machine that uses food calories as fuel. When the amount of fuel you take in equals the amount of fuel you need to run your body, your weight remains constant. There is no extra fuel to store and no deficit to make up. Eat too many calories, and your body uses what it needs and stores the leftovers for future use. You see this storage on your thighs, hips, and waist. Eat too few calories, and your body draws on its fuel reserves to meet demands. Your thighs, hips, and waist get slimmer as your fuel surplus is depleted.

You can think of the extra pounds you are carrying around as a warehouse of stored fuel. Empty the warehouse and you lose weight. Fill up the warehouse and you gain.

Again and again, studies have shown that if you cut calories, you lose weight. It doesn't matter if those calories come from bread, meat, or salad dressing. When you eat too many calories, even from healthy foods, you gain weight.

The key to long-term weight control is to burn as many calories as you eat. In order to do that effectively, you need to know how many calories you need, and how many calories you burn in activity. Then, you can see if the two balance each other.

And the Numbers Are?

On average, we eat 300 more calories a day than we ate 35 years ago and we weigh 24 pounds more. Women eat 1880 calories a day; men eat 2620.

UNDERSTANDING PORTIONS

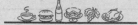

Smaller portions = a smaller you.

With the exception of a slice of bread, the portion sizes of commonly eaten foods have steadily grown over the last 20 years. Even the average restaurant dinner plate is 2 inches larger! We've gotten so used to these exaggerated amounts that we think of them as normal.

What Research Has Shown

Larger portions encourage people to overeat, even foods that they don't like or that don't taste good.

Serving large portions encourages people to eat up to 40% more calories at a meal.

After eating a large portion or a regular portion, people rated their feelings of fullness the same, though they ate more of the large portion.

Twenty years ago, the muffin or bagel you bought with your morning coffee weighed 2 ounces. Today, 4 to 6 ounces is more the norm. When burger shops first opened, an average soda was 8 ounces, regular french fries were 2.5 ounces, and the burger plus bun weighed less than 4 ounces. Today, a medium soda averages 20 ounces, and the french fries and burger have been supersized: they're 2 to 5 times larger than the original, adding up to a 1000 calorie meal.

You may think larger portions are bargains without appreciating how many extra calories you're eating. According to a government survey, Americans typically eat 2½ times the standard serving of potatoes, 4 times the standard serving of pasta, and 2 times the standard serving of rice. We even eat large portions of good-for-you fruits and vegetables. Many people don't realize that larger portions have more calories. They figure a soda is a soda, no matter how big—until you stop and calculate that a 32-ounce soda has 400 calories. Next time you order, think small—soda, coffee, movie theater popcorn, ice cream cones, french fries, even medium-size fruits.

Seeing Is Believing—

These visual cues will help you keep portion sizes reasonable.

computer mouse	=	*4-ounce portion of meat, chicken, seafood*
		or
		1 medium baked potato
yo-yo	=	*a mini bagel or 100 calories. How many yo-yo's fit into your bagel, muffin, or pastry?*
tennis ball	=	*medium piece of fresh fruit*
ping-pong ball	=	*2 ounces cheese*
		or
		2 tablespoons salad dressing, gravy, sour cream
thumbnail	=	*1 pat butter*

When you snack, pick single serving packages. How many times have you opened a bag of chips just to have a few, and before you knew it, the bag was empty? A one-ounce, snack-size bag of chips allows you to enjoy a favorite treat without sabotaging your weight loss goals. Single serving pudding, ice cream, pretzels, peanuts, cookies, and snack-size yogurt will help you keep overindulging under control.

CALORIES YOU NEED

Obesity may soon replace smoking as the country's leading
cause of preventable death.

Most of us eat more than we admit and exercise less than we
should. The consequence is that we weigh more than we
want and blame it all on our metabolism—even if we're not
quite sure what that is.

Metabolism is all the chemical reactions that occur in your
body. Your body takes in foods, burns some to generate
power, uses some to produce new material, and routes the
rest into storage for future use. The chemical reactions that
occur either break down large compounds into smaller units
(the foods you eat, for example, are broken down into smaller
units of energy), or build complex structures from smaller
units (your muscles are made up of fragments that come from
the protein foods you eat, like eggs). Human metabolism is
the sum total of all the energy used to keep your body alive
and moving. This energy requirement can be translated into
the calories you need each day.

Approximately 60% to 75% of your daily calories are used
just to keep you alive. Energy is needed to maintain your
body's temperature, allow your nerves to work, let you
breathe, keep your heart beating, allow your organs to func-
tion, nourish your body tissues, and repair and replace body

fluids and parts. It's a pretty big job that goes on 24 hours a day.

An interesting thing about this basic energy requirement is that different tissues in the body have different levels of activity. Fat tissue is less active and needs less energy. Muscle tissue, even at rest, is more active and uses up more energy. If you exercise and develop more muscle tissue, your body burns more calories every day just keeping your muscles healthy.

The rest of the calories you need each day are used to support your level of activity. Obviously, you need less if you are relatively inactive and more if you are very active.

To find out how many calories you need each day, you need to do two things. First, how much do you want to weigh? Not your current weight, but what is your target weight? Then, select an activity factor that fits your current activity level.

1. Your target weight is: _____
2. Your activity factor is: _____
   20 = Very active men
   15 = Moderately active men or very active women
   13 = Inactive men, moderately active women, and people over 55
   10 = Inactive women, repeat dieters, and seriously overweight people
3. Target weight × activity factor = calories needed each day.

For example, if your target weight is 130 and you are a moderately active woman (factor 13), you need about 1600 to 1700 calories a day.

130 pounds × 13 = 1690 calories

Eating this amount of calories each day would guarantee weight loss, because you are getting only enough calories to support your target weight, not your current heavier weight. Couple this calorie intake with some added exercise and the weight will come off even faster.

THE TRUTH, AND NOTHING BUT THE TRUTH

People who wear belts stop eating sooner
than people who don't.

French women do get fat.

Nearly 40% of the French are overweight and over 11% are obese; the rate is increasing yearly by 6% in adults and 11% in children. Experts blame the nation's weight gain on the loss of leisurely French-style eating, more snacking, more convenience foods, and less walking.

Repeated dieting does not slow down your metabolism.

You've probably heard over and over again that yo-yo dieting (repeatedly losing and regaining weight) slows down your metabolism and makes it harder to burn calories. It's just not true. Repeat dieters do not have slower metabolisms; they can and do burn calories just as efficiently as everyone else. So no matter how many times you have tried to lose weight in the past, you can succeed if you try again.

Sugar and fast food do not make you fat.

There is no specific food that causes weight gain. The only thing that makes you fat is eating too many calories. If you eat too much sugar and too many fast foods, you will gain weight. If you eat both in moderation, you won't. People who eat a lot of sugar or fast food also frequently eat larger portions, eat more often, and eat fewer good-for-you foods, like fruits, vegetables, and whole grains.

Smoking is not an effective weight loss strategy.

As a matter of fact, research has shown that smoking increases the accumulation of belly fat. Smokers, even lean ones, have thicker waists than nonsmokers.

Skipping meals does not help you cut calories.

People who eat many small amounts of food during the day are slimmer than those who eat fewer, larger meals. Regular breakfast skippers are 450% more likely to be overweight. *Eat when you're hungry, stop when you're full* is a simple rule that is difficult to follow. But those who do, usually eat fewer calories than people who sit down to a big lunch or dinner simply because the clock says it's time to eat.

Nighttime calories are no more fattening than daytime calories.

Time of day doesn't matter; the calorie count does. You can eat all the calories you need for a entire day between midnight and 6 A.M., if you wish. As long as you don't eat any more during the rest of the day, you won't gain weight. The warning against late-night eating *does* have value if the calories eaten watching TV or coping with stress are on top of the calories you've already eaten during the day.

One package does not always equal one serving.

Read food labels carefully to see if a package—even a small one—contains more than 1 serving. Many foods and snacks are currently packaged as single servings, and that's exactly what you are getting: 1 serving. But other "smaller"-size packages may hold more that 1 serving. For example, a small bag of chips may hold 2½ servings. Eat the whole bag and you've eaten 2½ times the calories listed as a serving.

Fat-free is not calorie free.

Buying fat-free foods seems virtuous and can seduce you into eating larger amounts. But beware: some brands of fat-free cookies, cakes, and crackers have the same number of calories as the regular versions. No reduced-fat choices are calorie free. If a fat-free salad dressing has half of the calories of a regular version and you use twice as much, there's no calorie benefit.

You won't burn fat faster if you exercise harder.

The intensity of your exercise makes no difference, as long as you burn more calories than you eat. It doesn't matter how long it takes you to go a distance: the more ground you cover, the more calories you burn. For each pound you weigh, you burn 1 calorie per mile. So whether walking, hiking, jogging, or sprinting, a 100-pound person burns 100 calories a mile on a flat surface, a 200-pound person uses 200 calories, and so on. Keep in mind that the time you exercise is only a small part of the day. A daily active lifestyle may actually burn more calories than a single exercise session—take the stairs, don't use the drive-thru, play with the kids at the park.

Water is a powerful calorie burner.

Seventy-five percent of people don't drink enough water. When you have too little water in your body, your metabolism slows down and you burn fewer calories. Exercising, running errands, and staying out in the sun can all make you mildly dehydrated. Water, juice, seltzer, mineral water, milk, and caffeine-free coffee, tea, and soda all contribute to your fluid intake. If you don't urinate at least every 4 hours when you are awake, you probably need to be drinking more.

Sleep Too Little, Weigh Too Much

People who sleep more weigh less. Getting too little sleep triggers hormonal changes that lead to increased appetite. Plus, more hours awake means more time to eat, and if you're tired, you're less likely to exercise—all adding up to extra pounds.

CALORIES YOU USE

There is less risk in activity than continuous inactivity.

Activity burns calories. Activity also builds muscles, which burn calories 70 times faster than fat. Someone who has been relatively inactive will see health benefits from using up just 500 extra calories a week through activity. If you're a true couch potato, this may be the level at which to start. Real weight loss and fitness benefits start to kick in when you use up 1,000 calories a week through activity. Consider 2,000 calories as a great goal to strive for over time.

Everything you do counts, planned activities as well as real-life fitness: walking, gardening, golf, tennis, even housework. The more active you are, the more calories you burn. And, the really good news is that research has shown you benefit from exercise whether the activity is continuous or done in small bursts. Being active for as little as 10 minutes at a time not only burns calories, but has a positive impact on your health. The key is to *move* every day.

Real-life Fitness

- Pace while you're talking on the phone
- Deliver memos and messages in person rather than by e-mail or phone

- Go window-shopping
- Clean your house—washing floors, vacuuming carpets, washing windows, and scrubbing bathrooms equal vigorous exercise
- Garden—weeding, hoeing, cutting the lawn, raking or trimming bushes burns as many calories as playing a game of tennis
- Turn your lunch break into an hour-long excursion
- Carry a basket when shopping for a few items—it's like a free weight that keeps getting heavier and heavier; switch arms for a maximum workout
- Sign up for a charity walk, bike, or run
- Turn off the TV one night a week and plan something active
- Make exercise a hobby—take golf, tennis, or skating lessons
- Park your car at the farthest end of the parking lot
- Take the stairs—you burn 10 calories for every flight you climb; over a lifetime that uses up thousands of calories
- Dance—salsa, polka, or tango; square dancers can cover 5 miles in an evening
- Grocery shop—one hour of pushing, lifting, and bending in the supermarket uses as many calories as a half hour on a treadmill
- Spend rainy weekend afternoons walking around a museum; when the sun shines, go to the zoo
- Wash the car
- Go bowling instead of to the movies

- Walk the dog
- Push the baby in a stroller or take the kids to the play-ground
- Be an active spectator—walk around the soccer field while the kids are playing
- Play games as a family—badminton, volleyball, stickball, croquet
- Practice yoga

Don't Sit Your Life Away

Americans average 23 hours a week in front of the TV. That adds up to almost 10 years over an average life-time!

Daily activity helps you reach your target weight faster. Depending on your current level of activity, aim to use up 500 to 1,000 calories a week. Your ultimate goal is to double this amount as you become more fit. In the table "Using Up Calories," page 19, find the activity you've done and the weight column closest to your current weight. Multiply the calories burned in 1 minute by the number of minutes you were active.

For example, if you weigh 150 pounds and you weeded your flowerbed for 15 minutes, you used up almost 89 calories.

Gardening (weeding)
5.9 (calories burned in 1 minute) × 15 minutes = 88.5 calories

If your activity goal for the week is to burn 500 calories, you've already burned 89 with one simple chore.

Keep track of the calories you burn each day, and total the amount you burn in a week.

USING UP CALORIES

POUNDS	100	125	150	175	200
ACTIVITY	CALORIES USED PER MINUTE				
Archery	3.1	4.0	4.8	5.6	6.4
Auto repair	2.8	3.5	4.2	4.8	5.5
Badminton	3.6	4.6	5.4	6.4	7.3
Baseball	3.1	4.0	4.7	5.5	6.3
Basketball	4.9	6.2	9.9	11.5	13.2
Bicycling					
5 mph	1.9	2.4	2.9	3.4	3.9
10 mph	4.2	5.3	6.4	7.4	8.5
Bowling	2.7	3.4	4.1	4.5	5.5
Boxing	6.2	7.8	9.3	10.9	12.4
Calisthenics, light	3.4	4.3	5.2	6.1	7.0
Canoeing, 4 mph	4.4	5.5	6.7	7.8	8.9
Card playing	1.0	1.6	1.9	2.2	2.5
Carpentry	2.6	3.2	3.8	4.6	5.3
Chopping wood	4.8	6.0	7.2	8.4	9.6
Croquet	2.7	3.4	4.1	4.7	5.4
Dancing					
Active (square, disco)	4.5	5.6	6.8	7.9	9.1
Aerobic dance	6.0	7.6	9.1	10.8	12.1
Moderate (waltz)	3.1	4.0	4.8	5.6	6.4
Fencing, moderate	3.3	4.1	5.0	5.8	6.7
Fishing	2.8	3.5	4.2	4.9	5.6
Football, touch	5.5	6.9	8.3	9.7	11.1
Gardening					
Lawn mowing, manual	3.0	3.8	4.6	5.2	5.9
Lawn mowing, power	2.7	3.4	4.1	4.7	5.4
Light gardening	2.4	3.0	3.6	4.2	4.8
Weeding	3.9	4.9	5.9	6.8	7.8
Golf					
Twosome (carry clubs)	3.6	4.6	5.4	6.4	7.3
Foursome (carry clubs)	2.7	3.4	4.1	4.5	5.4
Gymnastics	3.0	3.8	4.5	5.3	6.0

(continued)

POUNDS	100	125	150	175	200
ACTIVITY	CALORIES USED PER MINUTE				
Handball	6.5	6.2	9.9	11.5	13.2
Hiking, 3 mph	4.5	5.5	6.8	7.9	9.1
Hockey, field	5.0	7.6	9.1	10.8	12.1
Hockey, ice	6.6	8.3	10.0	11.7	13.4
Horseback riding					
Walk	1.9	2.4	2.9	3.4	3.9
Trot	2.7	3.4	4.1	4.8	5.4
Gallop	5.7	7.2	8.7	10.1	11.6
Horseshoes	2.5	3.1	3.8	4.4	5.2
House painting	2.3	2.9	3.5	4.0	4.6
Housework					
Dusting	1.8	2.3	2.6	3.1	3.5
Making beds	2.6	3.2	3.8	4.6	5.3
Washing floors	3.0	3.8	4.6	5.3	6.1
Washing windows	2.8	3.5	4.2	4.8	5.5
Ice Skating	4.2	5.2	6.4	7.4	8.5
Judo	8.5	10.6	12.8	14.9	17.1
Karate	8.5	10.6	12.8	14.9	17.1
Lacrosse	9.5	11.9	14.3	16.6	19.0
Motorcycling	2.4	3.0	3.6	4.2	4.8
Mountain climbing	6.5	8.2	9.8	11.5	13.1
Paddle ball	5.7	7.2	8.7	10.1	11.6
Pool (billiards)	1.5	1.9	2.2	2.6	3.0
Racquetball	6.5	8.1	9.8	11.4	13.0
Rollerblading, 9 mph	4.2	5.3	6.4	7.4	8.5
Rowing	3.4	4.2	5.0	5.9	6.7
Rowing machine	9.1	11.4	13.7	16.0	18.2
Running, steady rate					
5 mph	6.0	7.6	9.1	10.8	12.2
7 mph	9.7	12.1	14.6	17.1	19.5
Sailing, small boat	4.2	5.2	6.4	7.4	8.5
Shoveling snow	5.2	6.5	7.8	8.9	10.2
Skiing, alpine downhill	6.4	8.0	9.6	11.2	12.8

POUNDS	100	125	150	175	200
ACTIVITY	**CALORIES USED PER MINUTE**				
Skiing, cross-country					
2.5 mph	5.0	6.2	7.5	8.8	10.0
4 mph	6.5	8.2	9.9	11.5	13.2
Skindiving, moderate	9.4	11.8	14.1	16.5	18.8
Soccer	5.9	7.4	8.9	10.3	11.8
Squash	6.7	8.4	10.1	11.8	13.5
Swimming					
Backstroke	2.5	3.1	3.8	4.4	5.1
Breaststroke	3.1	4.0	4.8	5.6	6.4
Front crawl	4.0	5.0	6.0	7.0	8.0
Table tennis	3.4	4.3	5.2	6.3	7.2
Tennis					
Singles	5.0	6.2	7.5	6.8	10.0
Doubles	3.4	4.3	5.2	6.1	7.0
Typing	1.5	1.9	2.3	2.7	3.1
Volleyball	2.9	3.6	4.4	5.1	5.9
Walking					
1 mph	1.5	1.9	2.3	2.7	3.1
2 mph	2.1	2.6	3.2	3.7	4.3
4 mph	4.2	5.3	6.4	7.4	8.5
Water skiing	5.0	6.2	7.5	8.8	10.0
Weight training					
Free weights	3.9	4.9	5.9	6.8	7.8
Nautilus	4.2	5.3	6.3	7.4	8.4
Universal	5.3	6.6	8.0	9.3	10.6

Calorie Cost of Love

A kiss = 6 to 12 calories, depending on the intensity.
Lovemaking = 125 to 300 calories, depending on the
level of passion.

MINIMIZE MINDLESS EATING

Each of us makes over 112 food decisions a day.

You're thinking that's not possible. But it is. Each morning, you decide to eat or not. Cereal or toast? Toast with butter? Or butter and jelly? One slice or two? Coffee, tea, or coke? Milk or sugar? One spoonful or two? Fruit or juice? Large or small glass? Seconds?

These choices are considered *low involvement* decisions and often you're not even aware you're making them. They are mindless choices, but over time they can make a significant impact on what and how much you eat.

Your home and office are full of hidden persuaders, but there are a number of things you can do to become a more mindful eater.

Put distance between you and food.
The greater the distance you have to travel to get food, the less you eat. Empty the candy dish on your desk. At home, leave all food in the kitchen cabinets. Don't stock a mini refrigerator in the family room. Putting distance between you and food gives you enough time to pause and say, "Do I really want that?"

Use small plates, serving spoons, and bowls.

Large serving bowls encourage overeating. People take over 50% more food when given a large plate or when served from a large bowl. The next time you eat ice cream, use a dessert dish instead of a soup bowl. You generally eat whatever you serve yourself, so if you over-serve, you overeat. Shapes also affect consumption. You drink less from tall, slim glasses and more out of short, fat ones.

Don't be seduced by the "health halo."

Low fat, reduced calorie, low carb, sugar free, and *light* are all terms used to make you think a food is good for you. But too much of *any* food equals too many calories. A restaurant-size salad served in a huge bowl, slathered in dressing is more than anyone needs to eat at one sitting. Even healthy foods need to be eaten in moderation.

Buying bulk adds bulk.

Warehouse stores encourage you to buy bigger sizes, which leads to eating more, and eating more frequently. People take larger helpings out of larger packages. Single servings and individual packs are smarter purchases. Or, repack larger amounts into smaller sizes to discourage overeating.

Order small.

Regardless of the choice, go for the smallest option. At a restaurant, order a lunch or half portion. Select the small or regular coffee, even if it's called "tall." Try a "kid's" meal. Eat medium-size apples, oranges, and baked potatoes. Order a one-scoop cone. Remember, *smaller sizes = a smaller you.*

Rework your eating environment so it works *for* you, not against you. Counteract mindless eating with mindful solutions. Start small, easy, and doable—success, no matter how small, breeds success.

When Do You Eat Too Much?

Asked when they were most likely to overeat, 57% of people said at night, 25% said afternoon, and only 3% noted morning. Simply knowing this can help you cut calories and avoid temptation.

TRACKING CALORIES

People cut calories by 10% when they simply write down what they eat; 30% to 50% of those who keep a food diary change their eating habits.

We know it's a chore to write down everything you eat and keep track of the calories, but it's worth it. After a week of writing down calories, most people have a good idea of how many calories are in 75% of what they usually eat. And, people who keep a food diary are more successful at losing weight, even during difficult times like holidays.

"Your Daily Food Diary," on page 27, will tell you a lot about how you eat, why you eat, and what you eat. Research has shown that men are more likely to omit items than women, both sexes are more likely to omit snack items, and meat items are more likely to be underestimated than other foods. No one will ever see what you write down, so be honest.

Why is the day of the week important? Some days, like on weekends, you may eat more. Some people eat more on Friday, celebrating the end of a work week. Others eat more on Monday in response to the stress of a new week. If you find that some days trigger you to overeat, it will be easier to change the pattern.

We appreciate that many people eat on a crazy schedule, so the day is broken into 3 periods. It will help you figure out when you do the most eating.

A.M. is from midnight till noon. Many people eat in the middle of the night, so A.M. includes middle-of-the-night noshing, breakfast, coffee break, or morning snack.

Midday is from noon until dinner. It includes lunch and any afternoon or pre-dinner snack, like a drink after work.

P.M. is dinnertime through midnight. It includes your evening meal and after-dinner, TV, and bedtime snacks.

After a few days, you'll begin to see patterns in your eating habits. Ideally you want your calories to be spaced fairly evenly throughout the day. But we know that isn't always possible. Going too long without food or eating too frequently can both lead to eating too much.

By subtotaling your calories 3 times during the day, you can make adjustments for unexpected situations. For example, if a client comes in for lunch, you can skip your afternoon snack and eat a lighter dinner to compensate for the extra calories eaten at lunch.

Why does it matter if you eat alone or with company? Because many of us eat more when we are alone. Most people eat more with family and less with co-workers. Learning this about yourself can help you change habits that may be sabotaging your efforts to lose weight.

And finally, you'll want to note how many calories you burned through activity every day. Some days you may be more active than others, but if you start to fall into an inactive pattern, noting it will help you break the cycle quickly.

One meal or one day does not make a success or failure. But being totally honest with yourself can help keep you on the right track most of the time. Before you realize it, you'll be slimmer and fitter than ever before.

*It takes knowledge, motivation, action, and time
to create change.*

DAILY FOOD DIARY

Your Target Calorie Zone _____

Day _____ Date _____

Food	Portion	Calories	Ate Alone	With Company
AM				

AM Calorie Total _____

MIDDAY				

Midday Calorie Total _____

PM				

PM Calorie Total _____

Day's Calorie Total _____

Activity	Minutes Active	Calories Burned

Total Calories Burned _____

USING YOUR
CALORIE COUNTER

The Calorie Counter lists the calories and portion size for more than 20,000 foods. Now you can compare the values in your favorite foods and, when necessary, choose substitutes when you go out to shop or eat. This will save time and help you decide what to buy.

The counter section of the book is divided into two parts: Part One: Brand Name, Nonbranded (Generic), and Take-Out Foods (page 35); and Part Two: Restaurant Chains (page 511). Each part lists foods or restaurant chains alphabetically.

In Part One, for each category, you will find nonbranded (generic) foods listed first, in alphabetical order, followed by an alphabetical listing of brand name foods. The nonbranded listings will help you estimate calorie values when you don't see your favorite brand. They can also help you to evaluate store brands. Large categories are divided into subcategories, such as canned, fresh, frozen, and ready-to-eat, to make it easier to find what you're looking for. Some categories have "see" and "see also" references, to help you find related items.

Because we eat out so often, more than 600 take-out foods are listed in Part One. These are found in the take-out subcategory in many categories throughout this section. Look there for foods you take out or order in, since they are not nutrition labeled.

Most foods are listed alphabetically. In some cases, though, foods are grouped by category. For example, a tuna salad sandwich is found in the SANDWICH category. Other group categories include:

ASIAN FOOD   Page 42
 includes all types of Asian foods except
 egg rolls and sushi, which are found in
 separate categories

DELI MEATS/COLD CUTS   Page 211
 includes all sandwich meats except
 chicken, ham, and turkey, which are
 found in separate categories

DINNER   Page 213
 includes all by brand name, except
 pasta dinners, which are found in a
 separate category

LIQUOR/LIQUEUR   Page 310
 includes all alcoholic beverages and
 mixed drinks except beer, champagne,
 and wine, which are found in separate
 categories

NUTRITION SUPPLEMENTS   Page 337
 includes all dieting aids, meal
 replacements, and drinks except
 energy bars and energy drinks, which
 are found in separate categories

SANDWICHES   Page 415
 includes popular sandwich, calzone,
 and panini choices

SNACKS   Page 431

includes a variety of miscellaneous
snack items such as trail mix, pork
rinds, and cheese puffs

SPANISH FOOD   Page 459

includes all types of Spanish and
Mexican foods except salsa and
tortillas, which are found in separate
categories

In Part Two, Restaurant Chains, beginning on page 511, 97 national and regional restaurant, candy, coffee, doughnut, ice cream, pizza, and sandwich chains are listed. Brand name foods are required by federal law to have nutrition information on their labels, but restaurants provide this information only voluntarily.

With *The Calorie Counter* as your guide, you will never again wonder how many calories are in the food you eat.

DEFINITIONS

as prep (as prepared): refers to food that has been prepared according to package directions

lean and fat: describes meat with some fat on its edges that is not cut away before cooking, or poultry prepared with skin and fat as purchased

lean only: refers to lean meat that is trimmed of all visible fat, or poultry without skin

shelf-stable: refers to prepared products found on the supermarket shelf that are ready-to-eat or are ready to be heated and do not require refrigeration

take-out: describes prepared dishes that you purchase ready-to-eat; those included serve as a guide to the calories in products you may purchase.

ABBREVIATIONS

avg	=	average
diam	=	diameter
fl	=	fluid
frzn	=	frozen
g	=	gram
in	=	inch
lb	=	pound
lg	=	large
med	=	medium
mg	=	milligram
oz	=	ounce
pkg	=	package
pt	=	pint
prep	=	prepared
qt	=	quart
reg	=	regular
sec	=	second
serv	=	serving
sm	=	small
sq	=	square
tbsp	=	tablespoon
tr	=	trace
tsp	=	teaspoon
w/	=	with
w/o	=	without
<	=	less than

NOTES

0 (zero) indicates there are no calories in that food.

Discrepancies in figures are due to rounding, product reformulation, and reevaluation. Labeling law allows rounding of values. Some of the data listed is analysis data, obtained directly from manufacturers, not from labels. Therefore, some values may differ from those on labels because they have not been rounded.

PART ONE

Brand Name, Nonbranded (Generic), and Take-Out Foods

Eating 100 fewer calories each day can help you lose 10 pounds in a year! It can be done with small changes:

- Use mustard, salsa, or fat-free mayonnaise in place of 1 tablespoon regular mayonnaise
- Eat 1 slice of toast for breakfast instead of 2
- Order a cup of soup instead of a bowl
- Try a plain baked potato with pepper instead of sour cream
- Eat cereal with skim milk instead of whole milk
- Swap breaded and fried chicken fingers for broiled
- Use tuna packed in water rather than in oil
- Swap regular soda for diet soda
- Enjoy a glass of wine instead of a martini
- Have a chocolate kiss instead of a chocolate bar

FOOD	PORTION	CALS
ABALONE		
breaded & fried	1 serv (5 oz)	270
steamed	1 serv (3 oz)	177
ACAI JUICE		
Zola Acai		
Juice	1 box (11 oz)	170
ACEROLA		
fresh	1 (5 g)	2
ACEROLA JUICE		
juice	1 cup	56
ADZUKI BEANS		
canned sweetened	½ cup	351
dried cooked w/o salt	½ cup	147
AKEE		
fresh	3.5 oz	223
ALCOHOL (see BEER AND ALE, CHAMPAGNE, LIQUOR/LIQUEUR, MALT, WINE)		
ALE (see BEER AND ALE)		
ALFALFA		
sprouts	½ cup	40
ALLIGATOR		
cooked	3 oz	126
ALLSPICE		
ground	1 tsp	5
ALMONDS		
almond butter w/ salt	2 tbsp	203
almond butter w/o salt	2 tbsp	203
almond extract	1 tsp	38
almond paste	¼ cup	260
chocolate covered	6 pieces (0.6 oz)	102
dry roasted w/ salt	¼ cup	206
dry roasted w/o salt	¼ cup	206
honey roasted	¼ cup	214
jordan almonds	6 (0.7 oz)	99
oil roasted w/ salt	¼ cup	238

FOOD	PORTION	CALS
oil roasted w/o salt	¼ cup	238
praline	17 pieces (1.4 oz)	210
yogurt covered	6 pieces (0.8 oz)	122
American Almond		
Almond Paste	2 tbsp	140
Marzipan	2 tbsp	130
Roasted Butter	2 tbsp	180
Blue Diamond		
Almond Roca Buttercrunch	3 pieces (1.3 oz)	210
Honey Roasted	¼ cup	170
Jalapeno Smokehouse	28 pieces (1 oz)	170
Jordon Pastels	15 pieces (1.4 oz)	180
Lime 'N Chili	28 pieces (1 oz)	170
Maui Onion & Garlic	28 pieces (1 oz)	170
Milk Chocolate Covered	9 pieces (1.4 oz)	230
Salted	¼ cup	170
Smokehouse	28 pieces (1.3 oz)	170
Wasabi & Soy Sauce	28 pieces (1 oz)	170
Whole Natural	¼ cup	180
Yogurt Covered	12 pieces (1.4 oz)	210
Brach's		
Chocolate Coated	11 pieces	220
Judy's		
Sugar Free Coconut Almond Brittle	¼ piece (1 oz)	90
Keto		
Chocolatey Covered	1 oz	169
Low Carb Creations		
Soft Almond Brittle	2 pieces (1 oz)	170
Mama Mellace's		
Butter Rum	1 oz	150
Cinnamon Roasted	1 oz	140
Maranatha		
Almond Butter	2 tbsp	220
Raw Almond Butter	2 tbsp	190
Tamari Almonds	¼ cup	160
Odense		
Almond Paste	2 tbsp (1.4 oz)	170
Sweet Delights		
Almond Roasters	⅓ pkg (1 oz)	190

FOOD	PORTION	CALS
AMARANTH		
leaves cooked	½ cup	14
uncooked	½ cup (3.4 oz)	365
ANCHOVY		
boneless	1 oz	60
canned in oil drained	1 can (2 oz)	94
fresh	1 (4 g)	8
fresh fillets	3 (0.4 oz)	21
CANNED		
Brunswick		
Flat Fillets	1 can (2 oz)	25
ANGLERFISH		
raw	3.5 oz	72
ANISE		
seed	1 tsp	7
ANTELOPE		
roasted	4 oz	215
APPLE		
CANNED		
sliced sweetened	½ cup	68
Luck's		
Fried Apples	½ cup (4.7 oz)	130
DRIED		
chopped	½ cup	104
cooked w/o sugar	½ cup	73
rings	5	78
Crispy Green		
Crispy Apples	1 pkg (0.36 oz)	35
Del Monte		
Dried Apples	¼ cup	110
FRESH		
apple	1 lg	110
apple	1 med	72
apple	1 sm	55
candied	1 sm (4.9 oz)	179
candied	1 med (6.5 oz)	234
candied	1 lg (9.8 oz)	357

FOOD	PORTION	CALS
w/ skin sliced	1 cup	57
w/o skin sliced	1 cup	53
Chiquita		
Apple	1 med (5.4 oz)	80
Cool Cut		
Apples & Caramel Dip	1 pkg (4.25 oz)	180
TreeTop		
Slices Red or Green	1 pkg (2 oz)	35
FROZEN		
sliced w/o sugar	½ cup	42
TAKE-OUT		
baked	1 (6 oz)	128
baked no sugar	1 (5.6 oz)	136
fried apple rings	1 serv (2.7 oz)	91
APPLE JUICE		
cider	1 cup	117
drink	8 oz	125
frzn + vitamin C as prep	1 cup	112
frzn + vitamin C not prep	1 can (6 oz)	350
juice + vitamin C & calcium	1 cup	117
mulled cider	1 serv	265
unsweetened w/o vitamin C	1 cup	117
Apple & Eve		
100% Juice	8 fl oz	110
Cider	8 fl oz	110
Eden		
Organic Juice	8 oz	80
Hansen's		
Junior Juice 100%	1 box (4.23 oz)	60
Hi-C		
Sour Blast Green Apple	1 pkg	100
Kedem		
100% Juice	8 oz	110
Langers		
100% Cider	8 oz	120
100% Juice	8 oz	120
Diet Cocktail	8 oz	60
Low Carb Creations		
Apple Cider as prep	1 serv	10

FOOD	PORTION	CALS
Minute Maid		
100% Juice	8 oz	100
Mott's		
100% Juice	1 box (8 oz)	120
100% Juice	8 fl oz	120
100% Natural	8 fl oz	120
Naked Juice		
Just Apple	8 oz	120
NutraBalance		
Plus Fibre	1 pkg (8 oz)	120
Ocean Spray		
100% Juice	8 oz	110
Odwalla		
Spiced Harvest Cider	8 fl oz	130
Red Cheek		
100% Juice	8 oz	120
Robert & James		
100% Juice	8 oz	110
Seneca		
100% Juice	8 oz	110
Snapple		
Diet	8 oz	15
Snapple Apple	8 fl oz	120
Swiss Miss		
Hot Apple Cider Mix	1 serv	84
Hot Apple Cider Mix Low Calorie	1 serv	14
TreeTop		
100% Juice	8 oz	120
Cider 100% Juice No Sugar Added	8 oz	120
Tropicana		
Season's Best	8 oz	110
Turkey Hill		
Herbal Cider w/ Chamomile & Lemongrass	1 cup	100
Zeigler's		
Old Fashioned Cider	8 oz	120
APPLESAUCE		
sweetened	½ cup	97
unsweetened	½ cup	52

FOOD	PORTION	CALS
Eden		
Organic	½ cup	50
Organic Sweet Cinnamon	½ cup	50
Jok'n'Al		
Low Carb	1 tbsp	10
Mott's		
Single-Serve Cinnamon	1 pkg (4 oz)	100
Single-Serve Natural	1 pkg (4 oz)	50
Single-Serve Original	1 pkg (4 oz)	100
Musselman's		
Apple Sauce	1 pkg (4 oz)	80
Vermont Village		
Organic Unsweetened	½ cup	80
White House		
Apple Sauce	1 pkg (4 oz)	90

APRICOT JUICE

nectar	6 oz	106
Ceres		
Apricot	8 oz	120

APRICOTS
CANNED

heavy syrup	½ cup	91
juice pack	½ cup	59
light syrup	½ cup	80
water pack	½ cup	33
Del Monte		
Halves In Heavy Syrup	½ cup	100
Orchard Select Halves	½ cup	80

DRIED

halves	6	51
halves cooked w/o sugar	½ cup	106
Crispy Green		
Crispy Apricots	1 pkg (0.36 oz)	40

FRESH

apricots	1	17
sliced	½ cup	40
Chiquita		
Apricots	3 med (4 oz)	60

FOOD	PORTION	CALS
FROZEN		
sweetened	½ cup	119
ARROWHEAD		
corm boiled	1 med	9
flour	1 cup	457
ARROWROOT		
flour	1 cup	457
raw	1 root (1.2 oz)	21
raw root sliced	1 cup	78
ARTICHOKE		
CANNED		
hearts in oil	1 serv (3 oz)	100
Progresso		
Hearts	1 piece	15
Hearts Marinated	2 pieces (1.1 oz)	170
S&W		
Marinated Hearts	2 pieces (1 oz)	20
FRESH		
cooked	1 med	60
hearts cooked	½ cup	42
FROZEN		
cooked	1 cup	42
cooked w/o salt	1 pkg (9 oz)	108
Birds Eye		
Hearts	½ cup	40
TAKE-OUT		
stuffed	1 (8.8 oz)	397
ARUGULA		
fresh	1 cup	3
ASIAN FOOD (see also DINNER, EGG ROLLS, SUSHI)		
CANNED		
chow mein chicken	1 cup	95
Chun King		
Beef Pepper Oriental BiPack	1 cup (8.8 oz)	98
Chow Mein Beef BiPack	1 cup (8.6 oz)	78
Chow Mein BiPack Chicken	1 cup (8.8 oz)	98
Chow Mein Pork BiPack	1 cup (8.6 oz)	78

FOOD	PORTION	CALS
Hot & Spicy Chicken BiPack	1 cup (8.6 oz)	98
Sweet & Sour Chicken BiPack	1 cup (8.9 oz)	161
La Choy		
Beef Pepper Oriental BiPack	1 cup (8.8 oz)	98
Chow Mein Beef BiPack	1 cup (8.6 oz)	78
Chow Mein Chicken PiBack	1 cup (8.9 oz)	98
Chow Mein Shrimp BiPack	1 cup (8.6 oz)	52
Main Entree Chow Mein Chicken	1 cup (9.3 oz)	80
Oriental Beef w/ Noodles BiPack	1 cup (8.8 oz)	156
Oriental Chicken w/ Noodles BiPack	1 cup (8.7 oz)	154
Sweet & Sour Chicken BiPack	1 cup (8.9 oz)	161
Teriyaki Chicken BiPack	1 cup (8.6 oz)	109
FRESH		
wonton wrappers	1	23
Azumaya		
Round Wraps	10	160
Wrappers Large Square	8	160
Frieda's		
Won Ton Wrappers	4 (1 oz)	80
Nasoya		
Won Ton Wrappers	8	160
FROZEN		
Amy's		
Bowls Teriyaki	1 pkg (10 oz)	300
Skillet Meals Teriyaki Stir Fry	1 cup	320
Stir Fry Asian Noodle	1 pkg (10 oz)	240
Stir Fry Thai	1 pkg (9.5 oz)	270
Banquet		
Fried Rice w/ Chicken & Egg Rolls	1 meal (8.5 oz)	330
Birds Eye		
Easy Recipe Creations Oriental Lo Mein	2¼ cups	230
Easy Recipe Creations Sesame Ginger Teriyaki	2¼ cups	140
Easy Recipe Creations Spicy Szechuan Cashews	2¼ cups	180
La Choy		
Beef Pepper Oriental	1 cup (7.1 oz)	151
Chow Mein Vegetable	1 cup (8.9 oz)	108
Lean Cuisine		
Cafe Classics Asian Style Beef w/Ginger & Soy	1 pkg (9.25 oz)	210
Cafe Classics Bowl Chicken Fried Rice	1 pkg (10 oz)	310
Cafe Classics Bowl Chicken Teriyaki	1 pkg (11 oz)	320

FOOD	PORTION	CALS
Cafe Classics Bowl Teriyaki Steak	1 pkg (10.5 oz)	340
Cafe Classics Chicken Teriyaki Stir Fry	1 pkg (10 oz)	300
Cafe Classics Hunan Beef & Broccoli	1 pkg (8.5 oz)	230
Cafe Classics Thai-Style Chicken	1 pkg (9 oz)	230
One Dish Favorites Asian Style Pot Stickers	1 pkg (9 oz)	320
One Dish Favorites Chicken Chow Mein	1 pkg (9 oz)	200
Skillet Asian Style Chicken & Vegetables	1 serv	160
MIX		
Annie Chun's		
Meal Kit Black Bean	1 serv	230
Meal Kit Garlic Scallion	1 serv	230
Meal Kit Soy Ginger	1 serv	220
TAKE-OUT		
buddha's delight w/ cellophane noodles fat choi jai	1 serv (7.6 oz)	211
cashew chicken	1 serv	406
cha siu bao steamed buns w/ chicken filling	1 (2.3 oz)	160
chop suey cantonese chicken	1 serv	570
chop suey w/ beef & pork	1 cup	300
chop suey w/ pork	1 cup	375
chow mein chicken	1 cup	255
chow mein pork	1 cup	425
chow mein shrimp	1 cup	221
chow mein vegetable	1 serv (8 oz)	90
dim sum meat filled	3 pieces (4 oz)	124
egg foo yung beef	1 patty (6 oz)	243
egg foo yung chicken	1 patty (3 oz)	121
egg foo yung pork	1 patty (3 oz)	125
egg foo yung shrimp	1 patty (3 oz)	153
filipino chicken adobo	1 serv (15 oz)	555
fried rice chicken	1 serv	314
fried rice vegetable	1 cup	210
fried rice w/ egg	6.7 oz	395
general tsao's chicken	1 serv	723
kung pao chicken	1 cup	409
kung pao chicken w/ rice	1 serv (1.75 cups)	240
lo mein pork	1 serv	323
moo goo gai pan chicken	1 cup	272
phad thai	1 serv (9.2 oz)	232
sesame seed paste bun	1 (2.5 oz)	220

FOOD	PORTION	CALS
shrimp & snow peas	1 cup	220
shrimp chips	1¼ cups (1 oz)	140
shu mai chicken & vegetable dumplings	6 (3.6 oz)	160
soba noodles w/ vegetables	1 serv	276
spring roll	1 (3.5 oz)	112
stir fry beef & broccoli	2 cups	512
stir fry garlic green beans	1 serv	68
stir fry vegetable	1 serv	235
sweet & sour chicken w/o rice	1 serv	416
sweet & sour pork	1 serv (8 oz)	250
sweet red bean bun	1 (2.5 oz)	130
szechuan chicken w/ lo mein	1 cup (5.3 oz)	190
szechuan cold noodles	1 serv	334
tempura seafood & vegetable	1 serv	590
tempura vegetables	5 pieces (4 oz)	270
teriyaki beef w/ sticky rice	1 serv	664
teriyaki chicken plain	¾ cup	399
teriyaki chicken w/ rice	1 serv (11 oz)	430
wonton fried	½ cup (1 oz)	111

ASPARAGUS
CANNED
spears	1 cup	46
spears	1	3

Del Monte
Cuts & Tips	½ cup	20
Spears	½ cup	20
Tips	½ cup	20

S&W
Green	6 pieces (4.5 oz)	15

FRESH
cooked	½ cup	20
cooked	4 spears	13
raw	4 spears	10

Frieda's
White	⅔ cup	20

FROZEN
cooked	4 spears	11
cooked	1 pkg (10 oz)	53

FOOD	PORTION	CALS
Birds Eye		
Cuts	½ cup	25
Jumbo Spears	3 oz	20
ATEMOYA		
fresh	½ cup	94
AVOCADO		
california mashed	¼ cup	96
california peeled & pitted	1	289
florida mashed	¼ cup	69
florida peeled & pitted	1	365
Brooks Tropical		
Lite SlimCado	1 tbsp	35
Calavo		
Fresh	⅕ med (1 oz)	55
Chiquita		
Fresh	⅕ med (1 oz)	55
Frieda's		
Fresh Cocktail	1 (1.4 oz)	60
TAKE-OUT		
guacamole	1 serv (2.2 oz)	105
BACON		
bacon grease	1 tbsp	116
beef breakfast strips cooked	3 strips	153
gammon lean & fat grilled	4.2 oz	274
pan fried	3 strips	109
Health Is Wealth		
Uncured Sliced	2 slices (0.5 oz)	70
Oscar Mayer		
Center Cut cooked	2 slices (0.4 oz)	50
Cooked	2 slices (0.5 oz)	70
Ready Crisp		
Fully Cooked	3 slices (0.5 oz)	70
BACON SUBSTITUTES		
bacon bits meatless	1 tbsp	33
meatless	1 strip	16
Lightlife		
Organic Tempeh Smokey Strips	3 slices (2 oz)	80
Smart Bacon	2 strips (0.8 oz)	45

FOOD	PORTION	CALS
Morningstar Farms		
Breakfast Strips	2 (0.5 oz)	60
BAGEL		
cinnamon raisin	1 mini	71
cinnamon raisin	1 lg (4 in)	244
egg	1 lg (4.5 in)	364
mini onion	1 (1.4 oz)	100
oat bran	1 lg (4 in)	227
plain	1 lg (4.5 in)	360
plain	1 med (3.5 in)	289
plain	1 sm (3 in)	190
Alvarado Street Bakery		
Sprouted Wheat Cinnamon Raisin	1 (3.3 oz)	280
Atkins		
Cinnamon Raisin	1	200
Onion	1	190
Plain	1	190
Natural Ovens		
Blueberry	1 (3 oz)	190
Brainy	1 (3 oz)	170
Cinnamon Raisin	1 (3 oz)	180
Golden Crunch	1 (3 oz)	190
Hearty Grains & Onion	1 (3 oz)	190
Raspberry	1 (3 oz)	180
Whole Grain	1 (3 oz)	170
Otis Spunkmeyer		
Barnstormin' Blueberry	1 (3.6 oz)	250
Barnstormin' Cinnamon Raisin	1 (3.6 oz)	230
Barnstormin' Onion	1 (3.6 oz)	230
Barnstormin' Plain	1 (3.6 oz)	240
Pepperidge Farm		
100% Whole Wheat	1	250
Mini 100% Whole Wheat	1	100
Sara Lee		
Heart Healthy 100% Whole Wheat	1 (3.3 oz)	220
Heart Healthy Cinnamon Raisin	1 (3.3 oz)	250
Whole Grain Plain	1 (3.3 oz)	240
Thomas'		
Carb Consider Plain	1	150

FOOD	PORTION	CALS
Carb Consider Whole Wheat	1	140
Everything	1 (3.6 oz)	300
Multi-Grain	1 (3.6 oz)	280
Plain	1 (3.6 oz)	280
Uncle B's		
Plain	1 (2.8 oz)	210
Weight Watchers		
Original	1 (2.8 oz)	190
Wonder		
Blueberry	1 (3 oz)	210
Cinnamon Raisin	1 (3 oz)	210
Onion	1 (3 oz)	210
Plain	1 (3 oz)	210
Rye	1 (3 oz)	220
Wheat	1 (3 oz)	210

BAKING POWDER

baking powder	1 tsp	2
low sodium	1 tsp	5
Clabber Girl		
Baking Powder	1 tsp	0
Davis		
Baking Powder	1 tsp	0
Rumford		
Aluminum Free	⅛ tsp	0

BAKING SODA

baking soda	1 tsp	0

BALSAM PEAR (BITTER GOURD)

leafy tips cooked w/o salt	1 cup	20
leafy tips raw	1 cup	14
pods raw sliced	1 cup	16
pods sliced cooked w/ salt	1 cup	24

BAMBOO SHOOTS

canned sliced	½ cup	12
fresh sliced cooked w/ salt	½ cup	7
raw sliced	½ cup	20
Chun King		
Bamboo Shoots	2 tbsp (0.8 oz)	3

FOOD	PORTION	CALS
La Choy		
Bamboo Shoots	2 tbsp (0.8 oz)	3
BANANA		
banana chips	1 oz	147
fresh	1 med (7 in)	105
fresh	1 extra sm (<6 in)	72
fresh	1 sm (6 in)	90
fresh	1 lg (8 in)	121
fresh mashed	½ cup	100
fresh sliced	1 cup	134
powder	1 tbsp	21
whole dried	1 piece (1.2 oz)	130
Chiquita		
Fresh	1 med (4.4 oz)	110
Frieda's		
Burro	1 (3 oz)	80
Dried	1 piece (1.2 oz)	130
BARBECUE SAUCE		
barbecue	1 cup	188
Atkins		
Barbecue Sauce	1 tbsp	15
Bull's Eye		
Original	2 tbsp	50
Carb Options		
Original	2 tbsp	10
Consorzio		
Organic Original	1 tbsp	50
Organic Spicy	1 tbsp	50
Hunt's		
Hickory	2 tbsp	45
Hickory & Brown Sugar	2 tbsp	70
Honey Hickory	2 tbsp	50
Honey Mustard	2 tbsp	50
Hot & Spicy	2 tbsp	45
Mesquite	2 tbsp	40
Original	2 tbsp	50
Original Bold	2 tbsp	45
Muir Glen		
Garlic Mesquite	2 tbsp (1.3 oz)	40

FOOD	PORTION	CALS
Hot & Smoky	2 tbsp (1.2 oz)	40
Original	2 tbsp (1.2 oz)	40
Nando's		
Barbecue	1 tbsp	7
Steel's		
Sugar Free	2 tbsp	15
BARLEY		
flour	1 cup	511
pearled cooked	1 cup (5.5 oz)	193
pearled uncooked	¼ cup	176
Mother's		
Quick Cooking	⅓ cup	170
BARRACUDA		
broiled	4 oz	239
cooked flaked	1 cup	287
fresh	3 oz	122
poached	4 oz	227
TAKE-OUT		
breaded & fried	4 oz	282
BASIL		
fresh chopped	1 tbsp	1
ground	1 tsp	4
leaves fresh	5	1
BASS		
freshwater raw	3 oz	97
sea cooked	3 oz	105
sea raw	3 oz	82
striped baked	3 oz	105
striped bass farm raised	4 oz	110
BAY LEAF		
crumbled	1 tsp	2
BEANS (see also individual names)		
CANNED		
baked beans plain	½ cup	119
baked beans vegetarian	½ cup	119
baked beans w/ franks	½ cup	184
baked beans w/ pork	½ cup	134

FOOD	PORTION	CALS
baked beans w/ pork & tomato sauce	½ cup	119
refried beans	½ cup	134
Amy's		
Vegetarian Baked	½ cup	120
B&M		
Barbeque Baked Beans	½ cup (4.6 oz)	210
Maple Baked	½ cup	150
Vegetarian 99% Fat Free	½ cup	150
Bush's		
Barbecue	½ cup	150
Country Style	½ cup	170
Homestyle	½ cup	140
Maple Cured Bacon	½ cup	150
Onion 98% Fat Free	½ cup	140
Original	½ cup	150
Vegetarian Fat Free	½ cup (4.6 oz)	130
Campbell's		
Pork & Beans	½ cup	140
Eden		
Organic Baked w/ Sorghum & Mustard	½ cup (4.6 oz)	150
Gebhardt		
Chili	½ cup (4.6 oz)	134
Refried Jalapeno	½ cup (4.5 oz)	105
Refried No Fat	½ cup (4.5 oz)	92
Refried Traditional	½ cup (4.5 oz)	109
Refried Vegetarian	½ cup (4.5 oz)	118
Heinz		
Vegetarian	1 cup	250
Hunt's		
Big John's Beans & Fixin's	½ cup (4.7 oz)	127
Homestyle Country Kettle	½ cup (4.6 oz)	152
Homestyle Special Recipe	½ cup (4.7 oz)	185
Mix & Serve	½ cup (4.7 oz)	125
Pork & Beans	½ cup (4.5 oz)	130
Old El Paso		
Refried Fat Free	½ cup	100
Open Range		
Ranch	½ cup (4.4 oz)	124
Pringles		
Vegetarian	1 cup (7.9 oz)	250

FOOD	PORTION	CALS
Ranch Style		
Original Texas	½ cup	138
Rosarita		
3 Bean Recipe Bacon & Jalapeno	½ cup (4.6 oz)	117
3 Bean Recipe Chiles & Chicken	½ cup (4.6 oz)	115
3 Bean Recipe Chilies & Chorizo	½ cup (4.6 oz)	111
3 Bean Recipe Onions & Peppers	½ cup (4.6 oz)	104
Fiesta Beans Bacon & Jalapenos	½ cup (4.6 oz)	117
Fiesta Beans Chicken & Chilies	½ cup (4.6 oz)	115
Fiesta Beans Chilies & Chorizo	½ cup (4.6 oz)	110
Fiesta Beans Onions & Peppers	½ cup (4.6 oz)	104
Refried Bacon	½ cup (4.5 oz)	116
Refried Green Chile	½ cup (4.5 oz)	110
Refried Low Fat Black	½ cup (4.5 oz)	107
Refried Nacho Cheese	½ cup (4.5 oz)	108
Refried No Fat	½ cup	90
Refried No Fat Green Chiles & Lime	½ cup (4.5 oz)	101
Refried No Fat w/ Zesty Salsa	½ cup (4.5 oz)	105
Refried Onion	½ cup (4.5 oz)	114
Refried Spicy	½ cup (4.5 oz)	118
Refried Traditional	½ cup (4.5 oz)	108
Refried Vegetarian	½ cup (4.5 oz)	237
S&W		
Barbecue Beans Ranch Recipe	½ cup (4.5 oz)	100
Van Camp's		
Baked Fat Free	½ cup (4.6 oz)	132
Baked Original	½ cup	140
Baked Southern Style Sauteed Onion	½ cup (4.8 oz)	145
Baked Sweet Hickory & Bacon	1 can (4.8 oz)	143
Beanee Weenee Baked	1 cup (9.1 oz)	410
Beanee Weenee BBQ	1 cup (7.7 oz)	290
Beanee Weenee Microwave	1 cup (7.5 oz)	260
Beanee Weenee Original	1 cup (9.1 oz)	320
Beanee Weenee Zestful	1 cup (7.7 oz)	300
Brown Sugar	½ cup (4.6 oz)	170
Pork And Beans	½ cup	110
Vegetarian	½ cup (4.6 oz)	110
FROZEN		
Lean Cuisine		
Cafe Classics Sante Fe Style Rice & Beans	1 pkg (10.4 oz)	290

FOOD	PORTION	CALS
Natural Touch		
Nine Bean Loaf	1 in slice (3 oz)	160
TAKE-OUT		
baked beans	½ cup	191
barbecue beans	3.5 oz	120
four bean salad	3.5 oz	100
frijoles w/ cheese	1 cup	225
refried beans	½ cup	43
three bean salad	¾ cup	230

BEAN SPROUTS (see ALFALFA, SPROUTS)

BEAR

polar bear raw	3.5 oz	130
simmered	3 oz	220

BEAVER

roasted	3 oz	140
simmered	3 oz	141

BEECHNUTS

dried	1 oz	164

BEEF (see also BEEF DISHES, VEAL)

CANNED		
corned beef	1 oz	71
Armour		
Chopped Beef	2 oz	170
Corned Beef	2 oz	120
Potted Meat	1 can (3 oz)	120
Tripe	3 oz	90
Treet		
Luncheon Loaf	2 oz	130
Luncheon Loaf 50% Less Fat	2 oz	110
DRIED		
Armour		
Sliced	7 slices (1 oz)	60
FRESH		
arm pot roast trim 0 fat braised	3.5 oz	297
arm pot roast trim ⅛ in fat braised	3.5 oz	302
bottom round roast trim 0 in fat braised	4 oz	253
bottom round roast trim 0 in fat roasted	3.5 oz	187

FOOD	PORTION	CALS
bottom round roast trim ½ in fat braised	4 oz	337
bottom round roast trim ⅛ in fat braised	4 oz	280
bottom round roast trim ⅛ in fat roasted	4 oz	247
bottom sirloin butt roast trim 0 in roasted	3.5 oz	182
brisket flat half trim ⅛ in fat braised	3.5 oz	298
brisket flat trim 0 fat braised	3.5 oz	221
brisket point half trim 0 fat braised	3.5 oz	358
brisket point half trim ¼ in fat braised	3.5 oz	404
brisket point half trim ⅛ in fat braised	3.5 oz	349
chuck boston cut roast trim 0 fat roasted	3.5 oz	207
chuck boston cut roast trim ¼ in fat roasted	3.5 oz	242
chuck bottom roast trim 0 fat braised	3.5 oz	334
chuck bottom roast trim ¼ in fat braised	3.5 oz	345
chuck fillet steak trim 0 fat broiled	4 oz	181
chuck top roast trim 0 fat broiled	4 oz	245
club steak trim ½ in fat broiled	4 oz	384
corned beef brisket cooked	3 oz	213
crosscut shank trim ¼ in fat stewed	1 serv (6.8 oz)	510
crumbles 70% lean pan browned	3 oz	230
delmonico steak trim ¼ in fat broiled	4 oz	409
entrecote steak trim ½ in fat broiled	4 oz	413
eye round roast trim 0 in fat roasted	4 oz	190
eye round roast trim ⅛ in fat roasted	4 oz	236
filet mignon roast trim ¼ in fat roasted	4 oz	376
filet mignon roast trim ⅛ in fat roasted	4 oz	367
filet mignon trim 0 in fat broiled	4 oz	247
filet mignon trim ⅛ in fat broiled	4 oz	303
ground 70% lean broiled	3.5 oz	273
ground 75% lean broiled	2.5 oz	195
ground 80% lean broiled	3 oz	234
ground 85% lean pan fried	3 oz	197
ground 90% lean pan fried	3 oz	173
ground 95% lean pan fried	3 oz	139
ground 97% fat free irradiated	4 oz	160
ground low-fat w/ carrageenan raw	4 oz	160
london broil trim 0 fat broiled	3.5 oz	188
london broil trim ¼ in fat broiled	4 oz	260
new york strip steak trim 0 fat broiled	4 oz	219
porterhouse steak trim 0 in fat broiled	1 lb	1252
porterhouse steak trim ¼ in fat broiled	1 lb	1284

FOOD	PORTION	CALS
porterhouse steak trim ⅛ in fat broiled	4 oz	337
porterhouse steak trim ⅛ in fat broiled	1 lb	1346
rib eye roast trim ¼ in fat roasted	3.5 oz	365
rib eye steak trim ⅛ in fat broiled	4 oz	221
rib roast trim ¼ in fat roasted	4 oz	406
rib steak trim ¼ in fat broiled	4 oz	388
round tip roast trim 0 in fat roasted	4 oz	213
sandwich steaks thinly sliced	1 serv (2 oz)	173
shell steak trim ¼ in fat broiled	4 oz	366
shortribs lean & fat braised	1 serv (7.8 oz)	1060
skirt steak trim 0 fat broiled	4 oz	289
t-bone steak trim 0 fat broiled	4 oz	280
t-bone steak trim ¼ in fat broiled	1 lb	1388
t-bone steak trim ⅛ in fat broiled	1 lb	804
tip round roast trim ⅛ in fat roasted	4 oz	248
top loin steak boneless trim ⅛ in fat broiled	4 oz	299
top round roast trim 0 fat braised	4 oz	237
top round roast trim ¼ in fat braised	4 oz	281
top round roast trim ¼ in fat roasted	4 oz	265
top round steak trim ¼ in fat pan fried	4 oz	314
top sirloin steak trim ⅛ in fat broiled	4 oz	275
top sirloin steak trim ⅛ in fat pan fried	4 oz	355
tri-tip roast trim 0 fat roasted	3.5 oz	218
tri-tip steak trim 0 fat broiled	4 oz	300
Laura's Lean		
Eye Of Round Steak Or Roast	4 oz	140
Flank Steak	4 oz	140
Ground 92% Lean	4 oz	160
Ground Round 96% Lean	4 oz	140
Ribeye Steak	4 oz	145
Sirloin Steak	4 oz	140
Sirloin Tip Steak Or Roast	4 oz	120
Strip Steak	4 oz	140
Tenderloin Filet	4 oz	140
Top Round Steak Or Roast	4 oz	130
Maverick Ranch		
Filet Mignon	4 oz	120
Ground	4 oz	130
Ground Round	4 oz	130
Ground Sirloin & Chuck	4 oz	130

FOOD	PORTION	CALS
NY Strip Steak	4 oz	150
Rib Eye Steak	4 oz	170
Top Round Steak & Roast	4 oz	110
Top Sirloin	4 oz	160
Organic Valley		
Extra Lean Ground	3 oz	130
Extra Lean Patties	1 (3.2 oz)	130
FROZEN		
patty broiled medium	3 oz	240
Soy Lean		
Beef Patty	1 (2.5 oz)	90
READY-TO-EAT		
dried beef smoked chopped	1 oz	37
roast beef spread	¼ cup	127
smoked beef cooked	1 sausage (1.4 oz)	134
Alpine Lace		
Roast Beef 97% Fat Free	2 oz	70
Boar's Head		
Corned Beef Brisket	2 oz	80
Eye Round Pepper Seasoned	2 oz	90
Italian Style Oven Roasted Top Round	2 oz	80
Roast Beef Cajun	2 oz	80
Top Round Deluxe	2 oz	90
Top Round Oven Roasted No Salt Added	2 oz	90
TAKE-OUT		
roast beef rare	2 oz	70

BEEF DISHES

CANNED		
corned beef hash	3 oz	155
Armour		
Corned Beef Hash	1 cup (8.3 oz)	440
Corned Beef Hash w/ Peppers & Onions	1 cup (8.3 oz)	270
Roast Beef Hash	1 cup (8.4 oz)	400
Roast Beef In Gravy	½ cup (4.6 oz)	150
Stew	1 cup (8.6 oz)	220
Hormel		
Corned Beef Hash 50% Reduced Fat	1 cup	290
Libby's		
Hash Corned Beef	1 cup	420

FOOD	PORTION	CALS
FROZEN		
Banquet		
Sandwich Toppers Creamed Chipped Beef	1 pkg (4 oz)	120
Sandwich Toppers Gravy & Salisbury Steak	1 pkg (5 oz)	210
Sandwich Toppers Gravy & Sliced Beef	1 pkg (4 oz)	70
Boston Market		
Meatloaf w/ Mashed Potatoes & Gravy	1 pkg (16 oz)	880
MIX		
Hamburger Helper		
Fettuccine Alfredo as prep	1 cup	300
REFRIGERATED		
Hormel		
Beef Roast Au Jus	1 serv (5 oz)	200
Beef Tips w/ Gravy	½ cup	160
Morton's Of Omaha		
Beef Pot Roast w/ Gravy	1 serv (3 oz)	160
Smithfield		
Beef Tips w/ Gravy	½ cup	170
Tyson		
Roast Beef In Brown Gravy	1 serv + gravy (3.5 oz)	160
SHELF-STABLE		
Lunch Bucket		
Beef Stew	1 pkg (7.5 oz)	170
TastyBite		
Beef Roganjosh	1 pkg (9.5 oz)	270
Meatballs Vindaloo	1 pkg (9.5 oz)	270
TAKE-OUT		
beef bourguignon	1 serv (7 oz)	254
beef curry	1 cup	432
bool kogi korean marinated beef ribs	4 oz	190
bubble & squeak	5 oz	186
bulgoghi korean grilled beef	1 serv (5.2 oz)	256
cornish pasty	1 (8 oz)	847
greek moussaka	1 serv (8.5 oz)	450
irish stew	1 cup (7 oz)	280
kebab indian	1 (5.4 oz)	553
kheena	6.7 oz	781
koftas	5	280
peppered steak	1 cup	331
pot roast w/ gravy	1 serv (6 oz)	320

FOOD	PORTION	CALS
samosa	2 (4 oz)	652
shepherds pie	1 serv (7 oz)	282
steak & kidney pie w/ top crust	1 slice (5 oz)	400
stew w/ vegetables	1 serv (8 oz)	218
stroganoff	¾ cup	260
swiss steak	4.6 oz	214
toad in the hole	1 (4.7 oz)	383

BEEFALO

roasted	4 oz	213

BEER AND ALE

alcohol free beer	7 fl oz	50
ale brown	10 oz	77
ale pale	10 oz	88
beer light	12 oz can	103
beer regular	12 oz can	139
black & tan	1 serv (12 oz)	146
boilermaker	1 serv	216
lager	10 oz	80
mead	1 serv	250
pilsener lager	7 fl oz	85
shandy	1 serv	125
stout	10 oz	102
Amstel		
Light	1 bottle (12 oz)	95
Anchor		
Liberty Ale	1 bottle (12 oz)	188
Porter	1 bottle (12 oz)	205
Steam	12 oz	152
Beamish		
Stout	12 oz	131
Beck's		
Beer	1 bottle (12 oz)	143
Premium Light	1 bottle	64
Blue Moon		
White	1 bottle (12 oz)	171
Bud		
Ice Light	1 bottle (12 oz)	110
Budweiser		
Beer	1 bottle (12 oz)	143

FOOD	PORTION	CALS
Ice	1 bottle (12 oz)	148
Light	1 bottle (12 oz)	110
Busch		
Beer	1 bottle (12 oz)	133
Ice	1 bottle (12 oz)	173
Light	1 bottle (12 oz)	110
Clausthaler		
Beer	1 bottle (12 oz)	96
Colt 45		
Malt Liquor	1 bottle (12 oz)	172
Coors		
Extra Gold	1 bottle (12 oz)	147
Light	1 bottle (12 oz)	102
Nonalcoholic	1 bottle (12 oz)	73
Original	1 bottle (12 oz)	148
Corona		
Extra	1 bottle (12 oz)	148
Light	1 bottle (12 oz)	109
Deschutes		
Bachelor ESB	1 bottle (12 oz)	180
Black Butt Porter	1 bottle (12 oz)	185
Cascade Ale	1 bottle (12 oz)	140
Mirror Pond Pale	1 bottle (12 oz)	175
Edison		
Light	1 bottle	109
Genessee		
12 Horse	1 bottle (12 oz)	152
Genny Light	1 bottle (12 oz)	96
Guiness		
Draught	1 bottle (12 oz)	125
Foreign Extra Stout	1 bottle (12 oz)	176
Hamm's		
Beer	1 bottle (12 oz)	144
Light	1 bottle (12 oz)	110
Heineken		
Beer	1 bottle (12 oz)	166
I.C.		
Light	1 bottle (12 oz)	96

FOOD	PORTION	CALS
Icehouse		
5.0	1 bottle (12 oz)	132
5.5	1 bottle (12 oz)	149
J.W. Dundee		
Honey Brown	1 bottle (12 oz)	150
Keystone		
Light	1 bottle (12 oz)	100
Kilarney's		
Red Lager	1 bottle (12 oz)	197
Killian's		
Beer	1 bottle (12 oz)	163
Lowenbrau		
Beer	1 bottle (12 oz)	160
Michelob		
Ultra Low Carbohydrate	1 bottle (12 oz)	95
Weinhard's		
Ale	1 bottle (12 oz)	147
Amber Ale	1 bottle (12 oz)	169
Dark	1 bottle (12 oz)	150
Hefeweizen	1 bottle (12 oz)	128
BEET JUICE		
juice	7 oz	72
BEETS		
CANNED		
harvard	½ cup	90
pickled	½ cup	74
sliced	½ cup	37
Del Monte		
Pickled Sliced	½ cup	35
Sliced	½ cup	35
Greenwood		
Harvard	1 serv (4.4 oz)	100
Pickled	1 oz	25
S&W		
Julienne	½ cup (4.3 oz)	30
Pickled Sliced	1 oz	15
Pickled Whole	1 oz	15
Sliced	½ cup (4.3 oz)	30
Whole Small	½ cup (4.3 oz)	30

FOOD	PORTION	CALS
Veg-All		
Small Sliced	½ cup	40
FRESH		
greens cooked w/o salt	½ cup	19
sliced cooked	½ cup	37
whole cooked	2 med (3.5 oz)	44
Frieda's		
Beets	½ cup	35

BEVERAGES *(see BEER AND ALE, CHAMPAGNE, COFFEE, DRINK MIXERS, ENERGY DRINKS, FRUIT DRINKS, ICED TEA, LIQUOR/LIQUEUR, MALT, MILKSHAKE, SMOOTHIES, SODA, TEA/HERBAL TEA, WATER, WINE, YOGURT DRINKS)*

BISCUIT

FOOD	PORTION	CALS
MIX		
plain as prep	1 (2 oz)	190
Bisquick		
Buttermilk	½ cup	150
Cheese Garlic	½ cup	160
Cinnamon Swirl	½ cup	150
Mix	⅓ cup (1.4 oz)	160
Reduced Fat	⅓ cup	150
Jiffy		
Buttermilk as prep	1	170
Kentucky Kernel		
Biscuit	¼ cup (1 oz)	171
MiniCarb		
Buttery as prep	1	255
REFRIGERATED		
plain baked	1 (1 oz)	93
1869 Brand		
Buttermilk	1 (1.1 oz)	100
Hungry Jack		
Butter Tastin' Flaky	1 (1.2 oz)	100
Cinnamon & Sugar	1 (1.2 oz)	110
Flaky	1 (1.2 oz)	100
Flaky Buttermilk	1 (1.2 oz)	100
Pillsbury		
Big Country Butter Tastin'	1 (1.2 oz)	100
Big Country Buttermilk	1 (1.2 oz)	100
Big Country Southern Style	1 (1.2 oz)	100

FOOD	PORTION	CALS
Buttermilk	1 (2.2 oz)	150
Country	1 (2.2 oz)	150
Grands Blueberry	1 (2.1 oz)	210
Grands Butter Tastin'	1 (2.1 oz)	200
Grands Buttermilk	1 (2.1 oz)	200
Grands Buttermilk Reduced Fat	1 (2.1 oz)	190
Grands Extra Rich	1 (2.1 oz)	220
Grands Flaky	1 (2.1 oz)	200
Grands Golden Corn	1 (1.2 oz)	210
Grands HomeStyle	1 (2.1 oz)	210
Grands Southern Style	1 (2.1 oz)	200
Southern Style Flaky	1 (1.2 oz)	100
Tender Layer Buttermilk	1 (2.2 oz)	160
TAKE-OUT		
buttermilk	1 lg (2.7 oz)	280
oatcakes	2 (4 oz)	115
plain	1 sm (1.2 oz)	127
tea biscuit	1 (3 oz)	210
w/ egg	1 (4.8 oz)	373
w/ egg & bacon	1 (5.3 oz)	458
w/ egg & ham	1 (6.7 oz)	442
w/ egg & sausage	1 (6.3 oz)	581
w/ egg & steak	1 (5.2 oz)	410
w/ egg cheese & bacon	1 (5.1 oz)	477
w/ ham	1 (4 oz)	386
w/ sausage	1 (4.4 oz)	485

BISON
roasted	3 oz	122

BITTERMELON
Frieda's
Foo Qua	1 cup	15

BLACK BEANS
dried cooked	1 cup	227

Bean Cuisine
Pasta & Beans Mediterranean Black Beans & Fusilli	1 serv	210

Eden
Organic	½ cup (4.6 oz)	100

FOOD	PORTION	CALS
Progresso		
Black Beans	½ cup (4.6 oz)	110
BLACKBERRIES		
canned in heavy syrup	½ cup	118
fresh	½ cup	31
unsweetened frzn	½ cup	48
BLACKBERRY JUICE		
canned	6 oz	65
Clear Fruit		
Blackberry Rush	8 oz	90
Everfresh		
Clear Fruit Blackberry Rush	8 oz	90
BLACKEYE PEAS		
catjang dried cooked	1 cup (2.9 oz)	200
cowpeas canned	1 cup	184
cowpeas frozen cooked	½ cup	112
cowpeas leafy tips chopped cooked	1 cup	12
cowpeas leafy tips raw chopped	1 cup	10
CANNED		
w/pork	½ cup	199
Eden		
Organic	½ cup (4.6 oz)	90
DRIED		
cooked	1 cup	198
FROZEN		
Birds Eye		
Blackeye Peas	½ cup	110
BLINTZE		
Cohen's & Wilton		
Cheese	1	80
Golden		
Cheese	1 (2.1 oz)	80
Potato	1	90
Vegetable	1	110
Ratner's		
Cheese	1 (2.2 oz)	90
TAKE-OUT		
cheese	1 (2.7 oz)	160

FOOD	PORTION	CALS
BLUEBERRIES		
canned in heavy syrup	½ cup	113
fresh	½ cup	41
fresh	1 pt	229
frzn unsweetened	½ cup	40
A&L Farms		
Bleuets Fresh	1 pt	80
Frieda's		
Dried	¼ cup (1.4 oz)	140
Tree Of Life		
Organic	1 cup (5 oz)	80
BLUEBERRY JUICE		
Hi-C		
Blazin' Blueberry	1 box	100
Van Dyk's		
100% Juice	6 oz	74
BLUEFIN		
fillet baked	4.1 oz	186
BLUEFISH		
fresh baked	3 oz	135
BOAR		
wild roasted	3 oz	136
BOK CHOY (see CABBAGE)		
BONITO		
fresh	3 oz	117
BORAGE		
fresh chopped	1 cup	19
BOTTLED WATER (see WATER)		
BOYSENBERRIES		
frzn unsweetened	½ cup	33
in heavy syrup	½ cup	113
BRAINS		
beef pan-fried	3 oz	167
beef simmered	3 oz	123
lamb braised	3 oz	124

FOOD	PORTION	CALS
lamb fried	3 oz	232
pork braised	3 oz	117
veal braised	3 oz	115
veal fried	3 oz	181
Armour		
Pork Brains In Milk Gravy	⅔ cup (5.5 oz)	150

BRAN

corn	1 cup (2.7 oz)	170
oat	½ cup (1.6 oz)	116
oat cooked	½ cup (3.8 oz)	44
rice	½ cup (2.1 oz)	187
wheat	½ cup (2 oz)	63
Hodgson Mill		
Oat	¼ cup	120
Wheat Unprocessed	¼ cup	30

BRAZIL NUTS

dried unblanched	1 oz	186

BREAD
CANNED

boston brown	1 slice (1.6 oz)	88

FROZEN
Marie Callender's

Cornbread & Honey Butter	1 piece + butter	210
Original Garlic	1 piece	190
Parmesan & Romano Garlic	1 piece	200
Pepperidge Farm		
Whole Grain Garlic	1 serv (2.5 inch)	170
Whole Grain Garlic Texas Toast	1 slice	150

MIX

cornbread	1 piece (2 oz)	188
Atkins		
Caraway Rye as prep	1 slice	150
Country White as prep	1 slice	70
Sourdough as prep	1 slice	70
Buitoni		
Focaccia Rosemary & Garlic	1 piece (1 oz)	110
Foccacia Italian Herb & Cheese	1 slice	110

FOOD	PORTION	CALS
Carbolite		
Bread Mix as prep	1 slice	45
Hodgson Mill		
European Cheese & Herb	¼ cup (1.2 oz)	130
Honey Whole Wheat	¼ cup (1.2 oz)	120
Keto		
Quick Bread All Flavors as prep	1 slice	55
MiniCarb		
Country White as prep	1 slice	80
Sassafras		
12 Grain & Sunflower	1 slice (1.4 oz)	150
READY-TO-EAT		
anadama	1 (1.1 oz)	87
baguette parisian	2 oz	120
baguette whole wheat	2 oz	140
challah	1 slice (1.4 oz)	115
cinnamon	1 slice (0.9 oz)	69
cracked wheat	1 slice (1.1 oz)	78
cuban bread	1 slice (1.1 oz)	83
french	1 slice (1.1 oz)	88
italian	1 loaf (1 lb)	1255
navajo fry	1 piece	281
oat bran	1 slice (1.1 oz)	71
oatmeal	1 slice (0.9 oz)	73
pan criollo	1 piece (0.9 oz)	69
pannetone	1 slice (0.9 oz)	86
pita	1 lg (2 oz)	165
pita	1 sm (1 oz)	77
pita whole wheat	1 sm (1 oz)	74
pita whole wheat	1 lg (2.2 oz)	170
potato scallion	1 slice (2 oz)	120
pumpernickel	1 slice (0.9 oz)	65
raisin	1 slice (1.1 oz)	88
rye	1 slice (1.1 oz)	83
seven grain	1 slice (1.1 oz)	80
wheat berry	1 slice (0.9 oz)	65
wheat bran	1 slice (1.3 oz)	89
wheat germ	1 slice (1 oz)	73
white cubed	1 cup	93
whole wheat	1 slice (1 oz)	69

FOOD	PORTION	CALS
Alvarado Street Bakery		
Diabetic Lifestyle	1 (1.2 oz)	80
Arnold		
Bakery Light 100% Whole Wheat	1 slice	80
Carb Counting Multigrain	1 slice	60
Country Classics Buttermilk	1 slice	110
Country Classics Wheat	1 slice	100
Raisin Cinnamon	1 slice (1 oz)	80
Smart & Healthy Omega-3 100% Whole Wheat	1 slice	80
Smart & Healthy Sugar Free 100% Whole Wheat	1 slice	80
Atkins		
Rye	1 slice	60
White	1 slice	60
Beefsteak		
Rye Soft	1 slice	70
Bread Du Jour		
French	3 in slice (2 oz)	140
Cedar's		
Wraps Whole Wheat	1 (2 oz)	180
Damascus		
Pita	1 (2 oz)	130
Pita Whole Wheat	1 (2 oz)	160
Roll-Up Flax	1 (2 oz)	110
Roll-Up Whole Wheat	1 (2 oz)	110
Wraps Honey Wheat	½ wrap (2 oz)	130
Wraps Plain	½ wrap (2 oz)	130
Wraps Spinach	1 (4 oz)	280
Ecce Panis		
Country Wheat	1 slice (2 oz)	150
European Baguette	2 oz	150
Enjoy Life		
Rye-Less Rye	1 slice	80
Food For Life		
Brown Rice Bread Yeast Free	1 slice	100
Rice Bread Fruit & Seed Yeast Free	1 slice	140
Rice Bread Multi Seed Yeast Free	1 slice	120
White Rice Bread Yeast Free	1 slice	100
Freihofer's		
100% Whole Wheat	1 slice	90
Whole Wheat Light	2 slices	80

FOOD	PORTION	CALS
French Meadow Bakery		
Health Seed	1 slice	110
Healthy Hemp	1 slice	92
Men's Bread	1 slice	89
Woman's Bread	1 slice	81
Gold Medal		
100% Whole Wheat	1 slice	70
Home Pride		
Carb Action Multigrain	1 slice	60
Carb Action White Fiber	1 slice	60
Wheat	1 slice (1 oz)	80
Kangaroo		
Bread Wraps	1 (2.6 oz)	140
Greek Pita Flat	1 (2.6 oz)	200
Greek Pita Flat Wheat	1 (2.4 oz)	145
Pita Pockets Onion	½ (1.2 oz)	90
Pita Pockets Wheat N'Honey	½ (1.2 oz)	90
Pita Pockets White	½ (1.2 oz)	90
Salad Pockets	1 (1.2 oz)	90
Sandwich Pockets Whole Grain	1 (1.2 oz)	80
La Mexicana		
Wraps Chocolate	1 (1.3 oz)	120
Wraps Southwestern Mild Chili	1 (1.3 oz)	120
Wraps Spinach	1 (1.3 oz)	120
Wraps Tomato Basil	1 (1.3 oz)	120
Matthew's		
All Natural Cinnamon Raisin	1 slice	80
Milton's		
Healthy Multi-Grain	1 slice (1.4 oz)	110
Natural Ovens		
100% Whole Grain	1 slice	60
7 Grain Herb	1 slice	70
Better White	1 slice	80
Cracked Wheat	1 slice	80
English Muffin Bread	1 slice	80
Glorious Cinnamon Raisin	1 slice	70
Happiness Raisin Pecan	1 slice	70
Health Max	1 slice	80
Hunger Filler	1 slice	60
Lo Carb Golden Crunch	1 slice	70

FOOD	PORTION	CALS
Lo Carb Original	1 slice	60
Mild Rye	1 slice	70
Multi-Grain Stay Slim	1 slice	60
Nutty Natural	1 slice	70
Right Wheat	1 slice	60
Soft Wheat	1 slice	70
Sunny Millet	1 slice	60
Nature's Path		
Manna Carrot Raisin	1 slice	130
Manna Millet Rice	1 slice	130
Manna SunSeed	1 slice	160
Pepperidge Farm		
Deli Rye Seedless	1 slice	80
Farmhouse Soft 100% Whole Wheat	1 slice	110
Farmhouse Soft Oatmeal	1 slice	110
Hearty 100% Whole Wheat	1 slice	110
Hearty 15 Grain	1 slice	120
Jewish Rye Seeded	1 slice	80
Natural Whole Grain 100% Whole Wheat	1 slice	110
Natural Whole Grain 9 Grain	1 slice	110
Natural Whole Grain German Dark Wheat	1 slice	110
Natural Whole Grain Multi Grain	1 slice	120
Soft Honey Oat	1 slice	110
Soft Honey Whole Wheat	1 slice	110
Stoneground 100% Whole Wheat	1 slice	70
Swirl French Vanilla	1 slice	140
Whole Grain Cinnamon Raisin Swirl	1 slice	110
Whole Grain Cinnamon Swirl	1 slice	110
Sara Lee		
Blueberry Crumble	1 slice	180
Brown Sugar Cinnamon	1 slice	200
Cinnamon Raisin	1 slice	190
Delightful 100% Whole Wheat	1 slice	90
Delightful 100% Whole Wheat w/ Honey	1 slice	90
Delightful White	1 slice	90
Earth Grains Buttermilk	1 slice	220
Earth Grains Honey Whole Grain	1 slice	220
Earth Grains Oat & Nut	1 slice	230
Earth Grains Potato	1 slice	210
Earth Grains Wheat Berry	1 slice	200

FOOD	PORTION	CALS
Multigrain	1 slice	100
White Whole Grain	1 slice	150
Stroehmann		
100% Whole Wheat	1 slice (1.3 oz)	90
D'Italiano Italian No Seeds	1 slice (1 oz)	80
D'Italiano Italian Seeded	1 slice (1 oz)	80
Family Grains Twisted Bread	1 slice	70
Family White	1 slice (0.8 oz)	65
Homestyle Split Top White	1 slice (0.8 oz)	65
Honey Cracked Wheat	1 slice	90
King White	1 slice (0.8 oz)	65
New York Rye	1 slice (1 oz)	80
Potato	1 slice (1.2 oz)	100
Ranch White	1 slice (0.8 oz)	65
Rye	1 slice (1.1 oz)	80
Twelve Grain	1 slice (1.2 oz)	90
Super Bakery		
Athlete's Formula	1 slice (1.5 oz)	100
Fitness Formula	1 slice (1.5 oz)	90
Wrap Organic	1 (4 oz)	340
TastyBite		
Nan Kontos Massala	½ loaf (1.4 oz)	120
Nan Kontos Onion	½ loaf (1.4 oz)	120
Nan Kontos Roghani	½ loaf (1.4 oz)	125
Nan Kontos Tandoori	½ loaf (1.4 oz)	120
Roti Kontos Missy	½ loaf (1.4 oz)	125
Thomas'		
Toasting Cinnamon	1 slice	130
Toasting Cinnamon Raisin	1 slice	120
Toasting Corn	1 slice	110
Whole Grain Swirl Cinnamon Raisin	1 slice (1.3 oz)	110
Whole Grain Swirl Oatmeal Raisin	1 slice	110
Toufayan		
Wraps Sundried Tomato Basil	1 (2 oz)	183
Wraps Wheat	1 (2 oz)	183
REFRIGERATED		
Pillsbury		
Crusty French Loaf	⅕ loaf (2.2 oz)	150
Grands Wheat	1 (2.1 oz)	200

FOOD	PORTION	CALS
TAKE-OUT		
banana	1 slice (2 oz)	196
chapatis as prep w/ fat	1 bread (1.6 oz)	95
chapatis as prep w/o fat	1 (2.5 oz)	141
cornbread	1 piece (2.3 oz)	183
cornstick	1 (1.4 oz)	118
focaccia onion	1 piece (4.6 oz)	282
focaccia rosemary	1 piece (3.5 oz)	251
focaccia tomato olive	1 piece (4.7 oz)	270
garlic bread	1 slice (1 oz)	96
irish soda bread	1 slice (3 oz)	247
italian garlic	1 loaf (11 oz)	990
naan	1 bread (3.5 oz)	286
papadums fried	2 (1.5 oz)	81
paratha	1 bread (2.1 oz)	201
poori indian puffed bread	1 piece (1.3 oz)	112
zucchini	1 slice (1.4 oz)	150
BREAD COATING		
Don's Chuck Wagon		
Chicken Baking Mix	¼ cup (1 oz)	95
Fish & Chips Mix	¼ cup (1 oz)	100
Fish Mix	¼ cup (1 oz)	95
Mushroom Batter Mix	¼ cup (1 oz)	95
Onion Ring Mix	¼ cup (1 oz)	100
Seafood Bake & Fry Mix	¼ cup (1 oz)	95
Fryin' Magic		
Cornmeal	1 tbsp	30
Luzianne		
Cajun Chicken Coating Mix	2 tbsp (1 oz)	100
BREAD MACHINE MIX		
Betty Crocker		
Harvest Wheat	⅟₁₁ loaf	140
Home-Style White	⅟₁₁ loaf	130
Carbsense		
Harvest Wheat as prep	1 slice	60
Fleischmann's		
Apple Cinnamon	⅛ loaf	160
Cinnamon Raisin	⅛ loaf	160
Country White	⅛ loaf (1.6 oz)	170

FOOD	PORTION	CALS
Cranberry Orange	⅛ loaf	150
Honey Oatmeal	⅛ loaf	160
Italian Herb	⅛ loaf	160
Sourdough	⅛ loaf	150
Stoneground Wheat	⅛ loaf	160
Keto		
Cinnamon Raisin as prep	1 slice	79
French Loaf as prep	1 slice	79
Sourdough Rye as prep	1 slice	79
Ketogenics		
Low Carb Honey Wheat as prep	1 slice	80
Low Carb Original White as prep	1 slice	62
Low Carb Pumpernickel Rye as prep	1 slice	80

BREADCRUMBS

dry seasonsed	¼ cup	115
fresh	¼ cup	30
plain	¼ cup	107
4C		
Carb Careful Seasoned	⅓ cup	110
Arnold		
Italian	¼ cup	110
Keto		
Low Carb Cajun	½ cup	185
Low Carb Italian	½ cup	185
Low Carb Original	½ cup	185
Progresso		
Garlic & Herb	¼ cup (1 oz)	100
Italian Style	¼ cup	110
Parmesan	¼ cup (1 oz)	100
Plain	¼ cup (1 oz)	110
Rienzi		
Italian Style	¼ cup	120
Ronzoni		
Italian Flavored	¼ cup	120

BREADFRUIT

fresh	1 small (13.5 oz)	396
fried	1 cup	379
raw	1 cup	227

FOOD	PORTION	CALS
BREADNUTTREE SEEDS		
dried	1 oz	104
BREADSTICKS		
onion poppyseed	1	64
plain	1 sm	21
plain	1 lg	41
Angonoa		
Deli Style Sesame	3 (0.5 oz)	730
Bread Du Jour		
Original	1 (1.9 oz)	130
Sourdough	1 (1.9 oz)	130
John Wm Macy's		
CheeseSticks Original Cheddar	3 (1 oz)	130
Pepperidge Farm		
Snack Sticks Wheat	9 (1 oz)	130
Pillsbury		
Soft	1 (1.4 oz)	110
Soft Garlic & Herb	1 (2.1 oz)	180
Stella D'Oro		
Grissini Style Fat Free	3 (0.5 oz)	60
Mini Cracked Pepper	4 (0.5 oz)	70
Original	1 (0.4 oz)	40
Potato 'N Onion	1 (0.4 oz)	45
Roasted Garlic	1	45
Sesame	1 (0.4 oz)	50
Snack Stix Salted	4 (0.5 oz)	70
Sodium Free	1 (0.4 oz)	45
Wheat	1 (0.3 oz)	40
BREAKFAST BARS (see CEREAL BARS, ENERGY BARS)		
BREAKFAST DRINKS		
orange drink powder	3 rounded tsp	93
orange drink powder as prep w/ water	6 oz	86
Carnation		
Instant Breakfast Chocolate Malt as prep w/ fat free milk	1 serv	220
Instant Breakfast Classic French Vanilla as prep w/ fat free milk	1 serv	220

FOOD	PORTION	CALS
Instant Breakfast Junior Vanilla	1 box (8.8 oz)	250
Instant Breakfast Milk Chocolate as prep w/ fat free milk	1 serv	220
Instant Breakfast No Sugar Added Vanilla as prep w/ fat free milk	1 serv	150
Instant Breakfast Ready-To-Drink Carb Conscious French Vanilla	1 pkg	150
Instant Breakfast Ready-To-Drink Carb Conscious Milk Chocolate	1 pkg	150
Instant Breakfast Ready-To-Drink Creamy Milk Chocolate	1 pkg	250
Instant Breakfast Ready-To-Drink French Vanilla	1 pkg	240
Instant Breakfast Ready-To-Drink Strawberry Creme	1 pkg	250
Instant Breakfast Strawberry as prep w/ fat free milk	1 serv	220

BROAD BEANS
canned	½ cup	91
fava fresh cooked	½ cup	94
Progresso		
Fava Beans	½ cup (4.6 oz)	110

BROCCOFLOWER
fresh raw	½ cup (1.8 oz)	16

BROCCOLI
FRESH
chinese broccoli (gai lan) cooked	½ cup	10
raab cooked	½ cup	28
raw	1 bunch (1.3 lbs)	207
raw flower	1 piece	3
raw flowers	1 cup	20
River Ranch		
Broccoli Slaw	1 cup	25
Florets	1¼ cups	25
FROZEN		
chopped cooked	½ cup	26
spears cooked	1 pkg (10 oz)	70
spears cooked	½ cup	26

FOOD	PORTION	CALS
Birds Eye		
Chopped	⅓ cup	25
Cuts	½ cup	25
Florets	1 cup	25
In Cheese Sauce	½ cup	70
Fresh Like		
Spear	3.5 oz	26
Health Is Wealth		
Broccoli Munchees	2 (1 oz)	60
Tree Of Life		
Cuts	1 cup (3.1 oz)	25
TAKE-OUT		
batter dipped & fried	4 pieces	77
w/ cheese sauce	1 cup	242
BROWNIE		
FROZEN		
Greenfield		
Fat Free Homestyle	1 (1.3 oz)	110
Otis Spunkmeyer		
Blue Yonder w/ Walnuts	1 (2 oz)	230
MIX		
plain	1 (1.2 oz)	139
plain low calorie	1 (0.8 oz)	84
Atkins		
Kitchen Fudge as prep	1 (2 inch)	60
Aunt Paula's		
Low Carb Chef Fudge Brownie as prep	1 (2.5 inch)	89
Betty Crocker		
Chocolate Chunk as prep	1	180
Dark Chocolate Fudge as prep	1	170
Dark Chocolate w/ Syrup as prep	1	170
Fudge as prep	1	170
German Chocolate Coconut Pecan Filling as prep	1	200
Hot Fudge as prep	1	170
Original as prep	1	180
Peanut Butter as prep	1	180
Stir'n Bake w/ Mini Kisses as prep	1 serv	220

FOOD	PORTION	CALS
Turtle w/ Caramel & Pecans as prep	1	170
Walnut as prep	1	180
Big Train		
Low Carb Chocolate Chip as prep	1 (2 inch)	140
Jiffy		
Fudge as prep	1	160
Keto		
Chocolate Fudge as prep	1	59
MiniCarb		
Chocolate Brownie as prep	1	220
Nature's Path		
Organic Double Fudge	1/10 pkg	150
Organic HempPlus	1/10 pkg	140
No Pudge!		
All Flavors	1	100
Sweet Rewards		
Low Fat Fudge as prep	1	130
Reduced Fat Supreme as prep	1	140
READY-TO-EAT		
plain	1 lg (2 oz)	227
plain	1 sm (1 oz)	115
w/ nuts	1 (1 oz)	100
Dolly Madison		
Fudge	1 (3 oz)	330
Entenmann's		
Little Bites	3 (2.2 oz)	290
Ultimate Fudge	1 (1.6 oz)	220
Greenfield		
Blondie Fat Free Apple Spice	1 (1.3 oz)	110
Hostess		
Brownie Bites	3 (1.3 oz)	170
Fudge	1 (3 oz)	330
Light	1 (1.4 oz)	140
Laura's Wholesome Junk Food		
Gluten Free Better Brownie	2	120
Little Debbie		
Brownie Lights	1 (2 oz)	190
Brownie Loaves	1 (2.1 oz)	260
Fudge	1 pkg (2.1 oz)	270

FOOD	PORTION	CALS
Tastykake		
Fudge Walnut	1 (3 oz)	370
Tom's		
Fudge Nut	1 pkg (2.5 oz)	300
REFRIGERATED		
Toll House		
Brownie Dough	½ pkg (1.5 oz)	180
TAKE-OUT		
plain	2 in sq (2.1 oz)	243

BRUSSELS SPROUTS
FRESH

cooked	6 pieces	45
cooked	1 sprout	8
raw	1 sprout	8
FROZEN		
cooked	1 cup	65
Birds Eye		
Brussels Sprouts	11 sprouts	35

BUCKWHEAT

groats roasted cooked	½ cup	323
groats roasted uncooked	½ cup	292

BUFFALO

burger	4 oz	150
water buffalo roasted	3 oz	111

BULGUR

cooked	½ cup	76
uncooked	1¼ cups	239
TAKE-OUT		
tabbouleh	1 cup	198

BURBOT (FISH)

fresh baked	3 oz	98

BURDOCK ROOT

cooked w/o salt	1 root (5.8 oz)	146
cooked w/o salt	1 cup	110
Frieda's		
Gobo Root	¾ cup	60

FOOD	PORTION	CALS
BUTTER		
clarified butter	3½ oz	876
ghee cow's milk	1 tbsp	126
ghee vegetable oil	1 tbsp	126
stick	1 pat (5 g)	36
stick	1 stick (4 oz)	813
whipped	1 pat (4 g)	27
whipped	4 oz	542
whipped	1 tbsp	70
Breakstone's		
Salted	1 tbsp (0.5 oz)	100
Cabot		
Salted	1 tbsp	100
Unsalted	1 tbsp	100
Corman		
Light	1 tbsp	55
Hotel Bar		
Stick	1 tbsp (0.5 oz)	100
Keller's		
European	1 tbsp (0.5 oz)	100
Land O Lakes		
Salted	1 tbsp (0.5 oz)	100
Ultra Creamy Salted	1 tbsp (0.5 oz)	110
Unsalted	1 tbsp	100
Organic Valley		
Butter	1 tbsp (0.5 oz)	100
Unsalted	1 tbsp (0.5 oz)	110
BUTTER SUBSTITUTES		
stick	1 stick	811
Butter Buds		
Granules	1 pkg (2 g)	5
Keto		
Butta	1 tsp	43
Molly McButter		
Natural Butter	1 tsp	5
Natural Cheese	1 tsp	5
Roasted Garlic	1 tsp	5
Olivio		
Spread	1 tbsp	80

FOOD	PORTION	CALS
BUTTERBUR		
canned fuki chopped	1 cup	3
fresh fuki	1 cup	13
BUTTERFISH		
baked	3 oz	159
fillet baked	1 oz	47
BUTTERNUTS		
dried	1 oz	174
BUTTERSCOTCH *(see also* CANDY*)*		
Hershey's		
Chips	1 tbsp	80
Nestle		
Morsels	1 tbsp	80
CABBAGE *(see also* COLESLAW*)*		
chinese bok choy shredded cooked	½ cup	10
chinese pak-choi raw shredded	½ cup	5
chinese pe-tsai raw shredded	1 cup	12
chinese pe-tsai shredded cooked	1 cup	16
danish raw	1 head (2 lbs)	228
danish raw shredded	½ cup (1.2 oz)	9
danish shredded cooked	½ cup (2.6 oz)	17
green raw	1 head (2 lbs)	228
green raw shredded	½ cup (1.2 oz)	9
green shredded cooked	½ cup (2.6 oz)	17
napa cooked	1 cup (3.8 oz)	13
red raw shredded	½ cup	10
red shredded cooked	½ cup	16
savoy raw shredded	½ cup	10
savoy shredded cooked	½ cup	18
Frieda's		
Baby Bok Choy	⅔ cup	10
Bok Choy	1 cup	10
Gai Choy	1 cup (3 oz)	20
Napa	1 cup (3 oz)	15
Salad Savoy	⅔ cup (3 oz)	25
Tuscan	⅔ cup (3 oz)	20
Greenwood		
Sweet & Sour Red	½ cup	100

FOOD	PORTION	CALS
Lohmann		
Red Cabbage Sweet & Sour	¼ cup	40
River Ranch		
Angel Hair	1½ cups	20
TAKE-OUT		
korean kimchee	½ cup	22
northern white kimchi	½ cup	79
stuffed cabbage	1 (6 oz)	373
sweet & sour red cabbage	4 oz	61
CACTUS		
napoles fresh sliced	½ cup (1.5 oz)	7
pricklypear fresh	1 cup (5.3 oz)	56
Frieda's		
Cactus Pads	¾ cup (3 oz)	20
CAKE (*see also* CAKE MIX)		
angelfood	1 cake (11.9 oz)	876
battenburg cake	1 slice (2 oz)	204
boston cream pie frzn	⅙ cake (3.2 oz)	232
carrot w/ cream cheese icing	1 cake 10 in diam	6175
cheesecake	⅙ cake (2.8 oz)	256
cheesecake	1 cake 9 in diam	3350
cherry fudge w/ chocolate frosting	⅙ cake (2.5 oz)	187
coffeecake fruit	⅙ cake (1.8 oz)	156
cream puff shell	1 (2.3 oz)	239
crumpet	1 (2.3 oz)	131
devil's food cupcake w/ chocolate frosting	1	120
devil's food w/ creme filling	1 (1 oz)	105
eccles cake	1 slice (2 oz)	285
eclair	1 (1.4 oz)	149
fruitcake	1 piece (1.5 oz)	139
fruitcake dark home recipe	1 cake 7½ in x 2¼ in	5185
jelly roll lemon filled	1 slice (3 oz)	210
madeira cake	1 slice (1 oz)	98
pound	1 cake (8½ x 3½ x 3 in)	1935
pound	¹⁄₁₀ cake (1 oz)	117
pound fat free	1 cake (12 oz)	961
sheet cake w/ white frosting	1 cake 9 in sq	4020
sheet cake w/o frosting	1 cake 9 in sq	2830

FOOD	PORTION	CALS
sheet cake w/o frosting	1/9 cake	315
sour cream pound	1/10 cake (1 oz)	117
sponge	1/12 cake (1.3 oz)	110
sponge cake dessert shell	1 (0.8 oz)	70
sponge w/ creme filling	1 (1.5 oz)	155
tiramisu	1 cake (4.4 lbs)	5732
toaster pastry apple	1 (1¾ oz)	204
toaster pastry blueberry	1 (1¾ oz)	204
toaster pastry brown sugar cinnamon	1 (1¾ oz)	206
toaster pastry cherry	1 (1¾ oz)	204
toaster pastry strawberry	1 (1¾ oz)	204
treacle tart	1 slice (2.5 oz)	258
vanilla slice	1 slice (2.5 oz)	248
white w/ white frosting	1/16 cake	260
white w/ white frosting	1 cake 9 in diam	4170
yellow w/ chocolate frosting	1 cake 9 in diam	3895
yellow w/ chocolate frosting	1/8 cake (2.2 oz)	242
Amy's		
Toaster Pops Apple	1	140
Toaster Pops Strawberry	1	140
Arnold		
Date Nut Loaf	1 in slice (2 oz)	190
Baby Watson		
Cheesecake	1 slice (3 oz)	260
Boboli		
Mini Eclairs Custard Filled	4 (2.3 oz)	224
Dolly Madison		
Angel Food	1 slice (2.1 oz)	160
Apple Crumb	1 (1.6 oz)	160
Banana Dream Flip	1 (3.5 oz)	390
Bear Claw	1 (2.75 oz)	270
Carrot	1 (4 oz)	360
Chocolate Snack Squares	1 (1.6 oz)	210
Cinnamon Buttercrumb	1 (1.6 oz)	170
Cinnamon Buttercrumb Low Fat	1 (1.5 oz)	140
Cinnamon Stix	1 (1.3 oz)	170
Creme Cakes	2 (1.9 oz)	210
Cupcakes Chocolate	1 (2 oz)	210
Cupcakes Spice	1 (2 oz)	230
Dunkin' Stix	1 (1.3 oz)	170

FOOD	PORTION	CALS
Frosty Angel	1 (3.5 oz)	330
Holiday Cupcakes	1 (1.9 oz)	180
Honey Bun	1 (3.7 oz)	440
Koo Koos	1 (1.8 oz)	200
Mini Coconut Loaf	1 (3.5 oz)	350
Mini Pound Cake	1 (3.2 oz)	310
Raspberry Square	1 (1.8 oz)	190
Sweet Roll Apple	1 (2.2 oz)	200
Sweet Roll Cherry	1 (2.2 oz)	210
Sweet Roll Cinnamon	1 (2.2 oz)	230
Texas Cinnamon Bun	1 (4.2 oz)	440
Zingers Devil's Food	2 (2.6 oz)	270
Zingers Lemon	1 (1.4 oz)	150
Zingers Raspberry	1 (1.4 oz)	150
Zingers Yellow	2 (2.5 oz)	280
Drake's		
Coffee Cake Low Fat	1 (1.1 oz)	110
Coffee Cakes	1 (1.2 oz)	140
Yodel's	1 (1 oz)	150
Dutch Mill		
Dessert Shells Chocolate Covered	1 (0.5 oz)	80
Entenmann's		
Apple Puffs	1 (3 oz)	270
Coffee Cake Cheese Filled Crumb	1 serv (1.9 oz)	200
Coffee Cake Crumb	1 serv (2 oz)	260
Danish Twist Raspberry	⅛ cake	220
Light Loaf Cake Fat Free	⅛ cake (1.7 oz)	120
Loaf All Butter	⅙ cake (2.4 oz)	220
Louisiana Crunch	⅑ cake (2.9 oz)	330
Mini's Carrot Cake	1 (1.4 oz)	160
Ultimate Crumb Cake	¹⁄₁₀ cake	250
Fillo Factory		
Apple Turnovers Vegan	5 (5 oz)	270
Glenny's		
Cheesecake Vanilla	1 pkg (3 oz)	210
Goody Man		
Happy Birthday Cupcake Chocolate	1 (1.75 oz)	200
Happy Birthday Cupcake White	1 (1.75 oz)	190
Greenfield		
Blondie Fat Free Chocolate Chip	1 (1.3 oz)	110

FOOD	PORTION	CALS
Hostess		
Angel Food	⅛ cake (2 oz)	160
Chocodiles	1 (1.6 oz)	240
Chocolicious	1 (1.6 oz)	190
Coffee Crumb	1 (1.1 oz)	130
Crumb Cake Light	1 (1 oz)	100
Cupcakes Chocolate	1 (1.8 oz)	180
Cupcakes Orange	1 (1.5 oz)	160
Cupcakes Light Chocolate	1 (1.6 oz)	140
Ding Dongs	2 (2.7 oz)	360
Ho Ho's	2 (2 oz)	250
Honey Bun Glazed	1 (2.7 oz)	320
Honey Bun Iced	1 (3.4 oz)	410
Shortcake Dessert Cups	1 (1.1 oz)	100
Sno Balls	1 (1.8 oz)	180
Suzy Q's	1 (2 oz)	230
Sweet Roll Cherry	1 (2.2 oz)	210
Sweet Roll Cinnamon	1 (2.2 oz)	230
Twinkies	1 (1.5 oz)	150
Twinkies Light	1 (1.5 oz)	130
Jell-O		
Dessert Delights Cheesecake	1 bar (1.4 oz)	160
Dessert Delights Chocolate Fudge Pudding	1 bar (1.4 oz)	150
Little Debbie		
Angel Cakes Lemon	1 (1.6 oz)	130
Angel Cakes Raspberry	1 (1.6 oz)	130
Banana Nut Loaves	1 (1.9 oz)	220
Banana Twins	1 (2.2 oz)	250
Be My Valentine Chocolate	1 (2.2 oz)	280
Be My Valentine Vanilla	1 (2.2 oz)	290
Blueberry Loaves	1 (2 oz)	220
Chocolate Chip	1 (2.4 oz)	310
Christmas Tree Cake	1 pkg (1.5 oz)	190
Coconut Creme	1 (1.7 oz)	210
Coffee Cake Apple	1 (2.1 oz)	230
Cupcake Creme Filled Chocolate	1 (1.6 oz)	180
Cupcake Creme Filled Orange	1 (1.7 oz)	210
Cupcake Creme Filled Strawberry	1 (1.7 oz)	210
Devil Cremes	1 (1.6 oz)	190
Devil Squares	1 (2.2 oz)	270

FOOD	PORTION	CALS
Easter Basket Cake Chocolate	1 (2.4 oz)	300
Easter Basket Cake Vanilla	1 (2.5 oz)	320
Fall Party Cake Chocolate	1 (2.4 oz)	290
Fall Party Cake Vanilla	1 (2.5 oz)	310
Fancy Cakes	1 (2.4 oz)	300
Frosted Fudge	1 (1.5 oz)	200
Golden Cremes	1 (1.5 oz)	150
Holiday Cake Roll Cherry Creme	1 (2.1 oz)	260
Holiday Snack Cake Chocolate	1 (2.4 oz)	300
Holiday Snack Cake Vanilla	1 (2.5 oz)	320
Honey Bun	1 (1.8 oz)	220
Pecan Spinwheels	1 (1 oz)	110
Snack Cake Chocolate	1 (2.5 oz)	310
Strawberry Shortcake Roll	1 (2.1 oz)	230
Swiss Rolls	1 (2.1 oz)	270
Zebra Cakes	1 (2.6 oz)	330
Low Carb Creations		
Cheesecake Blueberry Swirl	1 slice (3 oz)	220
Cheesecake Chocolate	1 slice (3 oz)	250
Cheesecake Key Lime	1 slice (3 oz)	250
Cheesecake New York	1 slice (3 oz)	250
Cheesecake Pumpkin Swirl	1 slice (3 oz)	220
Marie Callender's		
Cobbler Apple	1 serv (4.25 oz)	370
Cobbler Berry	1 serv (4.25 oz)	370
Cobbler Cherry	1 serv (4.25 oz)	380
Cobbler Peach	1 serv (4.25 oz)	380
Natural Touch		
Toaster Square Blueberry	1 (2.8 oz)	180
Toaster Squares Date Walnut	1 (2.8 oz)	200
Nature's Path		
Organic Toaster Pastry Apple Cinnamon	1 (2 oz)	210
Organic Toaster Pastry Blueberry	1 (2 oz)	210
Organic Toaster Pastry Frosted Apple Cinnamon	1 (2 oz)	210
Organic Toaster Pastry Frosted Blueberry	1 (2 oz)	200
Organic Toaster Pastry Frosted Strawberry	1 (2 oz)	210
Pepperidge Farm		
Apple Turnover	1 (3.1 oz)	330
Blueberry Turnovers	1 (3.1 oz)	340
Cherry Turnover	1 (3.1 oz)	320

FOOD	PORTION	CALS
Large Layer Chocolate Fudge	⅛ cake (2.4 oz)	260
Large Layer Coconut	⅛ cake (2.4 oz)	260
Large Layer Vanilla	⅛ cake (2.4 oz)	250
Mini Turnover Apple	1 (1.4 oz)	140
Mini Turnover Cherry	1 (1.4 oz)	140
Mini Turnover Strawberry	1 (1.4 oz)	140
Peach Turnover	1 (3.1 oz)	340
Raspberry Turnovers	1 (3.1 oz)	330
Philadelphia		
Snack Bars Classic Cheesecake	1 (1.5 oz)	190
Snack Bars Strawberry Cheesecake	1 bar (1.5 oz)	190
Pillsbury		
Apple Turnovers	1 (2 oz)	170
Cherry Turnovers	1 (2 oz)	180
Sara Lee		
Cheesecake 25% Reduced Fat	¼ cake (4.2 oz)	310
Cheesecake Cherry Cream	¼ cake (4.7 oz)	350
Cheesecake Chocolate Chip	¼ cake (4.2 oz)	410
Cheesecake French	⅙ cake (3.9 oz)	350
Cheesecake French Strawberry	⅙ cake (4.3 oz)	320
Cheesecake Strawberry Cream	¼ cake (4.7 oz)	330
Coffee Cake Butter Streusel	⅙ cake (1.9 oz)	220
Coffee Cake Crumb	⅛ cake (2 oz)	220
Coffee Cake Pecan	⅙ cake (1.9 oz)	230
Coffee Cake Raspberry	⅙ cake (1.9 oz)	220
Coffee Cake Reduced Fat Cheese	⅙ cake (1.9 oz)	180
Layer Cake Coconut	⅛ cake (2.8 oz)	260
Layer Cake Double Chocolate	⅛ cake (2.8 oz)	260
Layer Cake Fudge Golden	⅛ cake (2.8 oz)	260
Layer Cake German Chocolate	⅛ cake (2.9 oz)	280
Layer Cake Vanilla	⅛ cake (2.8 oz)	260
Original Cheesecake	¼ cake (4.2 oz)	350
Pound Cake All Butter	¼ cake (2.7 oz)	320
Pound Cake Chocolate Swirl	¼ cake (2.9 oz)	330
Pound Cake Family Size	⅙ cake (2.7 oz)	310
Pound Cake Reduced Fat	¼ cake (2.7 oz)	280
Pound Cake Strawberry Swirl	¼ cake (2.9 oz)	290
Strawberry Shortcake	⅛ cake (2.5 oz)	180
Snack & Smile		
Mini Loaf Apple Cinnamon	1 loaf (2 oz)	190

FOOD	PORTION	CALS
Mini Loaf Banana	1 loaf (2 oz)	200
Mini Loaf Blueberry	1 loaf (2 oz)	190
Mini Loaf Carrot	1 loaf (2 oz)	200
SnackWell's		
Streusel Squares Apple Cinnamon	1 (1.5 oz)	150
Streusel Squares Cherry	1 (1.5 oz)	150
Tastykake		
Banana Creamie	1 (1.5 oz)	170
Bear Claw Apple	1 (3 oz)	280
Bear Claw Cinnamon	1 (3 oz)	300
Big Texas	1 (3 oz)	300
Breakfast Bun Chocolate Raisin	1 (3.2 oz)	330
Bunny Trail Treats	1 (1.3 oz)	150
Chocolate Creamie	1 (1.5 oz)	180
Chocolate Krimpies	2 (2.2 oz)	240
Coffee Roll Glazed	1 (3 oz)	300
Coffee Roll Vanilla	1 (3.2 oz)	320
Cupcakes	2 (2.1 oz)	200
Cupcakes Butter Cream Cream Filled Iced	2 (2.2 oz)	240
Cupcakes Chocolate Cream Filled Iced	2 (2.2 oz)	230
Cupcakes Low Fat Vanilla Cream Filled	2 (2.2 oz)	190
Cupid Kake	1 (1.3 oz)	150
Honey Bun Glazed	1 (3.2 oz)	350
Honey Bun Iced	1 (3.2 oz)	350
Junior Chocolate	1 (3.3 oz)	330
Junior Coconut	1 (3.3 oz)	310
Junior Koffee Kake	1 (2.5 oz)	270
Junior Pound Kake	1 (3 oz)	320
Kandy Kakes Chocolate	3 (2 oz)	250
Kandy Kakes Coconut	2 (2.7 oz)	330
Kandy Kakes Peanut Butter	2 (1.3 oz)	190
Koffee Kake	1 (2 oz)	210
Koffee Kake Cream Filled	2 (2 oz)	240
Koffee Kake Low Fat Apple	2 (2 oz)	170
Koffee Kake Low Fat Lemon	2 (2 oz)	180
Koffee Kake Low Fat Raspberry	2 (2 oz)	170
Kreepy Kakes	2 (2.2 oz)	240
Kreme Krimpies	2 (2 oz)	230
Krimpets Butterscotch Iced	2 (2 oz)	210
Krimpets Jelly Fillled	2 (2 oz)	190

FOOD	PORTION	CALS
Krimpets Strawberry	2 (2 oz)	210
Kringle Kake	1 (1.3 oz)	150
Santa Snacks	2 (2.2 oz)	240
Sparkle Kake	1 (1.3 oz)	150
Tasty Tweets	2 (2.2 oz)	240
Tropical Delight Coconut	2 (2 oz)	190
Tropical Delight Guava	2 (2 oz)	190
Tropical Delight Papaya	2 (2 oz)	200
Tropical Delight Pineapple	2 (2 oz)	200
Vanilla Creamie	1 (1.5 oz)	190
Witchy Treat	1 (1.3 oz)	150
Tom's		
Honey Bun	1 pkg (3 oz)	360
Honey Bun Jelly Filled	1 pkg (4 oz)	490
Marble Pound	1 pkg (2.5 oz)	300
Texas Cinnamon Roll	1 pkg (4 oz)	360
TAKE-OUT		
angelfood	1/12 cake (1 oz)	73
apple crisp	½ cup (5 oz)	230
baklava	1 oz	126
basbousa namoura	1 piece (1 oz)	60
boston cream pie	1/6 cake (3.3 oz)	293
cannoli w/ cannoli cream	1	369
carrot w/ cream cheese icing	1/12 cake (3.9 oz)	484
cheesecake w/ cherry topping	1/12 cake (5 oz)	359
chinese Moon cake	1 (4.8 oz)	458
chocolate w/ chocolate frosting	1/8 cake (2.2 oz)	235
coffeecake cheese	1/6 cake (2.7 oz)	258
coffeecake crumb topped cheese	1/6 cake (2.7 oz)	258
coffeecake crumb topped cinnamon	1/9 cake (2.2 oz)	263
cream puff w/ custard filling	1 (4.6 oz)	336
dutch honey cake	1 slice (0.8 oz)	70
eclair w/ chocolate icing & custard filling	1	205
french apple tart	1 (3.5 oz)	302
fruitcake	1/36 cake (2.9 oz)	302
gingerbread	1/9 cake (2.6 oz)	264
panettone	1/12 cake (2.9 oz)	300
petit fours	2 (0.9 oz)	120
pineapple upside down	1/9 cake (4 oz)	367
pound	1 slice (1 oz)	120

FOOD	PORTION	CALS
pound fat free	1 oz	80
sacher torte	1 slice (2.2 oz)	240
sacher torte chocolate + apricot jam	1 serv	430
sheet cake w/ white frosting	⅑ cake	445
strudel apple	1 piece (2.5 oz)	195
tiramisu	1 piece (5.1 oz)	409
torte chocolate ganache	1 slice (3.5 oz)	400
trifle w/ cream	6 oz	291
yellow w/ vanilla frosting	⅛ cake (2.2 oz)	239

CAKE ICING

FOOD	PORTION	CALS
chocolate ready-to-use	½ pkg (1.3 oz)	151
glaze home recipe	½ recipe (1 oz)	97
vanilla ready-to-use	½ pkg (1.3 oz)	159
Betty Crocker		
HomeStyle Mix Coconut Pecan as prep	2 tbsp	160
HomeStyle Mix White Fluffy as prep	6 tbsp	100
Party Frosting Chocolate w/ Stars	2 tbsp (1.2 oz)	140
Rich & Creamy Butter Cream	2 tbsp (1.3 oz)	140
Rich & Creamy Cherry	2 tbsp (1.2 oz)	140
Rich & Creamy Chocolate	2 tbsp (1.2 oz)	130
Rich & Creamy Cream Cheese	2 tbsp (1.2 oz)	140
Rich & Creamy Dark Chocolate	2 tbsp (1.3 oz)	130
Rich & Creamy French Vanilla	2 tbsp (1.2 oz)	140
Rich & Creamy Milk Chocolate	2 tbsp (1.3 oz)	130
Rich & Creamy Rainbow Chip	2 tbsp (1.2 oz)	140
Rich & Creamy Vanilla	2 tbsp (1.2 oz)	140
Toppers Milk Chocolate	2 tbsp (1.2 oz)	130
Toppers Vanilla	2 tbsp (1.2 oz)	140
Jiffy		
Fudge Frosting	¼ cup	150
White Frosting	¼ cup	150
Sweet Rewards		
Ready-To-Spread Reduced Fat Chocolate	2 tbsp (1.2 oz)	120
Ready-To-Spread Reduced Fat Vanilla	2 tbsp (1.2 oz)	130

CAKE MIX

FOOD	PORTION	CALS
angelfood	½ cake (1.8 oz)	129
angelfood	10 in cake (20.9 oz)	1535
carrot w/o frosting	½ cake (2.5 oz)	239
carrot w/o frosting	2 layers (29.6 oz)	2886

FOOD	PORTION	CALS
chocolate pudding type w/o frosting	2 layers (32.4 oz)	3234
chocolate pudding type w/o frosting	1/12 cake (2.7 oz)	270
chocolate w/o frosting	1/12 cake (2.3 oz)	198
chocolate w/o frosting	2 layers (26.8 oz)	2393
coffeecake crumb topped cinnamon	1/8 cake (2 oz)	178
devil's food w/o frosting	1/12 cake (2.3 oz)	198
devil's food w/ chocolate frosting	1/16 cake	235
devil's food w/ chocolate frosting	1 cake 9 in diam	3755
fudge w/o frosting	1/12 cake (2.3 oz)	198
gingerbread	1 cake 8 in sq	1575
gingerbread	1/9 cake (2.4 oz)	207
white w/o frosting	2 layer cake (26 oz)	2265
white w/o frosting	1/12 cake (2.2 oz)	190
yellow w/ chocolate frosting	1/16 cake	235
yellow w/o frosting	2 layers (26.5 oz)	2415
yellow w/o frosting	1/12 cake (2.2 oz)	202
yellow w/ chocolate frosting	1 cake 9 in diam	3895
Betty Crocker		
Angel Food Fat Free	1/12 cake	140
Angel Food Fat Free Confetti as prep	1/12 cake	150
Cheesecake Chocolate Chip as prep	1/8 cake	410
Cheesecake Original as prep	1/8 cake	400
Cheesecake Strawberry Swirl as prep	1/8 cake	380
Pineapple Upside Down as prep	1/6 cake	420
Quick Bread Banana	1/12 cake	170
Quick Bread Cinnamon Streusel as prep	1/14 cake	180
Quick Bread Cranberry Orange as prep	1/12 cake	170
Quick Bread Lemon Poppy Seed as prep	1/12 cake	170
Stir'n Bake Carrot Cake w/ Cream Cheese Frosting as prep	1/6 cake	260
Stir'n Bake Coffee Cake w/ Cinnamon Streusel as prep	1/6 cake	230
Stir'n Bake Devils Food w/ Chocolate Frosting as prep	1/6 cake	240
Stir'n Bake Yellow w/ Chocolate Frosting as prep	1/8 cake	240
SuperMoist Butter Pecan as prep	1/12 cake	240
SuperMoist Butter Yellow as prep	1/12 cake	260
SuperMoist Carrot as prep	1/10 cake	320
SuperMoist Cherry Chip	1/10 cake	300

FOOD	PORTION	CALS
SuperMoist Chocolate Fudge as prep	1/12 cake	270
SuperMoist Golden Vanilla as prep	1/12 cake	240
SuperMoist Lemon as prep	1/12 cake	240
SuperMoist Milk Chocolate as prep	1/12 cake	240
SuperMoist Pineapple as prep	1/12 cake	250
SuperMoist Spice as prep	1/12 cake	240
SuperMoist Strawberry as prep	1/12 cake	250
SuperMoist White as prep	1/12 cake	230
SuperMoist White Light as prep	1/10 cake	210
Bisquick		
Mix	1/3 cup (1.4 oz)	160
Reduced Fat	1/3 cup (1.4 oz)	140
Bob's Red Mills		
Gluten Free Chocolate as prep	1/6 cake	170
Carbolite		
Cheesecake Chocolate as prep	1/8 cake	260
Carbsense		
Zero Carb Baking Mix	1 oz	110
Dromedary		
Date Bread	1/11 cake (2 oz)	190
Date Nut Roll	1/2 in slice	80
Gingerbread	1 piece (2 in x 2 in)	100
Pound	1/2 in slice	150
Hodgson Mill		
Gingerbread Whole Wheat	1/4 cup (1 oz)	110
Jiffy		
Devil's Food as prep	1/5 cake	220
Golden Yellow as prep	1/5 cake	220
White Cake as prep	1/5 cake	210
MiniCarb		
Carrot as prep	1 slice	280
Chocolate as prep	1 slice	230
Zero Carb Baking Mix not prep	1/2 cup	55
Sweet Rewards		
Reduced Fat White as prep	1/12 cake	180
Reduced Fat Yellow as prep	1/12 cake	200

CALABAZA

fresh	1/2 cup	32

FOOD	PORTION	CALS
CALZONE (see SANDWICHES)		
CANADIAN BACON		
grilled	1 pkg (6 oz)	257
Boar's Head		
Canadian Bacon	2 oz	70
Hormel		
Sandwich Style	3 slices (2 oz)	70
Jones		
Slices	3	70
Real Canadian Bacon		
Peameal	4 oz	130
Yorkshire Farms		
Uncured	3 oz	100
CANADIAN BACON SUBSTITUTES		
Yves		
Canadian Veggie Bacon	1 serv (2 oz)	80
CANDY		
boiled sweets	¼ lb	327
butterscotch	1 piece (6 g)	24
candied cherries	1 (4 g)	12
candied citron	1 oz	89
candied lemon peel	1 oz	90
candied orange peel	1 oz	90
candied pineapple slice	1 slice (2 oz)	179
candy corn	1 oz	105
caramels	1 piece (8 g)	31
caramels chocolate	1 bar (2.3 oz)	231
caramels chocolate	1 piece (6 g)	22
carob bar	1 (3.1 oz)	453
crisped rice bar almond	1 bar (1 oz)	130
crisped rice bar chocolate chip	1 bar (1 oz)	115
dark chocolate	1 oz	150
fondant	1 piece (0.6 oz)	57
fondant chocolate coated	1 piece (0.4 oz)	40
fondant mint	1 oz	105
fruit pastilles	1 tube (1.4 oz)	101
fudge brown sugar w/ nuts	1 piece (0.5 oz)	56
fudge chocolate marshmallow	1 piece (0.7 oz)	84

FOOD	PORTION	CALS
fudge chocolate marshmallow w/ nuts	1 piece (0.8 oz)	96
fudge chocolate w/ nuts	1 piece (0.7 oz)	81
fudge peanut butter	1 piece (0.6 oz)	59
fudge vanilla w/ nuts	1 piece (0.5 oz)	62
gumdrops	10 sm (0.4 oz)	135
gumdrops	10 lg (3.8 oz)	420
hard candy	1 oz	106
jelly beans	10 sm (0.4 oz)	40
jelly beans	10 lg (1 oz)	104
lollipop	1 (6 g)	22
marzipan	1 oz	128
milk chocolate	1 bar (1.55 oz)	226
milk chocolate crisp	1 bar (1.45 oz)	203
milk chocolate w/ almonds	1 bar (1.45 oz)	215
nougat nut cream	0.5 oz	49
organic dark chocolate w/ raisins & pecans	1.4 oz	220
peanut bar	1 (1.4 oz)	209
peanut brittle	1 oz	128
peanuts chocolate covered	1 cup (5.2 oz)	773
peanuts chocolate covered	10 (1.4 oz)	208
praline	1 piece (1.4 oz)	177
pretzels chocolate covered	1 oz	130
pretzels chocolate covered	1 (0.4 oz)	50
sesame crunch	20 pieces (1.2 oz)	181
sweet chocolate	1 bar (1.45 oz)	201
sweet chocolate	1 oz	143
taffy	1 piece (0.5 oz)	56
toffee	1 piece (0.4 oz)	65
truffles	1 piece (0.4 oz)	59
100 Grand		
Bar	1 bar (1.5 oz)	200
3 Musketeers		
Bar	1 (2.1 oz)	260
Fun Size	2 (1.2 oz)	140
Miniatures	7 (1.4 oz)	180
5th Avenue		
Bar	1 (0.56 oz)	80
Almond Joy		
Bar	1 (0.68 oz)	90

FOOD	PORTION	CALS
Altoids		
All Flavors	3 pieces	10
Anastasia		
Coco Rhum Bites	2 pieces (1 oz)	110
At Last!		
Chocolate Almond	1 bar	120
Chocolate Crisp	1 bar	110
Chocolate Mint	1 bar	110
Chocolate Peanut Butter	1 bar	120
Atkins		
Endulge Caramel Nut Chew	1 bar (1.23 oz)	140
Endulge Chocolate Bar	1 bar (1.1 oz)	150
Endulge Chocolate Crunch	1 bar (1 oz)	150
Endulge Peanut Butter Cups	3 pieces	160
Baby Ruth		
Bar	1 bar (2.1 oz)	270
Fun Size	1 bar (0.7 oz)	100
Bittyfinger		
Bars	2	170
Body Smarts		
Chocolate Peanut Crunch	2 bars (1.8 oz)	210
Brach's		
Bridge Mix	16 pieces	190
Candy Corn	26 pieces	140
Caramel Clusters	3 pieces	210
Circus Peanuts	6 pieces	160
Fruit Rippers Berry Punch	1 pkg (0.5 oz)	60
Fruit Slices	3 pieces	150
Malts	15 pieces	190
Mellowcreme Pumpkins	6 pieces	130
Milk Maid Caramels	4 pieces	160
Mint Patties	3 pieces	140
Orange Slices	2 pieces	130
Peanut Butter Meltaways	3 pieces	200
Root Beer Barrels	3 pieces	70
Spearmint Leaves	5 pieces	130
Spice Drops	12 pieces	130
Sprinkles	17 pieces	200
Star Brites Butterscotch	3 pieces	60

FOOD	PORTION	CALS
Stars	10 pieces	200
Wild'N Fruity Gummi Bears	14 pieces	140
Breath Savers		
Sugar Free Peppermint	1 piece	5
Butterfinger		
Bar	1 (2.1 oz)	270
Crisps	1 bar (1.8 oz)	250
Crisps Minis	4 (1.5 oz)	220
Minis	4 (1.4 oz)	180
Cadbury		
Milk Chocolate Roast Almond	10 blocks (1.4 oz)	220
Royal Dark	10 blocks (1.4 oz)	220
Cape Cod Provisions		
Cranberry Bog Frogs	3 pieces (1.9 oz)	250
Carbolite		
Caramel	1 bar	100
CarbAway	1 bar	100
CarboSnack	1 bar	110
Chocolate Truffle	1 bar (1 oz)	122
Chocolate Almond	1 bar (1.75 oz)	298
Chocolate Crisp	1 bar (1.75 oz)	256
Chocolate Peanut Butter	1 bar (1.75 oz)	256
Crisy Caramel	1 bar (1 oz)	130
Milk Chocolate	1 bar (1.75 oz)	263
Peanut Butter Cup	1	170
Pecan Cluster	1 bar	120
CarbSlim		
Crunch Bites Chocolate Caramel	1 pkg	122
Crunch Bites Peanut Butter	1 pkg	171
Carmello		
Snack Size	1 (0.66 oz)	90
Cary's Of Oregon		
English Toffee Milk Chocolate Almond	1 piece (0.75 oz)	110
Charleston Chew		
Chocolate	½ bar	120
Strawberry	½ bar	120
Vanilla	½ bar	120
ChocoSoy		
Soy Milk Chocolate	1 piece (0.4 oz)	50

FOOD	PORTION	CALS
Chunky		
Bar	1 (1.4 oz)	210
Classic Caramels		
Chocolate Creme Filled	3 pieces	80
Soft & Chewy	3 pieces	80
Cloud Nine		
Australian Orange Peel	½ bar (1.5 oz)	220
Butter Nut Toffee	½ bar (1.5 oz)	230
Cool Mint Crisp	½ bar (1.5 oz)	220
Espresso Bean Crunch	½ bar (1.5 oz)	220
Malted Milk Crunch	½ bar (1.5 oz)	230
Milk Chocolate	½ bar (1.5 oz)	230
Oregan Red Raspberry	½ bar (1.5 oz)	230
Peanut Butter Brittle	½ bar (1.5 oz)	230
Sundried Cherry	½ bar (1.5 oz)	230
Toasted Coconut Crisp	½ bar (1.5 oz)	230
Vanilla Dark	½ bar (1.5 oz)	230
CocoaVia		
Blueberry & Almond Chocolate	1 bar	100
Chocolate	1 bar	80
Chocolate Almond	1 bar	80
Chocolate Blueberry	1 bar	80
Chocolate Cherry	1 bar	80
Chocolate Covered Almonds	1 bar	140
Crispy Chocolate	1 bar	90
Original Chocolate	1 bar	100
Coffee Rio		
Coffee Candy All Flavors	4 pieces	60
Crunch		
Fun Size	4 bars	210
Daboga		
Organic Milk Chocolate	1 bar (2 oz)	318
Del Monte		
Radical Raizins Cinnamon	1 pkg (0.7 oz)	70
Radical Raizins Rainbow	1 pkg (0.7 oz)	70
Doctor's CarbRite		
Sugar Free Dark Chocolate	1 oz	124
Sugar Free Dark Chocolate With Almonds	4 sq (1 oz)	132
Sugar Free Milk Chocolate	1 oz	128
Sugar Free Milk Chocolate With Peanuts	4 sq (1 oz)	132

FOOD	PORTION	CALS
Sugar Free Milk Chocolate With Soy Crisps	4 sq (1 oz)	120
Sugar Free Mint Chocolate	1 oz	128
Dove		
Dark Chocolate	1 bar (1.3 oz)	200
Dark Chocolate Miniatures	5 (1.4 oz)	210
Milk Chocolate	1 bar (1.3 oz)	200
Milk Chocolate Miniatures	5 (1.4 oz)	220
Eclipse		
Mints Sugarless All Flavors	3 pieces	5
Estee		
Fructose Sweetened Peanut Butter Cups	5	200
Fructose Sweetened Dark Chocolate	½ bar (1.4 oz)	200
Fructose Sweetened Milk Chocolate	½ bar (1.4 oz)	230
Fructose Sweetened Milk Chocolate w/ Almonds	½ bar (1.4 oz)	230
Fructose Sweetened Milk Chocolate w/ Crisp Rice	½ bar (1.2 oz)	370
Peanut Brittle	⅓ box (1.3 oz)	210
Sugar Free Assorted Fruit	3	15
Sugar Free Butterscotch	4	15
Sugar Free Gourmet Jelly Beans	26	70
Sugar Free Gum Drops Assorted Fruit	11	110
Sugar Free Gummy Bears Assorted Fruit	17	70
Sugar Free Peppermint	3	15
Sugar Free Sour Citrus Slices	9	60
Sugar Free Toffee	4	15
Sugar Free Tropical Fruit	3	15
Fauchon		
Assortment Truffles	3 pieces (1.3 oz)	160
Chocolate Assortment	3 pieces (1.1 oz)	170
Ferrero Rocher		
Candy	3 pieces (1.3 oz)	220
Godiva		
Chocolatier Dark Chocolate w/ Raspberry	1 bar (1.5 oz)	220
Chocolatier Milk Chocolate	1 bar (1.5 oz)	230
Chocolatier Milk Chocolate w/ Almonds	1 bar (1.5 oz)	230
Mochaccino Mousse	2 pieces (1.25 oz)	210
Sugar Free Chocolate	1 bar (1.5 oz)	190
Sugar Free Chocolate w/ Almonds	1 bar (1.5 oz)	200

FOOD	PORTION	CALS
Sugar Free Dark Chocolate	1 bar (1.5 oz)	190
Truffles Assorted	2 pieces (1.5 oz)	220
Goetze's		
Caramel Creams	3 pieces	130
Cow Tales	1 pkg (1 oz)	110
Gol D Lite		
Milk Chocolate Crisp	1 bar	125
Seashell Truffle	1 piece	54
Goldenberg's		
Peanut Chews	3 pieces	180
Golightly		
Sugar Free Caramels	5 pieces	150
Sugar Free Doublers Chews Peach & Creme	7 pieces	150
Sugar Free Fudgie Rolls	6 pieces	130
Sugar Free Hard Candy	4 pieces	45
Goobers		
Peanuts	1 pkg (1.38 oz)	210
Good & Plenty		
Snack Size	1 box (0.6 oz)	60
Good 'N Fruity		
Snack Size	1 box (0.6 oz)	60
Heath		
Snack Size	1 bar (0.3 oz)	50
Hershey's		
Bites Almond Joy	8 pieces	100
Bites Cookies 'N' Creme	8 pieces	90
Bites Milk Chocolate w/ Almond	7 pieces	90
Bites Reese's	7 pieces	90
Bites York	9 pieces	90
Candy Coated Milk Chocolate Eggs	4 pieces	90
Chocolate Miniatures Sugar Free	5 pieces (1.4 oz)	170
Chocolate w/ Almonds Miniatures Sugar Free	5 pieces (1.4 oz)	180
Dark Chocolate Miniatures Sugar Free	5 pieces (1.4 oz)	190
Hugs	1 piece	25
Kisses	1	25
Kisses w/ Almonds	1 piece	25
Milk Chocolate	1 bar (1.4 oz)	210
Milk Chocolate w/ Almonds	1 bar (1.4 oz)	230
Miniature Special Dark	1 (0.3 oz)	45
Nuggets Cookies 'N' Creme	4	190

FOOD	PORTION	CALS
Nuggets Dark Chocolate w/ Almonds	4	220
Nuggets Milk Chocolate	4	230
Nuggets Milk Chocolate w/ Almonds	1	60
Nuggets Milk Chocolate w/ Almonds & Toffee	1	50
Nuggets Milk Chocolate w/ Raisins & Almonds	1	50
Pot Of Gold	3 pieces	130
Sweet Escapes Caramel & Peanut Butter Crispy	1 bar	80
Sweet Escapes Crispy Caramel Fudge	1 bar	70
Sweet Escapes Crunchy Peanut Butter	1 bar (0.7 oz)	90
Sweet Escapes Triple Chocolate Wafer	1 bar	80
Take 5	2 pkg (1.5 oz)	220
Tastetations Butterscotch	3 pieces	60
Tastetations Caramel	3 pieces	60
Tastetations Chocolate	3 pieces	60
Hint Mint		
All Flavors	2 pieces	10
Jelly Belly		
Jelly Beans Sugar Free	35	80
Jolly Rancher		
All Flavors	4 pieces	60
Lollipops All Flavors	1 (0.6 oz)	60
Sugar Free	4 pieces (0.6 oz)	35
Joyva		
Halvah Chocolate Covered	1 serv (2 oz)	380
Halvah Marble	1 serv (2 oz)	390
Judy's		
Sugar Free Almond Caramel Cluster	1 piece (1.5 oz)	200
Sugar Free Cashew Caramel Cluster	1 pieces (1.5 oz)	190
Sugar Free English Toffee	1 piece (1.5 oz)	220
Sugar Free Macadamia Caramel Cluster	1 piece (1.5 oz)	220
Sugar Free Peanut Brittle	¾ cup	100
Sugar Free Pecan Almond Cluster	1 piece (1.5 oz)	220
Junior Mints		
Snack Size	1 box (0.7 oz)	80
Kit Kat		
Bar	1 (0.6 oz)	80
Klein		
Sugar Free Hard Candy All Flavors	3 pieces	12

FOOD	PORTION	CALS
Krackel		
Bar	1 (0.6 oz)	90
Miniature	1	45
Lambertz		
Petits Soleils Chocolate Coated Gingerbread	1 piece (0.4 oz)	47
Landies Candies		
Sugar Free Almond Clusters	2 pieces (1.5 oz)	240
Sugar Free Bon Bons Peanut Butter	2 (1.5 oz)	240
Sugar Free Coconut Clusters	2 pieces (1.5 oz)	250
Sugar Free Cookies & Cream	2 pieces (1.5 oz)	240
Sugar Free Dark Almond Bark	1 piece (1.5 oz)	230
Sugar Free Dark Miniature Bars	7 pieces (1.5 oz)	230
Sugar Free Milk Miniature Bars	7 pieces (1.5 oz)	240
Sugar Free Mint Discs	7 pieces (1.5 oz)	240
Sugar Free Peanut Clusters	2 (1.5 oz)	240
Sugar Free White Almond Bark	1 piece (1.5 oz)	230
Sugar Free White Caps	6 pieces (1.5 oz)	230
Lean Protein Bites		
Milk Chocolate	1 pkg (1 oz)	120
Peanut Butter	1 pkg (1 oz)	120
White Chocolate	1 pkg (1 oz)	120
Lifesavers		
Gummi Shapes Barnum's Animals	1 pkg (0.8 oz)	70
Lindt		
Dark Chocolate 70% Cocoa	4 blocks (1.4 oz)	220
Lindor Truffles Dark Chocolate	3 pieces	220
Lindor Truffles Milk Chocolate	3 pieces	220
Low Carb Chef		
Gummi Bears	14 pieces	138
Jelly Beans	37 pieces	120
Sugar Free Caramel Marshmallow Treats	3 pieces	140
Sugar Free Cherry Cordials	3 pieces	250
Sugar Free Coconut Clusters	4 pieces	210
Sugar Free Milk Chocolate Covered Vanilla Caramels	3 pieces	160
Sugar Free Peanut Butter Cups	1 piece	200
Sugar Free Peanut Butter Truffes	2 pieces	200
Sugar Free Peanut Clusters	4 pieces	210
Sugar Free Pecan Turtles	1 pieces	120
Sugar Free Peppermint Patties	3 pieces	150

FOOD	PORTION	CALS
M&M's		
Almond	1 pkg (1.3 oz)	200
Chewlicious	1 bar (0.8 oz)	100
Crispy	1 pkg (1.5 oz)	200
Crispy Fun Size	3 pkg (1.5 oz)	200
Crunchy M-Azing	1 bar (1.52 oz)	220
Mega	27 pieces	200
Mega Peanut	12 pieces	210
Minis	1 pkg (1.1 oz)	150
Peanut	1 pkg (1.7 oz)	250
Peanut Butter	1 pkg (1.6 oz)	240
Plain	1 pkg (1.7 oz)	240
Plain Fun Size	1 pkg (0.7 oz)	100
Maple Grove Farms		
Maple Sugar Candy	5 pieces (1.3 oz)	140
Mauna Loa		
Kona Coffee Crunch Chocolate	1 bar (1.8 oz)	270
Macadamia Crisp Milk Chocolate	1 bar (1.8 oz)	270
Macadamia Milk Chocolate	1 bar (1.8 oz)	280
Mentos		
Sugar Free Mixed Berries	1 piece	5
Milky Way		
Bar	1 (2 oz)	270
Bar	2 fun size (1.4 oz)	180
Caramel Dark Chocolate	5 pieces	200
Caramels Milk Chocolate	5 pieces	200
Midnight	2 fun size (1.4 oz)	170
Midnight	1 bar (1.8 oz)	220
Midnight Miniatures	5 (1.4 oz)	180
Miniature	5 (1.5 oz)	190
Mon Cheri		
Hazelnut	4 pieces	260
Mounds		
Bar	1 (0.7 oz)	90
Mr. Goodbar		
Bar	1 (0.6 oz)	100
Miniatures	1 (0.3 oz)	45
Mrs. Fields		
Decadent Chocolates	3 pieces (1.8 oz)	240

FOOD	PORTION	CALS
Munch		
Nut Bar	1 (1.42 oz)	220
Necco		
Bridge Mix	¼ cup (1.5 oz)	180
Chocolate Covered Raisins	30 pieces (1.5 oz)	170
Malted Milk Balls	11 pieces (1.5 oz)	180
Mint	1 piece	12
SkyBar	1 bar (1.5 oz)	190
Nestle		
Buncha Crunch	1 pkg (1.4 oz)	90
Crunch	1 bar (1.55 oz)	230
Crunch Disk	1 (1.2 oz)	180
Crunchkins	5 pieces	190
Jingles Milk Chocolate Butterfinger	5 pieces	180
Jingles Milk Chocolate Crunch	7 pieces	220
Jingles White Crunch	7 pieces	230
Milk Chocolate	1 bar (1.45 oz)	220
Nesteggs Milk Chocolate Butterfinger	5 pieces	210
Nesteggs Milk Chocolate Crunch	5 pieces	190
Nesteggs White Crunch	7 pieces	230
Pearson's Egg Nog	2 pieces	60
Toll House Brownie Bar	2 pieces (2 oz)	250
Toll House Cookie Bar	1 piece (1 oz)	130
Treasures Butterfinger	3 pieces	180
Treasures Crunch	4 pieces (1.4 oz)	210
Treasures Peanut Butter	4 pieces	250
Turtles Bite Size	1 piece (0.4 oz)	50
Turtles Original	3 pieces	240
White Crunch	1 bar (1.4 oz)	220
Newman's Own		
Organic Peanut Butter Cups Dark Chocolate	3 pieces (1.2 oz)	180
Organic Peanut Butter Cups Milk Chocolate	3 pieces (1.2 oz)	180
Organic Peppermint Cups	3 pieces (1.2 oz)	180
Nibs		
Licorice	9 pieces	35
Nips		
Butter Rum	2 pieces	60
Caramel	2 pieces	60
Chocolate	2 pieces	60
Chocolate Parfait	2 pieces	60

FOOD	PORTION	CALS
Coffee	2 pieces	50
Vanilla Almond Cafe	2 pieces	50
Odense		
Marzipan	2 tbsp (1.4 oz)	170
Oh Henry!		
Bar	1 (1.8 oz)	120
Payday		
Snack Size	1 (0.7 oz)	90
Pearson's		
Irish Cream Parfait	2 pieces	60
Mint Patties	1	30
Perlege		
Sugar Free	1 bar	532
Belgium Chocolate All Flavors	(3.5 oz)	
Sugar Free Cream Filled Belgian Chocolate All Flavors	1 bar (1.5 oz)	226
Pez		
Candy	1 roll (0.3 oz)	35
Candy Sugar Free	1 roll (0.3 oz)	30
Planters		
CarbWell Peanut Butter Crunch	1 bar (1.25 oz)	160
Original Peanut Bar	1 pkg (1.6 oz)	230
Pure De-Lite		
Caramel	1 bar	120
Caramel Crisp	1 bar	120
Caramel Nougat	1 bar	110
Caramel Peanut Butter	1 bar	120
Caramel Pecan	1 bar	130
Sugar Free Dark Chocolate	1 bar	173
Sugar Free Milk Choclate w/ Mint	1 bar	187
Sugar Free Milk Chocolate	1 bar	187
Sugar Free Milk Chocolate w/ Almonds	1 bar	190
Sugar Free Milk Chocolate w/ Coconut	1 bar	190
Sugar Free Milk Chocolate w/ Orange	1 bar	187
Sugar Free Milk Chocolate w/ Peanuts	1 bar	190
Sugar Free White Chocolate	1 bar	187
Truffle Bar Caramel	1 bar	140
Truffle Bar Dark Mint	1 bar	160
Truffle Bar Hazelnut	1 bar	160
Truffle Bar Peanut Butter	1 bar	160

FOOD	PORTION	CALS
Raisinets		
Candy	1 pkg (1.58 oz)	200
Fun Size	3 pkg	200
Reese's		
Bites	16 pieces	220
FastBreak	1 bar (0.7 oz)	90
Miniatures Peanut Butter Cups Sugar Free	5 pieces (1.4 oz)	170
Nutrageous	1 bar (0.6 oz)	95
Peanut Butter Cups	1 piece (1.4 oz)	210
Peanut Butter Cups Miniatures	5 (1.4 oz)	210
Peanut Butter Cups Sugar Free	1 piece (1.5 oz)	180
Peanut Butter Eggs	1	90
Pieces	25	90
White Miniatures Peanut Butter Cups	4 pieces (1.4 oz)	210
White Miniatures Peanut Butter Cups Sugar Free	5 pieces (1.4 oz)	180
Ritter Sport		
Dark Chocolate Whole Hazelnuts	6 pieces (1.3 oz)	210
Robin Eggs		
Large	2 pieces	70
Medium	4 pieces	90
Mini	10 pieces	70
Rokeach		
Cotton Candy	2 cups (1 oz)	110
Rolo		
Caramels In Milk Chocolate	3 pieces (0.64 oz)	90
Russell Stover		
Assorted	3 pieces (1.4 oz)	170
Low Carb Pecan Delights	1 pieces (1 oz)	130
Peanut Butter & Grape Jelly	1 piece (0.8 oz)	100
Peanut Butter & Red Raspberry	2 (1.2 oz)	140
Pecan Delights	1 pkg (2 oz)	280
Pecan Roll	1 (1.75 oz)	260
S'mores	3 (1.4 oz)	210
Sugar Free Peanut Butter Cups	4 pieces (1.3 oz)	200
Sugar Free Pecans & Caramel	2 pieces (1.2 oz)	170
Sixlets		
Sixlets	3 tubes	90
Smucker's		
Jelly Beans	25	150

FOOD	PORTION	CALS
Snickers		
Bar	1 bar (2.07 oz)	280
Cruncher	3 fun size (1.4 oz)	230
Cruncher	1 bar (1.6 oz)	230
Fun Size	2 bars (1.4 oz)	190
Miniatures	4 (1.3 oz)	170
Sno Caps		
Candies	1 pkg (2.3 oz)	300
Sour Patch		
Connectors	1.5 oz	150
Kids	1.5 oz	140
Speakeasy		
Organic Mints All Flaors	4 pieces (2 g)	10
Starburst		
Fruit Chew Pop	1	50
Fruit Chews	1 pkg (2.07 oz)	240
Hard Candies	3 pieces	50
Jellybeans	¼ cup	150
Steel's		
Salt Water Taffy Assorted	3 pieces (1 oz)	90
Sugar Babies		
Tidbits	1 pkg	180
Swedish Fish		
Aqua Life	1.5 oz	140
Original	20 pieces (1.5 oz)	140
Symphony		
Bar	1 (0.6 oz)	90
Take 5		
Snack Size	2 pieces	220
The Chocolate Traveler		
Carb Controlled Wedges Bittersweet	4 pieces	120
Carb Controlled Wedges Dark Chocolate Coffee	4 pieces	110
Carb Controlled Wedges Dark Chocolate Mint	4 pieces	110
Carb Controlled Wedges Milk Chocolate	4 pieces	120
Wedges Bittersweet	4 pieces	130
Wedges Dark Chocolate Coffee	4 pieces	130
Wedges Dark Chocolate Mint	4 pieces	130
Wedges Milk Chocolate	4 pieces	130

FOOD	PORTION	CALS
Tobler		
Orange Dark Chocolate	5 pieces (1.5 oz)	240
Toblerone		
Bittersweet Chocolate w/ Honey & Almond Nugget	⅓ bar (1.2 oz)	170
Milk Chocolate w/ Honey & Almond Nougat	⅓ bar (1.76 oz)	170
Tom's		
Cherry Sours	1 pkg (2.25 oz)	210
Jelly Beans	1 pkg (2.25 oz)	230
Tootsie		
Pop	1	60
Torras		
Sugar Free Dark Chocolate	1 oz	136
Sugar Free Milk Chocolate	1 oz	140
Sugar Free Milk Chocolate w/ Almonds	1 oz	146
Sugar Free Milk Chocolate w/ Hazelnuts	1 oz	148
Sugar Free White Chocolate	1 oz	138
Tropical Source		
Butterscotch Dream	4 pieces (0.5 oz)	60
Chocolate Dairy Free California Raisin & Currant	½ bar (1.5 oz)	230
Chocolate Dairy Free Hazelnut Espresso Crunch	½ bar (1.5 oz)	250
Chocolate Dairy Free Maple Almond Granola	½ bar (1.5 oz)	230
Chocolate Dairy Free Mint Candy Crunch	½ bar (1.5 oz)	220
Chocolate Dairy Free Red Raspberry Crush	½ bar (1.5 oz)	230
Chocolate Dairy Free Sundried Jungle Banana	½ bar (1.5 oz)	230
Chocolate Dairy Free Toasted Almond	½ bar (1.5 oz)	250
Chocolate Dairy Free Wild Rice Crisp	½ bar (1.5 oz)	230
Cool Peppermint	4 pieces (0.5 oz)	60
Lollipops All Flavors	1	24
Mango Papaya	4 pieces (0.5 oz)	60
Twix		
Caramel	1 bar	280
Peanut Butter	1 bar	280
Twizzlers		
Cherry	1 piece	30
Chocolate	1	25
Licorice	1 piece	30
Pull'N'Peel Cherry	1 piece	100

FOOD	PORTION	CALS
Strawberry Snack Size	3 pkgs	130
Sugar Free	4 pieces (1.5 oz)	130
Unique Origin		
Guaranda Dark Chocolate	1 piece (0.3 oz)	54
Weight Watchers		
English Toffee Squares	3 pieces	160
Mint Patties	2	100
Peanut Butter Crunch	4 pieces	180
Pecan Crowns	3 pieces	150
Werther's		
Original	3 pieces (0.5 oz)	60
Whatchamacallit		
Bar	1 (0.57 oz)	80
Whitman's		
Sampler	3 pieces (1.4 oz)	190
Whoppers		
Malted Milk Balls	18 pieces	190
Yamate Chocolatier		
No Sugar Almonds & Caramel	1 piece (0.6 oz)	70
York		
Peppermint Patty Sugar Free	3 pieces (1.3 oz)	110
Peppermint Patty	3 (1.4 oz)	150
Zagnut		
Snack Size	1 piece	70
Zero		
Bar	1	70
CANTALOUPE		
dried	3.5 pieces (1.4 oz)	140
fresh cubed	1 cup	57
fresh half	½	94
Chiquita		
Wedge	¼ med (4.7 oz)	50
CARAWAY		
seed	1 tsp	7
CARDAMOM		
ground	1 tsp	6
CARDOON		
fresh shredded	½ cup	36

FOOD	PORTION	CALS
Frieda's		
Cardoon	1 cup	15
CARIBOU		
roasted	3 oz	142
CARISSA		
fresh	1	12
CAROB		
carob mix	3 tsp	45
carob mix as prep w/ whole milk	9 oz	195
flour	1 tbsp	14
flour	1 cup	185
Sunspire		
Carob Chips Unsweetened	13 pieces (0.5 oz)	70
Carob Chips Vegan	13 pieces (0.5 oz)	70
CARP		
fresh	3 oz	108
fresh cooked	1 fillet (6 oz)	276
fresh cooked	3 oz	138
roe raw	1 oz	37
roe salted in olive oil	2 tbsp (1 oz)	40
CARROT JUICE		
canned	6 oz	73
Bolthouse Farms		
Carrot Juice	8 oz	70
Luvli Juices		
Zingy Carrot	1 bottle (10 oz)	145
Naked Juice		
Just Carrot	8 oz	80
CARROTS		
CANNED		
slices	½ cup	17
slices low sodium	½ cup	17
Del Monte		
Savory Sides Honey Glazed	½ cup	70
Sliced	½ cup	35
Glory		
Seasoned Honey	½ cup	50

FOOD	PORTION	CALS
S&W		
Julienne	½ cup (4.3 oz)	30
Sliced	½ cup (4.3 oz)	30
Whole Small	½ cup (4.3 oz)	30
FRESH		
baby raw	1 (½ oz)	6
raw	1 (2.5 oz)	31
raw shredded	½ cup	24
slices cooked	½ cup	35
Bolthouse Farms		
Baby	1 pkg (2.25 oz)	25
Matchstix	3 oz	35
Dole		
Shredded	1 cup (3 oz)	40
Earthbound Farms		
Organic Mini Peeled	½ cup	30
Frieda's		
Gold	⅔ cup (3 oz)	35
Nature's Gold		
Fresh	1 med (2.7 oz)	40
River Ranch		
Shredded	¾ cup	35
FROZEN		
slices cooked	½ cup	26
Birds Eye		
Baby Whole	½ cup	40
Sliced	½ cup	35
Fresh Like		
Carrots Slice	3.5 oz	42
CASABA		
cubed	1 cup	45
fresh	1/10	43
CASHEWS		
cashew butter w/o salt	1 tbsp	94
dry roasted salted	1 oz	163
dry roasted w/ salt	18 nuts (1 oz)	160
oil roasted	1 oz	163
oil roasted salted	1 oz	163

FOOD	PORTION	CALS
Bowlby's		
Bits Cashew	½ cup	200
Frito Lay		
Salted	3 tbsp	160
Maranatha		
Cashew Butter	2 tbsp	190
Tamari Cashews	¼ cup	160
Sweet Delights		
Cashew Roasters	⅓ pkg (1 oz)	170
CASSAVA		
fresh	3½ oz	120
CATFISH		
channel breaded & fried	3 oz	194
channel raw	3 oz	99
wolffish atlantic baked	3 oz	105
CAULIFLOWER		
FRESH		
cooked	½ cup (2.2 oz)	14
flowerets cooked	3 (2 oz)	12
flowerets raw	3 (2 oz)	14
green cooked	1½ cup (3.2 oz)	29
green raw	1 cup (2.2 oz)	20
green raw	1 head	158
	7 in diam (18 oz)	
green raw floweret	1 (0.9 oz)	8
raw	½ cup (1.8 oz)	13
River Ranch		
Florets	1 cup	20
FROZEN		
cooked	½ cup	17
Birds Eye		
Cauliflower	½ cup	20
Fresh Like		
Florets	3.5 oz	26
CAVIAR		
black	1 tbsp	40
red	1 tbsp	40

FOOD	PORTION	CALS
CELERY		
diced cooked	½ cup	13
fresh	1 stalk (1.3 oz)	6
raw diced	½ cup	10
seed	1 tsp	8
Dole		
Stalks	2 med (3 oz)	15
Frieda's		
Celery Root	¾ cup	35
River Ranch		
Sticks Fresh	4 (3 oz)	15
CELTUCE		
raw	3½ oz	22
CEREAL		
bran flakes	¾ cup	90
corn flakes	1¼ cups	110
farina as prep w/ water	¾ cup (6.1 oz)	88
granola	½ cup	285
oatmeal instant as prep w/ water	1 cup (8.2 oz)	138
oatmeal regular & quick as prep w/ water	¾ cup (6.1 oz)	149
oatmeal regular & quick not prep	⅓ cup (0.9 oz)	104
puffed rice	1 cup	56
puffed wheat	1 cup	44
shredded mini wheats	1 cup	107
shredded wheat rectangular	1 biscuit (0.8 oz)	85
Albers		
Hominy Quick Grits uncooked	¼ cup	140
Alpen		
Corn Flakes	1 serv (1 oz)	110
No Salt No Sugar	1 serv (2 oz)	200
Regular	1 serv (2 oz)	200
Alti Plano		
Hot Cereal Chai Almond	1 pkg	210
Hot Cereal Oaxacan Chocolate	1 pkg	170
Hot Cereal Orange Date	1 pkg	180
Hot Cereal Regular	1 pkg	190
Hot Cereal Spiced Apple Raisin	1 pkg	160
Alvarado Street Bakery		
Plain Grinola	½ cup	220

FOOD	PORTION	CALS
Atkins		
Banana Nut Harvest	⅔ cup	100
Blueberry Bounty w/ Almonds	⅔ cup	100
Crunchy Almond Crisp	⅔ cup	100
Aunt Paula's		
Hot Flax Cereal	1 serv (1½ oz)	100
Back To Nature		
Banana Nut Multibran	¾ cup	140
Flax & Fiber Crunch	1 cup	200
Granola Apple Blueberry	½ cup	200
Granola Apple Cinnamon	½ cup	180
Granola Classic	½ cup	180
Granola French Vanilla	½ cup	220
Hi Protein Crunch	½ cup	150
Hi-Fiber Multibran	½ cup	70
Muesli	¾ cup	230
Multigrain Harvest	1 cup	210
Oat & Soy Crisp	¾ cup	180
Strawberry & Seven Grains	1 cup	210
Barbara's Bakery		
Apple Cinnamon O's	¾ cup	110
Bite Size Shredded Oats	1¼ cups (2 oz)	220
Cinnamon Puffins	1¼ cup (2 oz)	100
Cocoa Crunch Stars	1 cup (1 oz)	110
Frosted Corn Flakes	1 cup (1 oz)	110
Fruit Juice Sweetened Breakfast O's	1 cup (1 oz)	120
Fruit Juice Sweetened Brown Rice Crisps	1 cup (1 oz)	120
Fruit Juice Sweetened Corn Flakes	1 cup (1 oz)	110
GrainShop	⅔ cup (1 oz)	90
Honey Crunch Stars	1 cup (1 oz)	110
Honey Nut Toasted O's	¾ cup	120
Organic Fruity Punch	1 cup (1 oz)	110
Organic Soy Essence	¾ cup (1 oz)	100
Puffins	¾ cup (0.9 oz)	90
Shredded Spoonfuls	¾ cup	120
Shredded Wheat	2 biscuits (1.4 oz)	140
Bear Naked		
Apple Cinnamon	¼ cup	140
Banana Nut	¼ cup	140

FOOD	PORTION	CALS
Fruit And Nut	¼ cup	140
Peak Protein	½ cup	200
Carbsense		
Hot Cereal Country Spice not prep	½ cup	130
Hot Cereal Roasted Hazelnut not prep	½ cup	140
CoCo Wheats		
Hot Cereal	⅓ cup	200
Country Choice Naturals		
Instant Oatmeal Apples 'N' Cinnamon	1 pkg	140
Instant Oatmeal Maple Syrup	1 pkg	170
Instant Oatmeal Organic Plus French Vanilla	1 pkg	180
Instant Oatmeal Organic Plus Golden Brown Sugar	1 pkg	180
Instant Oatmeal Regular	1 pkg	110
Oatmeal Steel Cut not prep	½ cup	150
Oats Old Fashioned not prep	½ cup	150
Oats Quick not prep	½ cup	150
Organic Multi Grain Hot Cereal not prep	½ cup	130
Deliciously Slim		
Granola Cranberry Cashew	¾ cup	230
Granola Strawberry Almond	¾ cup	230
Enjoy Life		
Cinnamon Crunch Nut & Gluten Free	¾ cup	160
EnviroKidz		
Organic Orangutan O's	¾ cup	120
Erewhon		
Apple Stroodles	¾ cup	110
Aztec	1 cup	110
Banana O's	¾ cup	110
Brown Rice Cream	¼ cup	170
Corn Flakes	1¼ cups	210
Crispy Brown Rice	1 cup	110
Crispy Brown Rice No Salt Added	1 cup	110
Fruit'n Wheat	¾ cup	170
Kamut Flakes	⅔ cup	110
Raisin Bran	1 cup	170
Rice Twice	¾ cup	120
Whole Wheat Flakes	1 cup	180
Expert Foods		
Low Carb Hot Cereal Sub	½ cup	24

FOOD	PORTION	CALS
General Mills		
Basic 4	1 cup (1.9 oz)	200
Boo Berry	1 cup (1 oz)	120
Cheerios	1 cup	110
Cheerios Apple Cinnamon	¾ cup	120
Cheerios Frosted	1 cup (1 oz)	120
Cheerios Honey Nut	1 cup (1 oz)	120
Cheerios Multi Grain	1 cup (1 oz)	110
Cheerios Yogurt Burst Vanilla	¾ cup	120
Chex Corn	1 cup (1 oz)	110
Chex Honey Nut	¾ cup	120
Chex Morning Mix Cinnamon	1 pkg (1.1 oz)	130
Chex Morning Mix Fruit & Nut	1 pkg (1.1 oz)	180
Chex Morning Mix Honey Nut	1 pkg (1.1 oz)	130
Chex Multi-Bran	1 cup (2 oz)	200
Chex Rice	1¼ cups (1.1 oz)	120
Cinnamon Grahams	¾ cup (1 oz)	120
Cinnamon Toast Crunch	¾ cup (1 oz)	130
Cocoa Puffs	1 cup (1 oz)	120
Cookie Crisp	1 cup (1 oz)	120
Count Chocula	1 cup (1 oz)	120
Country Corn Flakes	1 cup (1 oz)	120
Fiber One	½ cup (1 oz)	60
Fiber One Honey Clusters	1¼ cup	170
Franken Berry	1 cup (1 oz)	120
French Toast Crunch	¾ cup (1 oz)	120
Gold Medal Raisin Bran	1⅓ cups (1.9 oz)	170
Golden Grahams	¾ cup (1 oz)	120
Harmony	1¼ cups (1.9 oz)	200
Honey Nut Clusters	1 cup (1.9 oz)	210
Kix	1⅓ cups (1 oz)	120
Kix Berry Berry	¾ cup (1 oz)	120
Lucky Charms	1 cup (1 oz)	120
Newquick	¾ cup (1 oz)	120
Oatmeal Crisp Almond	1 cup (1.9 oz)	220
Oatmeal Crisp Apple Cinnamon	1 cup (1.9 oz)	210
Oatmeal Crisp Raisin	1 cup (1.9 oz)	210
Para Su Familia Cinnamon Stars	1 cup (1 oz)	120
Para Su Familia Fruitis	1 cup (1 oz)	120
Para Su Familia Raisin Bran	1¼ cups (2 oz)	170

FOOD	PORTION	CALS
Raisin Nut Bran	¾ cup (1.9 oz)	200
Reese's Puffs	¾ cup	130
Snack'N Dash Cinnamon Toast Crunch	1 pkg (1.2 oz)	140
Snack'N Dash Honey Nut Cheerios	1 pkg (1 oz)	110
Snack'N Dash Lucky Charms	1 pkg (1 oz)	110
Sunrise Organic	¾ cup (1 oz)	110
Total Brown Sugar & Oat	¾ cup (1 oz)	110
Total Protein	¾ cup	120
Total Raisin Bran	1 cup	170
Total Whole Grain	¾ cup (1 oz)	100
Trix	1 cup (1 oz)	120
Wheaties	1 cup (1 oz)	110
Wheaties Energy Crunch	1 cup (1.9 oz)	210
Wheaties Frosted	¾ cup (1 oz)	110
Wheaties Raisin Bran	1 cup (1.9 oz)	180
Grainfield's		
Brown Rice	1 serv (1 oz)	110
Crisp Rice	1 serv (1 oz)	112
Raisin Bran	1 serv (1 oz)	90
Wheat Flakes	1 serv (1 oz)	100
Gram's Gourmet		
Cream Of Flax not prep	½ cup	142
Crunch Granolas All Flavors	½ cup	349
Grandy Oats		
Organic Granola Classic	½ cup	252
Organic Granola Low Fat Cranberry Chew	½ cup	191
Organic Granola Mainely Maple	½ cup	204
Hansen's		
Orange & Chocolate	½ cup	230
Strawberry & Yogurt	½ cup	230
Toasted Nut Crunch	½ cup	230
Tropical Cluster	½ cup	210
Hi-Lo		
Low Carb Cereal	½ cup	90
Hodgson Mill		
Bulgur Wheat w/ Soy Grits	¼ cup	116
Cracked Wheat	¼ cup	110
Multi Grain w/ Flaxseed & Soy	⅓ cup	160
Kashi		
Go Apple Spice	½ cup (4.9 oz)	270

FOOD	PORTION	CALS
Go Banana Almond	½ cup (4.9 oz)	280
Go Blueberry Bliss	½ cup (4.9 oz)	260
Go Cherry Vanilla	½ cup (4.9 oz)	260
GoLean	1 cup	140
GoLean Crunch!	1 cup (1.9 oz)	190
Good Friends	1 cup	170
Heart To Heart	¾ cup	110
Mighty Bites All Flavors	1 cup	120
Organic Promise Cranberry Sunshine	1 cup	110
Pillows Apple	¾ cup (1.9 oz)	200
Pillows Chocolate	¾ cup (1.9 oz)	200
Pillows Strawberry Crisp	¾ cup (1.9 oz)	200
Kellogg's		
Raisin Bran	1 cup	190
Smart Start Antioxidants	1 cup	180
Smart Start Healthy Heart	1¼ cups	230
Special K Vanilla Almond	1 cup (1.1 oz)	110
Keto		
Cocoa Crisp	½ cup	110
Frosted Flakes All Flavors	¾ cup	110
Hot Cereal Apple Cinnamon	2 scoops	150
Hot Cereal Strawberry & Creme	2 scoops	150
Low Carb Crispy Soy	¾ cup	110
Oatmeal Old Fashioned	2 scoops	150
Liquid Cereal		
Apple & Cinnamon	1 can (11 oz)	160
Chocolate	1 can (11 oz)	170
Fruit	1 can (11 oz)	150
Peanut Butter	1 can (11 oz)	170
Lundberg		
Purely Organic Hot'n Creamy Rice	⅓ cup	190
McCann's		
Irish Oatmeal Instant Apples & Cinnamon	1 pkg (1 oz)	130
Irish Oatmeal Instant Maple & Brown Sugar	1 pkg (1 oz)	160
Irish Oatmeal Instant Regular	1 pkg (1 oz)	100
MiniCarb		
Milk Chocolate Hot Cereal not prep	½ cup	140
Mother's		
Cinnamon Oat Crunch	1 cup	230
Cocoa Bumpers	1 cup	120

FOOD	PORTION	CALS
Groovy Grahams	¾ cup	100
Honey Round-Ups	¾ cup	110
Multigrain Hot Cereal	½ cup	130
Oat Bran Hot Cereal	½ cup	150
Oatmeal Instant	½ cup	150
Peanut Butter Bumpers	1 cup	130
Rolled Oats	½ cup	150
Toasted Oat Bran	¾ cup	120
Whole Wheat Hot Cereal	½ cup	130
Natural Ovens		
Great Granola	¼ cup	110
Paul's Oatmeal not prep	⅓ cup	120
Nature's Path		
Optimum Organic ReBound	¾ cup	190
Organic Zen Instant Oatmeal Cranberry Ginger	1 pkg	150
Perky's		
Nutty Flax	¾ cup	230
PerkyO's Original	¾ cup	120
Post		
Alpha-Bits Marshmallow	1 cup (1 oz)	120
Grape-Nuts	½ cup	200
Grape-Nuts Flakes	¾ cup (1 oz)	100
Great Grains Raisins Dates Pecans	½ cup	210
Raisin Bran	1 cup (2 oz)	190
Selects Blueberry Morning	¾ cup (1.3 oz)	140
Shredded Wheat Spoon Size	1 cup	170
Quaker		
Instant Oatmeal Apples & Cinnamon	1 pkg	130
Instant Oatmeal Cinnamon & Spice	1 pkg	170
Instant Oatmeal Cinnamon Roll	1 pkg	160
Instant Oatmeal Lower Sugar Apples & Cinnamon	1 pkg	110
Instant Oatmeal Lower Sugar Maple & Brown Sugar	1 pkg	120
Instant Oatmeal Maple & Brown Sugar	1 pkg	160
Instant Oatmeal Nutrition For Women Golden Brown Sugar	1 pkg	170
Instant Oatmeal Nutrition For Women Vanilla Cinnamon	1 pkg	160
Instant Oatmeal Peaches & Cream	1 pkg	130

FOOD	PORTION	CALS
Instant Oatmeal Raisin & Spice	1 pkg	150
Instant Oatmeal Regular	1 pkg	100
Instant Oatmeal Strawberries & Cream	1 pkg	130
Instant Oatmeal Take Heart Blueberry	1 pkg	160
Instant Oatmeal Take Heart Golden Maple	1 pkg	160
Instant Oatmeal Weight Control Banana Bread	1 pkg	160
Instant Oatmeal Weight Control Cinnamon	1 pkg	160
Life	¾ cup	120
Life Cinnamon	¾ cup	120
Life Honey Graham	¾ cup	120
Life Vanilla Yogurt Crunch	1¼ cups	210
Ralston		
100% Hot Wheat	⅓ cup	150
Apple Dapples	1 cup	120
Cocoa Crumbles	1 cup	120
Confruity Crisp	¾ cup	110
Corn Biscuits	1 cup	110
Corn Flakes	1 cup	100
Crisp Crunch	¾ cup	120
Crisp Crunch Berry Treats	1 cup	120
Crisp Rice	1¼ cups	120
Enriched Bran Flakes	¾ cup	90
Farina	3 tbsp	120
Freaky Fruits	1 cup	120
Frosted Flakes	¾ cup	120
Fruit Rings	1 cup	120
Grits	¼ cup	140
Instant Oats Bananas & Cream	1 pkg	130
Magic Stars	¾ cup	120
Oats & More W/ Almonds	¾ cup	130
Oats Instant	1 pkg	100
Oats Instant Apples & Cinnamon	1 pkg	130
Oats Instant Blueberries & Cream	1 pkg	130
Oats Instant Cinnamon & Spice	1 pkg	170
Oats Instant For Kids Cinnawow	1 pkg	140
Oats Instant For Kids Maplicious & Brown Sugar	1 pkg	150
Oats Instant For Kids Roarin' Raspberry	1 pkg	150
Oats Instant For Kids Strawberries & Stars	1 pkg	140
Oats Instant Maple Brown Sugar	1 pkg	160
Oats Instant Peaches & Cream	1 pkg	130

FOOD	PORTION	CALS
Oats Instant Raisins & Spice	1 pkg	150
Oats Instant Strawberries & Cream	1 pkg	140
Oats Old Fashioned	½ cup	150
Oats Quick	½ cup	140
Raisin Bran	1 cup	200
Rice Biscuits	1¼ cups	120
Shredded Wheat Frosted Bite Size	1¼ cups	200
Silly Spheres	1½ cups	110
Tasteeos	1 cup	110
Tasteeos Apple Cinnamon	¾ cup	120
Tasteeos Honey Nut	1 cup	120
South Beach Diet		
Toasted Wheats	1¼ cups	210
Whole Grain Crunch	¾ cup	110
Sunbelt		
Berry Basic	½ cup (1.9 oz)	220
Granola Banana Nut	½ cup (1.9 oz)	250
Granola Cinnamon Raisins	½ cup (1.9 oz)	200
Granola Fruit & Nut	½ cup (1.9 oz)	240
Muesli 5 Whole Grains	½ cup (1.9 oz)	210
Uncle Sam		
Cereal	1 cup (1.9 oz)	190
Weetabix		
Cereal	2 biscuits (1.2 oz)	100
Wheatena		
Cereal	⅓ cup (1.4 oz)	150

CEREAL BARS *(see also* ENERGY BARS)
All Bran

Brown Sugar Cinnamon	1	130
Honey Oat	1	130
Oatmeal Raisin	1	130
Barbara's Bakery		
Nature's Choice Apple Cinnamon	1 bar (1.3 oz)	120
Nature's Choice Blueberry	1 bar (1.3 oz)	120
Nature's Choice Cherry	1 bar (1.3 oz)	120
Nature's Choice Granola Carob Chip	1 bar (0.7 oz)	80
Nature's Choice Granola Cinnamon & Raisin	1 bar (0.7 oz)	80
Nature's Choice Granola Oats 'N Honey	1 bar (0.7 oz)	80
Nature's Choice Granola Peanut Butter	1 bar (0.7 oz)	80

FOOD	PORTION	CALS
Nature's Choice Raspberry	1 bar (1.3 oz)	120
Nature's Choice Strawberry	1 bar (1.3 oz)	120
Nature's Choice Triple Berry	1 bar (1.3 oz)	120
Dolly Madison		
Apple	1 (1.3 oz)	120
Blueberry	1 (1.3 oz)	120
Raspberry	1 (1.3 oz)	120
Strawberry	1 (1.3 oz)	120
Enjoy Life		
Caramel Apple Nut & Gluten Free	1 (1 oz)	110
Entenmann's		
Apple Cinnamon	1 (1.3 oz)	140
Blueberry	1 (1.3 oz)	140
Multi-Grain Chocolate Chip	1	140
Multi-Grain Rainbow Chip	1	180
Multi-Grain Real Raspberry	1	140
Oatmeal Apple Cinnamon	1 (1.3 oz)	140
Oatmeal Apple Raisin	1 (1.3 oz)	140
Raspberry	1 (1.3 oz)	140
Strawberry	1 (1.3 oz)	140
EnviroKidz		
Crispy Rice Panda Peanut Butter	1 bar (1 oz)	110
Estee		
Rice Crunchy Chocolate	1 bar	60
Rice Crunchy Chocolate Chip	1 bar	70
Rice Crunchy Peanut Butter	1 bar	60
Rice Crunchy Vanilla	1 bar	70
General Mills		
Milk 'N Cereal Bars Chex	1 bar (1.6 oz)	160
Milk 'N Cereal Bars Cinnamon Toast Crunch	1 bar (1.6 oz)	180
Team Cheerios Strawberry	1	160
Trix	1	160
Glenny's		
Slim Carb Bars Peanut Caramel	1 bar	140
Hershey's		
Crispy Rice Peanut Butter	1 bar (0.5 oz)	60
Hostess		
Apple	1 (1.3 oz)	120
Banana Nut	1 (1.3 oz)	120
Blueberry	1 (1.3 oz)	120

FOOD	PORTION	CALS
Raspberry	1 (1.3 oz)	120
Strawberry	1 (1.3 oz)	120
Kashi		
Chewy Granola Honey Almond Flax	1 (1.2 oz)	140
Chewy Granola Peanut Peanut Butter	1 (1.2 oz)	130
Chewy Granola Trail Mix	1 (1.2 oz)	130
Kudos		
Granola Chocolate Chip	1	130
Granola Peanut Butter	1	130
Granola w/ M&M's	1	100
Granola w/ Snickers	1	100
Little Debbie		
Raspberry	1 (1.3 oz)	130
S'mores Granola Treats	1 (1 oz)	130
Strawberry	1 (1.3 oz)	130
Nabisco		
Nutter Butter Granola Bar	1 (1 oz)	120
Oreo Granola Bar	1 (1 oz)	120
Natural Ovens		
Great Granola Chocolate Almond	1 bar	150
Great Granola Fruit & Lemon	1 bar	130
Great Granola Mixed Fruit	1 bar	130
Nature Valley		
Chewy Trail Mix Fruit & Nut	1 bar	140
Healthy Heart Honey Nut	1 bar	160
Nutri-Grain		
Apple Cinnamon	1	140
Banana Muffin	1	170
Blueberry	1	140
Blueberry Muffin	1	170
Cherry	1	140
Chewy Granola Chocolatey Chunk	1	110
Chewy Granola Honey Oat & Raisin	1	110
Cinnamon Raisin Muffin	1	170
Mixed Berry	1	140
Raspberry	1	140
Strawberry	1	140
Strawberry Yogurt	1	140
Vanilla Yogurt	1	140

FOOD	PORTION	CALS
Quaker		
Breakfast Squares Brown Sugar Cinnamon	1 (2.1 oz)	220
Chewy Chocolate Chip	1 (1 oz)	120
Chewy Peanut Butter Chocolate Chunk	1 (1 oz)	120
Chewy Graham Slam Chocolate Chip	1 (1 oz)	110
Chewy Low Fat Chocolate Chunk	1 (1 oz)	110
Chewy Low Fat Maple Brown Sugar	1 (1 oz)	110
Chewy Low Fat S'mores	1 (1 oz)	110
Fruit & Oatmeal Bites Apple Crisp	1 pkg	140
Fruit & Oatmeal Bites Strawberry	1 pkg	140
Fruit & Oatmeal Bites Very Berry	1 pkg	140
Fruit & Oatmeal Low Fat Cherry Cobbler	1 (1.3 oz)	140
Fruit & Oatmeal Low Fat Strawberry	1 (1.3 oz)	140
Fruit & Oatmeal Low Fat Strawberry Banana	1 (1.3 oz)	130
Fruit & Oatmeal Low Fat Strawberry Cheesecake	1 (1.3 oz)	130
Oatmeal To Go Brown Sugar Cinnamon	1 bar (2.1 oz)	220
Old Fashioned Oats not prep	½ cup	150
Rice Krispies		
Split Stix Chocolatey	1 bar (1 oz)	130
Split Stix Original	1 bar (1 oz)	120
Treats Original	1 (0.8 oz)	90
Skippy		
Peanut Butter	1 bar	180
Peanut Butter & Fudge	1 bar	190
Peanut Butter & Marshmallow	1 bar	140
Peanut Butter & Strawberry	1 bar	170
SnackWell's		
Country Fruit Medley	1 (1.3 oz)	130
Fat Free Apple Cinnamon	1 (1.3 oz)	120
Fat Free Blueberry	1 (1.3 oz)	120
Fat Free Strawberry	1 (1.3 oz)	120
Hearty Fruit'n Grain Crisp Autumn Apple	1 (1.3 oz)	130
Hearty Fruit'n Grain Mixed Berry	1 (1.3 oz)	120
Hearty Fruit'n Grain Orchard Cherry	1 (1.3 oz)	130
South Beach Diet		
Chocolate	1 bar	140
Cinnamon Raisin	1 bar	140
Cranberry Almond	1 bar	140
Maple Nut	1 bar	140
Peanut Butter	1 bar	140

FOOD	PORTION	CALS
Special K		
Blueberry	1 bar	90
Chocolatey Drizzle	1	90
Cranberry Apple	1 bar	90
Peach Berry	1	90
Strawberry	1	90
Vanilla Crisp	1	90
Sunbelt		
Apple	1 (1.3 oz)	130
Blueberry	1 (1.3 oz)	130
Chewy Granola Almond	1 (1 oz)	130
Chewy Granola Apple Cinnamon	1 (1.2 oz)	140
Chewy Granola Chocolate Chip	1 (1.2 oz)	160
Chewy Granola Oatmeal Raisin	1 (1.2 oz)	130
Chewy Granola Oats & Honey	1 (1 oz)	120
Granola Fudge Dipped Chocolate Chip	1 (1.5 oz)	200
Granola Fudge Dipped Macaroon	1 (1.4 oz)	190

CHAMPAGNE

FOOD	PORTION	CALS
mimosa	1 serv	117
punch	1 serv	113
sekt german champagne	3.5 fl oz	84
Andre		
Blush	4 fl oz	88
Brut	4 fl oz	84
Cold Duck	4 fl oz	100
Extra Dry	4 fl oz	92
Ballatore		
Spumante	4 fl oz	92
Eden Roc		
Brut	4 fl oz	92
Brut Rosé	4 fl oz	99
Extra Dry	4 fl oz	84
Tott's		
Blanc de Noir	4 fl oz	88
Brut	4 fl oz	80
Extra Dry	4 fl oz	84

CHAYOTE

FOOD	PORTION	CALS
fresh cooked	1 cup	38

FOOD	PORTION	CALS
raw	1 (7 oz)	49
raw cut up	1 cup	32

CHEESE (see also CHEESE DISHES, CHEESE SUBSTITUTES, COTTAGE CHEESE, CREAM CHEESE, NEUFCHATEL)

FOOD	PORTION	CALS
american	1 oz	93
american cheese spread	1 oz	82
beaufort	1 oz	115
bel paese	1 oz	112
blue	1 oz	100
blue crumbled	1 cup (4.7 oz)	477
brick	1 oz	105
brie	1 oz	95
cacio di roma sheep's milk cheese	1 oz	130
caerphilly	1.4 oz	150
camembert	1 wedge (1.3 oz)	114
camembert	1 oz	85
cantal	1 oz	105
caraway	1 oz	107
chabichou	1 oz	95
chaource	1 oz	83
cheddar	1 oz	114
cheddar low fat	1 oz	49
cheddar low sodium	1 oz	113
cheddar reduced fat	1.4 oz	104
cheddar shredded	1 cup	455
cheshire	1 oz	110
cheshire reduced fat	1.4 oz	108
colby	1 oz	112
colby low fat	1 oz	49
colby low sodium	1 oz	113
comte	1 oz	114
coulommiers	1 oz	88
crottin	1 oz	105
derby	1.4 oz	161
edam	1 oz	101
edam reduced fat	1.4 oz	92
emmentaler	1 oz	115
feta	1 oz	75
fontina	1 oz	110

FOOD	PORTION	CALS
frais	1.6 oz	51
gjetost	1 oz	132
gloucester double	1.4 oz	162
goat fresh	1 oz	23
goat hard	1 oz	128
goat semisoft	1 oz	103
goat soft	1 oz	76
gorgonzola	1 oz	107
gouda	1 oz	101
grana padano parmesan shaved	1 tbsp	20
gruyere	1 oz	117
lancashire	1.4 oz	149
leicester	1.4 oz	160
limburger	1 oz	93
lymeswold	1.4 oz	170
maroilles	1 oz	97
monterey	1 oz	106
morbier	1 oz	99
mozzarella	1 oz	80
mozzarella	1 lb	1276
mozzarella fresh	1 oz	80
mozzarella low moisture	1 oz	90
mozzarella part skim	1 oz	72
muenster	1 oz	104
parmesan grated	1 oz	129
parmesan grated	1 tbsp (5 g)	23
parmesan hard	1 oz	111
picodon	1 oz	99
pimento	1 oz	106
pont l'eveque	1 oz	86
port du salut	1 oz	100
provolone	1 oz	100
pyrenees	1 oz	101
quark 20% fat	1 oz	33
quark 40% fat	1 oz	48
quark made w/ skim milk	1 oz	22
queso anego	1 oz	106
queso asadero	1 oz	101
queso chichuahua	1 oz	106
queso fresco	1 oz	41

FOOD	PORTION	CALS
queso manchego	1 oz	107
queso panela	1 oz	74
raclette	1 oz	102
reblochon	1 oz	88
ricotta part skim	½ cup (4.4 oz)	171
ricotta part skim	1 cup (8.6 oz)	340
ricotta whole milk	1 cup (8.6 oz)	428
ricotta whole milk	½ cup (4.4 oz)	216
romadur 40% fat	1 oz	83
romano	1 oz	110
roquefort	1 oz	105
rouy	1 oz	95
saint marcellin	1 oz	94
saint nectaire	1 oz	97
saint paulin	1 oz	85
sainte maure	1 oz	99
selles sur cher	1 oz	93
stilton blue	1.4 oz	164
stilton white	1.4 oz	145
swiss	1 oz	107
swiss processed	1 oz	95
tilsit	1 oz	96
tome	1 oz	92
triple creme	1 oz	113
vacherin	1 oz	92
wensleydale	1.4 oz	151
whey cheese	1 oz	126
yogurt cheese	1 oz	80
Alouette		
Garlic & Herbs	2 tbsp (0.8 oz)	70
Alpine Lace		
American Jalapeno Peppers	1 slice (1 oz)	80
American Less Fat Less Sodium White	1 slice (1 oz)	50
American Less Fat Less Sodium Yellow	1 slice (1 oz)	80
Cheddar Reduced Fat	1 slice (1 oz)	70
Colby Reduced Fat	1 slice (1 oz)	80
Fat Free Parmesan	2 tsp (5 g)	10
Feta Reduced Fat	1 oz	50
Feta Reduced Fat Sun Dried Tomato & Basil	1 oz	50
Goat Reduced Fat	1 oz	40

FOOD	PORTION	CALS
Mozzarella Reduced Fat	1 oz	70
Muenster Reduced Sodium	1 slice (1 oz)	100
Provolone Smoked Reduced Fat	1 slice (1 oz)	70
Swiss Reduced Fat	1 slice (1 oz)	90
Athenos		
Blue	1 oz	100
Feta	1 oz (1 in cube)	80
Feta Crumbled	¼ cup	90
Gorgonzola Crumbled	3 tbsp	110
Back To Nature		
Organic American Slices	1 slice (0.7 oz)	80
Organic Cheddar Cubes	8 pieces (1.1 oz)	130
Organic Cheddar Shredded	¼ cup	110
Organic Cream Cheese	⅛ pkg (1 oz)	100
Organic Mozzarella Shredded	¼ cup	80
Organic White Cheddar Slices Reduced Fat	1 slice (0.7 oz)	60
Boar's Head		
American	1 oz	100
Baby Swiss	1 oz	110
Canadian Cheddar	1 oz	110
Double Glouster Yellow	1 oz	110
Feta	1 oz	60
Havarti	1 oz	110
Havarti w/ Dill	1 oz	110
Havarti w/ Jalapeno	1 oz	110
Lacey Swiss	1 oz	90
Longhorn Colby	1 oz	110
Monterey Jack	1 oz	100
Monterey Jack w/ Jalapeno	1 oz	100
Mozzarella	1 oz	90
Muenster	1 oz	100
Muenster Low Sodium	1 oz	100
Provolone Picante Sharp	1 oz	100
Swiss	1 oz	110
Swiss No Salt Added	1 oz	110
Boursin		
Garlic & Fine Herbs	2 tbsp	120
Cabot		
American	1 slice (0.7 oz)	80
Cheddar	1 oz	110

FOOD	PORTION	CALS
Cheddar Smoked	1 oz	110
Cheddar Light 50% Reduced Fat	1 oz	70
Cheddar Light 50% Reduced Fat Jalapeno	1 oz	70
Cheddar Light 75% Reduced Fat	1 oz	60
Cheddar Shake	2 tsp	25
Colby Jack	1 oz	110
Fancy Blend Shredded	¼ cup	100
Monterey Jack	1 oz	110
Mozzarella Shredded	¼ cup	80
Pepper Jack	1 oz	110
Swiss Slices	1 slice (1 oz)	110
Cantare		
Baked Brie En Croute	1 oz	100
Cedar Grove		
Marble Colby	1 oz	110
Organic Tomato Basil Cheddar	1 oz	110
Chavrie		
Goat's Milk	2 tbsp	50
Connoisseur		
Asiago Spread	1 tbsp	90
Cracker Barrel		
Sharp Cheddar 2% Milk	1 oz	90
Fage		
Feta	1 oz	80
Finlandia		
Muenster	1 slice (1.1 oz)	120
Fleurs De France		
Brie	3.5 oz	311
Formaggio		
Fresh Mozzarella	1 oz	90
Heluva Good Cheese		
Cheddar Extra Sharp	1 oz	110
Hollow Road Farms		
Sheep's Milk	1 oz	45
Jordan's		
Provolone	1 slice (1 oz)	100
Kraft		
Cheddar Extra Sharp	1 oz	120
Land O Lakes		
American	1 slice (0.7 oz)	80

FOOD	PORTION	CALS
American Jalapeno	1 slice (0.6 oz)	70
American Light	1 oz	70
American Reduced Salt	1 oz	110
American Sharp	2 slices (1 oz)	100
American & Swiss	1 slice (0.6 oz)	70
Baby Swiss	1 oz	110
Chedarella	1 oz	100
Cheddar	1 oz	100
Cheddar Extra Sharp	1 oz	110
Cheddar Sharp	1 oz	110
Cheese Spread Golden Velvet	1 oz	80
Colby	1 oz	110
Jalapeno Light	1 oz	70
Monterey Jack	1 oz	110
Monterey Jack Hot Pepper	1 oz	110
Mozzarella	1 oz	80
Muenster	1 oz	100
Parmesan Grated	1 tbsp	35
Provolone	1 oz	100
Swiss	1 oz	110
Swiss Light	1 oz	80
Laughing Cow		
Cheese Bites Light	6 pieces (0.8 oz)	35
Creamy French Onion Light	1 wedge	35
Creamy Garlic & Herb Light	1 wedge (0.7 oz)	35
Creamy Swiss Light Original	1 wedge (0.7 oz)	35
Creamy Swiss Original	1 wedge (0.7 oz)	50
Mini Babybel Bonbel	1 piece (0.7 oz)	70
Mini Babybel Gouda	1 piece (0.7 oz)	80
Mini Babybel Light Original	1 piece (0.7 oz)	50
Mini Babybel Mild Cheddar	1 piece (0.7 oz)	70
Mini Babybel Original	1 piece (0.7 oz)	70
Meza		
Baked Brie In Pastry w/ Cranberries & Spiced Almonds	1 oz	110
Miller's		
Mozzarella	1 slice (1 oz)	81
Mont Chevre		
Assorted Crottins	1 oz	70

FOOD	PORTION	CALS
Northfield		
Naturally Slender	1 oz	90
Organic Valley		
Aged Swiss Unpasteurized	1 oz	100
Cheddar Reduced Fat Low Sodium	1 oz	90
Cheddar Sharp & Mild	1 oz	110
Cheddar Sharp & Mild Unpasteurized	1 oz	110
Colby	1 oz	110
Colby Unpasteurized	1 oz	110
Farmer Reduced Fat	1 oz	90
Feta	1 oz	90
Monterey Jack	1 oz	100
Monterey Jack Reduced Fat	1 oz	80
Mozzarella Part Skim	1 oz	80
Muenster	1 oz	100
Pepper Jack	1 oz	110
Provolone	1 oz	100
String Part Skim	1 oz	80
Wisconsin Raw Milk Cheese	1 oz	100
Polly-O		
Mozzarella Shredded	¼ cup	90
Mozzerella Part Skim	1 oz	70
Ricotta Part Skim	¼ cup	90
Ricotta Lite	¼ cup	70
String-Ums	1 stick (1 oz)	80
President		
Feta	1 in cube (1 oz)	90
Rouge Et Noir		
Breakfast	1 oz	86
Brie	1 oz	86
Camembert	1 oz	86
Schloss	1 oz	86
Sargento		
Blue Crumbled	¼ cup (1 oz)	100
Cheddar Extra Sharp	1 oz	110
Cheddar Shredded	¼ cup (1 oz)	110
Cheese For Nachos & Tacos Shredded	¼ cup (1 oz)	110
Cheese For Pizza Shredded	¼ cup (1 oz)	90
Cheese For Tacos Shredded	¼ cup (1 oz)	110
Colby	1 slice (1 oz)	110

FOOD	PORTION	CALS
Colby-Jack Shredded	¼ cup (1 oz)	110
Jarlsberg	1 slice (1.2 oz)	120
Monterey Jack	1 slice (1 oz)	100
Monterey Jack Shredded	¼ cup (1 oz)	100
MooTown Snackers Cheddar	1 piece (0.8 oz)	100
MooTown Snackers Cheddar Mild Light	1 piece (0.8 oz)	60
MooTown Snackers Cheese & Pretzels	1 pkg (0.9 oz)	90
MooTown Snackers Colby-Jack	1 piece (0.8 oz)	90
MooTown Snackers Pizza Cheese & Sticks	1 pkg (1 oz)	100
MooTown Snackers String Light	1 piece (0.8 oz)	60
Mozzarella	1 slice (1.5 oz)	130
Mozzarella Shredded	¼ cup (1 oz)	80
Muenster	1 slice (1 oz)	100
Parmesan Grated	1 tbsp (5 g)	25
Parmesan Shredded	¼ cup (1 oz)	110
Parmesan & Romano Grated	1 tbsp (5 g)	25
Parmesan & Romano Shredded	¼ cup (1 oz)	110
Pizza Double Cheese Shredded	¼ cup (1 oz)	90
Preferred Light Cheddar Mild Shredded	¼ cup (1 oz)	70
Preferred Light Mozzarella	1 slice (1.5 oz)	90
Preferred Light Mozzarella Shredded	¼ cup (1 oz)	70
Preferred Light Swiss	1 slice (1 oz)	80
Provolone	1 slice (1 oz)	100
Recipe Blend 4 Cheese Mexican Shredded	¼ cup (1 oz)	110
Recipe Blend 6 Cheese Italian Shredded	¼ cup (1 oz)	90
Reduced Fat 4 Cheese Mexican Shredded	¼ cup (1 oz)	80
Ricotta Light	¼ cup (2.2 oz)	60
Ricotta Old Fashioned	¼ cup (2.2 oz)	90
Ricotta Part-Skim	¼ cup (2.2 oz)	80
String	1 piece (0.8 oz)	70
Swiss	1 slice (0.7 oz)	80
Swiss Shredded	¼ cup (1 oz)	110
Swiss Wafer Thin	2 slices (1 oz)	110
Sorrento		
Mozzarella Fresh	1 oz	90
Mozzarella w/ Tomato & Basil Shredded	¼ cup	80
Pizza Cheese Shredded	¼ cup	90
Stringsters	1 stick (1 oz)	80
Suisse Delicat		
Healthy Swiss	1 oz	90

FOOD	PORTION	CALS
Tree Of Life		
Cheddar 33% Reduced Fat Organic Milk	1 oz	90
Colby	1 oz	110
Colby Organic Milk	1 oz	120
Farmer Part-Skim Organic Milk	1 oz	90
Jalapeno Organic Milk	1 oz	110
Monterey Jack 35% Reduced Fat Organic Milk	1 oz	80
Monterey Jack Organic Milk	1 oz	100
Mozzarella Organic Milk	1 oz	80
Muenster Organic Milk	1 oz	100
Provolone	1 oz	100
Wholesome Valley		
Organic American Reduced Fat	1 slice (0.7 oz)	50

CHEESE DISHES
FROZEN
Banquet

Mozzeralla Nuggets	6	260
Fillo Factory		
Tyropita Cheese Fillo Appetizers	5 (5 oz)	340
Health Is Wealth		
Mozzarella Stick	2 (1.3 oz)	120
TAKE-OUT		
fondue	½ cup (3.8 oz)	247
fried mozzarella sticks	3 (4.6 oz)	503
souffle	1 serv (7 oz)	504
welsh rarebit	1 slice	228

CHEESE SUBSTITUTES

mozzarella	1 oz	70
Sargento		
Cheddar Shredded	¼ cup (1 oz)	90
Mozzarella Shredded	¼ cup (1 oz)	80
Yves		
Good Slice American	1 slice (0.7 oz)	35
Good Slice Cheddar	1 slice (0.7 oz)	35
Good Slice Jalapeno Jack	1 slice (0.7 oz)	35
Good Slice Mozzarella	1 slice (0.7 oz)	30
Good Slice Swiss	1 slice (0.7 oz)	35

FOOD	PORTION	CALS
CHERIMOYA		
fresh	1	515
CHERRIES		
CANNED		
sour in heavy syrup	½ cup	232
sour in light syrup	½ cup	189
sour water packed	1 cup	87
sweet in heavy syrup	½ cup	107
sweet in light syrup	½ cup	85
sweet juice pack	½ cup	68
sweet water pack	½ cup	57
Del Monte		
Sweet Dark Pitted In Heavy Syrup	½ cup	100
DRIED		
bing unsulfured	¼ cup	130
montmorency tart pitted	⅓ cup	160
rainier unsulfured	⅓ cup	140
yogurt covered	¼ cup	170
Frieda's		
Bing	¼ cup (1.4 oz)	120
Tart	⅓ cup (1.4 oz)	150
FRESH		
sour	1 cup	51
sweet	10	49
Chiquita		
Cherries	21	90
Super Cherry		
Rainier	21	90
FROZEN		
dark sweet unsweetened	1 cup	110
sour unsweetened	1 cup	72
sweet sweetened	1 cup	232
CHERRY JUICE		
Eden		
Montmorency Juice	8 oz	140
Hi-C		
Sour Blast Wild Cherry	1 pkg	110
Wild Cherry	1 box	100

FOOD	PORTION	CALS
Juicy Juice		
Drink	1 box (4.23 oz)	70
Drink	1 box (8.5 oz)	140
Minute Maid		
Coolers Clear Cherry	1 pouch (7 oz)	100
Mott's		
Cherry	1 box (8 oz)	120
Ocean Spray		
Black Cherry	8 oz	140

CHERVIL
seed	1 tsp	1

CHESTNUTS
chinese steamed	3 (1 oz)	43
creme de marrons	1 oz	73
japanese roasted	1 oz	57
ready-to-eat vacuum packed	5 (1 oz)	40
roasted	3 (1 oz)	70

CHEWING GUM
bubble gum	1 block (8 g)	27
stick	1 (3 g)	10
Aquafresh		
Peppermint	2 pieces	5
Arm & Hammer		
Dental Care Spearmint or Peppermint	2 pieces (2.5 g)	5
Bazooka		
Bubble Gum	1 piece (4 g)	15
Big Red		
Gum	1 piece	10
Brach's		
Abra Cabubble	1 piece	45
CareFree		
Koolerz Lemonaide	1 piece	5
Dentyne		
Ice Peppermint	2 pieces (3 g)	5
Doublemint		
Gum	1 piece	10

FOOD	PORTION	CALS
Eclipse		
Flash All Flavors	1 piece	0
Sugarless All Flavors	2 pieces	5
Extra		
Sugar Free All Flavors	1 piece	5
Sugar Free Bubble Gum	1 piece	5
Glee Gum		
Peppermint	2 pieces (2.5 g)	5
Hubba Bubba		
Bubble Gum Cola	1 piece	23
Bubble Gum Sugarfree Grape	1 piece	13
Bubble Gum Sugarfree Original	1 piece	14
Original	1 piece	23
Strawberry Grape Raspberry	1 piece	23
Juicy Fruit		
Gum	2 pieces	10
Orbit		
All Flavors	1 piece	5
Sugarless All Flavors	2 pieces	5
Speakeasy		
Natural Rainforest All Flavors	2 pieces	10
SteviaDent		
Gum	2 pieces	3
Winterfresh		
Gum	1 stick	10
Thin Ice Mountain Rush	1 piece	0
Wrigley's		
Spearmint	1 stick	10
Xylichew		
Licorice	2 pieces	4

CHIA SEEDS
dried	1 oz	134

CHICKEN *(see also* CHICKEN DISHES, CHICKEN SUBSTITUTES, DINNER, HOT DOGS*)*
CANNED

breast meat in water	2 oz	70
chicken spread	1 tbsp	25
w/ broth	½ can (2.5 oz)	117

FOOD	PORTION	CALS
FRESH		
broiler/fryer breast w/ skin batter dipped & fried	½ breast (4.9 oz)	364
broiler/fryer breast w/ skin roasted	½ breast (3.4 oz)	193
broiler/fryer breast w/ skin stewed	½ breast (3.9 oz)	202
broiler/fryer breast w/o skin fried	½ breast (3 oz)	161
broiler/fryer breast w/o skin roasted	½ breast (3 oz)	142
broiler/fryer drumstick w/ skin batter dipped & fried	1 (2.6 oz)	193
broiler/fryer drumstick w/ skin floured & fried	1 (1.7 oz)	120
broiler/fryer drumstick w/ skin roasted	1 (1.8 oz)	112
broiler/fryer drumstick w/ skin stewed	1 (2 oz)	116
broiler/fryer drumstick w/o skin fried	1 (1.5 oz)	82
broiler/fryer drumstick w/o skin roasted	1 (1.5 oz)	76
broiler/fryer drumstick w/o skin stewed	1 (1.6 oz)	78
broiler/fryer leg w/ skin batter dipped & fried	1 (5.5 oz)	431
broiler/fryer leg w/ skin floured & fried	1 (3.9 oz)	285
broiler/fryer leg w/ skin roasted	1 (4 oz)	265
broiler/fryer leg w/ skin stewed	1 (4.4 oz)	275
broiler/fryer leg w/o skin fried	1 (3.3 oz)	195
broiler/fryer leg w/o skin roasted	1 (3.3 oz)	182
broiler/fryer leg w/o skin stewed	1 (3.5 oz)	187
broiler/fryer neck w/ skin stewed	1 (1.3 oz)	94
broiler/fryer neck w/o skin stewed	1 (.6 oz)	32
broiler/fryer skin floured & fried	from ½ chicken (2 oz)	281
broiler/fryer skin roasted	from ½ chicken (2 oz)	254
broiler/fryer skin stewed	from ½ chicken (2.5 oz)	261
broiler/fryer thigh w/ skin batter dipped & fried	1 (3 oz)	238
broiler/fryer thigh w/ skin floured & fried	1 (2.2 oz)	162
broiler/fryer thigh w/ skin roasted	1 (2.2 oz)	153
broiler/fryer thigh w/ skin stewed	1 (2.4 oz)	158
broiler/fryer thigh w/o skin fried	1 (1.8 oz)	113
broiler/fryer thigh w/o skin roasted	1 (1.8 oz)	109
broiler/fryer thigh w/o skin stewed	1 (1.9 oz)	107
broiler/fryer w/ skin floured & fried	½ chicken (11 oz)	844
broiler/fryer w/ skin fried	½ chicken (16.4 oz)	1347
broiler/fryer w/ skin roasted	½ chicken (10.5 oz)	715
broiler/fryer w/ skin stewed	½ chicken (11.7 oz)	730

FOOD	PORTION	CALS
broiler/fryer w/ skin neck & giblets batter dipped & fried	1 chicken (2.3 lbs)	2987
broiler/fryer w/ skin neck & giblets roasted	1 chicken (1.5 lbs)	1598
broiler/fryer w/ skin neck & giblets stewed	1 chicken (1.6 lbs)	1625
broiler/fryer w/o skin fried	1 cup	307
broiler/fryer w/o skin roasted	1 cup (5 oz)	266
broiler/fryer w/o skin stewed	1 cup (5 oz)	248
broiler/fryer wing w/ skin batter dipped & fried	1 (1.7 oz)	159
broiler/fryer wing w/ skin floured & fried	1 (1.1 oz)	103
broiler/fryer wing w/ skin roasted	1 (1.2 oz)	99
broiler/fryer wing w/ skin stewed	1 (1.4 oz)	100
capon w/ skin neck & giblets roasted	1 chicken (3.1 lbs)	3211
cornish hen w/ skin roasted	1 hen (8 oz)	595
cornish hen w/o skin & bone roasted	1 hen (3.8 oz)	144
cornish hen w/o skin & bone roasted	½ hen (2 oz)	72
cornish hen w/skin roasted	½ hen (4 oz)	296
roaster dark meat w/o skin roasted	1 cup (5 oz)	250
roaster light meat w/o skin roasted	1 cup (5 oz)	214
roaster w/ skin neck & giblets roasted	1 chicken (2.4 lbs)	2363
roaster w/ skin roasted	½ chicken (1.1 lbs)	1071
roaster w/o skin roasted	1 cup (5 oz)	469
stewing dark meat w/o skin stewed	1 cup (5 oz)	361
stewing w/ skin neck & giblets stewed	1 chicken (1.3 lbs)	1636
stewing w/ skin stewed	½ chicken (9.2 oz)	744
Amish Select		
Boneless Skinless Breast w/ Honey Dijon Mustard	1 serv (4 oz)	130
Murray's		
Breast Boneless & Skinless	4 oz	110
Ground	3 oz	130
Whole Lean	4 oz	170
Perdue		
Boneless Skinless Breasts Cooked	3 oz	110
Boneless Breast Roasted Garlic Herb	1 piece (3 oz)	90
Breaded Breast Strips Barbecue	3 oz	120
Breaded Breast Strips Hot & Spicy	3 oz	110
Breaded Breast Strips Original	3 oz	120
Burger Cooked	1 (3 oz)	160
Chicken Breast Seasoned Italian Cooked	1 piece (3 oz)	90
Chicken Breast Seasoned Teriyaki Cooked	1 piece (3 oz)	90

FOOD	PORTION	CALS
Ground Cooked	3 oz	170
Ground Breast Cooked	3 oz	80
Honey Rotisserie Dark Meat	3 oz	200
Honey Rotisserie White Meat	3 oz	140
Oven Stuffer Dark Meat Roasted	3 oz	210
Oven Stuffer Drumstick Roasted	1 (3.6 oz)	190
Oven Stuffer White Meat Roasted	3 oz	170
Oven Stuffer Wingette Roasted	3 (3.4 oz)	220
Ovenables Breast Lemon Pepper Cooked	1 piece (3 oz)	90
Seasoned Roasting Chicken Toasted Garlic Dark Meat	3 oz	190
Seasoned Roasting Chicken Toasted Garlic White Meat	3 oz	160
Seasoned Strips Parmesan Garlic Cooked	3 oz	100
Seasoned Strips Savory Classic Cooked	3 oz	90
Seasoned Strips Spicy Fiesta Cooked	3 oz	140
Split Breast Cooked	1 piece (6.8 oz)	370
Thin Sliced Breast Rosemary Garlic Thyme	1 piece (3 oz)	90
Thin Sliced Breast Tomato Herb	1 piece (3 oz)	90
Whole Dark Meat Cooked	3 oz	150
Whole White Meat Cooked	3 oz	170
Wings Roasted	2 (3.2 oz)	210
Wampler		
Breast Tenders	4 oz	130
FROZEN		
Banquet		
Breast Nuggets	7	280
Breast Patties Grilled Honey BBQ	1	110
Breast Patties Grilled Honey Mustard	1	120
Breast Tenders Our Original	3	250
Breast Tenders Southern	3 pieces	260
Country Fried	1 serv (3 oz)	270
Fat Free Baked Breast Patties	1	100
Fried Our Original	1 serv (3 oz)	280
Honey BBQ Skinless Fried	1 serv (3 oz)	230
Hot 'n Spicy Fried	1 serv (3 oz)	260
Nuggets Our Original	6	270
Nuggets Southern Fried	5	270
Patties Our Orignal	1	190
Patties Southern Fried	1	190

FOOD	PORTION	CALS
Skinless Fried	1 serv (3 oz)	220
Smokehouse Big Wings	2	200
Southern Fried	1 serv (3 oz)	280
Wings Firehouse Big	2	190
Wings Honey BBQ	4	380
Wings Hot & Spicy	4 pieces	280
Bell & Evans		
Breaded Breast	1 serv	190
Nuggets	(4 oz)	
Breaded Whole Breast Tenders	1 (4 oz)	190
Burgers	1 (3 oz)	120
Chicken Sandwich Steaks	1 serv (2 oz)	60
Country Skillet		
Bites	5	270
Breast Tenders	3	240
Chunks	5	270
Fried	3 oz	270
Nuggets	10	280
Patties	1	190
Southern Fried Chunks	5	270
Southern Fried Patties	1	190
Health Is Wealth		
Nuggets	4 (3 oz)	150
Patties	1 (3 oz)	150
Tenders	3 (3 oz)	130
Weaver		
Breast Strips	3 pieces	230
Breast Tenders	5 pieces	240
Buffalo Popcorn Chicken	7 pieces	230
Crispy Breast Strips	2 pieces	220
Crispy Mini Drums	5 pieces	250
Croquettes	2 + gravy	230
Honey Batter Breast Tenders	5 pieces	220
Hot Wings Buffalo Style	3 pieces	190
Nuggets	4 pieces	210
Patties Italian	1	210
Patties Breast	1	170
Patties Original	1	180
Wings Honey BBQ	3	200

FOOD	PORTION	CALS
READY-TO-EAT		
chicken roll light meat	2 oz	90
chicken roll light meat	1 pkg (6 oz)	271
chicken salad sandwich spread	¼ cup	104
Banquet		
Fat Free Baked Breast Tenders	3	120
Boar's Head		
Breast Hickory Smoked	2 oz	60
Breast Oven Roasted	2 oz	50
Breast Bar B Q Sauce Basted	2 oz	60
Butterball		
Crispy Baked Breasts Italian Style Herb	1 piece (0.5 oz)	190
Crispy Baked Breasts Lemon Pepper	1 piece (0.5 oz)	200
Crispy Baked Breasts Original	1 piece (0.5 oz)	180
Crispy Baked Breasts Parmesan	1 piece (0.5 oz)	200
Crispy Baked Breasts Southwestern	1 piece (0.5 oz)	170
Tenders Baked Breast	3 pieces	170
Tenders Hickory Smoked Grilled	4 pieces + sauce	160
Tenders Oriental Grilled	4 pieces + sauce	160
Carl Buddig		
Chicken Sliced	1 pkg (2.5 oz)	110
Lean Slices Honey Smoked Breast	1 pkg (2.5 oz)	70
Lean Slices Roasted Breast	1 pkg (2.5 oz)	60
Hillshire Farm		
Smoked Breast	6 slices (2 oz)	60
Perdue		
Breast Cutlets Homestyle	1 (2.9 oz)	110
Breast Cutlets Italian Style	1 (2.9 oz)	120
Breast Filets In Barbecue Sauce	1 piece + 3 tbsp sauce (5.9 oz)	200
Breast Strips In Garlic & Herb Sauce	1 serv (5 oz)	100
Breast Strips In Marinara Sauce	1 serv (5 oz)	120
Breast Strips In Teriyaki Sauce	1 serv (5 oz)	190
Carved Breast Honey Roasted	½ cup (2.5 oz)	100
Carved Breast Original Roasted	½ cup (2.5 oz)	90
Cutlets Cooked	1 (3.5 oz)	220
Nuggets	5 (3.4 oz)	210
Nuggets Chicken & Cheese	5 (3.4 oz)	230
Short Cuts Entrees In Teriyaki Sauce	5 oz	190
Short Cuts Grilled Italian	½ cup	80

FOOD	PORTION	CALS
Short Cuts Grilled Lemon Pepper	½ cup (2.5 oz)	80
Short Cuts Southwestern	½ cup (2.5 oz)	100
Tyson		
Grilled Breast Strips	1 serv (3 oz)	120
Roasted Whole Chicken w/ Skin	1 serv (3 oz)	160
TAKE-OUT		
oven roasted breast of chicken	2 oz	60

CHICKEN DISHES
FROZEN

FOOD	PORTION	CALS
Maple Leaf Farms		
Chicken Breast Stuffed Broccoli & Cheese	1 serv (6 oz)	340
REFRIGERATED		
salad low fat	⅓ cup	90
Lloyd's		
Barbecue Shredded Chicken	¼ cup (2 oz)	90
Old El Paso		
For Tacos Shredded Chicken	¼ cup	60
Oscar Mayer		
Lunchables Chicken Wraps	1 pkg	440
Tyson		
Chicken Breast Medallions In Tomato & Herb Sauce	1 serv (5 oz)	120
Wampler		
Cacciatore	1 cup	260
Fajitas	1 cup	210
Salad	⅓ cup	200
Salad Lite	½ cup	130
Smokey Barbecue Chicken	1 cup	430
Sweet-n-Sour	1 cup	250
SHELF-STABLE		
Lunch Bucket		
Dumplings'n Chicken	1 pkg (7.5 oz)	140
TastyBite		
Chicken Moglai	1 pkg (9.5 oz)	300
TAKE-OUT		
boneless breast w/ apple stuffing	1 serv (5 oz)	260
breast & wing breaded & fried	2 pieces (5.7 oz)	494
b'stilla chicken pie	1 serv	926
chicken & dumplings	¾ cup	256

FOOD	PORTION	CALS
chicken & noodles	1 cup	365
chicken a la king	1 cup	470
chicken cacciatore	¾ cup	394
chicken paprikash	1½ cups	296
chicken pie w/ top crust	1 slice (5.6 oz)	472
chicken cordon bleu	1 serv (5 oz)	280
chicken curry ½ breast	1 serv	160
chicken curry boneless	1 serv (6.2 oz)	219
chicken curry leg & thigh	1 serv	180
drumstick breaded & fried	2 pieces (5.2 oz)	430
grilled breast strips	4 strips (3 oz)	100
groundnut stew hkatenkwan	1 serv (15.7 oz)	576
jamaican jerk wings	4 wings (9.9 oz)	709
kobete turkish chicken w/ pastry	1 serv	513
sancocho de pollo dominican chicken stew	1 serv	702
souvlaki	1 serv	392
tandoori chicken breast	1 serv	260
tandoori chicken leg & thigh	1 serv	300
thigh breaded & fried	2 pieces (5.2 oz)	430

CHICKEN SUBSTITUTES
Health Is Wealth
Buffalo Wings	3 pieces (2.2 oz)	100
Chicken-Free Nuggets	3 pieces (2.25 oz)	90
Chicken-Free Patties	1 (3 oz)	120

Lightlife
Smart Cutlet Seasoned Chicken	1 (4 oz)	180
Smart Menu Chick'n Nuggets	4 pieces	220
Smart Menu Chick'n Patties	1 patty	160
Smart Menu Chick'n Strips	1 serv (3 oz)	80

Loma Linda
Chicken Supreme Mix not prep	⅓ cup (0.9 oz)	90
Chik Nuggets	5 pieces (3 oz)	240
Fried Chik'n w/ Gravy	2 pieces (2.8 oz)	160

Morningstar Farms
Chik Nuggets	4 pieces (3 oz)	160
Chik Patties	1 (2.5 oz)	150
Meatless Buffalo Wings	5 pieces (3 oz)	200

Quorn
Cutlets	1 (2.4 oz)	80

FOOD	PORTION	CALS
Nuggets	3–4 pieces (3 oz)	180
Patties	1 patty (2.6 oz)	160
Tenders	1 cup (3 oz)	90
Worthington		
Chicken Sliced or Roll	2 slices (2 oz)	80
Chic-Ketts	2 slices (1.9 oz)	120
ChikStiks	1 (1.6 oz)	110
CrispyChik Patties	1 (2.5 oz)	150
Cutlets	1 slice (2.1 oz)	70
Diced Chik	¼ cup (1.9 oz)	40
FriChik	2 pieces (3.2 oz)	120
FriChik Low Fat	2 pieces (3 oz)	80
Golden Croquettes	4 pieces (3 oz)	210
Yves		
Veggie Chicken Burgers	1 (3 oz)	120

CHICKPEAS
CANNED
chickpeas	1 cup	285
Progresso		
Chick Peas	½ cup (4.6 oz)	120
Garbanzo	½ cup (4.4 oz)	110

DRIED
cooked	1 cup	269

CHICORY
endive fresh	3.5 oz	9
endive fresh chopped	½ cup	4
greens raw chopped	½ cup	21
root raw	1 (2.1 oz)	44
roots raw cut up	½ cup (1.6 oz)	33
witloof head raw	1 (1.9 oz)	9
witloof raw	½ cup (1.6 oz)	8
Frieda's		
Belgian Endive	2 cups	115

CHILI
chile pepper paste	1 tbsp	6
chili w/ beans	1 cup	286
dried ancho	1 tsp	3
dried casabel	1 tsp	3

FOOD	PORTION	CALS
dried guajillo	1 tsp	3
dried mulato	1 tsp	3
dried pasilla	1 tsp	3
dried smoked chipotle	1 tsp	3
powder	1 tsp	8
Amy's		
Chili & Cornbread	1 pkg (10.5 oz)	320
Organic Black Bean	1 cup	200
Organic Medium	1 cup	190
Organic Medium w/ Vegetables	1 cup	190
Armour		
Chili No Beans	1 cup (8.7 oz)	390
Chili w/ Beans	1 cup (8.9 oz)	370
Chili w/ Beans Hot	1 cup (8.9 oz)	370
Chili W/ Beans Western Style	1 cup (8.8 oz)	370
Vienna Sausage & Chili	1 cup (8.7 oz)	410
Bush's		
Chili Beans Mild Sauce	½ cup	120
Original No Beans	1 cup	240
Carroll Shelby's		
Original Texas Chili Kit	2 tbsp	60
Chef Boyardee		
Chili Mac	½ can (7 oz)	260
Chili Man		
Seasoning Mix	1 tbsp (7 g)	25
Del Monte		
Sauce	1 tbsp	20
Frieda's		
California Dried	2 tbsp	15
Peppadew	⅓ cup	40
Gebhardt		
Chili Powder	¼ tsp (0.3 g)	i
Chili Quik Seasoning	1 tbsp (0.3 oz)	43
Plain	1 cup (9.4 oz)	232
With Beans	1 cup (9.4 oz)	322
Gringo Billy's		
Chili Mix	1 tbsp	24
Hunt's		
Chili Beans	½ cup (4.5 oz)	87
Family Favorites Chili	¼ cup (2.2 oz)	25

FOOD	PORTION	CALS
Instant India		
Chili Ginger Paste	2 tbsp (1 oz)	90
Just Rite		
With Beans	1 cup (9 oz)	379
Lean Cuisine		
Cafe Classics Three Bean Chili	1 pkg (10 oz)	260
Lightlife		
Smart Chili	1 pkg	200
Lunch Bucket		
Chili With Beans	1 pkg (7.5 oz)	260
Marie Callender's		
Chili & Cornbread	1 meal (16 oz)	560
McCormick		
Mexican Style Chili Powder	¼ tsp	0
Original Chili Seasoning	1⅓ tbsp (9 g)	30
Natural Choice		
Organic Vegan Three Bean	½ cup (4.6 oz)	140
Natural Touch		
Vegetarian	1 cup (8.1 oz)	170
Nature's Entree		
Texas Chili	1 pkg (12 oz)	320
Open Range		
Plain	1 cup (8.8 oz)	353
With Beans	1 cup (9 oz)	281
Pacific Foods		
Beef Steak w/ Beans	1 cup	250
Ro-Tel		
Chili Fixin's	½ cup	35
Soy7		
Chili Mix as prep	1 cup	150
Stagg		
Classic w/ Beans	1 cup	310
Country Blend	1 cup	330
Country Blend w/ Beans	1 cup	33
Ultimate		
No Beans Hot	1 cup (8.7 oz)	420
Turkey w/ Beans	1 cup (8.7 oz)	260
W/ Beans	1 cup (8.7 oz)	320
W/ Beans Hot	1 cup (8.7 oz)	320

FOOD	PORTION	CALS
Van Camp's		
Beanee Weenee Chilee	1 cup (7.7 oz)	240
Chili With Beans	1 cup (8.9 oz)	350
Mexican Style Chili Beans	½ cup (4.6 oz)	110
Wampler		
Turkey	1 cup	250
Wick Fowler's		
2 Alarm Chili Kit	3 tbsp	60
False Alarm Chili Kit	2 tbsp	50
Worthington		
Chili	1 cup (8.1 oz)	290
Low Fat	1 cup (8.1 oz)	170
Yves		
Veggie Chili	1 pkg (10.5 oz)	230

CHILI PEPPER (see PEPPERS)

CHINESE FOOD (see ASIAN FOOD)

CHINESE PRESERVING MELON

cooked	½ cup	11

CHIPS (see also SNACKS)

apple chips	10	101
barbecue	1 oz	139
barbecue	1 bag (7 oz)	971
corn	1 bag (7 oz)	1067
corn	1 oz	153
corn barbecue	1 oz	148
corn barbecue	1 bag (7 oz)	1036
corn cones	1 oz	145
corn cones nacho	1 oz	152
corn onion	1 oz	142
potato	1 bag (8 oz)	1217
potato	1 oz	152
potato cheese	1 bag (6 oz)	842
potato cheese	1 oz	140
potato light	1 bag (6 oz)	801
potato light	1 oz	134
potato sour cream & onion	1 bag (7 oz)	1051
potato sour cream & onion	1 oz	150
potato sticks	1 oz	148

FOOD	PORTION	CALS
potato sticks	½ cup (0.6 oz)	94
potato sticks	1 pkg (1 oz)	148
taco	1 oz	136
taco	1 bag (8 oz)	1089
taro	1 oz	141
taro	10 (0.8 oz)	115
tortilla	1 oz	142
tortilla	1 bag (7.5 oz)	1067
tortilla nacho	1 bag (8 oz)	1131
tortilla nacho	1 oz	141
tortilla nacho light	1 oz	126
tortilla nacho light	1 bag (6 oz)	757
tortilla ranch	1 bag (7 oz)	969
tortilla ranch	1 oz	139
Atkins		
Crunchers Barbeque	1 pkg (1 oz)	100
Crunchers Nacho Cheese	1 pkg (1 oz)	100
Crunchers Original	1 pkg (1 oz)	90
Crunchers Sour Cream & Onion	1 pkg (1 oz)	100
Bachman		
Golden Crisp	1 pkg (1 oz)	150
Barbara's Bakery		
Potato	1¼ cups (1 oz)	150
Potato No Salt Added	1¼ cups (1 oz)	150
Potato Ripple	1¼ cups (1 oz)	150
Potato Yogurt & Green Onion	1¼ cups (1 oz)	150
Tortilla Blue Corn	15 (1 oz)	140
Tortilla Blue Corn No Salt	15 (1 oz)	140
Tortilla Pinta Salsa	15 (1 oz)	130
Bruno & Luigi's		
Pasta Chips Garlic & Herb	1 oz	117
Cape Cod		
Potato 40% Reduced Fat	19	130
Potato Beachside BBQ	19	150
Potato Classic	19	150
Potato Fresh Garden Herb Reduced Fat	19	130
Potato Jalapeno & Cheddar	19	140
Potato No Salt	19	150
Potato Robust Russet	19	150
Potato Salt & Vinegar	19	150

FOOD	PORTION	CALS
Potato Sea Salt & Cracked Pepper	19	140
Tortilla Reduced Carb	10	140
Tortilla Veggie	12	140
Deliciously Slim		
Tortilla Black Bean & Sour Cream	1 oz	140
Tortilla Lightly Salted	1 oz	140
Tortilla Ranch	1 oz	140
Doritos		
Baked Cooler Ranch	15 (1 oz)	120
Baked Nacho Cheesier	15	120
Cooler Ranch	12	140
Four Cheese	12	140
Guacamole	12	150
Light Nacho Cheesier	11	90
Natural White Nacho Cheese	11	150
Ranchero	12	150
Rollitos Cooler Ranch	17	140
Rollitos Zesty Taco	17	150
Toasted Corn	13	140
Durangos		
Tortilla	15 (1 oz)	150
Eden		
Brown Rice Chips	1 oz	150
Sea Vegetable Chips	1 oz	140
Fritos		
Corn Chips King Size	12	160
Original	32	160
Scoops	10	160
Twists	23	150
GeniSoy		
Soy Crisps	1 oz	110
Soy Crisps Apple Cinnamon Crunch	1 oz	120
Soy Crisps Creamy Ranch	1 oz	110
Soy Crisps Deep Sea Salt	1 oz	110
Soy Crisps Rich Cheddar Cheese	1 oz	110
Soy Crisps Roasted Garlic & Onion	1 oz	100
Soy Crisps Zesty Barbeque	1 oz	110
Glenny's		
Soy Crisps Low Fat Lightly Salted	1 pkg (1.3 oz)	140
Soy Crispy Wispys Sour Cream & Onion	⅓ bag (0.5 oz)	60

FOOD	PORTION	CALS
Spud Delites Sea Salt	1 pkg (1.1 oz)	100
Veggie Fries	1 pkg (1.3 oz)	140
Guiltless Gourmet		
Guiltless Carbs Salsa Verde	1 oz	110
Guiltless Carbs Southwestern Ranch	1 oz	110
Guiltless Carbs Three Pepper	1 oz	110
Tortilla Blue Corn	18 (1 oz)	110
Tortilla Chili Lime	18 (1 oz)	110
Tortilla Chili Verde	18 (1 oz)	120
Tortilla Chipotle	18 (1 oz)	120
Tortilla Mucho Nacho	18 (1 oz)	110
Tortilla Organic Red Corn	18 (1 oz)	110
Tortilla Spicy Black Bean	18 (1 oz)	110
Tortilla Sweet White Corn	18 (1 oz)	110
Tortilla Yellow Corn	18 (1 oz)	110
Tortilla Yellow Corn Unsalted	18 (1 oz)	110
Herr's		
Potato	1 oz	140
Husman's		
Deli Style Tortilla	11	150
Potato	18 (1 oz)	160
Potato Sour Cream & Onion	18 (1 oz)	150
Potato Sweet N'Sassy	18 (1 oz)	155
Keto		
Low Carb Tortilla All Flavors	1 oz	150
Lay's		
Baked KC Masterpiece	11 (1 oz)	120
Baked Sour Cream & Onion	12 (1 oz)	120
Chile Limon	1 oz	150
Classic	1 pkg (1 oz)	150
Deli Style Original	17 (1 oz)	150
Dill Pickle	20 (1 oz)	160
Flamin' Hot	17 (1 oz)	160
KC Masterpiece BBQ	15 (1 oz)	150
Kettle Cooked Jalapeno	15 (1 oz)	140
Kettle Cooked Mesquite BBQ	18 (1 oz)	140
Kettle Cooked Original	22 (1 oz)	150
Kettle Cooked Sea Salt & Vinegar	18 (1 oz)	140
Light Fat Free KC Masterpiece	20 (1 oz)	75
Light Fat Free Original	20 (1 oz)	75

FOOD	PORTION	CALS
Limon	17 (1 oz)	150
Natural Country BBQ	14 (1 oz)	150
Natural Sea Salt & Vinegar	16 (1 oz)	150
Natural Sea Salted	16 (1 oz)	150
Original Baked	11 (1 oz)	110
Salt & Vinegar	17 (1 oz)	150
Sour Cream & Onion	17 (1 oz)	160
Stax	13 (1 oz)	160
Wavy	11 (1 oz)	150
Wavy Au Gratin	13 (1 oz)	150
Wavy Hickory Barbecue	13 (1 oz)	150
Wavy Ranch	12 (1 oz)	150
Manny's		
Organic Tortilla Blues	1 oz	150
Tortilla No Salt Added	1 oz	150
Maui		
Shrimp Chips	17	140
Met-Rx		
Pro Chips Bar-B-Que	1 pkg (2 oz)	260
Pro Chips Nacho	1 pkg (2 oz)	260
Old Dutch Foods		
Potato	12–15 (1 oz)	150
Potato BBQ	12–15 (1 oz)	150
Potato BBQ Ripple	12–15 (1 oz)	150
Potato Cajun Ripple	12–15 (1 oz)	150
Potato Cheddar & Sour Cream Ripple	12–15 (1 oz)	160
Potato Dill	12–15 (1 oz)	140
Potato Dutch Crunch	15–20 (1 oz)	130
Potato French Onion Ripple	12–15 (1 oz)	150
Potato Jalapeno & Cheddar Dutch Crunch	15–20 (1 oz)	130
Potato Jalapeno Cheese	12–15 (1 oz)	150
Potato Mesquite BBQ Dutch Crunch	15–20 (1 oz)	130
Potato Onion & Garlic	12–15 (1 oz)	140
Potato Outback Spicy BBQ	12–15 (1 oz)	150
Potato Ripples	12–15 (1 oz)	150
Potato Salt & Vinegar Dutch Crunch	15–20 (1 oz)	130
Potato Sour Cream & Onion	12–15 (1 oz)	150
Tortilla Bite Size White Corn	20 (1 oz)	150
Tortilla Nacho Cheese	15 (1 oz)	150
Tortilla Restaurant Style White	9 (1 oz)	140

FOOD	PORTION	CALS
Tostados White Corn	11 (1 oz)	140
Tostados Yellow	11 (1 oz)	140
Pita-Snax		
Cheddar Cheese	34 (1 oz)	110
Chili & Lime	34 (1 oz)	120
Cinnamon	34 (1 oz)	120
Dill Ranch	34 (1 oz)	120
Garlic	34 (1 oz)	120
Lightly Salted	34 (1 oz)	110
Pringles		
BBQ	14 (1 oz)	150
Cajun	14 (1 oz)	160
Cheese & Onion	14 (1 oz)	160
Cheez-ums	14 (1 oz)	150
Original	14 (1 oz)	160
Pizzalicious	14 (1 oz)	160
Ranch	14 (1 oz)	150
Salt & Vinegar	14 (1 oz)	160
Sour Cream & Onion	14 (1 oz)	160
Racquet		
Wheat Chips All Flavors	6 chips	30
Revival		
Baked Soy Pasta Chips Lightly Salted Sunshine	1 bag (0.9 oz)	100
Baked Soy Pasta Chips Naturally Nice	1 bag (0.9 oz)	80
Baked Soy Pasta Chips Rev It Up Ranch	1 bag (0.9 oz)	105
Ruffles		
Baked Original	10	120
Cheddar & Sour Cream	11	160
KC Masterpiece Mesquite BBQ	11	150
Light Cheddar & Sour Cream	15	75
Light Original	17	70
Original	12	160
Potato Crisps	16	160
Reduced Fat Sea Salted	15	140
Sour Cream & Onion	11	160
Santitas		
White Corn	9	130
Yellow Corn	9	130
Skinny		
BBQ	1½ cups	90

FOOD	PORTION	CALS
Corn	1½ cups	90
Nacho Cheese	1½ cups	90
Sour Cream & Onion	1½ cups	90
Sticks Garden Veggie	1 oz	140
Sticks Island Lime Chili	1 oz	140
Sticks Maui Wowie	1 oz	140
Sticks Original Spud	1 oz	140
Snyder's Of Hanover		
Barbeque Corn	1.5 oz	230
BBQ Rib	1 oz	140
Cheddar Bacon	1 oz	150
Corn Chips	1.5 oz	230
Grilled Steak & Onion	1 oz	140
Hot Buffalo	1 oz	150
Kosher Dill	1 oz	140
No Salt	1 oz	140
Potato	1 oz	140
Ripple	1 oz	140
Salt & Vinegar	1 oz	140
Sausage Pizza	1 oz	150
Sour Cream & Onion	1 oz	150
Tasty Veggie Potato Chips	1 oz	150
Tortilla Nacho	1 oz	140
Tortilla No Salt Yellow Corn	1 oz	140
Tortilla White Corn	1 oz	140
Tortilla Yellow Corn	1 oz	140
Tortilla Yellow Corn Mini	1 oz	160
Veggie Crisps	1 pkg (1.5 oz)	190
Soya King		
Soy Mongolian BBQ	23 (1 oz)	140
Soy Original	23 (1 oz)	140
Soy Sour Cream & Onion	23 (1 oz)	140
Soy Taco	23 (1 oz)	140
Stacy's		
Pita Chips Cinnamon Sugar	1 oz	130
Pita Chips Parmesan Garlic & Herb	1 oz	130
Pita Chips Simply Naked	1 oz	130
Twisted Pasta Low Fat	1 oz	110

FOOD	PORTION	CALS
Sunchips		
French Onion	10	140
Harvest Cheddar	10	140
Tastee		
Potato Yukon Gold	1 oz	130
Terra Chips		
Spiced Sweet Potato	1 pkg (½ oz)	190
Torengos		
Chips	13 (1 oz)	140
Tostitos		
Blue Corn	6	140
Crispy Rounds	13	140
Gold	6	140
Light Restaurant Style	6	90
Original Bite Size	20	110
Restaurant Style	6	130
Santa Fe	7	140
Scoops	13	140
Yellow Corn	6	140
Utz		
Baked Crisps	12 (1 oz)	110
Carolina Barbeque	20 (1 oz)	150
Cheddar & Sour Cream	20 (1 oz)	160
Corn Chips	24 (1 oz)	160
Corn Chips Barbecue	24 (1 oz)	160
Grandma	20 (1 oz)	140
Grandma BBQ	20 (1 oz)	140
Home Style Kettle	20 (1 oz)	140
Home Style Kettle BBQ	20 (1 oz)	140
Kettle Classics Crunchy	20 (1 oz)	150
Kettle Classics Crunchy Mesquite BBQ	20 (1 oz)	150
No Salt Added	20 (1 oz)	150
Onion & Garlic	20 (1 oz)	150
Potato	20 (1 oz)	150
Reduced Fat BBQ	22 (1 oz)	140
Reduced Fat Ripple	24 (1 oz)	140
Ripple	20 (1 oz)	150
Ripple Sour Cream & Onion	20 (1 oz)	160
Ripple Barbeque	20 (1 oz)	150
Salt'N Vinegar	20 (1 oz)	150

FOOD	PORTION	CALS
The Crab Chip	20 (1 oz)	150
Tortilla Black Bean & Salsa	13 (1 oz)	150
Tortilla Low Fat Baked	10 (1 oz)	120
Tortilla Nacho	13 (1 oz)	150
Tortilla Restaurant Style	6 (1 oz)	140
Tortilla Spicy Nacho	13 (1 oz)	150
Tortilla White Corn	12 (1 oz)	140
Wavy	20 (1 oz)	150
Yes! Fat Free	20 (1 oz)	75
Yes! Fat Free Barbeque	20 (1 oz)	75
Yes! Fat Free Ripple	20 (1 oz)	75

CHITTERLINGS

pork cooked	3 oz	258

CHIVES

freeze-dried	1 tbsp	1
fresh chopped	1 tbsp	1
fresh chopped	1 tsp	0

CHOCOLATE (see also CANDY, CHOCOLATE SPREAD, CHOCOLATE SYRUP, COCOA, HOT COCOA, ICE CREAM TOPPINGS, MILK DRINKS)

BAKING

baking	1 oz	145
grated unsweetened	¼ cup	165
liquid unsweetened	1 oz	134
mexican	1 sq (0.7 oz)	85
squares unsweetened	1 square (1 oz)	145

Nestle

Choco Bake	½ oz	80
Premier White Bar	½ oz	80
Premier White Morsels	1 tbsp	80
Semi-Sweet Bar	½ oz	70
Unsweetened Bar	½ oz	80

CHIPS

milk chocolate	1 cup (6 oz)	862
semisweet	1 cup (6 oz)	804
semisweet	60 pieces (1 oz)	136

Baker's

Chocolate Chunks	13 pices (0.5 oz)	70

FOOD	PORTION	CALS
Cloud Nine		
Double Dark Chocolate	13 pieces (0.5 oz)	80
Ghirardelli		
Semi-Sweet	33 pieces (0.5 oz)	70
Hershey's		
Holiday Baking Bits	1 tbsp	70
Milk Chocolate	1 tbsp	80
Mini Milk Chocolate	1 tbsp	80
Mini Kisses For Baking	11 pieces	80
Premier White Milk Chips	1 tbsp	80
Raspberry Chips	1 tbsp	80
Semi-Sweet	1 tbsp	80
Semi-Sweet Mini	1 tbsp	80
Skor English Toffee Baking Bits	1 tbsp	70
Nestle		
Crunch Baking Pieces	1½ tbsp	80
Milk Chocolate Morsels	1 tbsp	70
Mint Chocolate Morsels	1 tbsp	70
Morsels Semi-Sweet	1 tbsp	70
Semi-Sweet Mega Morsels	1 tbsp	70
Semi-Sweet Mini Morsels	1 tbsp	70
Sunspire		
Chocolate Sundrops	47 pieces (1.4 oz)	190
Dark Chocolate Grain Sweetened	13 pieces (0.5 oz)	70
Organic	13 pieces (0.5 oz)	70
Tropical Source		
Espresso Roast Dairy Free	13 pieces (1.5 oz)	70
Semi-Sweet Dairy Free	13 pieces (1.5 oz)	80
MIX		
powder	2–3 heaping tsp	75
powder as prep w/ whole milk	9 oz	226
Quik		
Chocolate Powder	2 tbsp (0.8 oz)	90
Chocolate Powder No Sugar	2 tbsp (0.4 oz)	40

CHOCOLATE MILK *(see MILK DRINKS)*

CHOCOLATE SPREAD
Twist

Sugar Free Chocolate Spread	2 tbsp	170

FOOD	PORTION	CALS
CHOCOLATE SYRUP		
chocolate fudge	1 tbsp (0.7 oz)	73
chocolate fudge	1 cup (11.9 oz)	1176
syrup	2 tbsp	82
syrup	1 cup	653
syrup as prep w/ whole milk	9 oz	232
Ah!Laska		
Organic	2 tbsp	85
Colac		
Chocolate Topping	1 tbsp	37
DaVinci Gourmet		
Sugar Free	2 tbsp	15
Hershey's		
Chocolate Fudge	1 tbsp	70
Double Chocolate	1 tbsp	50
Lite	2 tbsp	50
Syrup	2 tbsp	100
Nesquik		
Calcium Fortified	2 tbsp	100
Quik		
Chocolate	2 tbsp (1.3 oz)	100
Smucker's		
Sundae Syrup Chocolate	2 tbsp	110
Toll House		
Mint Chocolate	2 tbsp (1.5 oz)	130
Semi-Sweet	2 tbsp (1.5 oz)	130
Walden Farms		
Sugar Free	2 tbsp	0
Whoppers		
Chocolate Malt	2 tbsp	100
CHUTNEY		
apple	1.2 oz	68
apple cranberry	1 tbsp	16
coconut	¼ cup	74
mango	1 tbsp	54
tomato	1 tbsp	32
Wild Thyme Farms		
Apricot Cranberry Walnut	1 tbsp	15
Pineapple Peach Lime	1 tbsp	14

FOOD	PORTION	CALS
CINNAMON		
cinnamon sugar	1 tsp	16
ground	1 tsp	6
sticks	0.5 oz	39
Gringo Billy's		
Cinnamon Sweetener	½ tsp	0
CISCO		
raw	3 oz	84
smoked	3 oz	151
smoked	1 oz	50
CLAMS		
CANNED		
liquid only	3 oz	2
liquid only	1 cup	6
meat only	1 cup	236
meat only	3 oz	126
Brunswick		
Baby	2 oz	50
Bumble Bee		
Baby	¼ cup	50
Chopped Or Minced	¼ cup	25
Smoked	¼ cup	130
Chicken Of The Sea		
Chopped	¼ cup	30
Minced	¼ cup	30
Whole Baby	¼ cup	30
Orleans		
Clam Juice	1 tbsp	0
Progresso		
Creamy Clam Sauce	½ cup (4.2 oz)	110
Minced	¼ cup (2.1 oz)	25
Red Clam Sauce	½ cup (4.4 oz)	60
White Clam Sauce	½ cup (4.4 oz)	150
FRESH		
cooked	20 sm	133
cooked	3 oz	126
raw	3 oz	63
raw	9 lg (6.3 oz)	133
raw	20 sm (6.3 oz)	133

FOOD	PORTION	CALS
TAKE-OUT		
breaded & fried	20 sm	379
CLEMENTINES		
Haddon House		
In Light Syrup	½ cup	80
Sunkist		
Fresh	2	80
Tina		
Fresh	1	50
CLOVES		
ground	1 tsp	7
COCOA (*see also* HOT COCOA)		
powder unsweetened	1 tbsp (5 g)	11
powder unsweetened	1 cup (3 oz)	197
Ah!Laska		
Organic	2 tbsp	100
Organic Bakers Cocoa	1 tbsp	20
Hershey's		
Cocoa	1 tbsp	20
European Cocoa	1 tbsp	20
Nestle		
Cocoa	1 tbsp	15
COCONUT		
dried sweetened flaked	7 oz pkg	944
dried sweetened flaked	1 cup	351
dried sweetened flaked canned	1 cup	341
dried sweetened shredded	7 oz pkg	997
dried sweetened shredded	1 cup	466
dried toasted	1 oz	168
dried unsweetened	1 oz	187
fresh	1 piece (1.5 oz)	159
fresh shredded	1 cup	283
Frieda's		
White	¼ cup (1.4 oz)	140
COCONUT JUICE		
coconut water	1 tbsp	3
coconut water	1 cup	46

FOOD	PORTION	CALS
cream canned	1 tbsp	36
cream canned	1 cup	568
milk canned	1 tbsp	30
milk canned	1 cup	445
milk frozen	1 tbsp	30
milk frozen	1 cup	486
A Taste Of Thai		
Coconut Milk	⅓ cup	140
Lite Coconut Milk	⅓ cup	45
Amy & Brian		
Juice	8 oz	76
Thai Kitchen		
Milk	2 oz	124
Vita Coco		
Coconut Water	1 box (11 oz)	65
Coconut Water w/ Fruit Juice All Flavors	1 box (11 oz)	110
Zico		
Coconut Water Mango	11 oz	60
Coconut Water Natural	11 oz	60
Coconut Water Passion Fruit + Orange Peel	11 oz	60

COD

atlantic canned	3 oz	89
atlantic canned	1 can (11 oz)	327
atlantic dried	3 oz	246
atlantic fresh cooked	1 fillet (6.3 oz)	189
atlantic fresh cooked	3 oz	89
atlantic fresh raw	3 oz	70
pacific fresh baked	3 oz	95
roe canned	1 oz	34
roe raw	1 oz	37
roe tarama	3.5 oz	547
TAKE-OUT		
roe baked w/ butter & lemon juice	1 oz	36

COFFEE *(see also COFFEE BEVERAGES, COFFEE SUBSTITUTES)*
INSTANT

decaffeinated	1 rounded tsp	4
decaffeinated as prep	6 oz	4
regular as prep	1 cup (6 oz)	4

FOOD	PORTION	CALS
regular w/ chicory	1 rounded tsp	6
regular w/ chicory as prep	6 oz	6
Nescafe		
Decafe	1 tsp (2 g)	0
Decafe w/ Chicory	1 tsp (2 g)	0
French Vanilla	1 tsp (2 g)	5
French Vanilla Decaf	1 tsp (2 g)	5
Hazelnut	1 tsp (2 g)	5
Irish Creme	1 tsp (2 g)	5
Regular	1 tsp (2 g)	0
With Chicory	1 tsp (2 g)	5
REGULAR		
brewed	8 oz	2
roasted beans	1 oz	64
Nescafe		
Cafe Mocha	1 can (10 oz)	140
Caffe Latte	1 can (10 oz)	130
Caffe Latte Decaffeinated	1 can (10 oz)	130
Espresso	1 tsp (2 g)	0
Espresso Cafe Latte	1 pkg (0.6 oz)	70
Espresso Cafe Mocha	1 pkg (1 oz)	110
Espresso Cappuccino	1 pkg (0.6 oz)	80
Espresso Roast	1 can (10 oz)	90
French Vanilla	1 can (10 oz)	150
Hazelnut	1 can (10 oz)	130
Roasted Ground as prep	1 cup (6 oz)	0
Roasted Ground Decaffeinated as prep	1 cup (6 oz)	0
Revival		
Soy Caramal Corn	1 cup (8 oz)	0
Soy Hazelnut	1 cup (8 oz)	0
Soy Original Roast	1 cup (8 oz)	0
Soy Java		
All Flavors	1 tbsp	20
COFFEE BEVERAGES		
cappuccino mix as prep	7 oz	62
french mix as prep	7 oz	57
mocha mix as prep	7 oz	51
AchievONE		
All Flavors	1 bottle (9.5 oz)	120

FOOD	PORTION	CALS
America's Best Brew		
Iced Coffee All Flavors	8 oz	110
Arizona		
Iced Latte Supreme	8 oz	110
Iced Mocha Latte	8 oz	110
Big Train		
Low Carb Blended Ice Mocha as prep	1 serv (16 oz)	90
Chock full o'Nuts		
New York Cappuccino French Vanilla	1 pkg (0.9 oz)	90
New York Cappuccino Hazelnut	1 pkg. (0.9 oz)	90
Cinnabon		
Latte Caramel Nut	1 can (8 oz)	170
Latte Cinnamon Vanilla	1 can (8 oz)	170
Coffee House USA		
All Flavors	1 bottle (9.5 oz)	100
Double Bean Elixir		
Coffee Soda All Flavors	8 oz	90
Double Hit		
Maximum Energy Coffee Drink	1 can (12 oz)	80
Flavour Creations		
Coffee Flavoring Tablets All Flavors	1 tablet	0
Frappio		
Iced Coffee Energy Drink	1 can (15 oz)	260
Gehl's		
Iced Cappuccino	1 can (11 oz)	190
Jakada		
Latte Mocha	1 bottle (10.5 oz)	180
Latte Vanilla	1 bottle (10.5 oz)	180
Loco-Joe		
Iced Coffee	1 box (8.25 oz)	160
Low Carb Creations		
Cappuccino	1 cup	30
Shock		
Latte	8 oz	150
Triple Mocha	1 can (8 oz)	125
Silk		
Coffee Soylatte	1 bottle (11 oz)	220
Sipper Sweets		
Sugar Free Low Carb Cappuccino	1 serv	50

FOOD	PORTION	CALS
Starbucks		
Frappuccino	1 bottle (9.5 oz)	190
Frappuccino Mocha	1 bottle (9.5 oz)	190
Frappuccino Vanilla	1 bottle (9.5 oz)	190
Wolfgang Puck		
Gourmet Heated Lattes All Flavors	1 can (10 oz)	100
TAKE-OUT		
cafe amaretto w/ alcohol	1 serv	192
cafe au lait	1 cup (8 fl oz)	77
cafe brulot	1 cup	48
cafe brulot w/ alcohol	1 serv	130
cappuccino	1 cup (8 fl oz)	77
coffee con leche	1 cup (8 fl oz)	77
espresso	1 cup (3 fl oz)	2
irish coffee	1 serv	226
latte w/ skim milk	13 oz	88
latte w/ whole milk	13 oz	152
mocha	1 mug (9.6 fl oz)	202

COFFEE SUBSTITUTES

FOOD	PORTION	CALS
powder	1 tsp	9
powder as prep	6 oz	9
powder as prep w/ milk	6 oz	121
Natural Touch		
Kaffree Roma	1 tsp (2 g)	10
Roma Cappuccino	3 tbsp (0.4 oz)	50
Teecinno		
Herbal Coffee All Flavors	1 cup	15

COFFEE WHITENERS

FOOD	PORTION	CALS
liquid nondairy frzn	1 tbsp (0.5 oz)	20
powder nondairy	1 tsp	11
Coffee-Mate		
Half & Half Original	2 tbsp	40
Half & Half Vanilla	2 tbsp	60
Latte Classic	2 tbsp	100
Latte Mocha	2 tbsp	90
Latte Vanilla	2 tbsp	90
Liquid All Flavors	1 tbsp	40

FOOD	PORTION	CALS
Liquid French Vanilla Fat Free	1 tbsp	10
Liquid Original	1 tbsp	20
Liquid Original Fat Free	1 tbsp	10
Liquid Original Low Fat	1 tbsp	10
Original Powder	1 tsp	10
Original Lite Powder	1 tsp	10
Sugar Free All Flavors	1 tbsp	15
N-Rich		
Coffee Creamer	1 tsp (2 g)	10
Silk		
Creamer	1 tbsp	15
Creamer French Vanilla	1 tbsp	20
Creamer Hazelnut	1 tbsp	15

COLESLAW
Dole

Classic Cole Slaw no dressing	1½ cups (3 oz)	25
Fresh Express		
3 Color Deli	1½ cups	20
Cole Slaw Kit as prep	2 cups	120
River Ranch		
Country Homestyle Kit	1 cup	140
Honey Dijon Peppercorn Kit	1 cup	120
Mix	1¼ cups	25
TAKE-OUT		
coleslaw w/ dressing	¾ cup	147
vinegar & oil coleslaw	3.5 oz	150

COLLARDS

fresh cooked	½ cup	17
frzn chopped cooked	½ cup	31
raw chopped	½ cup	6
Birds Eye		
Chopped Greens frzn	1 cup	30

COOKIES
MIX

chocolate chip	1 (0.56 oz)	79
oatmeal	1 (0.6 oz)	74
oatmeal raisin	1 (0.6 oz)	74

FOOD	PORTION	CALS
Aunt Paula's		
Low Carb Chef Chocolate Chip as prep	1	66
Low Carb Chef Peanut Butter as prep	1	66
Betty Crocker		
Chocolate Peanut Butter as prep	1 bar	180
Date Bar as prep	1 bar	150
Oatmeal as prep	2	150
Big Train		
Low Carb Chocolate Chip as prep	2	140
Low Carb Peanut Butter as prep	2	140
Bob's Red Mill		
Gluten Free Chocolate Chip as prep	2	260
GoldnBrown		
Fat Free	1 (1.1 oz)	120
Keto		
Chocolate Chip as prep	1	47
Oatmeal Raisin as prep	2	59
MiniCarb		
All Flavors as prep	1	110
Nature's Path		
Organic Chocolate Chip	⅒ pkg	150
Pillsbury		
Ready To Bake Chocolate Chip Sugar Free	1	90
READY-TO-EAT		
animal	11 crackers (1 oz)	126
animal crackers	1 box (2.4 oz)	299
animal crackers	1 (2.5 g)	11
australian anzac biscuit	1	98
butter	1 (5 g)	23
chocolate chip	1 box (1.9 oz)	233
chocolate chip	1 (0.4 oz)	48
chocolate chip low fat	1 (0.25 oz)	45
chocolate chip low sugar low sodium	1 (0.24 oz)	31
chocolate chip soft-type	1 (0.5 oz)	69
chocolate w/ creme filling	1 (0.35 oz)	47
chocolate w/ creme filling chocolate coated	1 (0.60 oz)	82
chocolate w/ creme filling sugar free low sodium	1 (0.35 oz)	46
chocolate w/ extra creme filling	1 (0.46 oz)	65
chocolate wafer	1 (0.2 oz)	26
cream cheese	1 (1.1 oz)	141

FOOD	PORTION	CALS
digestive biscuits plain	2	141
fig bars	1 (0.56 oz)	56
fortune	1 (0.28 oz)	30
fudge	1 (0.73 oz)	73
gingersnaps	1 (0.24 oz)	29
graham	1 squares (0.24 oz)	30
graham chocolate covered	1 (0.49 oz)	68
graham honey	1 (0.24 oz)	30
hermits	1 (1 oz)	117
jumbles coconut	1 (1 oz)	121
ladyfingers	1 (0.38 oz)	40
macaroons	1 (0.8 oz)	97
madeleines	1 (0.8 oz)	86
marshmallow chocolate coated	1 (0.46 oz)	55
marshmallow pie chocolate coated	1 (1.4 oz)	165
meringue	1 (0.3 oz)	20
molasses	1 (0.5 oz)	65
neapolitan tri-color cookie	1 (0.6 oz)	79
oatmeal	1 (0.6 oz)	81
oatmeal soft-type	1 (0.5 oz)	61
oatmeal raisin	1 (0.6 oz)	81
oatmeal raisin low sugar no sodium	1 (0.24 oz)	31
oatmeal raisin soft-type	1 (0.5 oz)	61
peanut butter sandwich	1 (0.5 oz)	67
peanut butter sandwich sugar free low sodium	1 (0.35 oz)	54
peanut butter soft-type	1 (0.5 oz)	69
pinenut cookies	1 (1.1 oz)	134
raisin soft-type	1 (0.5 oz)	60
reginette queen's biscuit	1 (0.8 oz)	86
shortbread	1 (0.28 oz)	40
shortbread pecan	1 (0.49 oz)	79
spritz	1 (0.4 oz)	42
sugar	1 (0.52 oz)	72
sugar low sugar sodium free	1 (0.24 oz)	30
sugar wafers w/ creme filling	1 (0.12 oz)	18
sugar wafers w/ creme filling sugar free sodium free	1 (0.14 oz)	20
toll house original	1 (0.8 oz)	105
vanilla sandwich	1 (0.35 oz)	48

FOOD	PORTION	CALS
vanilla wafers	1 (0.21 oz)	28
zeppole	1 (0.8 oz)	78
Alex & Dani's		
Original Hazelnut	3 (1 oz)	130
Alternative Baking		
Vegan Chocolate Chip	1 serv (2.5 oz)	280
Vegan Expresso Chocolate Chip	1 serv (2 oz)	230
Vegan Lemon	1 serv (2.25 oz)	250
Vegan Oatmeal	1 serv (2.25 oz)	250
Vegan Peanut Butter	1 serv (2.25 oz)	270
Vegan Pumpkin	1 serv (2 oz)	200
Vegan Wheat Free Choco Cherry Chunk	1 serv (1.75 oz)	190
Vegan Wheat Free Hula Nut	1 serv (1.75 oz)	190
Vegan Wheat Free P-nut Fudge Fusion	1 serv (1.75 oz)	190
Vegan Wheat Free Snickerdoodle	1 serv (1.75 oz)	170
Amay's		
Chinese Style Almond	1 (0.5 oz)	80
Annie's Homegrown		
Bunny Grahams All Flavors	26	130
Archway		
Alpine Fudge	1 (1.3 oz)	160
Carrot Cake	1 (1 oz)	130
Chocolate Chip	1 (0.9 oz)	120
Chocolate Chip Sugar Free	1 (0.8 oz)	110
Coconut Macaroon	2 (1.4 oz)	180
Devils Food Chocolate Drop Fat Free	1 (0.7 oz)	60
Dutch Cocoa	1 (0.9 oz)	100
Frosty Lemon	1 (0.9 oz)	100
Fruit & Honey Bar	1 (0.9 oz)	110
Fruit Bar Fat Free	1 (0.9 oz)	90
Fruit Filled Apricot	1 (0.8 oz)	90
Fruit Filled Raspberry	1 (0.8 oz)	90
Ginger Snaps	5 (1 oz)	120
Homestyle Chocolate Chip	3 (1 oz)	130
Iced Spice	1 (1 oz)	120
Oatmeal	1 (0.9 oz)	100
Oatmeal Apple Filled	1 (0.9 oz)	90
Oatmeal Pecan	1 (0.9 oz)	110
Oatmeal Raisin	1	120
Oatmeal Raspberry Fat Free	1 (1.1 oz)	100

FOOD	PORTION	CALS
Oatmeal Sugar Free	1 (0.8 oz)	110
Oatmeal Raisin Fat Free	1 (1.1 oz)	100
Old Dutch Apple	1 (0.9 oz)	110
Peanut Butter	1 (1 oz)	150
Peanut Butter Fudge	1 (1.3 oz)	220
Peanut Butter Sugar Free	1 (0.8 oz)	110
Pecan Crunch	3 (1.2 oz)	180
Rocky Road	1 (0.8 oz)	110
Rocky Road Sugar Free	1 (0.8 oz)	100
Shortbread Sugar Free	1 (0.8 oz)	110
Windmill	1	90
Arico		
Gluten Free Casein Free	1 bar	150
Gluten Free Caesin Free Almond Cranberry	1 bar	150
Gluten Free Casein Free Double Chocolate	1 bar	150
Arnott's		
Raspberry Tartlets	2	100
Atkins		
Endulge Wafer Bars Chocolate Creme	2 bars (1 oz)	120
Endulge Wafer Bars Mint	2 bars (1 oz)	120
Endulge Wafer Bars Peanut Butter	2 bars (1 oz)	120
Back To Nature		
Chocolate Chunk	2	130
Crispy Oatmeal	2	120
Sandwich Chocolate & Mint Creme	2	130
Sandwich Classic Creme	2	130
Bahlsen		
Afrika	8 (1.1 oz)	170
Butter Leaves	7 (1 oz)	140
Choco Leibniz	2 (1 oz)	140
Choco Star Dark Chocolate	3 (1.1 oz)	170
Choco Star Milk Chocolate	3 (1.1 oz)	180
Chocolate Hearts	4 (1 oz)	160
Delice	6 (1 oz)	140
Deloba	4 (0.9 oz)	130
Hanover Waffelin	5 (1 oz)	160
Hit Chocolate Vanilla Filled	2 (1 oz)	140
Hit Vanilla Chocolate Filled	2 (1 oz)	140
Kipferl	4 (1 oz)	150

FOOD	PORTION	CALS
Leibniz	6 (1 oz)	130
Nuss Dessert	3 (1.1 oz)	180
Probiers	6 (1.1 oz)	150
Twingo	6 (1.1 oz)	170
Waffeletten	4 (1 oz)	160
Baker's Breakfast Cookie		
Apple Pie	1 (3 oz)	204
Banana Walnut	1 (3 oz)	274
Chocolate Chunk Raisin	1 (3 oz)	260
Double Chocolate Chunk	1 (3 oz)	250
Fruit & Nut	1 (3 oz)	270
Lemon Poppy Seed	1 (3 oz)	230
Mocha Chocolate Chunk	1 (3 oz)	250
Oatmeal Raisin	1 (3 oz)	250
Peanut Butter	1 (3 oz)	290
Peanut Butter & Jelly	1 (3 oz)	320
Pumpkin Spice	1 (3 oz)	230
Vegan Chocolate Chunk	1 (3 oz)	260
Vegan Peanut Butter Chocolate Chunk	1 (3 oz)	310
Baker's Harvest		
Animal	12 (0.9 oz)	130
Chocolate Graham	2 (0.9 oz)	130
Cinnamon Grahams	2 (0.9 oz)	130
Cinnamon Grahams Low Fat	2 (0.9 oz)	110
Fig Bars	2 (1.2 oz)	120
Graham	2 (0.9 oz)	120
Graham Low Fat	2 (0.9 oz)	110
Iced Oatmeal	1 (0.6 oz)	70
Pecan Shortbread	1 (0.5 oz)	80
Vanilla Wafers	7 (1.1 oz)	150
Barbara's Bakery		
Apple Cinnamon Bars Fat Free Whole Wheat	1 (0.7 oz)	60
Chocolate Chip	1 (0.6 oz)	80
Double Dutch Chocolate	1 (0.6 oz)	80
Fig Bars Fat Free Wheat Free	1 (0.7 oz)	60
Fig Bars Fat Free Whole Wheat	1 (0.7 oz)	60
Nature's Choice Coconut Almond	1 bar (1 oz)	120
Nature's Choice Expresso Bean	1 bar (1 oz)	120
Nature's Choice Lemon Yogurt	1 bar (1 oz)	120
Nature's Choice Roasted Peanut	1 bar (1 oz)	130

FOOD	PORTION	CALS
Old Fashioned Oatmeal	1 (0.6 oz)	70
Raspberry Bars Fat Free Wheat Free Raspberry	1 (0.7 oz)	60
Snackimals Chocolate Chip	8 (1 oz)	120
Snackimals Oatmeal Wheat Free	8 (1 oz)	120
Snackimals Vanilla	8 (1 oz)	120
Traditional Blueberry Low Fat	1 (0.7 oz)	60
Traditional Fig Low Fat	1 (0.7 oz)	60
Traditional Shortbread	1 (0.6 oz)	80
Bed & Breakfast		
Cranberry Orange Oatmeal	1 (0.8 oz)	110
Enrobed Shortbread	2 (1.4 oz)	190
Fruit Center Key Lime	2 (1.1 oz)	140
Fruit Center Raspberry	2 (1.1 oz)	140
Beigel's		
Black & White	1 (1 oz)	100
BP Gourmet		
Biscotti Fat Free Cinnamon Crunch	6 (1 oz)	110
Biscotti Fat Free Vanilla Crunch	4 (1 oz)	80
Chocolate Fudge Chip Sugar Free	5 (1 oz)	100
Dreams Chocolate	7 (1 oz)	120
Dreams Fat Free Chocolate Fudge	13 (1 oz)	100
Dreams Fat Free Vanilla	19 (1 oz)	100
Tangos Fat Free Chocolate Fudge Chip	4 (1 oz)	100
Breaktime		
Chocolate Chip	1 (0.3 oz)	37
Coconut	1 (0.3 oz)	35
Ginger	1 (0.3 oz)	34
Oatmeal	1 (0.3 oz)	35
Sprinkles	1 (0.3 oz)	36
Brent & Sam's		
Chocolate Chip Pecan	2 (0.5 oz)	80
Chocolate Chip Raspberry	2 (0.5 oz)	70
Chocolate Chips	2 (0.5 oz)	70
Key Lime White Chocolate	2 (0.5 oz)	70
Oatmeal Raisin Pecan	2 (0.5 oz)	70
Toffee Pecan	2 (0.5 oz)	80
White Chocolate Macadamia	2 (0.5 oz)	80
Bud's Best		
Cacoa Creme	7 (1 oz)	140
Chocolate Chip	6 (1 oz)	140

FOOD	PORTION	CALS
French Vanilla	7 (1 oz)	150
Oatmeal	6 (1 oz)	130
Cafe		
Cinnamony Twists Chocolate Chip	1 (0.5 oz)	40
Sugar Free California Almond	4 (1 oz)	110
Twists Cinnamony	1 (0.3 oz)	40
Carbolite		
Chocolate Chip	1 (1 oz)	120
Peanut Butter	1 (1 oz)	120
Shortbread	1 (1 oz)	180
Carriage Trade		
Finnish Ginger Snaps	3	60
Carr's		
Ginger Lemon Cremes	2 (1 oz)	140
Cookie Lover's		
Chocolate Chip	1 (0.8 oz)	90
Creme Supremes	2 (0.9 oz)	120
Creme Supremes Mint	2 (0.9 oz)	120
Grahams	2 (1 oz)	100
Grahams Cinnamon	2 (1 oz)	110
Peanut Butter	1 (0.8 oz)	100
Shortbread	1 (0.8 oz)	120
Country Choice Naturals		
Chocolate Chip Walnut	1	100
Double Fudge Brownie	1 (0.8 oz)	90
Ginger	1	90
Ginger Snaps	5	120
Lemon	1	90
Oatmeal Chocolate Chip	1 (0.8 oz)	100
Oatmeal Raisin	1 (0.8 oz)	100
Old Fashioned Oatmeal	1 (0.8 oz)	100
Peanut Butter	1	100
Sandwich Cremes Chocolate	1	130
Sandwich Cremes Duplex	2	130
Sandwich Cremes Ginger Lemon	2	130
Sandwich Cremes Mint Creme	2	130
Sandwich Cremes Vanilla	2	130
Vanilla Wafers	7	120
Dare		
Blueberry Cheesecake	1 (0.6 oz)	90

FOOD	PORTION	CALS
Butter Shortbread	1 (0.5 oz)	63
Butter Creme	1 (0.6 oz)	85
Carrot Cake	1 (0.6 oz)	92
Chocolate Chip	1 (0.5 oz)	77
Chocolate Fudge	1 (0.7 oz)	97
Cinnamon Danish	1 (0.4 oz)	47
Coconut Creme	1 (0.7 oz)	99
French Creme	1 (0.5 oz)	80
Harvest From The Rain Forest	1 (0.5 oz)	70
Key Lime Creme	1 (0.6 oz)	86
Lemon Creme	1 (0.7 oz)	95
Maple Leaf Creme	1 (0.6 oz)	83
Maple Walnut Fudge	1 (0.7 oz)	99
Milk Chocolate Fudge	1 (0.7 oz)	99
Oatmeal Raisin	1 (0.4 oz)	59
Social Tea	1 (0.2 oz)	26
Sun Maid Raisin Oatmeal	1 (0.5 oz)	52
David's		
Hamantash Raspberry	1 (0.7 oz)	85
De Beukelaer		
Pirouline	8 (1 oz)	130
Delarce		
Chocosprits	1 (0.6 oz)	90
Marquisettes	3 (0.9 oz)	140
Roules d'Or	4 (1 oz)	180
Doritos		
Barras De Coco	5	120
Dove		
Beyond Chocolate Chunk	1	110
Chocolate Walnut Oasis	1	110
Chocolate Walnut Rendezous	1	110
Milk Chocolate Moment	3	150
Mint Chocolate Serenade	3	160
Toffee Chocolate Tango	3	160
Dunkaroos		
Chocolate Graham	1 pkg	120
Cinnamon Graham	1 pkg	130
Honey Graham	1 pkg	120
Dutch Mill		
Chocolate Chip	3 (1.1 oz)	160

FOOD	PORTION	CALS
Coconut Macaroons	3 (1 oz)	120
Oatmeal Raisin	3 (1 oz)	130
Eddyleon		
Jelly Graham Raspberry	1 (0.9 oz)	134
Pudding Cookies	1 (0.9 oz)	134
Elite		
Tea Biscuits Chocolate	4	80
English Bay		
Strawberry Fruit Bar	1 (1.2 oz)	120
Enjoy Life		
Gingerbread Spice Nut & Gluten Free	2 (1 oz)	100
No-Oat Oatmeal Nut & Gluten Free	2 (1 oz)	110
Snickerdoodle Nut & Gluten Free	2 (1 oz)	130
Entenmann's		
Little Bites Chocolate Chip	8 (1.8 oz)	240
Original Chocolate Chip	3	140
Soft Baked Double Chocolate Chip	1 (0.7 oz)	100
Soft Baked White Chocolate Macadamia Nut	1 (0.7 oz)	100
Soft Baked Light Chocolately Chip	2 (1 oz)	120
Soft Baked Light Oatmeal Raisin	2 (1 oz)	100
Estee		
Fructose Sweetened Chocolate Chip	4	160
Fructose Sweetened Lemon	4	160
Fructose Sweetened Sandwich Chocolate	3	170
Fructose Sweetened Sandwich Original	3	170
Fructose Sweetened Sandwich Peanut Butter	3	190
Fructose Sweetened Vanilla	4	160
Fructose Sweetened Vanilla Sandwich	3	170
Sugar Free Chocolate Chip	3	110
Sugar Free Lemon	3	110
Sugar Free Wafer Chocolate Creme	4	150
Sugar Free Wafer Lemon Creme	4	150
Sugar Free Wafer Peanut Butter Creme	4	150
Sugar Free Wafer Strawberry Creme	4	150
Sugar Free Wafer Vanilla Creme	4	150
Falcone's		
Sorrentini	1 (1 oz)	100
Famous Amos		
Butter Shortie	1 (0.5 oz)	80
Chocolate Chip	4 (1 oz)	140

FOOD	PORTION	CALS
Chocolate Chip & Pecan	4 (1 oz)	140
Chocolate Chip Toffee	4 (1 oz)	130
Chocolate Creme Sandwich	3 (1.2 oz)	140
Chunky Chocolate Chip	1 (0.5 oz)	70
Fat Free Fig Bar	2 (1 oz)	90
Fat Free Strawberry Fruit Bar	2 (1 oz)	90
Fig Bar	2 (1.1 oz)	120
Oatmeal Chocolate Chip Walnut	4 (1 oz)	140
Oatmeal Raisin	4 (1 oz)	130
Oatmeal Macaroon Creme Sandwich	3 (1.2 oz)	160
Peanut Butter Chocolate Chunk	1 (0.5 oz)	80
Peanut Butter Creme Sandwich	3 (1.2 oz)	160
Pecan Shortie	1 (0.5 oz)	80
Vanilla Creme Sandwich	3 (1.2 oz)	160
Frieda's		
Asian Almond	2 (1 oz)	170
Frookie		
Animal Frackers	14 (1 oz)	130
Chocolate Chip Wheat & Gluten Free	3 (1.1 oz)	140
Double Chocolate Wheat & Gluten Free	3 (1.1 oz)	130
Dream Creams Strawberry	4 (1 oz)	140
Dream Creams Vanilla	4 (1 oz)	140
Funky Monkeys Chocolate	16 (1 oz)	120
Funky Monkeys Vanilla	16 (1 oz)	120
Graham Cinnamon	2 (1 oz)	100
Graham Honey	2 (1 oz)	110
Lemon Wafers	8 (1 oz)	110
Old Fashioned Ginger Snaps	8 (1 oz)	120
Organic Chocolate Chip	3 (1.1 oz)	150
Organic Double Chocolate Chip	3 (1.1 oz)	140
Organic Iced Lemon	3 (1.3 oz)	165
Organic Oatmeal Raisin	3 (1.1 oz)	140
Peanut Butter Chunk Wheat & Gluten Free	3 (1.1 oz)	140
Sandwich Chocolate	2 (0.7 oz)	100
Sandwich Lemon	2 (0.7 oz)	100
Sandwich Peanut Butter	2 (0.7 oz)	100
Sandwich Vanilla	2 (0.7 oz)	100
Shortbread	5 (1 oz)	130
Vanilla Wafers	8 (1 oz)	110

FOOD	PORTION	CALS
Gamesa		
Animalitos	14	110
Arcoiris Marshmallow	6	220
Arcoiris Marshmallow	2	120
Arcoiris Merengue	6	200
Emperador Chocolate	2	120
Emperador Fresa	2	120
Emperador Limon	6	270
Emperador Vanilla	2	120
Hawaianas	3	130
Marias	8	120
Ricanelas	8	140
Roscas	3	130
Sugar Wafers Chocolate	3	160
Sugar Wafers Strawberry	3	160
Sugar Wafers Vanilla	3	160
General Henry		
Fruit Bars Apple	1 (0.6 oz)	60
Fruit Bars Blueberry	1 (0.6 oz)	60
Fruit Bars Fig	1 (0.6 oz)	60
Girl Scout		
Apple Cinnamon Reduced Fat	3 (1 oz)	120
Lemon Drops	3 (1.2 oz)	160
Samoas	2 (1 oz)	160
Striped Chocolate Chip	3 (1.2 oz)	180
Tagalongs	2 (0.9 oz)	150
Thin Mints	4 (1 oz)	140
Trefoils	5 (1.1 oz)	160
Glenny's		
Light & Crispy Chocolate Chip Cookie Dough	1 bar (0.5 oz)	70
Soy Fudgies All Flavors	3	70
Godiva		
Biscotti Dipped In Milk Chocolate	1 (0.9 oz)	120
Gol D Lite		
Low Carb Pizzelle	1 (0.3 oz)	46
Golightly		
Fabulous Tastes Caramel Dulce De Leche	4	100
Goody Man		
Marshmallow Crispy Squares	1 (1.17 oz)	130

FOOD	PORTION	CALS
Gourmet		
Chocolate Chip	2 (1.1 oz)	160
Lemon Creme	2 (1.4 oz)	210
Oatmeal Raisin	2 (0.9 oz)	120
Peanut Butter Chip	2 (1 oz)	150
Raspberry Center	2 (1.1 oz)	140
Grandma's		
Homestyle Big Chocolate Chip	1 (1.4 oz)	190
Homestyle Big Fudge Chocolate Chip	1 (1.4 oz)	170
Homestyle Big Oatmeal Raisin	1 (1.4 oz)	180
Homestyle Big Peanut Butter	1 (1.4 oz)	200
Mini Vanilla Creme	9	150
Peanut Butter Sandwich	5	210
Rich N'Chewy Chocolate Chip	1 pkg	270
Vanilla Creme Sandwich	5	210
Granny Oats		
Low Carb Oatmeal	4	98
Heavenly		
Meringues All Flavors Sugar Free Fat Free	1	0
Hellema		
Almond	1 pkg (0.6 oz)	90
Hershey's		
Cripsy Rice Snacks Peanut Butter	1 (0.6 oz)	70
Jacques Gourmet		
Palmier Cinnamon	3 (1 oz)	140
Palmier Vanilla	3 (1 oz)	140
Joseph's		
Almond Sugar Free	2 (0.9 oz)	100
Chocolate Chip Sugar Free	2 (0.9 oz)	100
Chocolate Walnut Sugar Free	2 (0.9 oz)	100
Coconut Sugar Free	2 (0.9 oz)	105
Lemon Sugar Free	2 (0.9 oz)	95
Oatmeal Raisin Sugar Free	2 (0.9 oz)	100
Peanut Butter Sugar Free	2 (0.9 oz)	95
Pecan Shortbread Sugar Free	2 (0.9 oz)	100
Karen's		
Fabulous Tastes Heavenly Chocolate Chip	4	90
Fabulous Tastes Luscious Raspberry Almond	4	110
Fabulous Tastes Pecan Vanilla Pralines	4	120

FOOD	PORTION	CALS
Kedem		
Tea Biscuits Chocolate	2	32
Tea Biscuits Orange	2	32
Keebler		
Animal Crackers Chocolate Chip	7 (1 oz)	130
Animal Crackers Ernie's	1 box	250
Animal Crackers Iced	6 (1.1 oz)	150
Animal Crackers Sprinkled	6 (1.1 oz)	150
Butter	5 (1.1 oz)	150
Chips Deluxe	1 (0.5 oz)	80
Chips Deluxe Chocolate Lovers	1 (0.6 oz)	90
Chips Deluxe Coconut	1 (0.5 oz)	80
Chips Deluxe Rainbow	1 (0.6 oz)	80
Chips Deluxe Soft 'n Chewy	1 (0.6 oz)	80
Chips Deluxe w/ Peanut Butter Cups	1 (0.6 oz)	90
Classic Collection Chocolate Fudge Creme	1 (0.6 oz)	80
Classic Collection French Vanllia Creme	1 (0.6 oz)	80
Cookie Stix Butter	5 (1.2 oz)	160
Cookie Stix Chocolate Chip	4 (0.9 oz)	130
Cookie Stix Rainbow	5 (1.2 oz)	150
Danish Wedding	4 (0.9 oz)	120
Droxies	3 (1.1 oz)	140
Droxies Reduced Fat	3 (1.1 oz)	140
E.L. Fudge Butter w/ Fudge Filling	2 (0.9 oz)	120
E.L. Fudge Fudge w/ Fudge Filling	2 (0.9 oz)	120
E.L. Fudge w/ Peanut Butter Filling	2 (0.9 oz)	120
Fudge Shoppe Deluxe Grahams	3 (1 oz)	140
Fudge Shoppe Double Fudge 'n Caramel	2 (1 oz)	140
Fudge Shoppe Fudge Sticks	3 (1 oz)	150
Fudge Shoppe Fudge Sticks Peanut Butter	3 (1 oz)	150
Fudge Shoppe Fudge Stripes	3 (1.1 oz)	160
Fudge Shoppe Fudge Stripes Reduced Fat	3 (1 oz)	140
Fudge Shoppe Grasshoppers	4 (1 oz)	150
Fudge Shoppe S'mores	3 (1.2 oz)	160
Ginger Snaps	5 (1.1 oz)	150
Golden Fruit Cranberry	1 (0.7 oz)	80
Golden Fruit Raisin	1 (0.7 oz)	80
Graham Cinnamon Crisp	8 (1 oz)	140
Graham Cinnamon Crisp Low Fat	8 (1 oz)	110
Graham Honey	8 (1.1 oz)	140

FOOD	PORTION	CALS
Graham Honey Low Fat	8 (1.1 oz)	120
Graham Original	8 (1 oz)	130
Lemon Coolers	5 (1 oz)	140
Oatmeal Country Style	2 (0.8 oz)	120
Sandies Fruit Delights Lemon	1 (0.6 oz)	80
Sandies Pecan Shortbread	1 (0.5 oz)	80
Sandies Simply Shortbread	1 (0.5 oz)	80
Sandies Strawberry Shortcake	1 (0.6 oz)	80
Snack Size Chips Deluxe	1 pkg (2 oz)	300
Snack Size Chips Deluxe Chocolate Lovers	1 pkg (2 oz)	280
Snack Size Mini Fudge Stripes	1 pkg (2 oz)	280
Snack Size Rainbow Chips Deluxe	1 pkg (2 oz)	290
Snackin' Grahams Cinnamon	21 (1 oz)	130
Snackin' Grahams Honey	23 (1 oz)	130
Soft Batch Chocolate Chip	1 (0.6 oz)	80
Soft Batch Homestyle Chocolate Chunk	1 (0.9 oz)	130
Soft Batch Homestyle Double Chocolate	1 (0.9 oz)	130
Soft Batch Homestyle Oatmeal Raisin	1 (0.9 oz)	130
Soft Batch Oatmeal Raisin	1 (0.5 oz)	70
Sugar Wafers Creme	3 (0.9 oz)	130
Sugar Wafers Lemon	3 (0.9 oz)	130
Sugar Wafers Peanut Butter	4 (1.1 oz)	170
Vanilla Wafers	8 (1.1 oz)	150
Vanilla Wafers Reduced Fat	8 (1.1 oz)	130
Vienna Fingers	2 (1 oz)	140
Vienna Fingers Lemon	2 (1 oz)	140
Keto		
Low Carb Biscotti Chocolate	1 (1.2 oz)	157
Low Carb Biscotti Lemon Nut	1 (1.2 oz)	157
Low Carb Biscotti Vanilla Almond	1 (1.2 oz)	157
Knott's Berry Farm		
Shortbread Apricot	3 (1 oz)	120
Shortbread Boysenberry	3 (1 oz)	120
Shortbread Raspberry	3 (1 oz)	120
La Choy		
Fortune	4 (1 oz)	112
La Dolce Vita		
Biscotti Chocolate Passion	1 (1.2 oz)	130
Landies Candies		
Sugar Free Dark Royal Pecan Shortbread	2	167

FOOD	PORTION	CALS
Sugar Free Milk Chocolate Chip	2	173
Sugar Free Milk Chocolate Peanut Butter	2	171
Sugar Free White Chocolate Lemon	2	177
Larzaroni		
Arancelli	8 (1 oz)	160
Calypso	3 (1 oz)	150
Limonelli	5 (1 oz)	140
Malaika	5 (1 oz)	158
Nanette	4 (1.2 oz)	170
Okla	3 (1 oz)	186
Oskar	10 (1 oz)	150
Samba	5 (1 oz)	160
Velieri	3 (0.9 oz)	120
Laura's Wholesome Junk Food		
Anna Banana Split	1	105
Gluten Free Charlotte's Chocolate Chip	2	120
Gluten Free Sally's Raisin	2	110
Lemon Vanilla	2	120
Oatmeal Chocolate Chip	2	110
Oatmeal Raisin	2	100
Wheat Free X-Treme Chocolate Fudge	2	110
Leibniz		
Butter Biscuits	6	130
Linden's		
Lemon	1 (1 oz)	120
Little Debbie		
Apple Flips	1 (1.2 oz)	150
Caramel Bars	1 (1.2 oz)	160
Cherry Cordials	1 (1.3 oz)	170
Coconut Rounds	1 (1.2 oz)	150
Cookie Wreaths	1 (0.6 oz)	100
Easter Puffs	1 (1.2 oz)	140
Fig Bars	1 (1.5 oz)	150
Fudge Delights	1 (1.1 oz)	110
Fudge Rounds	1 (1.2 oz)	140
German Chocolate Ring	1 (1 oz)	140
Ginger	1 (0.7 oz)	90
Jelly Creme Pies	1 (1.2 oz)	160
Marshmallow Crispy Bar	1 (1.3 oz)	140
Marshmallow Supremes	1 (1.1 oz)	130

FOOD	PORTION	CALS
Marshmallow Pie Banana	1 pkg (1.5 oz)	180
Marshmallow Pie Chocolate	1 (1.4 oz)	160
Nutty Bar	1 (2 oz)	310
Oatmeal Raisin	1 (1.3 oz)	160
Oatmeal Creme Pie	1 (1.3 oz)	170
Oatmeal Delights	1 (1.1 oz)	110
Oatmeal Lights	1 (1.3 oz)	130
Peanut Butter Bars	1 (1.9 oz)	270
Peanut Butter & Jelly Oatmeal Pie	1 (1.1 oz)	130
Peanut Clusters	1 (1.4 oz)	190
Pumpkin Delights	1 (1.2 oz)	150
Raisin Creme Pie	1 (1.2 oz)	140
Star Crunch	1 (1.1 oz)	140
Sugar Free Chocolate Chip	3 (1.1 oz)	140
Yo-Yo's	1 (1.2 oz)	130
Low Carb Creations		
Chocolate Chip	1 (1 oz)	140
Coconut	1 (1 oz)	140
Lemon	1 (1 oz)	140
Snickerdoodle	1 (1 oz)	140
LU		
Chocolatier	3 (1 oz)	150
Le Bastogne	2 (0.8 oz)	120
Le Dore	4 (1 oz)	140
Le Fondant	4 (1.1 oz)	170
Le Petit Beurre	4 (1.2 oz)	150
Le Petit Ecolier Dark Chocolate	2 (0.9 oz)	130
Le Petit Ecolier Extra Dark Chocolate	2	120
Le Petit Ecolier Hazelnut Milk Chocolate	2 (0.9 oz)	130
Le Petit Ecolier Milk Chocolate	2 (0.9 oz)	130
Le Petit Fruit Strawberry	5 (1.2 oz)	110
Le Raisin Dore	4 (1.2 oz)	160
Le Truffe Coconut	4 (1.2 oz)	190
Le Truffe Praline Chocolate	4 (1.2 oz)	170
Pim's Orange	2 (0.9 oz)	90
Pim's Raspberry	2 (0.9 oz)	90
Pim's Sensation Bar Chocolate	1	110
Pim's Sensation Bar Hazelnut	1	110
Shortbread	2	140

FOOD	PORTION	CALS
Mamma Says		
Biscotti Almond Pistachio	1 (0.5 oz)	50
Biscotti Chocolate Macadamia	1 (0.5 oz)	45
Biscotti Orange Citrine	1 (0.5 oz)	60
Mauna Loa		
Macadamia Nut Chocolate Chip	2	130
Macadamia Nut Hawaiian Crunch	2	150
Macadamia Nut White Chocolate Chip	2	130
Milk Lunch Brand		
New England Biscuits	4 (1.1 oz)	140
Miss Meringue		
Minis Chocolate Raspberry	13 (1 oz)	80
Minis Chocolate Chip	13 (1 oz)	120
Minis Mint Chocolate Chip	13 (1 oz)	120
Minis Mochaccino	13 (1 oz)	80
Minis Orange	13 (1 oz)	80
Minis Rainbow Vanilla	13 (1 oz)	110
Minis Toasted Coconut	13 (1 oz)	90
Minis Very Chocolate	13 (1 oz)	80
Minis Very Minty	13 (1 oz)	80
Minis Very Vanilla	13 (1 oz)	80
MoonPie		
Chocolate	1 (2.75 oz)	330
Mini Banana	1 (1.2 oz)	152
Mini Chocolate	1 (1.2 oz)	152
Mini Vanilla	1 (1.2 oz)	152
Mother's		
Almond Shortbread	3	180
Checkerboard Wafers	8	150
Chocolate Chip	2	160
Chocolate Chip Angel	3	180
Chocolate Chip Parade	4	130
Circus Animals	6	140
Classic Assortments	2	140
Cocadas	5	150
Cookie Parade	4	140
Dinosaur Grrrahams	2	130
Double Fudge	2	180
English Tea	2	180
Flaky Flix Fudge	2	140

FOOD	PORTION	CALS
Flaky Flix Vanilla	2	140
Gaucho Peanut Butter	2	190
Iced Oatmeal	2	130
Iced Raisin	2	180
Macaroon	2	150
Marias	3	170
MLB Double Header Duplex	3	170
Oatmeal	2	110
Oatmeal Chocolate Chip	2	120
Oatmeal Raisin	5	150
Oatmeal Walnut Chocolate Chip	2	130
Rainbow Wafers	8	150
Striped Shortbread	3	170
Sugar	2	140
Taffy	2	180
Triplet Assortment	2	140
Vanilla Wafers	6	150
Wallops Boysenberry	1	80
Wallops Honey Crust Fig	1	80
Wallops Honey Graham Fig	1	80
Wallops Mixed Berry	1	80
Wallops Peach Apricot	1	80
Wallops Raspberry	1	80
Wallops Strawberry	1	80
Walnut Fudge	2	130
Zoo Pals	14	140
Mrs. Alison's		
Coconut Bar	2 (1 oz)	130
Creme Wafers	5 (1.1 oz)	170
Duplex Sandwich	3 (1 oz)	130
Fudge Fingers	3 (1 oz)	160
Ginger Snaps	4 (1 oz)	130
Jelly Tops	5 (1 oz)	140
Lemon Creme	3 (1 oz)	130
Macaroons	2 (1 oz)	140
Pecan	2 (1 oz)	140
Shortbread	5 (1 oz)	120
Vanilla Sandwich	3 (1 oz)	130
Murray's		
Sugar Free Double Fudge	3 (1.2 oz)	140

FOOD	PORTION	CALS
Sugar Free Ginger Snap	6 (1 oz)	110
Sugar Free Oatmeal	6 (1.1 oz)	120
Sugar Free Peanut Butter	6 (1 oz)	130
Sugar Free Vanilla Sandwich Creme	3 (1 oz)	120
Sugar Free Vanilla Wafers	9 (1.1 oz)	120
Nabisco		
Barnum's Animal Crackers	10 (1 oz)	130
Barnum's Animal Crackers Chocolate	10 (1 oz)	130
Biscos Sugar Wafers	8 (1 oz)	140
Cafe Cremes Cappuccino	2 (1.1 oz)	160
Cafe Cremes Vanilla	2 (1.1 oz)	160
Cafe Cremes Vanilla Fudge	2 (1.1 oz)	200
Cameo	2 (1 oz)	130
Chips Ahoy!	3 (1.1 oz)	160
Chips Ahoy! Chewy	3 (1.3 oz)	170
Chips Ahoy! Chunky	1 (0.5 oz)	80
Chips Ahoy! Munch Size	6 (1.1 oz)	160
Chips Ahoy! Reduced Fat	3 (1.1 oz)	140
Family Favorites Iced Oatmeal	1 (0.6 oz)	80
Family Favorites Oatmeal	1 (0.6 oz)	80
Famous Chocolate Wafers	5 (1.1 oz)	140
Honey Maid Chocolate	8 (1 oz)	120
Honey Maid Cinnamon Grahams	8 (1 oz)	120
Honey Maid Cinnamon Sticks	1 pkg (1 oz)	120
Honey Maid Honey Grahams	8 (1 oz)	120
Honey Maid Low Fat Cinnamon Grahams	8 (1 oz)	110
Honey Maid Low Fat Grahams	8 (1 oz)	110
Honey Maid Oatmeal Crunch	8 (1 oz)	120
Lorna Doone	4 (1 oz)	140
Mallomars	2	120
Marshmallow Twirls	1 (1 oz)	130
Mystic Mint	1 (0.5 oz)	90
National Arrowroot	1 (5 g)	20
Newton Fat Free Fig	2 (1 oz)	90
Newtons Fig	2 (1.1 oz)	110
Newtons Fat Free Apple	2 (1 oz)	90
Newtons Fat Free Cobblers Apple Cinnamon	1 (0.8 oz)	70
Newtons Fat Free Cobblers Peach Apricot	1 (0.8 oz)	70
Newtons Fat Free Cranberry	2 (1 oz)	100
Newtons Fat Free Raspberry	2 (1 oz)	100

FOOD	PORTION	CALS
Newtons Fat Free Strawberry	2 (1 oz)	90
Nilla Wafers	8 (1.1 oz)	140
Nilla Wafers Chocolate Reduced Fat	8 (1 oz)	110
Nilla Wafers Reduced Fat	8 (1 oz)	120
Nutter Butter Bites	10 (1 oz)	150
Nutter Butter Chocolate Peanut Butter Sandwich	2 (1 oz)	130
Nutter Butter Peanut Butter Sandwich	2 (1 oz)	130
Old Fashioned Ginger Snaps	4 (1 oz)	120
Oreo	3 (1.2 oz)	160
Oreo Double Stuff	2 (1 oz)	140
Oreo Mini	1 pkg (1.2 oz)	170
Oreo Reduced Fat	3 (1.1 oz)	130
Oreo Halloween	2 (1 oz)	140
Pecanz	1 (0.5 oz)	90
Pinwheels Chocolate Marshmallow	1 (1 oz)	130
Rugrats Chocolate Frosted	8 (1.1 oz)	150
Rugrats Vanilla Frosted	8 (1.1 oz)	150
Social Tea	6 (1 oz)	120
Sweet Crispers Chocolate	18 (1.1 oz)	130
Sweet Crispers Chocolate Chip	18 (1.1 oz)	130
Teddy Grahams Chocolate	24 (1 oz)	130
Teddy Grahams Chocolately Chip	24 (1 oz)	130
Teddy Grahams Cinnamon	24 (1 oz)	130
Teddy Grahams Honey	24 (1 oz)	130
Natural Ovens		
Carob Chip	1	90
Chocolate Raspberry	1	120
Oatmeal Raisin	1	90
Nature's Path		
Organic Signature Lemon Poppyseed	4	130
Organic Animal Vanilla	9	120
Nestle		
Flipz Crunchy Graham White Fudge Chocolate	8 (1 oz)	140
Nonni's		
Biscotti Cioccalati	1 (1 oz)	130
Biscotti Decadence	1 (1.1 oz)	130
Biscotti Original	1 (1 oz)	100
Biscotti Paradiso	1 (1.1 oz)	130
NutraBalance		
Fibre Oatmeal Raisin	1 (0.7 oz)	80

FOOD	PORTION	CALS
Protein Fortified	1 (2 oz)	260
ReNeph Spice	1 (2 oz)	210
Old Brussels		
Ginger Crisps	2 (0.9 oz)	140
Old London		
Coffee Toppers Chocolate Creme	3 (0.5 oz)	70
Coffee Toppers Vanilla Creme	3 (0.5 oz)	70
Olde World		
Pizzelle Almond	3 (1 oz)	90
Pizzelle Anise	3 (1 oz)	90
Pizzelle Chocolate	3 (1 oz)	100
Pizzelle Lemon	3 (1 oz)	90
Pizzelle Vanilla	3 (1 oz)	90
Otis Spunkmeyer		
Butter Sugar	1 med (1.3 oz)	160
Butter Sugar	1 (2 oz)	250
Carnival	1 med (1.3 oz)	170
Chocolate Chip	1 med (1.3 oz)	170
Chocolate Chip	1 bite size (0.75 oz)	100
Chocolate Chip	1 (2 oz)	250
Chocolate Chip Pecan	1 med (1.3 oz)	170
Chocolate Chip Walnut	1 med (1.3 oz)	180
Chocolate Chip Walnut	1 bite size (0.75 oz)	100
Chocolate Chip Walnut	1 (2 oz)	270
Double Chocolate Chip	1 bite size (0.75 oz)	100
Double Chocolate Chip	1 med (1.3 oz)	180
Oatmeal Raisin	1 med (1.3 oz)	160
Oatmeal Raisin	1 bite size (0.75 oz)	90
Otis Express Chocolate Chunk	1 (2 oz)	280
Otis Express Double Chocolate Chip	1 (2 oz)	270
Otis Express Oatmeal Raisin	1 (2 oz)	240
Otis Express Peanut Butter	1 (2 oz)	270
Peanut Butter	1 med (1.3 oz)	180
Pinnacle Checkpoint Chocolate Almond Coconut	1 (2.4 oz)	320
Pinnacle Mach One Mocha Chocolate Chunk	1 (2.4 oz)	300
Pinnacle Passport Peanut Butter Chocolate Chunk	1 (2.4 oz)	300
Pinnacle Ripcord Rocky Road	1 (2.4 oz)	310
Pinnacle Takeoff Triple Chocolate	1 (2.4 oz)	300

FOOD	PORTION	CALS
Pinnacle Transatlantic Turtle	1 (2.4 oz)	310
Travel Lite Low Fat Apple Cinnamon	1 (1.3 oz)	130
Travel Lite Low Fat Chocolate Chip	1 (1.3 oz)	130
Travel Lite Low Fat Ginger Spice	1 (1.3 oz)	130
Travel Lite Low Fat Oatmeal Rum Raisin	1 (1.3 oz)	130
White Chocolate Macadamia Nut	1 med (1.3 oz)	180
White Chocolate Macadamia Nut	1 (2 oz)	280
Pally		
Butter	5 (1 oz)	140
Carnival	5 (1 oz)	130
Cinnamon Biscuit	5 (1 oz)	130
Mariel Biscuit	6 (1 oz)	150
Tea Biscuits	5 (1 oz)	150
Pamela's		
Pecan Shortbread Rice Flour	1 (0.8 oz)	130
Parmalat		
Grisbi Lemon	1 (0.6 oz)	90
Peek Freans		
Arrowroot	4 (1.2 oz)	150
Assorted Creme	1 (1 oz)	130
Dream Puffs	2 (0.9 oz)	110
Fruit Creme	2 (0.9 oz)	130
Ginger Crisp	4 (1.2 oz)	150
Nice	4 (1.2 oz)	160
Petit Beret Creme Caramel	2 (0.8 oz)	110
Petit Beret Fudge Truffle	2 (0.8 oz)	110
Petit Beurre	4 (1 oz)	130
Rich Tea	4 (1.2 oz)	160
Shortcake	2 (0.9 oz)	140
Traditional Oatmeal	1 (0.7 oz)	90
Tropical Cremes Calypso Lime	2 (0.9 oz)	130
Pepperidge Farm		
Biscotti Almond	1 (0.7 oz)	90
Biscotti Chocolate Hazelnut	1 (0.7 oz)	90
Bordeaux	4	130
Brussels	2	100
Chantilly Raspberry	2 (1 oz)	120
Chessman	3	120
Chocoate Chunk Soft Baked Double Chocolate	1 (0.9 oz)	130
Chocolate Chip	3	140

FOOD	PORTION	CALS
Chocolate Chunk Chesapeake	1 (0.7 oz)	140
Chocolate Chunk Minis Nantauket	1 pkg (1.75 oz)	260
Chocolate Chunk Minis Sausalito	4 (1 oz)	160
Chocolate Chunk Montauk	1 (0.9 oz)	130
Chocolate Chunk Nantucket	1 (0.9 oz)	140
Chocolate Chunk Sausalito	1 (0.7 oz)	140
Chocolate Chunk Soft Baked	1	140
Chocolate Chunk Soft Baked Milk Chocolate Macademia	1	130
Chocolate Chunk Soft Baked Reduced Fat	1	110
Chocolate Chunk Soft Baked White Chocolate Pecan	1	120
Chocolate Chunk Tahoe	1 (0.9 oz)	130
Fruitful Apricot Raspberry Cup	3	140
Fruitful Strawberry Cup	3	140
Geneva	3	160
Ginger Man	4 (1 oz)	130
Goldfish Grahams Cinnamon	1 pkg (1.75 oz)	240
Lemon Nut Crunch	3	170
Lido	1	90
Milano	3	180
Milano Endless Chocolate	3	180
Milano Milk Chocolate	3	170
Milano Double Chocolate	2 (0.7 oz)	140
Milano Mint	2	130
Milano Orange	2	130
Pirouettes Chocolate Laced	5 (1.1 oz)	180
Pirouettes Traditional	5 (1.2 oz)	170
Shortbread	2	140
Soft Baked Chocolate Chunk	1 (1.1 oz)	140
Soft Baked Oatmeal Raisin	1 (0.9 oz)	130
Spritzers Cool Key Lime	6 (1.1 oz)	140
Spritzers Ripe Red Raspberry	5 (1.1 oz)	140
Spritzers Zesty Lemon	5 (1.1 oz)	140
Sugar	3	140
Verona Strawberry	3 (1.1 oz)	140
Whims Chocolate Cashew	9 (1 oz)	150
Pure De-Lite		
High Protein Chocolate Fudge	1 (2.2 oz)	210
High Protein Peanut Butter Crunch	1 (2.2 oz)	210

FOOD	PORTION	CALS
Ralston		
Animal	12 (0.9 oz)	130
Chocolate Graham	2 (0.9 oz)	130
Cinnamon Grahams	2 (0.9 oz)	130
Cinnamon Grahams Low Fat	2 (0.9 oz)	110
Fig Bars	2 (1.2 oz)	120
Vanilla Wafers	7 (1.1 oz)	150
Real Torino		
Lady Fingers	3 (1 oz)	110
Reko		
Pizzelle Maple	5 (1 oz)	150
Pizzelle Vanilla	1 (6 g)	30
Royal		
Apple Bars	1 (1.1 oz)	100
Apple Cake	1 (1.1 oz)	110
Brownie Rounds	1 (1.1 oz)	130
Chocolate Chip	1 (1.1 oz)	140
Devilfood	1 (1 oz)	110
Fig Bars	1 (1.1 oz)	100
Oatmeal	1 (1.1 oz)	130
Raisin	1 (1 oz)	110
Strawberry Bars	1 (1.1 oz)	100
Salerno		
Mini Butter	25 (1 oz)	180
Mini Dinosaur Chocolate Graham	16 (1.1 oz)	140
Scotter Pie	1 (1.2 oz)	140
Santa Fe Farms		
Chocolate Chocolate Chip Fat Free	2 (1 oz)	60
Chocolate Mint Fat Free	2 (1 oz)	60
Ginger Fat Free	2 (1 oz)	70
Sargento		
MooTown Snackers Honey Graham Sticks & Vanilla Creme w/ Sprinkles	1 pkg (1 oz)	140
MooTown Snackers Vanilla Sticks & Chocolate Fudge Creme	1 pkg (1 oz)	130
Savion		
Chocolate Biscuits	5 (1 oz)	120
Tea Biscuits	5 (1 oz)	120
Tea Biscuits Vanilla	5 (1 oz)	120

FOOD	PORTION	CALS
Scotto's		
Biscotti Fat Free French Vanilla	4 (1 oz)	80
Season		
Hamantashen Apricot	1 (1 oz)	150
Hamantashen Poppy	1 (1 oz)	150
Simple Pleasures		
Almond	1 (0.3 oz)	37
Cinnamon Snaps	1 (0.2 oz)	31
Digestive	1 (0.3 oz)	46
Encore Tea Cookie	1 (0.2 oz)	29
Lemon Social Tea	1 (0.2 oz)	29
Oatmeal	1 (0.5 oz)	74
Spice Snaps	1 (0.3 oz)	34
Sugar	1 (0.4 oz)	45
SnackWell's		
Bite Size Chocolate Chip	13 (1 oz)	130
Bite Size Double Chocolate Chip	13 (1 oz)	130
Chocolate Sandwich	2 (0.8 oz)	110
Creme Sandwich	1 pkg (1.7 oz)	210
Fat Free Devil's Food	1 (0.5 oz)	50
Golden Devil's Food	1 (0.5 oz)	50
Mint Creme	2	110
Oatmeal Raisin	2 (0.9 oz)	110
Sugar Free Chocolate Chip	3 (1.2 oz)	150
Sugar Free Oatmeal	1 (0.8 oz)	90
South Beach Diet		
Chocolate Chip	2	100
Peanut Butter	2	100
Soybite		
All Flavors	1	79
Stella D'Oro		
Almond Toast Mandel	2 (1 oz)	110
Angel Wings	2 (0.9 oz)	140
Angelica	1 (0.8 oz)	100
Anginetti	4 (1.1 oz)	140
Anisette Sponge	2 (0.9 oz)	90
Anisette Toast	3 (1.2 oz)	130
Biscotti Almond	1 (0.8 oz)	100
Biscotti Chocolate Almond	1 (0.8 oz)	90
Biscotti Chocolate Chunk	1 (0.8 oz)	90

FOOD	PORTION	CALS
Biscotti Hazelnut	1 (0.8 oz)	100
Biscottini Cashews	1 (0.7 oz)	110
Breakfast Treats	1 (0.8 oz)	100
Breakfast Treats Chocolate	1 (0.8 oz)	100
Breakfast Treats Viennese Cinnamon	1 (0.8 oz)	100
Chinese Dessert Cookies	1 (1.2 oz)	170
Chocolate Castelets	2 (1 oz)	130
Egg Jumbo	2 (0.8 oz)	90
Fruit Slices Fat Free	1 (0.6 oz)	50
Kichel Low Sodium	21 (1 oz)	150
Lady Stella	3	130
Margherite Chocolate	2 (1.1 oz)	140
Margherite Vanilla	2 (1.1 oz)	140
Roman Egg Biscuits	1 (1.2 oz)	140
Sesame Regina	3 (1.1 oz)	150
Swiss Fudge	2 (0.9 oz)	130
Stieffenhofer		
Choco Minis	4 (1 oz)	160
Snaky	3 (1 oz)	160
Streit's		
Wafers	3 (1 oz)	160
Suissette		
Swiss Chocolate Hearts	4 (1 oz)	170
Swiss Delight	4 (1 oz)	160
Swiss Praline	4 (1 oz)	150
Sunshine		
All American Butter	5 (1.1 oz)	140
All American Lemon Coolers	5 (1 oz)	140
All American Mini Chip-A-Roos	5 (1.1 oz)	160
Animal Crackers	14 (1.1 oz)	140
Ginger Snaps	7 (1 oz)	130
Golden Fruit Cranberry	1 (0.7 oz)	80
Golden Fruit Raisin	1 (0.7 oz)	80
Hydrox	3 (1.1 oz)	150
Hydrox Reduced Fat	3 (1.1 oz)	140
Oatmeal Country Style	2 (0.8 oz)	120
Sugar Wafers Peanut Butter Creme	4 (1.1 oz)	170
Sugar Wafers Vanilla Creme	3 (0.9 oz)	130
Vanilla Wafers	7 (1.1 oz)	150
Vienna Fingers	2 (1 oz)	140

FOOD	PORTION	CALS
Vienna Fingers Lemon	2 (1 oz)	140
Vienna Fingers Reduced Fat	2 (1 oz)	130
Super Chip		
Chocolate Chip	2 (0.9 oz)	100
Sweet'N Low		
Sugar Free Amaretto Biscotti	4 (1 oz)	120
Sugar Free Chocolate Chip	4 (1 oz)	135
Sugar Free Cinnamon Graham	7 (1 oz)	120
Sugar Free Morning Crunch Bars	2 (1 oz)	120
Sugar Free Vanilla Wafers	7 (1 oz)	120
Sweetzels		
Chocolate Chip	7 (1 oz)	160
Ginger Snaps	4 (1.2 oz)	140
Vanilla Wafers	7 (1.1 oz)	137
Tastykake		
Chocolate Chip	1 (1.4 oz)	180
Chocolate Chip Bar	1 (2 oz)	270
Chocolate Fudge Iced	1 (1.4 oz)	170
Fudge Bar	1 (2 oz)	250
Lemon Bar	1 (2 oz)	260
Oatmeal Raisin Bar	1 (2 oz)	260
Oatmeal Raisin Boxed	3 (0.4 oz)	130
Oatmeal Raisin Iced	1 (1.4 oz)	170
Strawberry Bar	1 (2 oz)	260
Sugar Boxed	3 (0.4 oz)	120
The Source		
Barry's Raspberry Palmiers	1 (0.7 oz)	80
Tom's		
Animal Crackers	½ pkg (1 oz)	120
Big Cookie Chocolate Chip	1 pkg (2.75 oz)	340
Big Cookie Peanut Butter Chocolate Chip	1 pkg (2 oz)	280
Chocolate Chip	1 pkg (2 oz)	280
Confetti Chip	1 pkg (2 oz)	300
Fat Free Apple Bar	1 pkg (1.75 oz)	160
Fat Free Fig Bar	1 pkg (1.75 oz)	160
Vanilla Wafers	½ pkg (1 oz)	130
Tree Of Life		
Fat Free Almond Butter	1 (0.8 oz)	60
Fat Free Carrot Cake	1 (0.8 oz)	60
Fat Free Devil's Food Chocolate	1 (0.8 oz)	70

FOOD	PORTION	CALS
Fat Free Oatmeal Raisin	1 (0.8 oz)	70
Fruit Bars Fat Free Fig	1 (0.8 oz)	70
Fruit Bars Fat Free Peach Apricot	1 (0.8 oz)	70
Fruit Bars Fat Free Wildberry	1 (0.8 oz)	70
Monster Carob Chip	1 (4.7 oz)	700
Monster Granola	1 (4.7 oz)	700
Monster Macaroon	1 (4.7 oz)	750
Monster Peanut Butter	1 (4.7 oz)	700
Monster Fat Free Carrot Cake	1 cookie (3.8 oz)	240
Monster Fat Free Devil's Food Chocolate	1 cookie (3.8 oz)	320
Monster Fat Free Gingerbread	1 cookie (3.8 oz)	320
Monster Fat Free Maple Pecan	1 cookie (3.8 oz)	360
Oatmeal	1 (0.8 oz)	100
Sandwich Royal Vanilla	2 (0.9 oz)	120
Wheat Free Carob	1 (0.8 oz)	100
Wheat Free Maple Walnut	1 (0.8 oz)	100
Wheat Free Oatmeal	1 (0.8 oz)	90
Wheat Free Peanut Butter	1 (0.8 oz)	109
Voortman		
Almonette	2 (1 oz)	150
Chocolate Chip	1 (0.7 oz)	100
Chocolate Wafers Sugar Free	3 (1 oz)	160
Coconut Delight	1 (0.6 oz)	90
Peanut Delight	1 (0.9 oz)	130
Strawberry Wafers Sugar Free	3 (1 oz)	160
Sugar	1 (0.6 oz)	80
Turnovers Blueberry	1 (0.9 oz)	100
Turnovers Cherry	1 (0.9 oz)	100
Turnovers Strawberry	1 (0.9 oz)	100
Vanilla Wafers Sugar Free	3 (1 oz)	160
Windmill	1 (0.7 oz)	90
White Eagle Bakery		
Chruscik	2 (1 oz)	140
Wortz		
Animal	9 (1.1 oz)	140
Chocolate Graham	2 (0.9 oz)	130
Cinnamon	2 (0.9 oz)	130
Vanilla Wafers	7 (1.1 oz)	150
REFRIGERATED		
chocolate chip	1 (0.42 oz)	59

FOOD	PORTION	CALS
chocolate chip unbaked	1 oz	126
oatmeal	1 (0.4 oz)	56
oatmeal raisin	1 (0.4 oz)	56
peanut butter	1 (0.4 oz)	60
peanut butter dough	1 oz	130
sugar	1 (0.42 oz)	58
sugar dough	1 oz	124
Pillsbury		
Bunny	2	130
Chocolate Chip	1 (1 oz)	130
Chocolate Chip Reduced Fat	1 (1 oz)	110
Chocolate Chip w/ Walnuts	1 (1 oz)	140
Chocolate Chunk	1 (1 oz)	130
Christmas Tree	2	130
Double Chocolate	1 (1 oz)	130
Flag	2	130
Frosty	2	130
M&M's	1 (1 oz)	130
Oatmeal Chocolate Chip	1 (1 oz)	120
One Step Pan Chocolate Chip	⅛ pan (1 oz)	130
One Step Pan M&M's	⅛ pan (1 oz)	130
Peanut Butter	1 (1 oz)	120
Pumpkin	2	130
Reeses	1 (1 oz)	130
Shamrock	2	130
Sugar	2	130
Sugar Holiday Red & Green	2	130
Valentine	2	130
White Chocolate Chunk	1 (1 oz)	130
TAKE-OUT		
biscotti with nuts chocolate dipped	1 (1.3 oz)	117
black & white	1 lg (3 oz)	302
finikia	1 (1.2 oz)	171
koulourakia butter cookie twist	1 (0.9 oz)	113
linzer tart	1 (2.4 oz)	280

CORIANDER

cilantro fresh	1 cup (1.6 oz)	11
cilantro fresh	1 tsp (2 g)	tr
leaf dried	1 tsp	2

FOOD	PORTION	CALS
leaf fresh	¼ cup	1
seed	1 tsp	5
Instant India		
Tomato Coriander Paste	2 tbsp (1 oz)	90

CORN
CANNED

FOOD	PORTION	CALS
cream style	½ cup	93
w/ red & green peppers	½ cup	86
white	½ cup	66
yellow	½ cup	66
Del Monte		
Cream Style	½ cup	60
Fiesta	½ cup	50
Gold & White	½ cup	80
Savory Sides In Butter Sauce	½ cup	90
Savory Sides Santa Fe	½ cup	70
Summer Crisp	½ cup	70
White	½ cup	60
Green Giant		
Mexicorn	⅓ cup	70
Yellow & White	⅓ cup	60
S&W		
Cream Style	½ cup (4.4 oz)	60
Whole Kernel	⅓ cup (3 oz)	70
Veg-All		
Whole Kernel	½ cup	80

FRESH

FOOD	PORTION	CALS
white cooked	½ cup	89
white raw	½ cup	66
yellow cooked	½ cup	89
yellow cooked	1 ear (2.7 oz)	83
yellow raw	1 ear (3 oz)	77
yellow raw	½ cup	66

FROZEN

FOOD	PORTION	CALS
cooked	½ cup	67
on-the-cob cooked	1 ear (2.2 oz)	59
Birds Eye		
Baby Gold & White	⅔ cup	100

FOOD	PORTION	CALS
Cob Big Ear	1 ear	120
Cut	⅓ cup	70
Fresh Like		
Cut	3.5 oz	85
On The Cob	1 ear (3 in)	96
Tree Of Life		
Corn	⅔ cup (3.2 oz)	80
TAKE-OUT		
fritters	1 (1 oz)	62
on-the-cob w/ butter cooked	1 ear	155
scalloped	½ cup	258

CORN CHIPS (see CHIPS)

CORNISH HEN (see CHICKEN)

CORNMEAL

FOOD	PORTION	CALS
corn grits cooked	1 cup	146
corn grits uncooked	1 cup	579
white	1 cup (4.8 oz)	505
whole grain	1 cup (4.3 oz)	442
yellow	1 cup (4.8 oz)	505
yellow self-rising	1 cup (4.3 oz)	407
Albers		
White	3 tbsp	110
Yellow	3 tbsp	110
Expert Foods		
Low Carb Grits Mix	1½ tsp	15
Hodgson Mill		
Cornbread Mix Jalapeno Mexican	¼ cup (1 oz)	100
Yellow Organic	¼ cup (1 oz)	100
Yellow Self Rising	¼ cup (1 oz)	90
Indian Head		
Stone Ground	¼ cup	100
Kentucky Kernal		
Sweet Cornbread Mix	¼ cup (1 oz)	120
McKenzie's		
Hush Puppies	1 serv (1.9 oz)	190
Quaker		
Old Fashioned Grits not prep	¼ cup	140

FOOD	PORTION	CALS
Quick Grits not prep	¼ cup	130
Yellow	3 tbsp (1 oz)	90
TAKE-OUT		
hush puppies	1 (0.75 oz)	74

CORNSTARCH

cornstarch	1 cup (4.5 oz)	488
Argo		
Cornstarch	1 tbsp	30
Armour		
Cream Cornstarch	1 tbsp (0.4 oz)	40
Kingsford's		
Cornstarch	1 tbsp	30

COTTAGE CHEESE

creamed	1 cup (7.4 oz)	217
creamed	4 oz	117
creamed w/ fruit	4 oz	140
dry curd	4 oz	96
dry curd	1 cup (5.1 oz)	123
lowfat 1%	1 cup (7.9 oz)	164
lowfat 1%	4 oz	82
lowfat 2%	1 cup (7.9 oz)	203
lowfat 2%	4 oz	101
Breakstone's		
Cottage Doubles Peach	1 pkg (5.5 oz)	140
Fat Free	½ cup	90
Cabot		
Cottage Cheese	½ cup	100
No Fat	½ cup	70
Horizon Organic		
Cottage Cheese	½ cup (3.9 oz)	110
Light N'Lively		
Lowfat	½ cup	80

COTTONSEED

kernels roasted	1 tbsp	51

COUSCOUS

cooked	1 cup (5.5 oz)	176
dry	1 cup (6.1 oz)	650

FOOD	PORTION	CALS
Near East		
Broccoli & Cheese as prep	1 cup	230
Curry as prep	1 cup	220
Herbed Chicken as prep	1 cup	220
Original as prep	1 cup	230
Parmesan as prep	1 cup	220
Roasted Garlic Olive Oil as prep	1 cup	230
Toasted Pine Nut as prep	1 cup	230
Tomato Lentil as prep	1 cup	220
Wild Mushroom Herb as prep	1 cup	230
CRAB		
CANNED		
blue	½ cup	67
blue drained	1 can (6.5 oz)	124
Brunswick		
Crabmeat 15% Leg	2 oz	40
Fancy Lump	2 oz	45
Bumble Bee		
Lump	¼ cup	40
Pink	¼ cup	35
White	¼ cup	40
Chicken Of The Sea		
Fancy	½ can (2 oz)	40
Lump	½ can (2 oz)	35
Madam		
Crab Meat	½ cup	40
Terry's		
Crabmeat	¼ cup	40
FRESH		
alaska king meat only steamed	3 oz	82
blue cooked flaked	1 cup (4 oz)	120
dungeness steamed	3 oz	94
queen steamed	3 oz	98
FROZEN		
Margaritaville		
Coral Reef Cakes + Sauce	1	200
TAKE-OUT		
alaska king leg steamed	1 leg (4.7 oz)	130

FOOD	PORTION	CALS
baked	1 (3.8 oz)	160
cakes	2 (4.2 oz)	186
crab imperial	1 crab (6.8 oz)	289
crab salad	1 serv (5.5 oz)	285
crab thermidor	1 serv (6.4 oz)	456
deviled	1 serv (4.5 oz)	254
dungeness steamed	1 crab (4.5 oz)	140
empanada de jueyes	1 (4.4 oz)	341
fried crab puffs	4 (3.2 oz)	323
kenagi korean crab cooked	1 serv (3 oz)	71
mousse	¼ cup	364
salmorejo de jueyes (in tomato sauce)	1 serv (4.5 oz)	215
soft-shell breaded & fried	1 med (2.3 oz)	216
taco de jueyes	1 (4.2 oz)	266

CRACKER CRUMBS

chocolate wafer cookie crumbs	½ cup (5.9 oz)	728
cracker meal	1 cup (4 oz)	440
graham cracker crumbs	½ cup (4.4 oz)	540
Baker's Harvest		
Graham	⅓ cup (1 oz)	130

CRACKERS

cheese	14 (½ oz)	71
cheese	1 (1 in sq) (1 g)	5
cheese low sodium	14 (½ oz)	71
cheese low sodium	1 (1 in sq) (1 g)	5
cheese w/ peanut butter filling	1 (0.24 oz)	34
crispbread	3	61
crispbread rye	1 (0.35 oz)	37
crispbread rye	3	77
melba toast plain	1 (5 g)	19
melba toast pumpernickel	1 (5 g)	19
melba toast rye	1 (5 g)	19
melba toast wheat	1 (5 g)	19
milk	1 (0.42 oz)	55
oyster cracker	1 (1 g)	4
peanut butter sandwich	1 (7 g)	34
rusk toast	1 (0.35 oz)	41
rye w/ cheese filling	1 (0.24 oz)	34
rye wafers plain	1 (0.9 oz)	84

FOOD	PORTION	CALS
rye wafers seasoned	1 (0.8 oz)	84
saltines	1 (3 g)	13
saltines fat free low sodium	3 (0.5 oz)	59
saltines fat free low sodium	6 (1 oz)	118
saltines low salt	1 (3 g)	13
snack cracker	1 (3 g)	15
snack cracker low salt	1 (3 g)	15
snack cracker w/ cheese filling	1 (7 g)	33
soup cracker	1 (1 g)	4
water biscuits	3	92
wheat w/ cheese filling	1 (0.24 oz)	35
wheat w/ peanut butter filling	1 (0.24 oz)	35
wheat thins	1 (2 g)	9
wheat thins	7 (0.5 oz)	67
wheat thins low salt	7 (0.5 oz)	67
whole wheat	1 (4 g)	18
whole wheat low salt	1 (4 g)	18
zwieback	1 oz	107
American Vintage		
Wine Biscuits All Flavors	5	140
Andre's		
CarboSave Crackerbread All Flavors	1 oz	140
Annie's Homegrown		
Cheddar Bunnies BBQ	50	130
Cheddar Bunnies Original	50	150
Cheddar Bunnies Ranch	50	130
Cheddar Bunnies Whole Wheat	50	130
Austin		
Cracker Sandwich Cheese On Cheese	6 (1.3 oz)	170
Cracker Sandwich Cheese Peanut Butter	6 (1.3 oz)	170
Cracker Sandwich Toasty Peanut Butter	6 (1.3 oz)	170
Cracker Sandwich Whole Wheat Cheese	6 (1.3 oz)	170
Back To Nature		
Classic Rounds	5	70
Crispy Wheats	17	130
Rice Thin Sesame Ginger	16	120
Rice Thin White Cheddar	16	120
Baker's Harvest		
Cheese	23 (1 oz)	150
Cheese Reduced Fat	29 (1 oz)	130

FOOD	PORTION	CALS
Oyster	35 (0.5 oz)	70
Saltines Unsalted	5 (0.5 oz)	70
Saltines Deluxe	5 (0.5 oz)	60
Snackers	9 (1.1 oz)	160
Snackers Reduced Fat	10 (1.1 oz)	140
Snackers Unsalted	9 (1.1 oz)	160
Wheat Snacks	16 (1 oz)	140
Wheat Snacks Reduced Fat	16 (1.1 oz)	140
Woven Wheats	7 (1.1 oz)	140
Woven Wheats Reduced Fat	8 (1.1 oz)	130
Barbara's Bakery		
Cheese Bites	26 (1 oz)	120
Right Lite Rounds Original	5 (0.5 oz)	55
Rite Lite Rounds Savory Poppy	5 (0.5 oz)	70
Rite Lite Rounds Tamari Sesame	5 (0.5 oz)	70
Wheatines All Flavors	1 lg sq (0.5 oz)	50
Blue Diamond		
Nut Thins Almond	16 (1 oz)	130
Nut Thins Hazelnut	16 (1 oz)	120
Nut Thins Pecan	16 (1 oz)	130
Bran-A-Crisp		
Low Carb Wheat Bran	1	20
Breton		
Cabaret	3 (5 g)	70
Garden Vegetable	3	60
Light	1 (5 g)	20
Minis	20 (0.6 oz)	89
Minis Cheddar Cheese	20 (0.6 oz)	87
Minis Garden Vegetable	20 (0.6 oz)	87
Multi Grain	3	70
Original	3	60
Reduced Fat & Sodium	3	60
Sesame	3	60
Cheeters		
Low Carb All Flavors	1 pkg (1 oz)	104
Cheetos		
Cheddar	1 pkgz	240
Cheez It		
Big	13 (1 oz)	150
Big Reduced Fat	15 (1 oz)	140

FOOD	PORTION	CALS
Heads & Tails	37 (1 oz)	140
Hot & Spicy	26 (1 oz)	150
Low Sodium	27 (1 oz)	160
Nacho	28 (1 oz)	150
Original	27 (1 oz)	160
Party Mix	½ cup (1 oz)	140
Party Mix Nacho	½ cup (1 oz)	130
Party Mix Reduced Fat	½ cup (1 oz)	130
Peanut Butter	1 pkg (1.3 oz)	190
Reduced Fat	29 (1 oz)	140
Snack Mix	½ cup (1 oz)	130
Snack Mix Big Crunch	¾ cup (1 oz)	110
Snack Mix Double Cheese	¾ cup (1 oz)	110
White Cheddar	26 (1 oz)	150
Courtney's		
Sun-Dried Tomato Organic	4 (0.5 oz)	60
Dare		
Cabaret	3	70
Vinta	1 (6 g)	30
Doritos		
Jalapeno Chesse	1 pkg	230
Nacho Cheesier	1 pkg	240
Dr. Kracker		
Flatbread Klassic 100% Whole Wheat 3 Seed	1	90
Flatbread Klassic Seed	1	100
Flatbread Pumpkin Seed	1	100
Flatbread Seeded Spelt	1	110
Flatbread Seedlander	1	100
Flatbread Spelt Sunflower Cheese	1	100
Kribbons Krispy Graham	5	120
Kribbons Muesli	5	120
Eden		
Nori Nori Rice	15 (1 oz)	110
Foods Alive		
Golden Flax Maple & Cinnamon	5	150
Golden Flax Mexican Harvest	5	150
Golden Flax Onion Garlic	5	140

FOOD	PORTION	CALS
Golden Flax Organic Hemp	5	130
Golden Flax Regular	5	150
Frito Lay		
Cheddar Snacks	1 pkg	200
Frookie		
Cheddar	17 (1 oz)	140
Cracked Pepper	8 (0.7 oz)	70
Garden Vegetable	13 (1 oz)	130
Garlic & Herb	8 (0.7 oz)	70
Pizza	17 (1 oz)	130
Snack & Party	10 (1 oz)	140
Water Crackers	8 (0.7 oz)	70
Wheat & Onion	12 (1 oz)	120
Wheat & Rye	13 (1 oz)	120
Gamesa		
Sabrisas	11	150
Gold'n Krackle		
Cheese	½ oz	65
Cheese & Oregano	½ oz	65
Hot & Spicy	½ oz	58
Onion & Garlic	½ oz	58
Plain	½ oz	58
Heavenly		
All Flavors Cholesterol Free Sugar Free	1	16
Kashi		
TLC Country Cheddar	15 (1 oz)	130
TLC Honey Sesame	15 (1 oz)	130
TLC Natural Ranch	15 (1 oz)	130
TLC Original 7 Grain	15 (1 oz)	130
Keebler		
Club 33% Reduced Fat	5 (0.6 oz)	70
Club 50% Reduced Sodium	4 (0.5 oz)	70
Club Original	4 (0.5 oz)	70
Elfin	23 (1 oz)	130
Export Soda	3 (0.5 oz)	60
Harvest Bakery Multigrain	2 (0.6 oz)	70
Munch'ems Cheddar	30 (1 oz)	130
Munch'ems Cheddar	39 (1 oz)	140
Munch'ems Chili Cheese	28 (1.1 oz)	130
Munch'ems Mexquite BBQ	40 (1 oz)	140

FOOD	PORTION	CALS
Munch'ems Ranch	33 (1 oz)	130
Munch'ems Ranch	40 (1 oz)	140
Munch'ems Salsa	28 (1.1 oz)	130
Munch'ems Seasoned Original 55% Reduced Fat	30 (1 oz)	130
Munch'ems Sour Cream & Onion	39 (1 oz)	140
Munch'ems Sour Cream & Onion 55% Reduced Fat	33 (1 oz)	130
Paks Cheese & Peanut Butter	1 pkg	190
Paks Club & Cheddar	1 pkg	190
Paks Toast & Peanut Butter	1 pkg	190
Sandwich Cracker Wheat & Cheddar	1 pkg	200
Toasteds Buttercrisp	9 (1 oz)	140
Toasteds Buttercrisp	5 (0.6 oz)	80
Toasteds Onion	9 (1 oz)	140
Toasteds Sesame	9 (1 oz)	140
Toasteds Sesame	5 (0.6 oz)	80
Toasteds Sesame Reduced Fat	10 (1 oz)	120
Toasteds Wheat	9 (1 oz)	140
Toasteds Wheat	5 (0.6 oz)	80
Toasteds Wheat Reduced Fat	10 (1 oz)	120
Toasteds Wheat Reduced Fat	5 (0.5 oz)	60
Town House	5 (0.6 oz)	80
Town House 50% Reduced Sodium	5 (0.6 oz)	80
Town House Reduced Fat	6 (0.6 oz)	70
Town House Wheat	5 (0.6 oz)	80
Wheatables Honey Wheat	12 (1 oz)	140
Wheatables Original	12 (1 oz)	140
Wheatables Seven Grain	12 (1 oz)	140
Zesta Saltine 50% Reduced Sodium	5 (0.5 oz)	60
Zesta Saltine Fat Free	5 (0.5 oz)	50
Zesta Saltine Original	5 (0.5 oz)	60
Zesta Saltine Unsalted Top	5 (0.5 oz)	70
Zesta Soup & Oyster	42 (0.5 oz)	80
Kitchen Table Bakers		
Aged Paramesan	3	80
Caraway Cheese	3	80
Sesame Cheese	3	80
Little Debbie		
Cheese Crackers With Peanut Butter	1 (0.9 oz)	140

FOOD	PORTION	CALS
Cheese On Cheese Crackers	1 (0.9 oz)	140
Cream Cheese & Chive	1 (0.9 oz)	140
Toasty Crackers With Peanut Butter	1 (0.9 oz)	140
Wheat Crackers With Cheddar Cheese	1 (0.9 oz)	140
Nabisco		
Royal Lunch	1 (0.4 oz)	60
Zwieback	1 (8 g)	35
Nature's Path		
Signature Tamari Flax	15	110
No-Carb Kitchen		
Cheese	1	25
No-No		
Flatbreads Tortilla Corn Low Fat Sugar Free Everything	3 (1 oz)	95
Old London		
Mediterranean Toast	3	60
Pepperidge Farm		
English Water Biscuits	4 (0.5 oz)	70
Giant Goldfish Peanut Butter Sandwich	1 pkg (1.4 oz)	190
Giant Goldfish Wheat	14	140
Goldfish Cheddar	55	140
Goldfish Cheddar 30% Less Sodium	60 (1.1 oz)	150
Goldfish Cheese Trio	58	140
Goldfish Colors On The Go	1 pkg	170
Goldfish Original	55	140
Goldfish Pizza Flavored	55 (1 oz)	140
Goldfish Pretzel	43	130
Goldfish Snack Mix Fat Free	⅔ cup (0.9 oz)	90
Goldfish w/ Whole Grain	55	140
Hearty Wheat	3 (0.6 oz)	80
Sesame	3 (0.5 oz)	70
Peter Pan		
Peanut Butter Cheese	1 pkg	210
Peanut Butter Toast	1 pkg	210
Premium		
Saltine Fat Free	5	60
Saltine Multigrain	5 (0.5 oz)	60
Saltine Unsalted Tops	5	70
Ralston		
Cheese	23 (1 oz)	150

FOOD	PORTION	CALS
Cheese Reduced Fat	29 (1 oz)	130
Oyster	35 (0.5 oz)	70
Rich & Crisp	1 (0.5 oz)	70
Saltines Fat Free	5 (0.5 oz)	60
Saltines Deluxe	5 (0.5 oz)	60
Snackers	9 (1.1 oz)	160
Snackers Reduced Fat	10 (1.1 oz)	140
Snackers Unsalted	9 (1.1 oz)	160
Wheat Snacks	16 (1 oz)	140
Wheat Snacks Reduced Fat	16 (1.1 oz)	140
Woven Wheats	7 (1.1 oz)	140
Woven Wheats Reduced Fat	8 (1.1 oz)	130
RedOval Farms		
Stoned Wheat Thins Cracked Pepper	4 (0.6 oz)	70
Ritz		
Reduced Fat	5	70
Rykrisp		
Seasoned	2	60
SnackWell's		
Cracked Pepper	5	60
South Beach Diet		
Whole Wheat	1 pkg (0.8 oz)	100
Sunshine		
Hi Ho	4 (0.5 oz)	70
Hi Ho Reduced Fat	5 (0.5 oz)	70
Krispy	5 (0.5 oz)	60
Krispy Fat Free	5 (0.5 oz)	50
Krispy Mild Cheddar	5 (0.5 oz)	60
Krispy Soup & Oyster	17 (0.5 oz)	60
Krispy Unsalted Tops	5 (0.5 oz)	60
Krispy Whole Wheat	5 (0.5 oz)	60
Tree Of Life		
Bite Size Fat Free Cracked Pepper	12 (0.5)	55
Bite Size Fat Free Garden Vegetable	12 (0.5 oz)	55
Bite Size Fat Free Garlic & Herb	12 (0.5 oz)	55
Bite Size Fat Free Toasted Onion	12 (0.5 oz)	55
Oyster	40 (0.5 oz)	60
Saltine Cracked Pepper Fat Free	4 (0.5 oz)	60
Saltine Fat Free	4 (0.5 oz)	50

FOOD	PORTION	CALS
Venus		
Fat Free Cracked Pepper	11 (0.5 oz)	60
Fat Free Garden Vegetable	5 (0.5 oz)	60
Fat Free Garlic & Herb	11 (0.5 oz)	60
Fat Free Multi-Grain	5 (0.5 oz)	60
Fat Free Spicy Chili	10 (0.5 oz)	60
Fat Free Toasted Onion	5 (0.5 oz)	60
Fat Free Toasted Wheat	5 (0.5 oz)	60
Fat Free Tomato & Basil	10 (0.5 oz)	60
Fat Free Zesty Italian	10 (0.5 oz)	60
Garden Vegetable	6 (1 oz)	150
Honey Wheat	1 oz	140
Low Fat Cracker Bread	5 (0.5 oz)	60
Low Fat Water Crackers	4 (0.5 oz)	60
Sesame & Flaxseed	1 oz	130
Soup Original	0.5 oz	60
Toasted Wheat	6 (1 oz)	150
Wine Cheese Caviar Original	0.5 oz	60
Wine Cheese Caviar Pepper & Poppy	0.5 oz	60
Wasa		
Crispbread Fiber Rye	1 (0.4 oz)	30
Wheat Thins		
Harvest Crisps Five-Grain	13	140
Wheatsworth		
Crackers	5	80
Wisecrackers		
Low Fat Roasted Garlic	10	110
Wortz		
Cheese	23 (1 oz)	150
Oyster	35 (0.5 oz)	70
Rich & Crisp	1 (0.5 oz)	70
Saltines Deluxe	5 (0.5 oz)	60
Saltines Fat Free	5 (0.5 oz)	60
Wheat Snacks	16 (1 oz)	140
Wheat Snacks Reduced Fat	16 (1.1 oz)	140
Woven Wheats	7 (1.1 oz)	140

CRANBERRIES

cranberry sauce sweetened	½ cup	209

FOOD	PORTION	CALS
dried organic	⅓ cup	120
fresh chopped	1 cup	54
Frieda's		
Dried	⅓ cup (1.4 oz)	110
Jok'n'Al		
Cranberry Sauce	1 tbsp	8
Ocean Spray		
Craisins	⅓ cup	130
Cranberry Sauce Jellied	¼ cup	110
Cranorange	¼ cup	120
Whole Berry Sauce	¼ cup	110
Steel's		
Spiced Cranberry Sauce	⅓ cup	20
Wild Thyme Farms		
Cranberry Sauce	1 tbsp	19

CRANBERRY BEANS

FOOD	PORTION	CALS
canned	½ cup	108
dried cooked w/o salt	½ cup	120

CRANBERRY JUICE

FOOD	PORTION	CALS
cranberry juice cocktail	6 oz	108
cranberry juice cocktail low calorie	6 oz	33
cranberry juice cocktail frzn	12 oz can	821
cranberry juice cocktail frzn as prep	6 oz	102
Keto		
Kooler	½ tsp	0
Langers		
Cocktail	8 oz	140
Diet	8 oz	30
White	8 oz	120
Mott's		
Cocktail	8 fl oz	150
Nantucket Nectars		
Big Cran	8 oz	140
Ocean Spray		
Cocktail	8 oz	140
Cocktail Reduced Calorie	8 oz	50
Cocktail Light Low Calorie	8 oz	40
Cranberry Spritzer	8 oz	160

FOOD	PORTION	CALS
Cranberry Drink	8 oz	130
Crantastic	8 oz	100
White Cranberry	8 oz	120
White Cranberry Peach	8 oz	120
White Cranberry Strawberry	8 oz	120
Tropicana		
Twister Ruby Red	1 bottle (10 oz)	160

CRAYFISH
cooked	3 oz	97
raw	3 oz	76
raw	8	24

CREAM *(see also* WHIPPED TOPPINGS*)*
clotted cream	2 tbsp (1 oz)	164
creme fraiche	2 tbsp (1 oz)	100
half & half	1 cup (8.5 oz)	315
half & half	1 tbsp (0.5 oz)	20
heavy whipping	1 tbsp (0.5 oz)	52
heavy whipping whipped	1 cup (4.1 oz)	411
light coffee	1 cup (8.4 oz)	496
light coffee	1 tbsp (0.5 oz)	29
light whipping	1 tbsp (0.5 oz)	44
light whipping cream whipped	1 cup (4.2 oz)	345
Cabot		
Whipped	2 tbsp	30
Coffee-Mate		
Half & Half Fat Free	2 tbsp	20
Land O Lakes		
Fat Free Half & Half	2 tbsp (1 oz)	20
Half & Half	2 tbsp (1 oz)	40
Heavy Whipping	1 tbsp (0.5 oz)	50
Organic Valley		
Half & Half	2 tbsp (1 oz)	40

CREAM CHEESE
cream cheese	1 oz	99
cream cheese	1 pkg (3 oz)	297

FOOD	PORTION	CALS
Alpine Lace		
Reduced Fat Roasted Garlic & Herbs	1 tsp (1 oz)	60
Reduced Fat Sundried Tomato & Basil	2 tsp (1 oz)	70
Boar's Head		
Cream Cheese	2 tbsp (1 oz)	100
Galaxy		
Slices	1 slice (1 oz)	50
Horizon Organic		
Spreadable	2 tbsp	100
Organic Valley		
Cream Cheese	1 oz	100
Philadelphia		
⅓ Less Fat	1 oz	70
Fat Free	1 oz	30

CREAM CHEESE SUBSTITUTE
WholeSoy & Co.

Soy Cream Cheese Organic Original & Flavored	2 tbsp	70

CREAM OF TARTAR

cream of tartar	1 tsp	8

CREAM SUBSTITUTES
ExpertExtras

RealCream	1 tsp	14

CREPES

basic crepe unfilled	1	75
Frieda's		
Ready-To-Use	1 (0.5 oz)	30

CROAKER

atlantic breaded & fried	3 oz	188
atlantic raw	3 oz	89

CROCODILE

cooked	3 oz	78

CROISSANT

apple	1 (2 oz)	145
cheese	1 (2 oz)	236
plain	1 (2 oz)	232
plain	1 mini (1 oz)	115

FOOD	PORTION	CALS
Sara Lee		
Broccoli & Cheese	1 (3.7 oz)	280
French Style	1 (1.5 oz)	170
Ham & Swiss	1 (3.7 oz)	300
Petite	2 (2 oz)	230
TAKE-OUT		
w/ egg & cheese	1 (4.5 oz)	368
w/ egg cheese & bacon	1 (4.5 oz)	413
w/ egg cheese & ham	1 (5.3 oz)	474
w/ egg cheese & sausage	1 (5.6 oz)	523

CROUTONS

FOOD	PORTION	CALS
plain	1 cup (1 oz)	122
seasoned	1 cup (1.4 oz)	186
Cardini's		
Italian	2 tbsp	30
Pepperidge Farm		
Whole Grain Caesar	6	35
Whole Grain Seasoned	6	30
Rothbury Farms		
Seasoned	2 tbsp	30
Up Country Naturals		
Organic Whole Wheat Garlic & Herb	¼ cup (0.3 oz)	35

CUCUMBER

FOOD	PORTION	CALS
fresh raw	1 (11 oz)	38
fresh raw sliced	½ cup (1.8 oz)	7
Chiquita		
Cucumber	⅓ med (3.5 oz)	15
Frieda's		
Japanese	⅔ cup	10
Seedless Hothouse	⅔ cup	110
TAKE-OUT		
cucumber salad	3.5 oz	50
kimchee	½ cup (1.8 oz)	36
tzatziki	½ cup (3.4 oz)	72

CUMIN

FOOD	PORTION	CALS
seed	1 tsp	8

FOOD	PORTION	CALS
CURRANT JUICE		
black currant nectar	7 oz	110
red currant nectar	7 oz	108
CURRANTS		
black fresh	½ cup	36
zante dried	½ cup	204
Sun-Maid		
Zante	¼ cup	130
CURRY		
curry powder	1 tsp	7
A Taste Of Thai		
Curry Paste Green	1 tsp	15
Curry Paste Panang	1 tsp	25
Curry Paste Red	1 tsp	20
Curry Paste Yellow	1 tsp	30
Instant India		
Curry Paste Cilantro Garlic	2 tbsp (1 oz)	110
Curry Paste Ginger Garlic	2 tbsp (1 oz)	90
CUSK		
fillet baked	3 oz	106
CUSTARD		
MIX		
as prep w/ 2% milk	½ cup (4.7 oz)	148
as prep w/ whole milk	½ cup (4.7 oz)	163
flan as prep w/ 2% milk	½ cup (4.7 oz)	135
flan as prep w/ whole milk	½ cup (4.7 oz)	150
Betty Crocker		
Flan w/ Caramel Sauce as prep	1 serv	330
READY-TO-EAT		
Kozy Shack		
Flan	1 pkg (4 oz)	145
Swiss Miss		
Egg Custard	1 pkg (4 oz)	153
TAKE-OUT		
baked	½ cup (5 oz)	148
flan	½ cup (5.4 oz)	220
tocino del cielo heaven's delight	1 cup	856
zabaione	½ cup (57.2 g)	135

FOOD	PORTION	CALS
CUTTLEFISH		
steamed	3 oz	134
DANDELION GREENS		
fresh cooked	½ cup	17
raw chopped	½ cup	13
Frieda's		
Dandelion Greens	2 cups	40
DANISH PASTRY		
FROZEN		
Morton		
Honey Buns	1 (2.28 oz)	270
Honey Buns Mini	1 (1.3 oz)	160
READY-TO-EAT		
plain ring	1 (12 oz)	1305
Dolly Madison		
Danish Rollers	3 (2.8 oz)	290
Tastykake		
Cheese	1 (3 oz)	290
Lemon	1 (3 oz)	290
Raspberry	1 (3 oz)	290
TAKE-OUT		
almond	1 (4¼ in) (2.3 oz)	280
apple	1 (4¼ in) (2.5 oz)	264
cheese	1 (4¼ in) (2.5 oz)	266
cinnamon	1 (4¼ in) (2.3 oz)	262
cinnamon nut	1 (4¼ in) (2.3 oz)	280
lemon	1 (4¼ in) (2.5 oz)	264
raisin	1 (4¼ in) (2.5 oz)	264
raisin nut	1 (4¼ in) (2.3 oz)	280
raspberry	1 (4¼ in) (2.5 oz)	264
strawberry	1 (4¼ in) (2.5 oz)	264
DATES		
deglet noor dried	10	240
dried chopped	1 cup	489
dried whole	10	228
jujube dried	1 oz	75
jujube fresh	1 oz	30

FOOD	PORTION	CALS
jujube preserved in sugar	1 oz	91
medjool	2–3 (1.4 oz)	120
Calavo		
Dried Pitted	5–6 (1.4 oz)	120
California Redi-Date		
Deglet Noor Dried	5–6 (1.4 oz)	120
Dromedary		
Chopped Dried	¼ cup	130
Frieda's		
Medjool	2 to 3 (1.4 oz)	120
SunDate		
Fancy Medjool	3	120

DEER *(see* VENISON*)*

DELI MEATS/COLD CUTS *(see also* BEEF, CHICKEN, HAM, MEAT SUBSTITUTES, TURKEY*)*

FOOD	PORTION	CALS
barbecue loaf pork & beef	1 slice (0.8 oz)	40
beerwurst beef	2 oz	155
beerwurst beef	1 slice (4 in x ⅛ in)	75
berliner pork & beef	1 slice (0.8 oz)	53
blood sausage	1 slice (0.9 oz)	95
bologna beef	1 slice (1 oz)	88
bologna beef low fat	1 slice (1 oz)	57
bologna beef reduced sodium	1 slice (1 oz)	88
bologna beef & pork	1 slice (1 oz)	87
bologna beef & pork low fat	1 slice (1 oz)	64
braunschweiger pork	1 slice (1 oz)	92
dutch brand loaf pork & beef	1 slice (1.3 oz)	104
headcheese pork	1 slice (1.6 oz)	71
honey loaf pork & beef	1 slice (1 oz)	35
lebanon bologna beef	2 slices (1 oz)	105
mortadella beef & pork	1 slice (0.5 oz)	47
olive loaf pork	2 slice (2 oz)	134
pastrami beef	1 slice (1 oz)	41
peppered loaf pork & beef	1 slice (1 oz)	41
pepperoni pork & beef	15 slices (1 oz)	135
picnic loaf pork & beef	1 slice (1 oz)	65
salami cooked beef & pork	1 slice (0.8 oz)	58
salami hard pork	3 slices (0.9 oz)	14
salami hard pork & beef less sodium	1 slice (1 oz)	113

FOOD	PORTION	CALS
sandwich spread pork & beef	¼ cup	141
summer sausage thuringer cervelat	2 oz	203
Boar's Head		
Bologna Beef	2 oz	150
Bologna Garlic	2 oz	150
Bologna Lowered Sodium	2 oz	150
Bologna Pork & Beef	2 oz	150
Braunschweiger Lite	2 oz	120
Head Cheese	2 oz	90
Liverwurst Strassburger	2 oz	170
Olive Loaf	2 oz	130
Pastrami	2 oz	90
Prosciutto	1 oz	60
Red Pastrami	2 oz	90
Salami Beef	2 oz	120
Salami Cooked	2 oz	130
Salami Genoa	2 oz	180
Salami Hard	1 oz	110
Spiced Ham	2 oz	120
Carl Buddig		
Beef	1 pkg (2.5 oz)	100
Corned Beef	1 pkg (2.5 oz)	100
Pastrami	1 pkg (2.5 oz)	100
Hebrew National		
Bologna Beef	1 slice (1 oz)	80
Bologna Lean Beef	4 slices (2 oz)	90
Salami Beef	3 slices (2 oz)	150
Salami Lean Beef	4 slices (2 oz)	90
Hormel		
Pepperoni Sliced	16 slices (1 oz)	140
TAKE-OUT		
corned beef brisket	2 oz	90
DILL		
seed	1 tsp	6
sprigs fresh	5	0
sprigs fresh	1 cup	4
weed dry	1 tsp	3

FOOD	PORTION	CALS

DINNER (see also ASIAN FOOD, PASTA DINNERS, POT PIES, SPANISH FOOD)
Amy's

FOOD	PORTION	CALS
Country Dinner Vegetable Salisbury Steak	1 pkg (11 oz)	380
Banquet		
Beef Patty w/ Country Style Vegetables	1 meal (9.5 oz)	310
Boneless Pork Rib	1 meal (10 oz)	400
Boneless White Fried Chicken	1 meal (8.25 oz)	540
Chicken Parmigiana	1 meal (9.5 oz)	320
Chicken Fingers Meal	1 meal (7.1 oz)	740
Chicken Fried Beef Steak	1 pkg (10 oz)	420
Chicken Nuggets Meal	1 meal (6.75 oz)	430
Extra Helping Boneless Pork Riblet	1 meal (15.25 oz)	720
Extra Helping Fried Beef Steak	1 meal (16 oz)	820
Extra Helping Fried Chicken	1 meal (14.7 oz)	910
Extra Helping Meatloaf	1 meal (16 oz)	610
Extra Helping Salisbury Steak	1 meal (16.5 oz)	740
Extra Helping Turkey & Gravy w/ Dressing	1 meal (17 oz)	620
Extra Helping White Fried Chicken	1 meal (13 oz)	690
Extra Helping Yankee Pot Roast	1 meal (14.5 oz)	410
Family Size Brown Gravy & Salisbury Steak	1 serv	240
Family Size Brown Gravy & Sliced Beef	1 serv	140
Family Size Chicken & Broccoli Alfredo	1 serv	270
Family Size Country Style Chicken & Dumplings	1 serv	290
Family Size Creamy Broccoli Chicken Cheese & Rice	1 serv	280
Family Size Hearty Beef Stew	1 cup	170
Family Size Homestyle Gravy & Sliced Turkey	2 slices	140
Family Size Mushroom Gravy & Charbroiled Beef Patties	1 patty	250
Family Size Potato Ham & Broccoli Au Gratin	⅔ cup	210
Family Size Savory Gravy & Meatloaf	1 slice	120
Fish Sticks	1 meal (6.6 oz)	290
Grilled Chicken	1 meal (9.9 oz)	330
Honey Roast Turkey Breast	1 meal (9 oz)	270
Meatloaf	1 meal (9.5 oz)	280
Our Original Fried Chicken	1 meal (9 oz)	470
Pork Cutlet Meal	1 meal (10.25 oz)	420
Sliced Beef	1 meal (9 oz)	270
Turkey Meal	1 meal (9.25 oz)	290

FOOD	PORTION	CALS
Veal Parmagiana	1 meal (8.75 oz)	330
Western Style Beef Patty	1 meal (9.5 oz)	360
White Meat Fried Chicken	1 meal (8.75 oz)	460
Yankee Pot Roast	1 meal (9.4 oz)	230
Birds Eye		
Easy Recipe Creations Sweet & Sour w/ Pineapple Tidbits	1⅔ cups	200
Voila! Beef Sirloin Steak And Garlic Potatoes	1 cup	240
Voila! Chicken Alfredo	1 cup	230
Voila! Garden Herb Chicken	1 cup	310
Voila! Grilled Salsa Chicken w/ Rice	1 cup	240
Voila! Homestyle Turkey w/ Roasted Potatoes	1 cup	200
Voila! Teriyaki	2 cups (6.4 oz)	240
Voila! Zesty Garlic Chicken	2 cups (6.2 oz)	260
Boston Market		
Glazed Rotisserie White Meat Chicken w/ Mashed Potatoes Gravy Carrots	1 pkg (16 oz)	380
Meatloaf w/ Mashed Potatoes & Gravy	1 pkg (16 oz)	880
Fillo Factory		
Fillo Pie Broccoli & Cheese	¼ pie (4 oz)	350
Fillo Pie Spinach & Cheese	⅕ pie (4.8 oz)	210
Golden Cuisine		
Beef Stew	1 pkg	350
Boneless Pork Patty	1 pkg	504
Breaded Baked Fish w/ Rice Pilaf	1 pkg	300
Chicken Cacciatore	1 pkg	417
Chicken & Noodles	1 pkg	331
Chicken Parmesan	1 pkg	430
Chicken w/ Marinara Sauce	1 pkg	329
Meatloaf Patty & Gravy	1 pkg	340
Mesquite Chicken	1 pkg	320
Pot Roast w/ Gravy	1 pkg	343
Salisbury Steak & Mushroom Sauce	1 pkg	350
Swedish Meatballs	1 pkg	440
Turkey Tetrazzini	1 pkg	304
Healthy Choice		
Beef Merlot	1 pkg	240
Beef Pot Roast	1 pkg	320
Beef Stroganoff	1 pkg	320
Beef Teriyaki	1 pkg	310

FOOD	PORTION	CALS
Beef Tips Portabello	1 pkg	280
Blackened Chicken	1 pkg	300
Boneless Beef Ribs w/ Classic BBQ Sauce	1 pkg	360
Charbroiled Beef Patty	1 pkg	310
Cheesy Rice & Chicken	1 pkg	250
Chicken Carbonara	1 pkg	290
Chicken Margherita	1 pkg	340
Chicken Parmigiana	1 pkg	320
Chicken Breast & Vegetables	1 pkg	260
Chicken Broccoli Alfredo	1 pkg	300
Chicken Piccata	1 pkg	260
Chicken Teriyaki	1 pkg	270
Chicken Tuscany	1 pkg	340
Country Breaded Chicken	1 pkg	370
Country Glazed Chicken	1 pkg	230
Country Herb Chicken	1 pkg	280
Creamy Herb Roasted Chicken	1 pkg	240
Grilled Basil Chicken	1 pkg	330
Grilled Chicken Breast & Pasta	1 pkg	250
Grilled Chicken Breast w/ Mashed Potatoes	1 pkg	190
Grilled Chicken Caesar	1 pkg	300
Grilled Chicken Marinara	1 pkg	270
Grilled Steak w/ Roasted Garlic Sauce	1 pkg	220
Grilled Turkey Breast	1 pkg	250
Grilled Whiskey Steak	1 pkg	280
Herb Baked Fish	1 pkg	360
Homestyle Chicken & Pasta	1 pkg	250
Honey Glazed Chicken	1 pkg	320
Lemon Pepper Fish	1 pkg	280
Mandarin Chicken	1 pkg	250
Mesquite Chicken BBQ	1 pkg	300
Mixed Grills Chicken Honey BBQ w/ Dipping Sauce	1 pkg	380
Mixed Grills Chicken Honey Mustard w/ Dipping Sauce	1 pkg	360
Mixed Grills Chicken Teriyaki w/ Dipping Sauce	1 pkg	340
Mixed Grills Chicken Tomato Garlic w/ Dipping Sauce	1 pkg	370
Mixed Grills Steak BBQ Sauce	1 pkg	420
Mixed Grills Steak Teriyaki w/ Dipping Sauce	1 pkg	350

FOOD	PORTION	CALS
Mixed Grills Steak w/ Zesty Steak Sauce	1 pkg	350
Oriental Style Beef	1 pkg	310
Oriental Style Chicken	1 pkg	240
Oven Roasted Beef	1 pkg	280
Princess Chicken	1 pkg	310
Roast Turkey Breast	1 pkg	220
Roasted Chicken Breast	1 pkg	280
Roasted Chicken Chardonnay	1 pkg	290
Salisbury Steak	1 pkg	360
Salisbury Steak w/ Red Skin Mashed Potatoes	1 pkg	200
Sesame Chicken	1 pkg	260
Slow Roasted Turkey Breast w/ Mashed Potatoes	1 pkg	210
Sweet & Sour Chicken	1 pkg	340
Traditional Meatloaf	1 pkg	300
Tradtional Turkey Breast	1 pkg	330
Tuna Casserole	1 pkg	270
Kid Cuisine		
All American Fried Chicken	1 meal	500
All Star Chicken Breast Nuggets	1 meal	460
Bug Safari Chicken Breast Nuggets	1 meal	450
Carnival Corn Dog	1 meal	430
Deep Sea Adventure Fish Sticks	1 meal	400
Fiesta Beef Taco Dippers	1 meal	370
Pop Star Popcorn Chicken	1 meal	410
Laura's Lifestyle		
Carb Conscious Chicken Chow Mein	1 pkg (9 oz)	260
Carb Conscious Chicken Puttanesca	1 pkg (9 oz)	270
Carb Conscious Chicken Santa Fe	1 pkg (9 oz)	280
Carb Conscious Thai Chicken	1 pkg (9 oz)	280
Lean Cuisine		
Cafe Classics Baked Chicken Florentine	1 pkg (8 oz)	200
Cafe Classics Baked Lemon Pepper Fish	1 pkg (9 oz)	220
Cafe Classics Beef Peppercorn	1 pkg (8.75 oz)	220
Cafe Classics Beef Portabello	1 pkg (9 oz)	200
Cafe Classics Beef Pot Roast	1 pkg (9 oz)	190
Cafe Classics Bowl Creamy Basil Chicken	1 pkg (10.5 oz)	310
Cafe Classics Bowl Grilled Chicken Caesar	1 pkg (9 oz)	270
Cafe Classics Chicken & Vegetables	1 pkg (10.5 oz)	240
Cafe Classics Chicken Carbonara	1 pkg (9 oz)	280

FOOD	PORTION	CALS
Cafe Classics Chicken L'Orange	1 pkg (9 oz)	230
Cafe Classics Chicken Marsala	1 pkg (8.1 oz)	140
Cafe Classics Chicken Parmesan	1 pkg (10.9 oz)	280
Cafe Classics Chicken Tuscan	1 pkg (12 oz)	300
Cafe Classics Chicken w/ Almonds	1 pkg (8.5 oz)	260
Cafe Classics Chicken w/ Basil Cream Sauce	1 pkg (8.5 oz)	270
Cafe Classics Fiesta Grilled Chicken	1 pkg (9.5 oz)	250
Cafe Classics Garlic Beef & Broccoli	1 pkg (9 oz)	170
Cafe Classics Glazed Chicken	1 pkg (8.5 oz)	220
Cafe Classics Glazed Turkey Tenderloins	1 pkg (9 oz)	260
Cafe Classics Grilled Chicken	1 pkg (9.4 oz)	160
Cafe Classics Grilled Chicken w/ Teriyaki Glaze	1 pkg (10 oz)	270
Cafe Classics Herb Roasted Chicken	1 pkg (8 oz)	190
Cafe Classics Honey Dijon Grilled Chicken	1 pkg (8 oz)	220
Cafe Classics Honey Mustard Chicken	1 pkg (8 oz)	250
Cafe Classics Honey Roasted Pork	1 serv (9.5 oz)	230
Cafe Classics Lemon Garlic Shrimp	1 pkg (12 oz)	280
Cafe Classics Mandarin Chicken	1 pkg (9 oz)	270
Cafe Classics Meatloaf w/ Gravy & Whipped Potatoes	1 pkg (9.4 oz)	280
Cafe Classics Orange Peel Chicken	1 pkg (12 oz)	390
Cafe Classics Oven Roasted Beef	1 pkg (9.25 oz)	210
Cafe Classics Roasted Garlic Chicken	1 pkg (8.8 oz)	200
Cafe Classics Roasted Turkey & Vegetables	1 pkg (8 oz)	150
Cafe Classics Roasted Turkey Breast	1 pkg (12 oz)	280
Cafe Classics Roasted Turkey Breast w/ Dressing	1 pkg (9.75 oz)	270
Cafe Classics Salisbury Steak	1 pkg (12.5 oz)	310
Cafe Classics Salisbury Steak w/ Mac & Cheese	1 pkg (9.5 oz)	280
Cafe Classics Sesame Chicken	1 pkg (9 oz)	330
Cafe Classics Southern Beef Tips	1 pkg (8.75 oz)	250
Cafe Classics Steak Tips Dijon	1 pkg (12 oz)	320
Cafe Classics Steak Tips Portobello	1 pkg (7.5 oz)	180
Cafe Classics Stuffed Cabbage	1 pkg (9.5 oz)	200
Cafe Classics Swedish Meatballs	1 pkg (9.1 oz)	290
Cafe Classics Sweet & Sour Chicken	1 pkg (10 oz)	290
Cafe Classics Three Cheese Chicken	1 pkg (8 oz)	230
Comfort Classics Baked Chicken	1 pkg (8.6 oz)	230
Dinnertime Selects Balsamic Glazed Chicken	1 pkg (12 oz)	400
Dinnertime Selects Chicken Florentine	1 pkg (13.25 oz)	420

FOOD	PORTION	CALS
Dinnertime Selects Chicken Portabello	1 pkg (12 oz)	370
Skillet Beef Teriyaki & Rice	1 serv	190
Spa Cuisine Chicken Mediterranean	1 pkg (10.5 oz)	240
Spa Cuisine Chicken In Peanut Sauce	1 pkg (9 oz)	280
Spa Cuisine Chicken Pecan	1 pkg (9 oz)	260
Spa Cuisine Lemon Chicken	1 pkg (9 oz)	290
Spa Cuisine Lemongrass Chicken	1 pkg (9.4 oz)	240
Spa Cuisine Pork w/ Cherry Sauce	1 pkg (8.25 oz)	260
Spa Cuisine Rosemary Chicken	1 pkg (8.25 oz)	230
Spa Cuisine Salmon w/ Beef	1 pkg (9.5 oz)	360
Luzianne		
Cajun Creole Dirty Rice	1 serv	160
Cajun Creole Etouffee	1 serv	200
Cajun Creole Gumbo	1 serv	160
Cajun Creole Jambalaya	1 serv	200
Marie Callender's		
Beef Stroganoff w/ Noodles	1 meal (13 oz)	600
Beef Tips In Mushroom Sauce	1 meal (13 oz)	430
Breaded Chicken Parmigiana	1 meal (16 oz)	860
Breaded Fish w/ Mac & Cheese	1 meal (12 oz)	550
Cheesy Rice w/ Chicken & Broccoli	1 meal (12 oz)	390
Chicken & Dumplings	1 meal (14 oz)	390
Chicken & Noodles	1 meal (13 oz)	520
Chicken Cordon Bleu	1 meal (13 oz)	610
Chicken Fried Beef Steak & Gravy	1 meal (15 oz)	650
Chicken Teriyaki	1 meal (13 oz)	510
Country Fried Chicken & Gravy	1 meal (16 oz)	620
Country Fried Pork Chop	1 meal (15 oz)	540
Escalloped Noodles & Chicken	1 meal (13 oz)	740
Glazed Chicken	1 meal (13 oz)	490
Grilled Chicken & Mashed Potatoes	1 meal (10 oz)	340
Grilled Chicken Breast & Rice Pilaf	1 meal (11.75 oz)	360
Grilled Chicken In Mushroom Sauce	1 meal (14 oz)	480
Grilled Southwestern Style Chicken	1 meal (14 oz)	410
Grilled Turkey Breast & Rice Pilaf	1 meal (11.75 oz)	310
Herb Roasted Chicken & Mashed Potatoes	1 meal (14 oz)	580
Homestyle Turkey & Noodles	1 meal (12 oz)	600
Honey Roasted Chicken	1 meal (14 oz)	440
Honey Smoked Ham Steak w/ Macaroni & Cheese	1 meal (14 oz)	490

FOOD	PORTION	CALS
Meatloaf & Gravy w/ Mashed Potatoes	1 meal (14 oz)	540
Old Fashioned Beef Pot Roast & Gravy	1 meal (15 oz)	500
Roast Beef	1 meal (14.5 oz)	390
Sirloin Salisbury Steak & Gravy	1 meal (14 oz)	550
Skillet Meal Au Gratin Potatoes	⅔ cup (5 oz)	190
Skillet Meal Beef Pot Roast	½ pkg	290
Skillet Meal Beef Stroganoff	½ pkg	310
Skillet Meal Chicken & Rice w/ Broccoli & Cheese	½ pkg	440
Skillet Meal Chicken Teriyaki	½ pkg	340
Skillet Meal Herb Chicken	½ pkg	290
Skillet Meal Roasted Chicken & Vegetables	½ pkg	260
Skillet Meal White & Wild Rice In Cheese Sauce	1 cup	300
Swedish Meatballs	1 meal (12.5 oz)	520
Sweet & Sour Chicken	1 meal (14 oz)	570
Turkey w/ Gravy & Dressing	1 meal (14 oz)	500
Morton		
Breaded Chicken Pattie	1 meal (6.75 oz)	290
Chicken Nuggets	1 meal (7 oz)	340
Chili Gravy w/ Beef Enchilada & Tamale	1 meal (10 oz)	270
Fried Chicken	1 meal (9 oz)	470
Gravy & Charbroiled Beef Patty	1 meal (9 oz)	310
Gravy & Salisbury Steak	1 meal (9 oz)	310
Gravy & Turkey w/ Stuffing	1 meal (9 oz)	240
Tomato Sauce w/ Meat Loaf	1 meal (9 oz)	250
Veal Parmagiana w/ Tomato Sauce	1 meal (8.75 oz)	290
Nature's Choice		
Broccoli Parmesan Alfredo	1 pkg (12 oz)	270
Nature's Entree		
Hearty Stew	1 pkg (12 oz)	290
Tuscany White Bean	1 pkg (12 oz)	330
Pacific Foods		
Beef Steak Stew	1 cup	250
Chicken Stew	1 cup	200
Patio		
Ranchera	1 pkg (13 oz)	470
Quorn		
Meat Free Simply Saute Indian	½ pkg	240
Meat Free Simply Saute Mexican	½ pkg	340
Meat Free Simply Saute Thai	½ pkg	240

FOOD	PORTION	CALS
Savvy Faire		
Baja Jack Scramble	1 pkg (8.2 oz)	370
Braised Beef	1 pkg (9.4 oz)	320
Herb Crusted Chicken	1 pkg (9.7 oz)	430
South Beach Diet		
Beef & Broccoli & Asian Style Noodles	1 pkg	320
Caprese Style Chicken w/ Cauliflower & Broccoli	1 pkg	250
Cashew Chicken w/ Sugar Snap Peas	1 pkg	360
Garlic Herb Chicken w/ Green Beans	1 pkg	250
Mediterranean Style Chicken w/ Couscous	1 pkg	330
Savory Beef w/ Cheesy Broccoli	1 pkg	240
Savory Pork w/ Pecans & Green Beans	1 pkg	260
Swanson		
Beef Pot Roast	1 pkg (14 oz)	320
Chicken Parmigiana w/ Spaghetti	1 pkg (11 oz)	380
Turkey Breast & Stuffing Dinner	1 pkg (11.7 oz)	350
Tamarind Tree		
Alu Chole	1 pkg (9.25 oz)	320
Channa Dal Masala	1 pkg (9.25 oz)	290
Dal Makhani	1 pkg (9.25 oz)	350
Navratan Korma	1 pkg (9.25 oz)	370
Palak Paneer	1 pkg (9.25 oz)	350
Saag Chole	1 pkg (9.25 oz)	330
Vegetable Jalfrazi	1 pkg (9.25 oz)	280
Weight Watchers		
Smart Ones Swedish Meatballs	1 pkg (9 oz)	280
Yves		
Veggie Country Stew	1 pkg (10.5 oz)	170
DIP		
Blue Bunny		
IncreDiples	2 tbsp	30
IncreDiples Taco Fiesta	2 tbsp	30
Spicy Buffalo	2 tbsp	30
Cabot		
Bac'n Horseradish	2 tbsp	50
Clam	2 tbsp	50
French Onion	2 tbsp	50
Ranch	1 tbsp	50

FOOD	PORTION	CALS
Salsa Grande	2 tbsp	50
Veggie	2 tbsp	50
Fritos		
Bean	2 tbsp	40
Chili Cheese	2 tbsp	45
Hot Bean	2 tbsp	40
Jalapeno Cheddar Cheese	2 tbsp	50
Mild Cheddar	2 tbsp	60
Gringo Billy's		
Guacamole Mix	1 tsp	10
Guiltless Gourmet		
Black Bean Mild	2 tbsp	30
Black Bean Spicy	2 tbsp	30
Marzetti		
Veggie Fat Free Ranch	2 tbsp	35
Veggie Dip Light Veggie	1 pkg (3.25 oz)	170
Racquet		
Hot Cheddar Jalapeno	2 tbsp	30
Ruffles		
French Onion	¼ cup	200
Ranch	2 tbsp	60
Snyder's Of Hanover		
Microwavable Hot Nacho Cheese	2 tbsp	48
Microwavable Mild Cheese	2 tbsp	45
Mustard Pretzel	2 tbsp	60
Sour Cream & Onion	2 tbsp	60
Utz		
Fat Free Sour Cream & Onion	2 tbsp (1.1 oz)	30
Jalapeno & Cheddar	2 tbsp (1 oz)	30
Low Fat Desert Garden	2 tbsp (1.1 oz)	40
Low Fat Salsa Con Queso	2 tbsp (1 oz)	40
Mild Cheddar	2 tbsp (1 oz)	45
Sour Cream & Onion	2 tbsp (1 oz)	60
Walden Farms		
Low Carb Bruschetta	2 tbsp	35
Low Carb Pesto Bruschetta	1 tsp	10
DOCK		
fresh cooked	3½ oz	20
raw chopped	½ cup	15

FOOD	PORTION	CALS
DOLPHINFISH		
fresh baked	3 oz	93
fresh fillet baked	5.6 oz	174
DOUGHNUTS		
cake type unsugared	1 (1.6 oz)	198
chocolate glazed	1 (1.5 oz)	175
chocolate sugared	1 (1.5 oz)	175
chocolate coated	1 (1.5 oz)	204
creme filled	1 (3 oz)	307
french cruller glazed	1 (1.4 oz)	169
frosted	1 (1.5 oz)	204
honey bun	1 (2.1 oz)	242
jelly	1 (3 oz)	289
old fashioned	1 (1.6 oz)	198
sugared	1 (1.6 oz)	192
wheat glazed	1 (1.6 oz)	162
wheat sugared	1 (1.6 oz)	162
yeast glazed	1 (2.1 oz)	242
Dolly Madison		
Chocolate Frosted	1 (1.1 oz)	140
Donut Gems Chocolate	4 (2 oz)	260
Donut Gems Crunch	3 (2 oz)	220
Donut Gems Powdered	4 (2 oz)	230
English Cruller	1 (2 oz)	250
Glazed Whirl	1 (1.6 oz)	210
Glazed Yeast	1 (1.5 oz)	190
Old Fashioned	1 (2.1 oz)	280
Plain	1 (1.2 oz)	140
Powdered	1 (1 oz)	120
Dutch Mill		
Cider	1 (2.1 oz)	240
Cinnamon	1 (1.8 oz)	210
Donut Holes Double-Dipped Chocolate	3 (1.4 oz)	220
Donut Holes Shootin' Stars	3 (1.4 oz)	190
Double-Dipped Chocolate	1 (2.1 oz)	280
Glazed	1 (2.1 oz)	250
Glazed Chocolate	1 (2.4 oz)	270
Plain	1 (1.8 oz)	210
Sugared	1 (1.8 oz)	220

FOOD	PORTION	CALS
Entenmann's		
Crumb	1	260
Frosted Mini	1 (1 oz)	150
Glazed	1	260
Plain Old Fashion	1	230
Rich Frosted	1	280
Hostess		
Blueberry	1 (1.7 oz)	210
Donettes Crumb	3 (1.5 oz)	170
Donettes Frosted	3 (1.5 oz)	200
Donettes Powdered	3 (1.5 oz)	180
Frosted	1 (1.4 oz)	180
Old Fashioned Glazed	1 (2.1 oz)	260
O's Raspberry Filled	1 (2.2 oz)	230
Plain	1 (1.1 oz)	140
Powdered	1 (1.3 oz)	150
Little Debbie		
Donut Sticks	1 (1.6 oz)	210
Mini Powdered	1 pkg (2.5 oz)	290
Snack & Smile		
Mini Donuts Chocolate	6	370
Mini Donuts Glazed	6	340
Mini Donuts Powdered Sugar	6	320
Super Bakery		
Daily Donut	1 (2.2 oz)	250
Proballs Slam Powdered Baseballs	1 (1.3 oz)	130
Tastykake		
Mini Plain Glaze	1 pkg (2.5 oz)	260
Mini Powdered Sugar	1 pkg (2.5 oz)	260
Mini Rich Frosted	1 pkg (3 oz)	370
Tom's		
Chocolate Gem	1 pkg (2.5 oz)	320
Dunkin' Sticks	1 pkg (2.5 oz)	370
Powdered Gems	1 pkg (2.5 oz)	320
DRINK MIXERS		
whiskey sour mix not prep	1 pkg (0.6 oz)	64
whiskey sour mix	2 oz	55
Baja Bob's		
Bloody Mary Mix Lean & Mean	4 oz	20

FOOD	PORTION	CALS
Pina Colada	4 oz	30
Sugar Free Margarita Mix	4 oz	10
Sugar Free Margarita Mix Desert Lime	4 oz	10
Sugar Free Margarita Mix Wild Strawberry	4 oz	10
Sweet-n-Sour Mix	4 oz	10
Daily's		
Bloody Mary Original	1 serv (6 oz)	50
Margarita Daiquiri Strawberry	1 serv (4 oz)	180
Margarita Green Demon	1 serv (3 oz)	80
Pina Colada	1 serv (3 oz)	160
Ocean Spray		
Bloody Mary Mix	4 oz	40
Margarita Mix	4 oz	160
Sour Mix	4 oz	140
DRUM		
freshwater fillet baked	5.4 oz	236
freshwater baked	3 oz	130
DUCK		
w/ skin roasted	1 cup (4.9 oz)	472
w/ skin w/ bone leg roasted	3 oz	184
w/ skin w/o bone breast roasted	3 oz	172
w/o skin roasted	1 cup (4.9 oz)	281
w/o skin w/ bone leg braised	1 cup (6.1 oz)	310
w/o skin w/o bone breast broiled	1 cup (6.1 oz)	244
wild w/ skin raw	½ duck (9.5 oz)	571
wild w/o skin breast raw	½ breast (2.9 oz)	102
Grimaud Farms		
Muscovy Duck Confit	1 serv (3 oz)	170
Maple Leaf Farms		
Breast Filet	4 oz	360
Leg Quarters	4 oz	420
Orange Breast Filet	4 oz	320
DUMPLING		
Health Is Wealth		
Potstickers Chicken Free	2 (1.6 oz)	80
Potstickers Pork Free	2 (1.6 oz)	80
Potstickers Vegetable	2 (1.6 oz)	90
Steamed Dumpling	2 (1.6 oz)	50

FOOD	PORTION	CALS
Pepperidge Farm		
Apple	1 (3 oz)	230
Peach	1 (3 oz)	320
TAKE-OUT		
bread dumpling	1 lg	330
DURIAN		
fresh	3.5 oz	141
EEL		
fresh cooked	3 oz	200
fresh cooked	1 fillet (5.6 oz)	375
raw	3 oz	156
smoked	3.5 oz	330
EGG (see also EGG DISHES, EGG SUBSTITUTES)		
CHICKEN		
hard or soft cooked	1	77
pickled	1	72
poached	1	73
white cooked	1	17
yolk cooked	1	55
Egg-Land's Best		
Organic Brown	1	70
Eggology		
100% Organic Egg Whites	¼ cup	30
Gold Circle Farms		
Cage Free	1 large	70
Horizon Organic		
Medium	1 (1.5 oz)	70
Land O Lakes		
Brown Extra Large	1 (2 oz)	80
Organic Valley		
Brown Extra Large	1 (2.2 oz)	90
Brown Large	1 (2 oz)	80
Brown Medium	1 (1.8 oz)	70
Sunny Fresh		
Eggs ASAP!	2	140
OTHER POULTRY		
duck 100 year old	1 (1 oz)	49
duck cooked	1 (2.5 oz)	129

FOOD	PORTION	CALS
duck preserved hard core	1 (1.8 oz)	80
duck preserved soft core	1 (1.8 oz)	80
duck salted	1 (1 oz)	54
goose cooked	1 (5 oz)	265
quail canned	1 (0.3 oz)	14
turkey raw	1 (2.8 oz)	135

EGG DISHES
TAKE-OUT

FOOD	PORTION	CALS
deviled	1 half	62
eggs benedict	2	825
omelet cheese	3 eggs	387
omelet mushroom	3 eggs	251
omelet mushroom & onion	3 eggs	294
omelet plain	3 eggs	338
omelet spanish	3 eggs	496
omelet spinach	3 eggs	279
omelet western	3 eggs	355
salad	½ cup	353
scotch egg	1 (4.2 oz)	301
scrambled plain	2	199
sunny side up	2	155
tortilla de amarillo omelet w/ plantain	3 eggs	536

EGG ROLLS

FOOD	PORTION	CALS
egg roll wrapper fresh	1	83
Chun King		
Chicken Mini	6	210
Chicken Restaurant Style	1 (3 oz)	190
Pork & Shrimp Mini	6	210
Shrimp Mini	6	190
Shrimp Restaurant Style	1 (3 oz)	180
Frieda's		
Egg Roll Wrappers	2 (1.6 oz)	130
Health Is Wealth		
Broccoli	1 (3 oz)	150
Oriental Vegetable	1 (3 oz)	160
Oriental Chicken Free	1 (3 oz)	120
Pizza	1 (3 oz)	200

FOOD	PORTION	CALS
Spinach	1 (3 oz)	180
Spring Rolls	1 (1.6 oz)	70
Veggie	1 (3 oz)	130
La Choy		
Chicken Mini	6	210
Chicken Restaurant Style	1 (3 oz)	210
Pork Restaurant Style	1 (3 oz)	220
Pork & Shrimp Bite Size	12	210
Pork & Shrimp Mini	6	210
Shrimp Mini	6	190
Shrimp Restaurant Style	1 (3 oz)	180
Sweet & Sour Chicken Restaurant Style	1 (3 oz)	220
Vegetable w/ Lobster Mini	6	190
Lean Cuisine		
Cafe Classics Vegetable	1 pkg (9 oz)	310
Loompya		
Lumpia Chicken & Vegetables	2	170
Nasoya		
Egg Roll Wrapper	3	170
Pagoda		
Sweet & Sour Chicken	1 (2.7 oz)	170
TAKE-OUT		
chicken	1 (3 oz)	140
lobster	1 (4.8 oz)	270
lumpia vegetable & shrimp	2 (3 oz)	120
meat & shrimp	1 (4.8 oz)	320
pork & shrimp	1 (5 oz)	300
shrimp	1 (3 oz)	170
spicy pork	1 (3 oz)	200
vegetable	1 (3 oz)	170

EGG SUBSTITUTES
Better'n Eggs
Fat Free Cholesterol Free	¼ cup (2 oz)	30

Deb-El
Just Whites	2 tsp	12

Egg Beaters
Original	¼ cup	30

FOOD	PORTION	CALS
Morningstar Farms		
Breakfast Sandwich Bagel Scramblers Pattie Cheese	1 (5.9 oz)	320
Scramblers	¼ cup (2 oz)	35
Quick Eggs		
Fat Free Cholesterol Free	¼ cup	30

EGGNOG

eggnog	1 qt	1368
eggnog	1 cup	342
eggnog flavor mix as prep w/ milk	9 oz	260
Oberweis		
Egg Nog	½ cup	240
TAKE-OUT		
eggnog	1 cup	306

EGGNOG SUBSTITUTES
Silk

Nog	½ cup	90

EGGPLANT

cubed cooked w/ oil	1 cup	133
pickled	½ cup	33
slices grilled	1 (2 oz)	36
Frieda's		
Chinese	⅔ cup (3 oz)	20
Japanese Nasu	⅔ cup (3 oz)	20
Progresso		
Caponata	2 tbsp (1 oz)	25
TastyBite		
Punjab Eggplant	½ pkg (5 oz)	130
TAKE-OUT		
baba ghannouj	¼ cup	55
caponata	2 tbsp (1 oz)	30
iman bayildi eggplant w/ onion & tomato	1 serv (15.6 oz)	345
indian eggplant runi	1 serv	180
moussaka	1 cup	237
papoutsakis little shoes	1 serv (15.5 oz)	245

ELDERBERRIES

fresh	1 cup	105

FOOD	PORTION	CALS
ELDERBERRY JUICE		
elderberry	7 oz	76
ELK		
roasted	4 oz	215
EMU		
cooked	3 oz	130
ENERGY BARS (see also CEREAL BARS, NUTRITION SUPPLEMENTS)		
All In One		
All Flavors	1 bar (1.8 oz)	180
AllGoode Organics		
Amazin' Peanut Raisin	1 bar	210
Banana Nut Nirvana	1 bar	190
Cashew Almond Passion	1 bar	210
Chocolate Peanut Pleasure	1 bar	200
Honey Nut Harvest	1 bar	210
Nutty Chocolate Apricot	1 bar	200
Atkins		
Advantage Almond Brownie	1 bar (1.6 oz)	220
Advantage Chocolate Coconut	1 bar (1.6 oz)	230
Advantage Chocolate Decadence	1 bar (1.6 oz)	220
Advantage Chocolate Mocha Crunch	1 bar (1.6 oz)	220
Advantage Chocolate Peanut Butter	1 bar (1.6 oz)	240
Advantage Cookies 'N Creme	1 bar (1.6 oz)	220
Advantage S'mores	1 bar (1.6 oz)	220
Morning Start Apple Crisp	1 bar	170
Morning Start Blueberry Muffin	1 bar	160
Morning Start Chocolate Chip Crisp	1 bar	160
Balance		
Big Bar Honey Peanut	1 bar	310
Chocolate Banana + Antioxidants	1 bar	200
Chocolate Mint + Antioxidants	1 bar	200
Gold Caramel Nut Blast	1 bar	210
Gold Chocolate Peanut Butter	1 bar	210
Gold Rocky Road	1 bar	210
Gold Triple Chocolate Chaos	1 bar	200
Gold Crunch Chocolate Chocolate	1 bar	210
Gold Crunch Chocolate Mint Cookie	1 bar	210
Gold Crunch S'mores	1 bar	210

FOOD	PORTION	CALS
Honey Peanut + Ginseng	1 bar	200
Lemon Meringue + Calcium	1 bar	190
Original Almond Brownie	1 bar	200
Original Chocolate	1 bar	200
Original Chocolate Raspberry Fudge	1 bar	200
Original Honey Peanut	1 bar	200
Original Mocha Chip	1 bar	200
Original Peanut Butter	1 bar	200
Original Yogurt Honey Peanut	1 bar	200
Outdoor Chocolate Crisp	1 bar	200
Outdoor Crunchy Peanut	1 bar	200
Outdoor Honey Almond	1 bar	200
Outdoor Nut Berry	1 bar	200
Satisfaction Apple Cinnamon Oatmeal	1 bar	280
Satisfaction Chocolate Crisp	1 bar	280
Satisfaction Chocolate Peanut	1 bar	280
Satisfaction Peanut Butter Crisp	1 bar	280
Yogurt Berry + Antioxidants	1 bar	200
Be Natural		
Almond & Apricot	1 bar	218
Almond & Coconut	1 bar	248
Banana & Wheat Bran	1 bar	201
Fruit & Nut Delight	1 bar	225
Macadamia & Apricot	1 bar	224
Nut Delight	1 bar	266
Sesame Nut Split	1 bar	256
Walnut & Date	1 bar	147
Yogurt Coated Almond & Apricot	1 bar	233
Yogurt Coated Fruit & Nut	1 bar	190
Benecol		
Chocolate Crisp	1 bar (1.2 oz)	130
Peanut Crisp	1 bar (1.2 oz)	140
Better Bar		
Chocolate Coated Caramel Pecan	1 bar (1.8 oz)	180
Chocolate Coated Peanut	1 bar (1.8 oz)	180
Yogurt Coated Raspberry	1 bar (1.8 oz)	180
Boost		
Chocolate Crunch	1 bar (1.5 oz)	190

FOOD	PORTION	CALS
Carb Options		
Chocolate Chip	1 bar	200
Chocolate Peanut	1 bar	200
Cinnamon Delight	1 bar	200
Carbolite		
Chocolate Peanut Butter Sugar Free	1 bar (1 oz)	144
CarbWise		
Chocolate S'Mores Crunch	1 bar	240
Centrum		
Energy Chocolate Nougat	1 (1.98 oz)	220
Energy Chocolate Peanut Butter	1 (1.98 oz)	220
Choice		
Berry Almond Crispy	1 bar	50
Fudge Brownie	1 bar	140
Peanut Butter Crispy	1 bar	60
Peanutty Chocolate	1 bar	140
Clif Bar		
Apricot	1 bar (2.4 oz)	220
Carrot Cake	1 bar (2.4 oz)	240
Chocolate Brownie	1 bar (2.4 oz)	240
Chocolate Almond Fudge	1 bar (2.4 oz)	230
Chocolate Chip	1 bar (2.4 oz)	240
Chocolate Chip Peanut Crunch	1 bar (2.4 oz)	240
Cookies'N Cream	1 bar (2.4 oz)	230
Cranberry Apple Cherry	1 bar (2.4 oz)	220
Crunchy Peanut Butter	1 bar (2.4 oz)	240
GingerSnap	1 bar (2.4 oz)	230
Deliciously Slim		
Chocolate Fudge Cake	1 bar (2.1 oz)	200
DrSoy		
Double Chocolate	1 bar (1.76 oz)	180
Ensure		
All Flavors	1 bar (2.1 oz)	230
Extend		
Chocolate Chip Crunch	1 bar (1.4 oz)	160
Peanut Butter Crunch	1 bar (1.4 oz)	160
Fast Fuel Up		
Natural Chocolate Espresso	1 bar (2.3 oz)	300
Natural Chocolate Crunch	1 bar (2.3 oz)	300

FOOD	PORTION	CALS
Organic Chocolate Espresso	1 bar (1.8 oz)	230
Organic Chocolate Crunch	1 bar (1.8 oz)	230
Gatorade		
All Flavors	1 bar (2.3 oz)	260
GeniSoy		
Soy Protein Artic Frost Crispy Chocolate Mint	1 bar (2.2 oz)	230
Soy Protein Dutch Crunch Sour Apple Crisp	1 bar (2.2 oz)	230
Soy Protein Fair Trade Arabica Cafe Mocha Fudge	1 bar (2.2 oz)	220
Soy Protein New York Style Blueberry Cheesecake	1 bar (2.2 oz)	220
Soy Protein Obsession Fudge Cookies & Cream	1 bar (2.2 oz)	230
Soy Protein Pure Golden Honey Creamy Peanut Yogurt	1 bar (2.2 oz)	230
Soy Protein Southern Style Chunky Peanut Butter Fudge	1 bar (2.2 oz)	240
Soy Protein Ultimate Chocolate Fudge Brownie	1 bar (2.2 oz)	230
Xtreme Carrot Cake Quake	1 bar (1.6 oz)	190
Xtreme Peanut Butter Fix	1 bar (1.6 oz)	200
Xtreme Raspberry Rush	1 bar (1.6 oz)	190
Xtreme Rocky Roadtrip	1 bar (1.6 oz)	190
Glucerna		
All Flavors	1 bar (1.3 oz)	140
Hansen's		
Chocolate Banana Crunch	1 bar	180
Chocolate Orchard Crunch	1 bar	170
Natural Bar Tropical Fruit Crunch	1 bar	170
Natural Bar Yogurt Strawberry Crunch	1 bar	190
HeartBar		
Cranberry	1 bar (1.8 oz)	190
Original	1 bar (1.76 oz)	180
Hi-Lo		
Chocolate Caramel	1 bar (1.76 oz)	200
Chocolate Mint	1 bar (2.1 oz)	200
Chocolate Peanut Butter	1 bar (2.1 oz)	210
Chocolate Raspberry	1 bar (2.1 oz)	200
Hooah!		
Chocolate Crisp	1 bar (2.29 oz)	280
Ideal		
Mixed Berry Tart	1 bar (1.7 oz)	200

FOOD	PORTION	CALS
Jenny Craig		
Meal Bar Chocolate Peanut	1 bar (2 oz)	220
Meal Bar Lemon Meringue	1 bar (2 oz)	210
Meal Bar Milk Chocolate	1 bar (2 oz)	210
Meal Bar Oatmeal Raisin	1 bar (1.97 oz)	210
Meal Bar Yogurt Peanut	1 bar (2 oz)	220
Kashi		
GoLean Chocolate Almond Toffee	1 (2.7 oz)	290
GoLean Cookies 'N Cream	1 (2.7 oz)	290
GoLean Crunchy Chocolate Caramel Karma	1 (1.6 oz)	140
GoLean Crunchy Chocolate Peanut Bliss	1 (1.8 oz)	270
GoLean Crunchy Sublime Lemon Lime	1 (1.8 oz)	670
GoLean Frosted Spice Cake	1 (2.7 oz)	290
GoLean Honey Vanilla Yogurt	1 (2.7 oz)	290
GoLean Malted Chocolate Chip	1 (2.7 oz)	290
GoLean Mocha Java	1 (2.7 oz)	290
GoLean Oatmeal Raisin Cookie	1 (2.7 oz)	280
GoLean Peanut Butter & Chocolate	1 (2.7 oz)	290
GoLean Strawberries 'N Cream	1 (2.7 oz)	290
GoLean Strawberry Vanilla Yogurt	1 (2.7 oz)	280
LaraBar		
Apple Pie	1	190
Banana Cookie	1	210
Cashew Cookie	1	230
Cherry Pie	1	190
Chocolate Coconut Chew	1	220
Cocoa Mule	1	200
Ginger Snap	1	220
Lean Body For Her		
Chocolate Honey Peanut	1 bar (1.76 oz)	190
Luna		
Chai Tea	1 bar (1.7 oz)	180
Chocolate Pecan Pie	1 bar (1.7 oz)	180
Key Lime Pie	1 bar (1.7 oz)	180
LemonZest	1 bar (1.7 oz)	180
Nutz Over Chocolate	1 bar (1.7 oz)	180
Sesame Raisin Crunch	1 bar (1.7 oz)	170
Toasted Nuts 'n Cranberry	1 bar (1.7 oz)	170
Tropical Crisp	1 bar (1.7 oz)	180

FOOD	PORTION	CALS
Met-Rx		
Big 100 Gram Bar Peanut Butter	1 bar (3.5 oz)	340
Source/One Chocolate Cheesecake	1 bar (2.1 oz)	160
Momentum		
Chocolate Caramel Nut	1 bar	150
Chocolate Peanut Butter	1 bar	150
Double Chocolate	1 bar	150
Moto Bar		
Bodacious Banana Split	1 bar	300
Charming Cherry Almond	1 bar (2.9 oz)	300
Cozy Pumpkin Pie	1 bar	300
Jazzy Peanut Butter & Jelly	1 bar	300
Kooky Cappuccino	1 bar	300
Luscious Lemon Blueberry	1 bar	300
Saucy Apple Cinnamon	1 bar	280
Zany Cranberry Orange	1 bar	300
Nature's Path		
Optimum Blueberry Flax & Soy	1 bar (2 oz)	200
Optimum Cranberry Ginger & Soy	1 bar (2 oz)	200
Optimum Peanut Butter	1 bar (2 oz)	230
Optimum ReBound	1 bar (2 oz)	190
New You		
Chocolate Crisp	1 bar (1.65 oz)	180
NuGo		
Banana Chocolate Protein	1 bar	190
Blue Berry Boom	1 bar	180
Chocolate Blast	1 bar	180
Coffee Break	1 bar	180
Orange Smoothie Protein	1 bar	190
Peanut Butter Pleaser	1 bar	180
Nutiva		
Flaxseed & Raisin Organic	1 bar (1.4 oz)	280
Hempseed Bar Organic	1 bar (1.4 oz)	210
Organic Flax & Raisin	1	200
Original Organic Hempseed	1	210
Nutribar		
Chocolate Covered Belgian Chocolate	1 bar (2.3 oz)	252
Chocolate Covered Caramel	1 bar (2.3 oz)	261
Chocolate Covered Chocolate Fudge	1 bar (2.3 oz)	267
Chocolate Covered Hazelnut	1 bar (2.3 oz)	261

FOOD	PORTION	CALS
Chocolate Covered Mocha Almond	1 bar (2.3 oz)	261
Chocolate Covered Peanut	1 bar (2.3 oz)	262
Yogurt Covered Peach Apricot	1 bar (2.3 oz)	261
Yogurt Covered Raspberry	1 bar (2.3 oz)	261
Yogurt Covered Wildberry	1 bar (2.3 oz)	261
Odwalla Bar!		
Peanut Crunch	1 bar (2.2 oz)	260
Peacekeeper		
Nuts About Peace All Flavors	1 bar (1.4 oz)	180
PermaLean		
Protein Crunch Chocoholic Chocolate	1 bar (1.8 oz)	170
Protein Crunch Chocolate Raspberry	1 bar (1.8 oz)	180
Protein Crunch Stark Raving Peanutz	1 bar (1.8 oz)	180
PowerBar		
Harvest Apple Cinnamon Crisp	1 bar (2.3 oz)	240
Harvest Chunky Cherry Crunch	1 bar (2.3 oz)	240
Harvest Dipped Double Chocolate Crisp	1 bar (2.3 oz)	250
Harvest Dipped Oatmeal Raisin Cookie	1 bar (2.3 oz)	250
Harvest Dipped Toffee Chocolate Chip	1 bar (2.3 oz)	250
Harvest Peanut Butter Chocolate Chip	1 bar (2.3 oz)	240
Harvest Strawberry Crunch	1 bar (2.3 oz)	230
Performance Apple Cinnamon	1 bar (2.3 oz)	230
Performance Banana	1 bar (2.3 oz)	230
Performance Cappuccino	1 bar (2.3 oz)	230
Performance Chocolate	1 bar (2.3 oz)	230
Performance Chocolate Peanut Butter	1 bar (2.3 oz)	240
Performance Cookies & Cream	1 bar (2.3 oz)	240
Performance Malt Nut	1 bar (2.3 oz)	230
Performance Oatmeal Raisin	1 bar (2.3 oz)	230
Performance Peanut Butter	1 bar (2.3 oz)	230
Performance Strawberry Cream	1 bar (2.3 oz)	230
Performance Vanilla Crisp	1 bar (2.3 oz)	230
Performance Wild Berry	1 bar (2.3 oz)	230
Protein Plus Carb Select Chocolate	1 bar (2.5 oz)	260
Protein Plus Carb Select Chocolate Caramel Crunch	1 bar (2.6 oz)	270
Protein Plus Carb Select Chocolate Peanut Butter	1 bar (2.5 oz)	270
Protein Plus Carb Select Peanut Caramel	1 bar (2.6 oz)	270
Protein Plus Chocolate Fudge Brownie	1 bar (2.7 oz)	270

FOOD	PORTION	CALS
Protein Plus Chocolate Peanut Butter	1 bar (2.7 oz)	290
Protein Plus Cookies & Cream	1 bar (2.7 oz)	290
Protein Plus Vanilla Yogurt	1 bar (2.7 oz)	290
Triple Treat Caramel Peanut Crisp	1 bar (1.9 oz)	220
Triple Treat Caramel Peanut Fusion	1 bar (1.9 oz)	230
Triple Treat Chocolate Caramel Fusion	1 bar (1.9 oz)	230
Triple Treat Chocolate Peanut Butter Crisp	1 bar (1.9 oz)	220
Pria		
Carb Select Caramel Nut Brownie	1 bar (1.7 oz)	170
Carb Select Chocolate Mocha Crisp	1 bar (1.7 oz)	130
Carb Select Chocolate Peanut Butter Crisp	1 bar (1.7 oz)	130
Carb Select Cookies N' Caramel	1 bar (1.7 oz)	170
Carb Select Peanut Butter Caramel Nut	1 bar (1.7 oz)	170
Chocolate Peanut Crunch	1 bar (1 oz)	110
Complete Nutrition Chocolate Mint Crisp	1 bar (1.6 oz)	170
Complete Nutrition Chocolate Peanut Butter Crisp	1 bar (1.6 oz)	170
Complete Nutrition French Vanilla Crisp	1 bar (1.6 oz)	170
Creme Carmel Crisp	1 bar (1 oz)	110
Double Chocolate Cookie	1 bar (1 oz)	110
French Vanilla Crisp	1 bar (1 oz)	110
Mint Chocolate Cookie	1 bar (1 oz)	110
Strawberry Shortcake	1 bar (1 oz)	110
Pure Protein		
Blueberry Cheesecake	1 bar	190
Resource		
Mini Nutrition Bar	1 bar	90
Revival		
Soy Apple Cinnamon Celebration	1 bar	200
Soy Autumn Frost Low Carb	1 bar	200
Soy Chocolate Raspberry Zing Low Carb	1 bar	200
Soy Chocolate Temptation	1 bar	220
Soy Marshmallow Krunch	1 bar	220
Soy Peanut Butter Chocolate Pal	1 bar	240
Soy Peanut Butter Pal	1 bar	240
Slim-Fast		
Classic Meal Bar Chocolate Cookie Dough	1 bar	220
Classic Meal Bar Milk Chocolate Peanut	1 bar	220
High Protein Granola Bar Peanut	1 bar	200
High Protien Granola Bar Chocolate Chip	1 bar	190

FOOD	PORTION	CALS
Low Carb Breakfast Bar Apple Cobbler	1 bar	180
Low Carb Breakfast Bar Peanut Butter	1 bar	190
Low Carb Snack Bar Caramel Nut	1 bar	120
Low Carb Snack Bar Coconut Almond	1 bar	120
Low Carb Snack Bar Peanut Butter Crunch	1 bar	120
Optima Meal Bar Apple Crisp	1 bar	180
Optima Meal Bar Caramel Crispy Peanut	1 bar	220
Optima Meal Bar Chewy Granola Trail Mix	1 bar	210
Optima Snack Bar Banana Nut Muffin	1 bar	150
Optima Snack Bar Blueberry Muffin	1 bar	140
Optima Snack Bar Chocolate Peanut Nougat	1 bar	120
Optima Snack Bar Oatmeal Raisin Cookie	1 bar	120
Snickers Marathon		
Energy Chewy Chocolate Peanut	1 (1.9 oz)	220
Energy Multi Grain Crunch	1 (1.9 oz)	220
For Women Double Chocolate Nut	1 (2.8 oz)	150
For Women Honey Nut Oat	1 (2.8 oz)	150
Low Carb Chocolate Fudge Nut	1 (1.8 oz)	170
Low Carb Peanut Butter	1 (1.8 oz)	170
Protein Caramel Nut Surge	1 (2.8 oz)	290
Protein Chocolate Nut Burst	1 (2.8 oz)	290
SoBe		
Milk Chocolate	1 bar (1.75 oz)	240
Solo GI		
Berry Bliss	1 bar (1.6 oz)	190
Chocolate Charger	1 bar (1.6 oz)	190
Mint Mania	1 bar (1.6 oz)	190
Peanut Power	1 bar (1.6 oz)	200
South Beach Diet		
Chocolate Crisp	1 bar	210
Chocolate Peanut Butter	1 bar	210
Cinnamon Creme	1 bar	220
Strive		
Crunchy Chocolate Smores	1 bar (2.1 oz)	200
Sweet Success		
Chewy Chocolate Brownie	1 bar (1.2 oz)	120
T.H.E. Bar		
Granola Raisin	1 (1.8 oz)	200
Think!		
Apple Spice	1 bar (2 oz)	205

FOOD	PORTION	CALS
Chocolate Almond Coconut Raisin	1 bar (2 oz)	243
Chocolate Fruit Harvest	1 bar (2 oz)	217
Zoe		
Flax & Soy Apple Crisp	1 bar (1.83 oz)	180
ZonePerfect		
Honey Peanut	1 bar (1.8 oz)	200

ENERGY DRINKS
Accelerade
All Flavors	8 oz	80

AMP
Energy Drink	1 can (8.4 oz)	120

Arizona
Extreme Energy Shot	1 bottle (8.3 oz)	130

Atkins
Cafe Au Lait	1 can (11 oz)	170
Chocolate	1 can (11 oz)	170
Chocolate Royale	1 can (11 oz)	170
Strawberry	1 can (11 oz)	170
Vanilla	1 can (11 oz)	170

Balance
Chocolate as prep w/ 2% milk	1 serv	310
Vanilla as prep w/ 2% milk	1 serv	310

Banzai
Energy Drink	8 oz	120

Bawls
Guarana	1 bottle (10 oz)	120
Guaranexx Sugar Free	1 bottle (10 oz)	0

Beaver Buzz
Cirus	1 can	140

Bliss
Energy Drink	1 can (8.4 oz)	110
Low Carb	1 can (8.4 oz)	26

Blu Fuel
Energy Drink	1 can (10 oz)	133

BooKoo
Energy Drink	8 oz	110
Shot All Flavors	1 can (5.57 oz)	80
Zero Carb	8 oz	0

FOOD	PORTION	CALS
Boost		
High Protein Vanilla	1 can (8 oz)	240
Vanilla	8 oz	240
Bossa Nova		
Acai Juice Mango	1 bottle (10 oz)	132
Acai Juice Original	1 bottle (10 oz)	138
Acai Juice Passion Fruit	1 bottle (10 oz)	132
Brain Twist		
Flu & Cold Defense All Flavors	8 oz	70
Cascabel		
Energy Drink	1 çan (8.4 oz)	110
Sugar Free	1 can (8.4 oz)	10
Cheetah		
Energy Drink	1 can (12 oz)	80
Choice		
Chocolate	1 can (8 oz)	220
Chocolate Fudge Sugar Free	1 pkg (11 oz)	125
French Vanilla Sugar Free	1 pkg (11 oz)	100
Strawberries'n Cream Sugar Free	1 pkg (11 oz)	100
Vanilla	1 can (8 oz)	220
Crunk		
Energy Drink	1 can	120
Cytomax		
Sport Drinks All Flavors	1 bottle (20 oz)	130
Defcon3		
Healthy Energy Soda	1 can (12 oz)	45
Defense		
Effervescent Supplement	1 can	150
Diablo		
Energy Drink	1 can (8.7 oz)	151
Double Hit		
Maximun Energy Coffee Drink Sugar Free	1 can (12 oz)	0
Energy 69		
Energy Drink	1 can	110
Sugar Free	1 can	0
Everlast		
High Energy Citrus Blast	1 can (8.3 oz)	140
Full Throttle		
Energy Drink	8 oz	100
Fury	8 oz	110

FOOD	PORTION	CALS
Fuze		
Energize Blackberry Grape	8 oz	100
Energize Exotic Punch	8 oz	100
Energize Mojo Mango	8 oz	100
Essential Cranberry Grapefruit	8 oz	90
Focus Orange Carrot	8 oz	90
Refresh Banana Colada	8 oz	90
Refresh Mixed Berry	8 oz	90
Refresh Peach Mango	8 oz	90
Replenish Agave Cactus	8 oz	90
Stamina Grape & Aronia Punch	8 oz	80
Vitaboost Citrus Starfruit Punch	8 oz	90
Gatorade		
All Flavors	1 cup (8 oz)	50
Lemonade All Flavors	8 oz	50
Nutrition Shake All Flavors	1 can (11 oz)	370
X-Factor All Flavors	8 oz	50
GeniSoy		
Soy Protein Shake Chocolate	1 scoop (1.2 oz)	120
Soy Protein Shake Vanilla	1 scoop (1.2 oz)	130
Soy Protein Shake Strawberry Banana	1 scoop	130
Go Fast		
Energy Drink	1 can (8.4 oz)	90
Light	1 can (8.4 oz)	20
Sportsman's	1 can (8.4 oz)	90
Guaraviton		
Energy Drink	8 oz	98
Guru		
Energy Drink	1 can (8.3 oz)	100
Lite	1 can (8.3 oz)	5
Hansen's		
Energy Kiwi Strawberry	8 oz	120
Energy Peach	8 oz	130
Energy Punch	8 oz	120
Healthy Start Carrot Orange Antioxidant Blend	8 oz	130
Healthy Start Citrus Punch Focus Blend	8 oz	130
Healthy Start Cranberry Grape Defense Blend	8 oz	110

FOOD	PORTION	CALS
Healthy Start Tropical Orange Vitamix Blend	8 oz	110
Happy Bunny		
Spaz Juice	1 can (8.4 oz)	110
Healthy Pleasures		
Chocolate Irish Cream	1 bottle (10.5 oz)	260
Her Energy		
Pink Lemonade	1 can (8.4 oz)	130
Pink Lemonade Sugar Free	1 can (8.4 oz)	0
Hiball		
All Flavors	1 bottle (10 oz)	10
High Voltage		
Sugar Free	8 oz	5
Hype		
Classic Energy	1 can (8.3 oz)	110
Impulse		
Energy Drink	1 can (8.3 oz)	110
Sugar Free	1 can (8.3 oz)	5
Invigor8		
Energy Boost	1 can	110
Nutrition Boost	1 can	110
Iron Energy		
All Flavors	8 oz	90
Jet Set		
Club Soda	1 can (12 oz)	0
Ginger Ale	1 can (12 oz)	150
Original	1 can (12 oz)	105
Tonic Water	1 can (12 oz)	150
Jones Soda		
Big Energy	8 oz	120
Lemon Lime Energy	1 can (8.4 oz)	140
Mixed Berry Energy	1 can (8.4 oz)	140
Orange Energy	1 can (8.4 oz)	140
Sugar Free Energy	1 can (8.4 oz)	10
Jugular		
Energy Drink	1 can (8.3 oz)	49
Kabbalah		
Original	1 can (12 oz)	174
Sugar Free	1 can (12 oz)	<3

FOOD	PORTION	CALS
KaBoom		
All Flavors	8 oz	105
Kashi		
GoLean Shake Mix Vanilla	2 scoops	220
GoLean Shake Mix Woman Chocolate	2 scoops	220
Shake Chocolate	1 can	230
Shake Vanilla	1 can	220
Kindercal		
Vanilla	1 can (8 oz)	250
Krank'd		
All Flavors	1 bottle (16 oz)	80
Lolli's Pop		
Cheery Energy Drink	1 bottle	170
Passion Stimulating Elixir	1 bottle	140
Lost		
Big Gun	6 oz	100
Five-O	8 oz	70
Perfect 10	8 oz	10
Monster		
Energy Assault	8 oz	100
Energy Drink	8 oz	100
Khaos Energy Juice	8 oz	90
Lo Carb	8 oz	10
Natural Ovens		
Ultra Omega Balance	1 tbsp	75
Zesty Flax Energy Mix	1 tbsp	40
New York Minute		
Energy Drink	1 can (8.4 oz)	130
Nexcite		
Herbal Fizz	1 bottle	72
Nitro2Go		
High Energy	1 can	110
High Energy Lite	1 can	20
NOS		
High Performance	8 oz	110
NutraShake		
Citrus	1 pkg (4 oz)	200
Citrus Free	1 serv (4 oz)	200
Vanilla	1 serv (8 oz)	400
Vanilla No Added Sugar	1 serv (4 oz)	200

FOOD	PORTION	CALS
Odwalla		
Blueberry B Monster	8 fl oz	140
C Monster	8 fl oz	150
Femme Vitale	8 fl oz	130
Glorious Morning	8 fl oz	130
Mango Tango	8 fl oz	150
Mo Beta	8 fl oz	140
Serious Energy	8 fl oz	150
Strawberry C Monster	8 fl oz	150
Super Protein	8 fl oz	170
Superfood	8 fl oz	140
Wellness	8 fl oz	150
Orange County Choppers		
High Octane Fuel	1 can (8.4 oz)	110
Peep One		
Erotic Drink	1 can (8.3)	109
Pimp Juice		
Energy Drink	1 can (8 oz)	140
Tight	1 can (8 oz)	140
Pink		
Diet	1 can	10
Piranha		
Phunky Fruit Punch	1 can (8.4 oz)	140
Pit Bull		
Energy Drink	1 can (8.4 oz)	110
Sugar Free	1 can (8.4 oz)	0
Pounds Off		
Dark Chocolate Ecstasy	1 can (11 oz)	200
French Vanilla	1 can (11 oz)	220
Powerade		
Arctic Shatter	8 oz	64
Flava 23	8 oz	63
Fruit Punch	8 oz	65
Green Squall	8 oz	64
Jagged Ice	8 oz	65
NASCAR Grape	8 oz	64
Olympic Citrus	8 oz	63
Option All Flavors	8 oz	10

FOOD	PORTION	CALS
PowerBar		
Endurance Sport Drink	1 pkg (0.6 oz)	70
Performance Recovery Drink	1 pkg (0.8 oz)	90
Pure Power		
Energy Drink	1 can (8.4 oz)	110
Shotz	1 can (5.75 oz)	80
Raw Dawg		
Energy Drink	8 oz	110
Sugar Free	8 oz	0
Rawlings EX2		
Sustained Energy	1 can (8.4 oz)	132
Red Bull		
Energy Drink	1 can (8.3 oz)	110
Sugar Free	1 can	10
Red Eye		
Classic	1 bottle (12 oz)	208
Extreme	1 bottle (12 oz)	140
Gold	1 bottle (12 oz)	208
Passion	1 bottle (12 oz)	149
Platinum	1 bottle (12 oz)	149
RESQ		
Energy Drink	1 can (8 oz)	126
Rip It		
Citrus X	8 oz	130
Citrus X Sugar Free	8 oz	0
Energy Fuel	8 oz	130
Energy Lite	8 oz	0
Rockstar		
Energy Cola	8 oz	120
Energy Drink	8 oz	110
Juiced	8 oz	90
Rox		
Energy Drink	1 can	110
Zero	1 can	10
Slim-Fast		
Classic Ready-To-Drink Creamy Milk Chocolate	1 can	220
Classic Ready-To-Drink French Vanilla	1 can	220
High Protein Ready-To-Drink All Flavors	1 can	190
Low Carb Diet Ready-To-Drink All Flavors	1 can	190

FOOD	PORTION	CALS
Snapple A Day		
Meal Replacement All Flavors	1 bottle (11.5 oz)	210
SoBe		
Adrenaline Rush	1 can (8.3 oz)	140
Black & Blue Berry Brew	8 oz	120
Courage Cherry Citrus	8 oz	110
Drive	8 oz	120
Elixir Cranberry Grapefruit	8 oz	110
Elixir Orange Carrot 3C	8 oz	90
Elixir Pomegranate Cranberry	8 oz	100
Energy	8 oz	120
Fuerte	8 oz	130
Karma	8 oz	120
Lean Diet Citrus	8 oz	5
Long John Lizard's Grape Grog	8 oz	120
Power	8 oz	120
Synergy All Flavors	1 can (11.5 oz)	120
Tsunami	8 oz	110
Wisdom	8.5 oz	110
Zen Blend	8.5 oz	90
Source Burn		
2	8 oz	130
Energy Drink	8 oz	140
Sugar Free	8 oz	10
Speed Zone		
Energy Drink	1 can (8.4 oz)	110
Stevita		
All Flavors	2 tsp	0
Stewie's		
Domination Serum	1 can (8.45 oz)	110
Mind Erase Elixir	1 can (8.45 oz)	100
Stinger		
All Flavors	1 can (8.4 oz)	130
Sugar Free All Flavors	1 can (8.4 oz)	0
Sweet Success		
Creamy Milk Chocolate	1 can	200
Creamy Milk Chocolate as prep w/ skim milk	1 serv	180
Tab		
Energy Drink	1 can (10.5 oz)	5

FOOD	PORTION	CALS
Tantra		
Erotic	1 can (8.4 oz)	130
The Beast		
Energy Drink	1 can (8.3 oz)	120
Tornado		
Energy Drink	8 oz	110
TwinLab		
Hydra Fuel	16 oz	132
Nitro Fuel	16 oz	460
Ultra Fuel	16 oz	400
Vipa		
Energy Drink	1 can (12 oz)	0
Wide Open Performance		
Energy Drink	1 can (8.3 oz)	120
Wired		
Energy Drink	8 oz	110
Sugar Free	8 oz	5
X 3000 Taurine	8 oz	110
Xcyto		
Sugar Free	1 can (12.5 oz)	10
XO		
Balance	8 oz	50
Berry	1 bottle	90
Citrus	1 bottle	90
Defense	8 oz	40
Diet	1 bottle	15
Endurance	8 oz	50
Energy	8 oz	40
Essential	8 oz	40
Focus	8 oz	40
Grape	1 bottle	90
Multi-V	8 oz	40
Original	1 bottle	110
Peach	1 bottle	90
Power-C	8 oz	40
Rescue	8 oz	40
Revive	8 oz	50
Stress-B	8 oz	40
Vanilla	1 bottle	90

FOOD	PORTION	CALS
XS Energy		
Citrus Blast	1 can (8.4 oz)	8
Cranberry Grape	1 can (8.4 oz)	8
Electric Lemon Blast	1 can (8.4 oz)	16
Tropical Blast	1 can (8.4 oz)	8
Xtazy		
All Flavors	1 can	160
YET		
Your Energy Drink	1 can	8

ENGLISH MUFFIN
READY-TO-EAT

FOOD	PORTION	CALS
apple cinnamon	1	138
crumpets	1 (1.5 oz)	80
granola	1	155
mixed grain	1	155
plain	1	134
plain toasted	1	133
raisin cinnamon	1	138
sourdough	1	134
wheat	1	127
whole wheat	1	134
Food For Life		
7 Sprouted Grains	1	160
Ezekiel 4:9 Sprouted Grain	1	160
Ezikiel 4:9 Cinnamon Raisin	1	160
Genesis 1:29 Original	1	180
Milton's		
Multi-Grain	1 (2 oz)	150
Pepperidge Farm		
100% Whole Wheat	1	140
7 Grain	1	130
Sara Lee		
Heart Healthy Wheat w/ Honey	1	140
Original w/ Whole Grain	1	140
Thomas'		
Blueberry	1	140
Carb Consider	1	100
Hearty Grains 100% Whole Wheat	1	120
Hearty Grains Honey Wheat	1	130

FOOD	PORTION	CALS
Original	1	120
Raisin Bran	1	150
Raisin Cinnamon	1	140
Sourdough	1	120
Super Size	1	190
Super Size Multi Grain	1	240
Wonder		
Cinnamon Raisin	1 (2.1 oz)	140
Original	1 (2 oz)	130
Sourdough	1 (2 oz)	130
TAKE-OUT		
w/ butter	1 (2.2 oz)	189
w/ cheese & sausage	1 (4 oz)	393
w/ egg cheese & canadian bacon	1 (4.8 oz)	289
w/ egg cheese & sausage	1 (5.8 oz)	487

EPAZOTE

FOOD	PORTION	CALS
fresh	1 tbsp (1 g)	tr
fresh sprig	1 (2 g)	1

EPPAW

FOOD	PORTION	CALS
raw	½ cup	75

FALAFEL

Near East

FOOD	PORTION	CALS
Falafel as prep	2½ patties	230
TAKE-OUT		
falafel	1 (1.2 oz)	57

FAT (see also BUTTER, BUTTER SUBSTITUTES, MARGARINE, OIL)

FOOD	PORTION	CALS
bacon grease	1 tbsp	116
beef shortening	1 tbsp	115
beef suet	1 oz	242
chicken	1 cup	1846
chicken	1 tbsp	115
cocoa butter	1 tbsp	120
duck	1 tbsp (13 g)	115
goose	1 tbsp	115
goose	1 oz	257
lamb new zealand	1 oz	182

FOOD	PORTION	CALS
lard	1 tbsp (13 g)	115
lard	1 cup (205 g)	1849
meat pan drippings	½ tbsp	124
nutmeg butter	1 tbsp	120
pork backfat	1 oz	230
pork cooked	1 oz	178
salt pork	1 oz	212
shortening	1 tbsp	113
shortening	1 cup	1812
turkey	1 tbsp	115
ucuhuba butter	1 tbsp	120
Spectrum		
Organic Shortening	1 tbsp	110

FEIJOA
fresh	1 (1.75 oz)	25
puree	1 cup	119

FENNEL
fresh bulb	1 (8.2 oz)	72
fresh sliced	1 cup	27
leaves	1 oz	7
seed	1 tsp	7

FENUGREEK
seed	1 tsp	12

FIBER
apple fiber	0.5 oz	40
Apple Fiber		
Pure	2 tbsp (7 g)	16
Benefiber		
Supplement	1 pkg (4 g)	20
Choice		
Fiber Burst Lemon Lime	3 pieces	45
Fiber Burst Tropical Fruit	3 pieces	45
Metamucil		
Fiber Wafers Apple Crisp	2	120
Natural Fiber Regular Flavor	1 rounded tsp (7 g)	25

FOOD	PORTION	CALS
ND Labs		
Pure Apple Fiber	1 tbsp (7 g)	16
FIDDLEHEAD FERNS		
fresh	3.5 oz	34
FIGS		
calimyrna	3 (5.4 oz)	120
canned in heavy syrup	3	75
canned in light syrup	3	58
canned water pack	3	42
dried california	½ cup (3.5 oz)	200
dried cooked	½ cup	140
dried whole	10	477
fresh	1 med	50
Jenny		
Sundried Kalamata	4	120
Trucco		
Kalamata	2	100
FIREWEED		
leaves chopped	1 cup (0.8 oz)	24
FISH (see also individual names, FISH SUBSTITUTES, SUSHI)		
CANNED		
Beach Cliff		
Fish Steaks In Louisiana Hot Sauce	1 can (3.7 oz)	160
Fish Steaks In Mustard Sauce	1 can (3.7 oz)	160
Fish Steaks In Soybean Oil	1 can (3.7 oz)	200
Fish Steaks w/ Hot Green Chilies	1 can (3.7 oz)	160
Fish Steaks w/ Jalapeno Peppers	1 can (3.7 oz)	130
Brunswick		
Fish Steaks In Louisiana Hot Sauce	1 can (3.7 oz)	160
Fish Steaks In Mustard Sauce	1 can (3.7 oz)	160
Fish Steaks In Soybean Oil	1 can (3.7 oz)	200
Fish Steaks In Spring Water	1 can (3.7 oz)	150
Fish Steaks w/ Hot Tabasco Peppers	1 can (3.7 oz)	220
Seafood Snacks Golden Smoked	1 can (3.2 oz)	170
Seafood Snacks In Lemon & Cracked Pepper	1 can (3.2 oz)	160
Seafood Snacks In Louisiana Hot Sauce	1 can (3.2 oz)	140
Seafood Snacks In Teriyaki Sauce	1 can (3.2 oz)	160

FOOD	PORTION	CALS
Seafood Snacks In Tomato & Basil Sauce	1 can (3.2 oz)	140
Seafood Snacks Kippered	1 can (3.2 oz)	160
Chicken Of The Sea		
Fish Steaks	½ can (2 oz)	70
FROZEN		
breaded fillet	1 (2 oz)	155
sticks	1 stick (1 oz)	76
Gorton's		
Baked Au Gratin	1 piece (4.6 oz)	130
Baked Broccoli Cheddar	1 piece (4.6 oz)	130
Baked Primavera	1 piece (4.6 oz)	120
Batter Dipped Portions	1 piece (2.5 oz)	170
Crunchy Golden Fillets Breaded	2 (3.8 oz)	250
Crunchy Golden Sticks	6 (3.8 oz)	250
Garlic & Herb	2 pieces (3.6 oz)	220
Garlic Butter Crumb	1 piece (4.6 oz)	170
Grilled Cajun Blackened	1 piece (3.8 oz)	120
Grilled Garlic Butter	1 piece (3.8 oz)	120
Grilled Italian Herb	1 piece (3.8 oz)	100
Grilled Lemon Butter	1 piece (3.8 oz)	120
Grilled Lemon Pepper	1 piece (3.8 oz)	120
Parmesan	2 pieces (3.6 oz)	260
Ranch	1 piece (3.6 oz)	240
Southern Fried Country Style	2 pieces (3.6 oz)	230
Tenders	3.5 pieces (4 oz)	250
Tenders Extra Crunchy	3.5 pieces (4 oz)	270
TAKE-OUT		
fish cake	1 (4.7 oz)	166
jamaican brown fish stew	1 serv	426
kedgeree	5.6 oz	242
mousse	1 serv (3.5 oz)	185
stew	1 cup (7.9 oz)	157
taramasalata	2 tbsp	124
FISH OIL		
cod liver	1 tbsp	123
herring	1 tbsp	123
menhaden	1 tbsp	123
salmon	1 tbsp	123
sardine	1 tbsp	123

FOOD	PORTION	CALS
shark	1 oz	270
whale	1 oz	270
Cormega		
Omega-E Orange	1 pkg	20
Spectrum		
Cod Liver Oil w/ Lemon	1 tsp	40

FISH PASTE
fish paste	2 tsp	15

FISH SUBSTITUTES
Loma Linda		
Ocean Platter not prep	⅓ cup (0.9 oz)	90
Worthington		
Fillets	2 (3 oz)	180

FLAXSEED
Arrowhead		
Organic Flax Seeds	¼ cup	140
Bite Me		
Flax Bar	1 bar (1.8 oz)	242
Bob's Red Mill		
Flax Seed Meal	2 tbsp	60
Cracker Flax		
Organic Apple Raisin	1 oz	130
Hodgson Mill		
Milled	2 tbsp	60

FLOUNDER
FRESH		
cooked	3 oz	99
cooked	1 fillet (4.5 oz)	148
TAKE-OUT		
breaded & fried	3.2 oz	211
stuffed w/ crab	1 piece (7.6 oz)	332

FLOUR
buckwheat	1 cup	402
whole groat		
corn masa	1 cup (4 oz)	416
cottonseed lowfat	1 oz	94
peanut defatted	1 cup	196

FOOD	PORTION	CALS
peanut lowfat	1 cup	257
potato	1 cup (6.3 oz)	628
rice brown	1 cup (5.5 oz)	574
rice white	1 cup (5.5 oz)	578
rye dark	1 cup (4.5 oz)	415
rye light	1 cup (3.6 oz)	374
rye medium	1 cup (3.6 oz)	361
sesame lowfat	1 oz	95
triticale whole grain	1 cup (4.6 oz)	439
white all-purpose	1 cup (4.4 oz)	455
white bread	1 cup (4.8 oz)	495
white cake unsifted	1 cup (4.8 oz)	496
white self-rising	1 cup (4.4 oz)	443
white unbleached	1 cup (4.4 oz)	455
whole wheat	1 cup (4.2 oz)	407
All Trump		
Flour	¼ cup (1 oz)	100
Arrowhead		
Whole Grain Oat	⅓ cup	120
Gold Medal		
All Purpose	¼ cup (1 oz)	100
Better For Bread	¼ cup (1 oz)	100
Organic All Purpose	¼ cup (1 oz)	100
Self Rising	¼ cup (1 oz)	100
Unbleached	¼ cup (1 oz)	100
Wondra	¼ cup	100
Heckers		
All Purpose Unbleached	¼ cup	100
Whole Wheat	¼ cup	100
Hodgson Mill		
White Unbleached Organic	¼ cup (1 oz)	100
Whole Wheat Graham Organic	¼ cup (1 oz)	100
King Arthur		
All Purpose Unbleached	¼ cup	100
La Pina		
Flour	¼ cup (1 oz)	100
Red Band		
All Purpose	¼ cup (1 oz)	100
Self-Rising	¼ cup (1 oz)	100

FOOD	PORTION	CALS
Robin Hood		
Whole Wheat	¼ cup (1 oz)	90
FOOD COLORS		
blue	1 tsp	0
orange	1 tsp	0
red	1 tsp	tr
yellow	1 tsp	tr
FRENCH BEANS		
dried cooked	1 cup	228
FRENCH FRIES *(see POTATOES)*		
FRENCH TOAST		
FROZEN		
french toast	1 slice (2 oz)	126
TAKE-OUT		
plain	1 slice	151
sticks	5 (4.9 oz)	513
w/ butter	2 slices	356
FROG LEGS		
frog legs	3 oz	175
TAKE-OUT		
as prep w/ seasoned flour & fried	1 (0.8)	70
FRUCTOSE		
Estee		
Fructose	1 tsp	15
Packet	1 pkg	10
FRUIT DRINKS *(see also individual names, SMOOTHIES, YOGURT DRINKS)*		
READY-TO-DRINK		
fruit punch	6 fl oz	87
Apple & Eve		
Apple Cranberry	8 oz	120
Bolthouse Farms		
Berry Blast	8 oz	110
Green Goodness	8 oz	140
Passion Fruit Apple Carrot Juice	8 oz	120

FOOD	PORTION	CALS
Ceres		
Cranberry & Kiwi	8 oz	110
Medley	8 oz	130
Youngberry	8 oz	120
Champion Lyte		
All Flavors	1 bottle	0
Citrus Squeeze		
California Punch	8 oz	130
Florida Punch	8 oz	120
Del Monte		
Peach Raspberry	5.5 fl oz	160
Pineapple Banana Orange	5.5 fl oz	170
Strawberry Peach Banana	5.5 fl oz	150
Dole		
Apple Berry Burst	8 fl oz	120
Cranberry Apple	8 fl oz	120
Fruit Fiesta	8 fl oz	140
Fruit Punch	1 carton (10 oz)	160
Mountain Cherry	8 fl oz	150
Orange Peach Mango	8 oz	120
Orange Strawberry Banana	8 oz	120
Orchard Peach	8 oz	140
Pineapple Orange	8 oz	120
Pineapple Orange Strawberry	8 oz	130
Tropical Fruit	8 oz	160
Eden		
Organic Apple Cherry Juice	8 oz	120
Feel Good Drinks		
Spritz Cranberry & Lime No Sugar Added	1 bottle	159
Spritz Orange & Passionfruit No Sugar Added	1 bottle	151
Spritz Pink Citrus No Sugar Added	1 bottle	159
Firefly		
Chill Out De-stress Drink	1 bottle (11.2 oz)	100
De-tox Morning After Drink	1 bottle (11.2 oz)	104
Five Alive		
Citrus	8 oz	120
Fresh Samantha		
Banana Strawberry	1 cup (8 oz)	130
Carrot Orange	1 cup (8 oz)	100
Desperately Seeking C	1 cup (8 oz)	110

FOOD	PORTION	CALS
Protein Blast	1 cup (8 oz)	160
Super Juice	1 cup (8 oz)	140
The Big Bang	1 cup (8 oz)	100
Guzzler		
Citrus Punch	8 fl oz	140
Island Punch	8 fl oz	140
Hansen's		
Fruit Punch 100% Juice	1 box (4.23 oz)	60
Juice Slam Wild Berry	1 box	120
Hawaiian Punch		
Bodacious Berry	8 oz	110
Fruit Juicy Red	8 oz	120
Green Berry Rush	8 oz	120
Mazin Melon Mix	8 oz	110
Tropical Vibe	8 oz	110
Wild Purple Smash	8 oz	110
Hi-C		
Blast Berry Blue	1 bottle	170
Blast Fruit Pow	1 bottle	180
Blast Wild Berry	1 pkg	100
Flashin' Fruit Punch	1 box	90
Shoutin' Orange Tangergreen	1 box	90
Strawberry Kiwi Kraze	1 box	100
Hog Wash		
All Flavors	1 bottle (10 oz)	37
Juici		
Sparkling All Flavors	1 bottle (12 oz)	105
Juicy Juice		
Apple Grape	1 box (8.45 oz)	140
Berry	1 box (8.45 oz)	130
Punch	1 box (8.45 oz)	140
Punch	1 box (4.23 oz)	70
Tropical	1 box (8.45 oz)	140
Kool-Aid		
Jammers 10 All Flavors	1 pouch (6.75 oz)	10
Langers		
100% Juice Pineapple Coconut	8 oz	140
Blueberry Cranberry	8 oz	135
Cranberry Berry	8 oz	135
Cranberry Fuji	8 oz	160

FOOD	PORTION	CALS
Cranberry Grape	8 oz	165
Cranberry Grape Cocktail	8 oz	165
Cranberry Orange	8 oz	130
Diet Cranberry Berry	8 oz	30
Diet Cranberry Grape	8 oz	30
Fruit Punch Cocktail	8 oz	120
Kiwi Raspberry Cocktail	8 oz	120
Kiwi Strawberry Cocktail	8 oz	120
Mango Orange	8 oz	130
Mixed Berry 100% Juice	8 oz	120
Pineapple Orange Guava	8 oz	130
Ruby Orange	8 oz	130
Tropical Ruby	8 oz	135
White Cranberry Raspberry	8 oz	120
Minute Maid		
Berry Kiwi	1 can (12 oz)	160
Cranberry Grape	8 oz	150
Light Guava Citrus	8 oz	5
Light Mango Tropical	8 oz	5
Light Orange Tangerine	8 oz	15
Orange Passion	8 oz	130
Orange Tangerine	8 oz	110
Tropical Punch Chilled	8 oz	110
Mott's		
Berry	1 box (8 oz)	100
Fruit Punch	1 box (8 oz)	110
Fruit Punch	8 fl oz	130
Naked Juice		
Berry Blast	8 oz	120
Blue Machine	8 oz	170
Green Machine	8 oz	130
Mango Acai	8 oz	190
Power C	8 oz	120
Protein Zone	8 oz	210
Red Machine	8 oz	160
Strawberry Banana C	8 oz	120
Very Berry	8 oz	130
Very Pro Berry	8 oz	190
Well Being	8 oz	140

FOOD	PORTION	CALS
Nantucket Nectars		
Organic Banana Mango Carrot	8 oz	120
Organic Blueberry Banana	8 oz	120
Organic Cranberry Orange	8 oz	130
Peach Orange	8 oz	130
Pomegranate Pear	8 oz	110
Northland		
Cranberry Blueberry	1 cup (8 oz)	140
Oberweis		
Fruit Punch	8 oz	120
Ocean Spray		
Citrus Splash Spritzer	8 oz	160
Cran*Grape	8 oz	170
Cran*Raspberry	8 oz	140
Cran*Strawberry	8 oz	140
Cranapple	8 oz	160
Grape Cranberry	8 oz	170
Kiwi Strawberry	8 oz	120
Mandarin Magic	8 oz	120
Orange Citrus Spritzer	8 oz	160
Ruby Tangerine Spritzer	8 oz	160
White Cranberry Apple Juice	8 oz	120
Wildberry Spritzer	8 oz	160
Odwalla		
Carrot Orange Apple	8 fl oz	100
Rooty Fruity	8 fl oz	110
Strawberry Banana	8 fl oz	120
Purity Organic		
Citrus Punch	8 oz	123
Snapple		
Cranberry Raspberry	8 oz	120
Diet Carrot Apple	8 oz	10
Diet Plum-A-Granate	8 oz	0
Fruit Punch	8 fl oz	110
Go Bananas	8 oz	120
Kiwi Strawberry	8 oz	110
Snapricot Orange	8 oz	120
Soy20		
All Flavors	1 bottle (12 oz)	90

FOOD	PORTION	CALS
TreeTop		
Apple Grape No Sugar Added	8 oz	130
Tropicana		
Berry Punch	8 fl oz	130
Citrus Punch	8 fl oz	140
Fruit Punch	8 oz	130
Just 10 Fruit Punch	1 pouch (6.75 oz)	10
Tropics Orange Strawberry Banana	8 fl oz	110
Tropics Orange Kiwi Passion	8 fl oz	100
Tropics Orange Peach Mango	8 fl oz	110
Tropics Orange Pineapple	8 fl oz	110
Twister Apple Raspberry Blackberry	1 bottle (10 fl oz)	160
Twister Citrus Punch	1 bottle (10 oz)	180
Twister Cranberry Punch	1 bottle (10 oz)	170
Twister Fruit Punch	1 bottle (10 oz)	170
Twister Light Orange Strawberry Banana	1 bottle (10 oz)	45
Twister Orange Cranberry	1 bottle (10 fl oz)	160
Twister Orange Strawberry Banana Burst	8 oz	130
Twister Ruby Red Tangerine	1 bottle (10 oz)	160
Twister Strawberry Kiwi	1 bottle (10 oz)	160
V8		
Splash Berry Blend	8 oz	110
Wadda Juice		
All Flavors	8 oz	50
FRUIT MIXED (see also individual names)		
CANNED		
fruit cocktail in heavy syrup	½ cup	93
fruit cocktail juice pack	½ cup	56
fruit cocktail water pack	½ cup	40
fruit salad in heavy syrup	½ cup	94
fruit salad in light syrup	½ cup	73
fruit salad juice pack	½ cup	62
fruit salad water pack	½ cup	37
mixed fruit in heavy syrup	½ cup	92
tropical fruit salad in heavy syrup	½ cup	110
Del Monte		
Carb Clever Fruit Cocktail	½ cup	40
Fruit Cocktail In 100% Juice	½ cup	60
Fruit Cocktail In Extra Light Syrup	½ cup	60

FOOD	PORTION	CALS
Fruit Cocktail In Heavy Syrup	½ cup	100
Fruit Cup Mixed In Extra Light Syrup	1 pkg (4 oz)	50
Fruit Naturals Tropical Medley	½ cup	70
Orchard Select Premium Mixed	½ cup	80
Snack Cups Strawberry Banana Peaches	1 pkg	70
SunFresh Citrus Salad	½ cup	80
Dole		
FruitBowls Tropical Fruit	1 pkg (4 oz)	60
Tropical Fruit Salad	½ cup (4.3 oz)	80
Mott's		
Fruitsations Banana	1 pkg (4 oz)	90
Fruitsations Cherry	1 pkg (4 oz)	70
Fruitsations Mango Peach	1 pkg (4 oz)	70
Fruitsations Mixed Berry	1 pkg (4 oz)	90
Fruitsations Pear	1 pkg (4 oz)	90
Fruitsations Strawberry	1 pkg (4 oz)	80
Fruitsations Tropical Fruit	1 pkg (4 oz)	70
Healthy Harvest Peach Medley	1 pkg (3.9 oz)	50
DRIED		
mixed	11 oz pkg	712
Paradise		
Old English Fruit & Peel Mix	1 tbsp (0.8 oz)	70
Sun-Maid		
Tropical Medley	¼ cup (1.4 oz)	130
FROZEN		
mixed fruit sweetened	1 cup	245
Birds Eye		
Mixed Fruit	½ cup	90
Tree Of Life		
Organic Mixed Berries	¾ cup (5 oz)	60

FRUIT SNACKS

FOOD	PORTION	CALS
fruit leather	1 bar (0.8 oz)	81
fruit leather pieces	1 pkg (0.9 oz)	92
fruit leather pieces	1 oz	97
fruit leather rolls	1 sm (0.5 oz)	49
fruit leather rolls	1 lg (0.7 oz)	73
Betty Crocker		
Fruit By The Foot All Flavors	1 roll	80

FOOD	PORTION	CALS
CoolFruits		
Apple Grape	1 bar (0.5 oz)	51
Apple Strawberry	1 bar (0.5 oz)	51
Wild Blueberry	1 bar (0.5 oz)	51
Sunbelt		
Fruit Jammers	1 pkg (1 oz)	100
Sunkist		
100% Fruit Roll All Flavors	1 (0.5 oz)	50
Welch's		
White Grape Peach	20 pieces	110
GARLIC		
clove	1	4
fresh chopped	1 tbsp	18
powder	1 tsp	9
Dorot		
Frozen Crushed Cubes	1 cube (4 g)	5
Frieda's		
Elephant	1 tbsp	5
Vinegar Marinated	1 oz	30
McCormick		
Garlic Salt	¼ tsp	0
GEFILTE FISH		
sweet	1 piece (1.5 oz)	35
Mrs. Adler's		
Pike'n Whitefish	1 piece (1.8 oz)	50
GELATIN		
READY-TO-EAT		
Del Monte		
Mandarin Orange In Lite Orange Gel	1 pkg (4.5 oz)	60
Mixed Fruit In Cherry Gel	1 pkg (4.5 oz)	90
Peaches In Lite Strawberry Banana Gel	1 pkg (4.5 oz)	60
Peaches In Peach Gel	1 pkg (4.5 oz)	90
Peaches In Raspberry Gel	1 pkg (4.5 oz)	90
Hunt's		
Snack Pack Juicy Gels Raspberry Mixed Berry	1 serv (3.5 oz)	100
Snack Pack Juicy Gels Strawberry	1 serv (3.5 oz)	100
Snack Pack Juicy Gels Strawberry Orange	1 serv (3.5 oz)	100
Snack Pack Tropical Punch	1 serv (3.5 oz)	100

FOOD	PORTION	CALS
Jell-O		
Sugar Free Tropical Berry	1 serv (3.2 oz)	10
Kozy Shack		
Gel Treats Cherry	1 pkg (4 oz)	85
Gel Treats Lemon Lime	1 pkg (4 oz)	85
Gel Treats Orange	1 pkg (4 oz)	85
Gel Treats Strawberry	1 pkg (4 oz)	85
Gel Treats Sugar Free Orange	1 pkg (4 oz)	11
Gel Treats Sugar Free Strawberry	1 pkg (4 oz)	11
Swiss Miss		
Gels Berry Strawberry	1 pkg (3.5 oz)	79
Gels Berry Lemon	1 pkg (3.5 oz)	79
Gels Raspberry Orange	1 pkg (3.5 oz)	79
Gels Strawberry Raspberry	1 pkg (3.5 oz)	79
GIBLETS		
capon simmered	1 cup (5 oz)	238
chicken floured & fried	1 cup (5 oz)	402
chicken simmered	1 cup (5 oz)	228
turkey simmered	1 cup (5 oz)	243
GINGER		
ground	1 tsp	6
pickled	0.5 oz	5
root fresh	5 slices	9
root fresh sliced	¼ cup	19
Eden		
Pickled w/ Shiso Leaves	1 tbsp	15
Frieda's		
Crystallized	9 pieces (1.1 oz)	100
Galanga Thai Ginger	⅔ cup	60
McCormick		
Crystallized	¼ tsp	15
GINKGO NUTS		
canned	1 oz	32
dried	1 oz	99
raw	1 oz	52
GINSENG		
dried	1 oz	90
fresh	1 oz	28

FOOD	PORTION	CALS
GIZZARDS		
chicken simmered	1 cup (5 oz)	222
turkey simmered	1 cup (5 oz)	236
GNOCCHI		
Bellino		
W/ Potato	1 cup	240
GOAT		
roasted	3 oz	122
GOOSE		
w/ skin roasted	6.6 oz	574
w/ skin roasted	½ goose (1.7 lbs)	2362
w/o skin roasted	5 oz	340
w/o skin roasted	½ goose (1.3 lbs)	1406
GOOSEBERRIES		
canned in light syrup	½ cup	93
fresh	1 cup	67
GRAPE JUICE		
bottled	1 cup	155
frzn sweetened as prep	1 cup	128
frzn sweetened not prep	6 oz	386
grape drink	6 oz	84
Ceres		
Hanepoot White Grape	8 oz	130
Daily		
Drink	8 oz	110
Hansen's		
White Grape 100% Juice	1 box (4.23 oz)	90
Juicy Juice		
Drink	1 box (4.23 oz)	70
Drink	1 box (8.45 oz)	140
Keto		
Kooler	½ tsp	0
Langers		
Cocktail	8 oz	160
Mott's		
100% Juice	1 box (8 oz)	130
Grape Juice	8 fl oz	130

FOOD	PORTION	CALS
Nantucket Nectars		
Organic Concord Grape	8 oz	130
Welch's		
100% Juice	8 oz	170
100% White	8 oz	160
Light White Grape	8 oz	70
GRAPE LEAVES		
canned	1 (4 g)	3
fresh raw	1 (3 g)	3
TAKE-OUT		
dolmas	5 (4.2 oz)	200
GRAPEFRUIT		
CANNED		
juice pack	½ cup	46
unsweetened	1 cup	93
water pack	½ cup	44
Del Monte		
Fruit Naturals Red	½ cup	60
SunFresh Red	½ cup	80
SunFresh White In Real Fruit Juice	½ cup	45
FRESH		
pink	½	37
pink sections	1 cup	69
red	½	37
red sections	1 cup	69
white	½	39
white sections	1 cup	76
Sunkist		
Fresh	½ med	60
Oroblanco	½	100
GRAPEFRUIT JUICE		
fresh	1 cup	96
frzn as prep	1 cup	102
frzn not prep	6 oz	302
sweetened	1 cup	116
Fresh Samantha		
Juice	1 cup (8 oz)	90

FOOD	PORTION	CALS
Langers		
Diet Ruby Red	8 oz	40
Ruby Red	8 oz	130
Minute Maid		
Frozen + Calcium	8 oz	100
Ruby Red	8 oz	130
Mott's		
100% Juice	8 fl oz	110
Ocean Spray		
100% Juice Pink	8 oz	110
100% White Juice	8 oz	100
Ruby Drink	8 oz	120
Ruby Red Drink	8 oz	130
Odwalla		
Juice	8 fl oz	90
Tao Tea		
Grapefruit Lemon Fusion	8 oz	72
Tropicana		
Ruby Red	8 oz	90
Season's Best	8 oz	90
Twister Pink	1 bottle (10 oz)	140
GRAPES		
fresh	10	36
thompson seedless in heavy syrup	½ cup	94
thompson seedless water pack	½ cup	48
Chiquita		
Grapes	1½ cups (4.8 oz)	90
Frieda's		
Champagne	½ cup (3 oz)	50
GRAVY		
CANNED		
au jus	1 cup	38
beef	1 cup	124
beef	1 can (10 oz)	155
chicken	1 cup	189
mushroom	1 cup	120
turkey	1 cup	122
Campbell's		
Beef	¼ cup	29

FOOD	PORTION	CALS
Brown	¼ cup	46
Chicken	¼ cup	42
Turkey	¼ cup	29
Heinz		
Home Style Chicken	¼ cup	25
Pacific Foods		
Natural Beef	1 cup	20
Natural Chicken	¼ cup	25
Natural Mushroom	¼ cup	20
Natural Turkey	¼ cup	25
MIX		
au jus as prep w/ water	1 cup	32
brown as prep w/ water	1 cup	75
chicken as prep	1 cup	83
mushroom as prep	1 cup	70
onion as prep w/ water	1 cup	77
pork as prep	1 cup	76
turkey as prep	1 cup	87
Bournvita		
Extract	2 heaping tsp	34
Bovril		
Extract	1 heaping tsp	9
Durkee		
Au Jus as prep	¼ cup	5
Brown as prep	¼ cup	10
Brown Mushroom as prep	¼ cup	15
Brown Onion as prep	¼ cup	15
Chicken as prep	¼ cup	20
Country as prep	¼ cup	35
Homestyle as prep	¼ cup	15
Onion as prep	¼ cup	10
Pork as prep	¼ cup	10
Sausage as prep	¼ cup	35
Swiss Steak as prep	¼ cup	15
Turkey as prep	¼ cup	20
French's		
Au Jus as prep	¼ cup	5
Brown as prep	¼ cup	10
Chicken as prep	¼ cup	25
Country as prep	¼ cup	35

FOOD	PORTION	CALS
Herb Brown as prep	¼ cup	15
Homestyle as prep	¼ cup	10
Mushroom as prep	¼ cup	10
Onion	¼ cup	15
Pork as prep	¼ cup	10
Sausage as prep	¼ cup	35
Turkey as prep	¼ cup	20
Loma Linda		
Gravy Quik Brown	1 tbsp (5 g)	20
Gravy Quik Chicken	1 tbsp (5 g)	20
Quik Gravy Country	1 tbsp (5 g)	25
Quik Gravy Mushroom	1 tbsp (5 g)	15
Quik Gravy Onion	1 tbsp (5 g)	20
Marmite		
Extract	1 heaping tsp	9
McCormick		
Au Jus Natural as prep	¼ cup	5
Beef & Herb as prep	¼ cup	30
Brown as prep	¼ cup	20
Chicken as prep	¼ cup	20
Onion as prep	¼ cup	20
Pork as prep	¼ cup	20
Turkey as prep	¼ cup	20

GREAT NORTHERN BEANS

canned	1 cup	299
dried cooked	1 cup	209
Eden		
Organic	½ cup (4.6 oz)	110

GREEN BEANS
CANNED

green beans w/o salt	½ cup	18
Del Monte		
Cut	½ cup	20
Cut Italian	½ cup	30
Cut w/ Potatoes & Ham Flavor	½ cup	30
French Style	½ cup	20
Savory Sides Green Bean Casserole	½ cup	70
Whole	½ cup	20

FOOD	PORTION	CALS
S&W		
Blue Lake Cut	½ cup (4.2 oz)	20
French Style	½ cup (4.2 oz)	20
Whole Small	½ cup (4.2 oz)	20
Veg-All		
French Style	½ cup	20
FRESH		
raw	½ cup	17
raw whole beans	10	17
GreenLine		
Fresh Trimmed	3 oz	25
FROZEN		
cooked	½ cup	20
italian cooked	½ cup	18
Birds Eye		
Cut	½ cup	25
Italian	½ cup	35
Fresh Like		
Cut	3.5 oz	29
French Cut	3.5 oz	29
Tree Of Life		
Cut	⅔ cup (2.8 oz)	25

GREENS
Ready Pac

Microwave Leafy Greens as prep	½ cup	15

GROUNDCHERRIES

fresh	½ cup	37

GROUPER

cooked	1 fillet (7.1 oz)	238
cooked	3 oz	100
raw	3 oz	78

GUAR GUM
Bob's Red Mill

Guar Gum	1 tbsp	20

GUAVA

fresh	1	45
guava sauce	½ cup	43

FOOD	PORTION	CALS
Frieda's		
Fresh	1 (3 oz)	45
GUAVA JUICE		
Ceres		
Guava	8 oz	120
Nantucket Nectars		
Guava	8 oz	130
GUINEA HEN		
w/ skin raw	½ hen (12.1 oz)	545
w/o skin raw	½ hen (9.3 oz)	292
HADDOCK		
fresh cooked	3 oz	95
fresh cooked	1 fillet (5.3 oz)	168
fresh raw	3 oz	74
roe raw	1 oz	37
smoked	1 oz	33
smoked	3 oz	99
TAKE-OUT		
breaded & fried	1 piece (3.5 oz)	187
HALIBUT		
atlantic & pacific cooked	3 oz	119
atlantic & pacific cooked	½ fillet (5.6 oz)	223
atlantic & pacific raw	3 oz	93
greenland baked	5.6 oz	380
greenland baked	3 oz	203
HALVA (see SESAME)		
HAM		
canned extra lean roasted	3 oz	116
center slice country style lean roasted	4 oz	220
chopped canned	1 oz	68
ham & cheese loaf	1 oz	73
ham & cheese spread	1 tbsp	37
ham salad spread	1 tbsp	32
minced	1 oz	75
patty cooked	1 patty (2 oz)	203
prosciutto	4 slices (1.3 oz)	72

FOOD	PORTION	CALS
sliced extra lean 5% fat	1 oz	37
sliced regular 11% fat	1 oz	52
steak boneless extra lean	1 (2 oz)	69
westphalian smoked	1 oz	105
Alpine Lace		
Boneless Cooked 98% Fat Free	2 slices (2 oz)	60
Honey Ham 98% Fat Free	2 slices (2 oz)	60
Smoked Virginia 98% Fat Free	2 slices (2 oz)	60
Armour		
Chopped Ham canned	2 oz	130
Deviled Ham Spread	1 pkg (3 oz)	210
Lean Slices Brown Sugar	1 pkg (2.5 oz)	90
Boar's Head		
Black Forest Smoked	2 oz	60
Cappy	2 oz	60
Deluxe	2 oz	60
Deluxe Lowered Sodium	2 oz	50
Maple Glazed Honey	2 oz	60
Pepper	2 oz	60
Rosemary & Sundried Tomato	2 oz	70
Sweet Slice Smoked	3 oz	100
Virgina	2 oz	60
Virginia Smoked	2 oz	60
Carl Buddig		
Ham Sliced w/ Natural Juices	1 pkg (2.5 oz)	120
Honey Ham Sliced w/ Natural Juice	1 pkg (2.5 oz)	120
Lean Slices Oven Roasted Honey Ham	1 pkg (2.5 oz)	90
Lean Slices Smoked	1 pkg (2.5 oz)	80
Hillshire		
Deli Select Honey Ham	6 slices (2 oz)	60
Oscar Mayer		
Brown Sugar	3 slices (1.8 oz)	60
Lunchables Ham Bagels	1 pkg	410
Lunchables Ham Wraps	1 pkg	430
Smoked	3 slices (2.2 oz)	60
Wampler		
Black Forest	2 oz	60

FOOD	PORTION	CALS
HAM DISHES		
TAKE-OUT		
croquettes	1 (3.1 oz)	217
salad	½ cup	287
HAM SUBSTITUTES		
Yves		
Veggie Ham Deli Slices	1 serv (2.2 oz)	80
HAMBURGER		
Kid Cuisine		
Cheeseburger Builder	1 meal	390
Lean Pockets		
Cheeseburger	1 (4.5 oz)	280
TAKE-OUT		
double patty w/ bun	1 reg	544
double patty w/ cheese & bun	1 reg	457
double patty w/ cheese & double bun	1 reg	461
double patty w/ cheese ketchup mayonnaise onion pickle tomato & bun	1 reg	416
double patty w/ ketchup mayonnaise onion pickle tomato & bun	1 reg	649
double patty w/ ketchup cheese mayonnaise mustard pickle tomato & bun	1 lg	706
double patty w/ ketchup mustard mayonnaise onion pickle tomato & bun	1 lg	540
double patty w/ ketchup mustard onion pickle & bun	1 reg	576
single patty w/ bacon ketchup cheese mustard onion pickle & bun	1 lg	609
single patty w/ bun	1 lg	400
single patty w/ bun	1 reg	275
single patty w/ cheese & bun	1 reg	320
single patty w/ cheese & bun	1 lg	608
single patty w/ ketchup cheese ham mayonnaise pickle tomato & bun	1 lg	745
single patty w/ ketchup mustard mayonnaise onion pickle tomato & bun	1 reg	279
triple patty w/ cheese & bun	1 lg	769
triple patty w/ ketchup mustard pickle & bun	1 lg	693

FOOD	PORTION	CALS
HAMBURGER SUBSTITUTES (see also MEAT SUBSTITUTES)		
Amy's		
All American Burger	1 (2.5 oz)	120
California Burger	1 (2.5 oz)	130
Chicago Burger	1 (2.5 oz)	160
Boca Burgers		
Flamed Grilled	1	90
Dr. Praeger's		
California Burger	1 (2.7 oz)	100
Franklin Farms		
Veggiburger Portabella	1 (3 oz)	120
Gardenburger		
Classic Greek	1 (2.5 oz)	120
Fire Roasted Vegetable	1 (2.5 oz)	120
Harmony Farms		
Soy Burger Onion	1 (2.5 oz)	90
Soy Burgers Garlic	1 (2.5 oz)	110
Soy Burgers Mushroom	1 (2.5 oz)	110
Soy Burgers Original	1 (2.5 oz)	110
Lightlife		
Light Burgers	1 (3 oz)	120
Smart Menu Burger	1	80
Loma Linda		
Patty Mix not prep	⅓ cup (0.9 oz)	90
Redi-Burger	⅝ in slice (3 oz)	120
Vege-Burger	¼ cup (1.9 oz)	70
Morningstar Farms		
Better'n Burger	1 (2.7 oz)	80
Garden Grille	1 patty (2.5 oz)	120
Garden Veggie Patties	1 patty	100
Hard Rock Cafe Veggie Burger	1 (3 oz)	170
Harvest Burger	1	140
Harvest Burger Italian Style	1 patty (3.2 oz)	140
Harvest Burger Southwestern	1 (3.2 oz)	140
Spicy Black Bean Burger	1 (2.7 oz)	110
Natural Touch		
Garden Veggie Pattie	1 (2.4 oz)	110
Okara Pattie	1 (2.2 oz)	110
Original Veggie Burger Kit not prep	¼ pkg (0.8 oz)	80

FOOD	PORTION	CALS
Southwestern Veggie Burger Kit not prep	¼ pkg (0.9 oz)	90
Spicy Black Bean Burger	1 (2.7 oz)	100
Vegan Burger	1 (2.7 oz)	70
Superburgers		
Vegan Organic Original	1 (3 oz)	98
Vegan Organic Smoked	1 (3 oz)	98
Vegan Organic TexMex	1 (3 oz)	110
V'dora		
Vegetable BurgerLites	1 (3.3 oz)	58
Worthington		
Granburger not prep	3 tbsp (0.6 oz)	60
Prosage Patties	1 (1.3 oz)	80
Yves		
Black Bean & Mushroom Burgers	1 (3 oz)	100
Garden Vegetable Patties	1 (3 oz)	90
Veggie Burger	1 (3 oz)	119
HAZELNUTS		
dried blanched	1 oz	191
dried unblanched	1 oz	179
dry roasted unblanched	1 oz	188
oil roasted unblanched	1 oz	187
Low Carb Creations		
Soft Hazelnut Brittle	2 pieces (1 oz)	160
Torras		
Hazelnut Chocolate Spread	1 tsp	27
Twist		
Sugar Free Chocolate Hazelnut Spread	2 tbsp	180
HEART		
beef simmered	3 oz	140
chicken simmered	1 cup (5 oz)	268
lamb braised	3 oz	158
pork braised	1	191
pork braised	1 cup	215
turkey simmered	1 cup (5 oz)	257
veal braised	3 oz	158
HEARTS OF PALM		
canned	1 cup (5.1 oz)	41
canned	1 (1.2 oz)	9

FOOD	PORTION	CALS
Del Monte		
Hearts Of Palm	2–3 pieces	20
HEMP		
HempNut		
Shelled Hempseed	1 oz	162
Nutiva		
Hempseed	1½ tbsp (0.5 oz)	70
Organic Protein Powder	2 scoops (1 oz)	120
Shelled Hempseed	2 tbsp	110
HERBAL TEA *(see TEA/HERBAL TEA)*		
HERBS/SPICES *(see also individual names)*		
cajun seasoning	1 tbsp	19
chinese five spice	1 tsp	7
garam masala	1 tsp	8
poultry seasoning	1 tsp	5
pumpkin pie spice	1 tsp	6
A Taste Of Thai		
Chicken & Rice Seasoning	¼ pkg (6 g)	15
Cut N Clean		
Greens Seasoning	1½ tsp	20
Eden		
Furikake Seasoning	½ tsp	5
Gringo Billy's		
Meat Rubs Chipotle	¼ tsp	0
Meat Rubs Montreau	¼ tsp	0
Meat Rubs Ultimate	¼ tsp	0
Tuna Seasoning	1 tsp	5
McCormick		
Big'n Season Buffalo Wings	1 tbsp (8 g)	30
Big'n Season Chicken	1 tbsp (6 g)	20
Big'n Season Pot Roast	1 tsp	10
Blends Bon Appetit	¼ tsp	0
Cajun Seasoning	¼ tsp	0
Greek Seasoning	¼ tsp	0
Jamaican Jerk Seasoning	¼ tsp	0
Meat Loaf Seasoning	1 tsp (4 g)	15
Seafood Seasoning	¼ tsp	0

FOOD	PORTION	CALS
Mrs. Dash		
Classic Italian	¼ tsp	0
Extra Spicy	¼ tsp	0
Garlic & Herb	¼ tsp	0
Grilling Blend Mesquite	¼ tsp	0
Grilling Blend Original Chicken	¼ tsp	0
Grilling Blend Original Steak	¼ tsp	0
Lemon Pepper	¼ tsp	0
Minched Onion Medley	¼ tsp	0
Original Blend	¼ tsp	0
Table Blend	¼ tsp	0
Tomato Basil Garlic	¼ tsp	0
Nueva Cocina		
Picadillo	2 tsp	15
Taco Fresco	2 tsp	15
HERRING		
atlantic cooked	1 fillet (5 oz)	290
atlantic cooked	3 oz	172
atlantic raw	3 oz	134
pacific baked	3 oz	213
pacific fillet baked	5.1 oz	360
roe canned	1 oz	34
roe raw	1 oz	37
smoked	3.5 oz	210
Beach Cliff		
Kippered Snacks	1 can (4 oz)	220
TAKE-OUT		
atlantic kippered	1 fillet (1.4 oz)	87
atlantic pickled	½ oz	39
fried	1 serv (3.5 oz)	233
HICKORY NUTS		
dried	1 oz	187
HOMINY		
CANNED		
white	1 cup (5.6 oz)	482
Van Camp's		
Golden	½ cup (4.3 oz)	80
White	½ cup (4.3 oz)	80

FOOD	PORTION	CALS
HONEY		
honey	1 tbsp (0.7 oz)	64
honey	1 cup (11.9 oz)	1031
orange blossom	1 tbsp	60
wild honey	1 tbsp	60
Frieda's		
Honeycomb	½ cup (3 oz)	260
Steel's		
Sugar Free	1 tbsp	24
SueBee		
Clover	1 tbsp	60
HONEYDEW		
FRESH		
cubed	1 cup	60
wedge	⅟₁₀	46
Chiquita		
Wedge	⅟₁₀ melon (4.7 oz)	50
HORSE		
roasted	3 oz	149
HORSERADISH		
japanese wasabi	¼ tsp	1
wasabi root raw	1 (5.9 oz)	184
wasabi root raw sliced	1 cup (4.6 oz)	142
Boar's Head		
Horseradish	1 tsp (5 g)	5
Eden		
Wasabi Powder	1 tsp	10
HOT CHOCOLATE		
mix as prep w/ water	7 oz	103
mix w/ equal as prep w/ water	7 oz	48
Carnation		
Hot Cocoa 70 Calorie	1 pkg (0.7 oz)	70
Hot Cocoa Double Chocolate Meltdown	1 pkg (1.2 oz)	150
Hot Cocoa Fat Free Raspberry	1 pkg (0.3 oz)	30
Hot Cocoa Fat Free w/ Marshmallows	1 pkg (0.4 oz)	45
Hot Cocoa Lactose Free	1 pkg (1 oz)	120
Hot Cocoa Marshmallow Blizzard	1 pkg (1.5 oz)	180

FOOD	PORTION	CALS
Hot Cocoa Milk Chocolate	3 tbsp (1 oz)	110
Hot Cocoa Rich Chocolate as prep w/ 2% milk	1 pkg	200
Hot Cocoa Rich Chocolate Fat Free	1 pkg (0.3 oz)	25
Hot Cocoa Rich Chocolate No Sugar Added	3 tbsp (0.5 oz)	50
Hot Cocoa Rich Chocolate w/ Marshmallows	3 tbsp (1 oz)	110
Country Choice Naturals		
Irish Chocolate Mint Cocoa	1 pkg	100
Royal Chocolate Cocoa	1 pkg	100
Soy Cocoa Irish Chocolate Mint	1 pkg	100
Soy Cocoa Royal Chocolate	1 pkg	100
Keto		
Hot Cocoa	1 tsp	12
Low Carb Creations		
Cocoa as prep	1 cup	30
White Hot Chocolate	1 cup	25
Nestle		
Hot Cocoa Rich Chocolate	1 pkg (1 oz)	110
Hot Cocoa Rich w/ Marshmallows	1 pkg (1 oz)	110
Sipper Sweets		
Sugar Free Low Carb Mix	1 serv	50
Swiss Miss		
Caramel Cream	1 serv	110
Hot Cocoa And Cream	1 serv	153
Hot Cocoa Chocolate Sensation	1 serv	148
Hot Cocoa Diet	1 serv	22
Hot Cocoa Fat Free	1 serv	52
Hot Cocoa Fat Free Marshmallow Lovers	1 serv	65
Hot Cocoa Lite	1 serv	76
Hot Cocoa Marshmallow Lovers	1 serv	142
Hot Cocoa Milk Chocolate No Sugar Added	1 serv	55
Hot Cocoa Rich Chocolate	1 serv	110
Hot Cocoa w/ Marshmallows No Sugar Added	1 serv	56
Hot Cocoa White Chocolate	1 serv	109
Milk Chocolate	1 pkg	120
Milk Chocolate w/ Marshmallows	1 pkg	120
Premiere Hot Cocoa Almond Mocha	1 serv	144
Premiere Hot Cocoa Raspberry Truffle	1 serv	144
Premiere Hot Cocoa Suisse Truffle	1 serv	142
Rich Hot Cocoa No Sugar Added	1 serv	54

FOOD	PORTION	CALS
Sidewalk Cafe Cappuccino	1 serv	119
Sidewalk Cafe Cinnamon	1 serv	126
Sidewalk Cafe French Vanilla	1 serv	121
Sidewalk Cafe Mocha	1 serv	120
TAKE-OUT		
hot cocoa	1 cup	218
mexican hot chocolate	1 cup	173

HOT DOG

FOOD	PORTION	CALS
beef	1 (1.5 oz)	149
beef & pork	1 (1.5 oz)	137
beef low fat	1 (2 oz)	133
chicken	1 (1.5 oz)	116
fat free	1 (2 oz)	62
low fat	1 (2 oz)	88
low sodium	1 (2 oz)	180
pork and beef cheese smokie	1 (1.5 oz)	141
turkey	1 (1.5 oz)	102
Boar's Head		
Beef Lite	1 (1.6 oz)	90
Beef Cocktail	5 (2 oz)	170
Pork & Beef	1 (2 oz)	150
Health Is Wealth		
Uncured Beef	1 (1.5 oz)	80
Uncured Chicken	1 (1.5 oz)	100
Healthy Choice		
Beef Low Fat	1 (1.8 oz)	70
Low Fat Turkey Pork Beef	1 (1.4 oz)	60
Hebrew National		
97% Fat Free Beef	1 (1.7 oz)	45
Beef	1 (1.7 oz)	150
Cocktail Franks	5 (2 oz)	180
Dinner Frank	1 (4 oz)	350
Franks In A Blanket	5 (2.8 oz)	290
Reduced Fat Beef	1 (1.7 oz)	120
Organic Valley		
All-Natural Beef	1 (1.6 oz)	90
Oscar Mayer		
Corn Dogs	1 (3.2 oz)	260
Fat Free Turkey & Beef	1 (1.8 oz)	40

FOOD	PORTION	CALS
State Fair		
Corn Dogs	1 (2.67 oz)	180
Wampler		
Chicken	1 (2 oz)	120
TAKE-OUT		
corndog	1	460
w/ bun chili	1	297
w/ bun plain	1	242

HOT DOG SUBSTITUTES
Lightlife		
Smart Dogs	1	45
Smart Franks	1 (2 oz)	110
Tofu Pups	1 (1.5 oz)	60
Loma Linda		
Big Franks	1 (1.8 oz)	110
Big Franks Low Fat	1 (1.8 oz)	80
Corn Dogs	1 (2.5 oz)	150
Morningstar Farms		
America's Original Veggie Dog	1 (2 oz)	80
Meatfree Corn Dog	1 (2.5 oz)	150
Meatfree Mini Corn Dog	4 (2.7 oz)	170
Natural Touch		
Vege Frank	1 (1.6 oz)	100
Quorn		
Meat-Free Dogs	1 (1.5 oz)	70
Yves		
Good Dog	1 (1.8 oz)	70
Tofu Dogs	1 (1.3 oz)	45
Veggie Dogs	1 (1.6 oz)	60
Veggie Dogs Chili	1 (1.6 oz)	50
Veggie Dogs Jumbo	1 (2.7 oz)	100
Veggie Dogs Jumbo Hot N' Spicy	1 (2.7 oz)	106

HUMMUS
hummus	1 cup	420
Athenos		
Black Olive	2 tbsp	50
Original	2 tbsp	50
Travelers Hummus & Pita	1 pkg	325

FOOD	PORTION	CALS
Guiltless Gourmet		
Original	2 tbsp	35
Roasted Garlic	2 tbsp	35
TAKE-OUT		
hummus	⅓ cup	140

HYACINTH BEANS
dried cooked	1 cup	228

ICE CREAM AND FROZEN DESSERTS (see also ICES AND ICE POPS, SHERBET, YOGURT FROZEN)
chocolate	½ cup (4 fl oz)	143
dixie cup chocolate	1 (3.5 fl oz)	125
dixie cup strawberry	1 (3.5 fl oz)	112
dixie cup vanilla	1 (3.5 fl oz)	116
strawberry	½ cup (4 fl oz)	127
vanilla	½ cup (4 fl oz)	132
vanilla soft serve	½ cup	111
Atkins		
Endulge Bars Chocolate Fudge	1 bar	130
Endulge Bars Chocolate Fudge Swirl	1 bar	180
Endulge Bars Peanut Butter Swirl	1 bar	180
Endulge Bars Vanilla Fudge Swirl	1 bar	180
Endulge Butter Pecan	½ cup	170
Endulge Chocolate	½ cup	140
Endulge Chocolate Peanut Butter Swirl	½ cup	170
Endulge Vanilla	½ cup	140
Endulge Vanilla Fudge	½ cup	140
Better Than Ice Creme		
Soy Vanilla as prep	½ cup	110
Bon Bons		
Dark Chocolate	5 pieces	190
Milk Chocolate	5 pieces	200
Breyers		
Almond Joy	½ cup	140
Banana Fudge Chunk	½ cup	170
Bar Light Creamy Vanilla Chocolate Coated	1	160
Butter Almond	½ cup	160
Butter Pecan	½ cup	170
Butter Pecan Homemade	½ cup	170

FOOD	PORTION	CALS
Butter Pecan No Sugar Added	½ cup	120
Caramel Praline Crunch	½ cup	180
Caramel Toffee Crunch	½ cup	180
CarbSmart Chocolate	½ cup	130
CarbSmart Strawberry	½ cup	130
CarbSmart Vanilla	½ cup	130
Cherry Chocolate Chip	½ cup	150
Cherry Vanilla	½ cup	140
Chocolate	½ cup	150
Chocolate 98% Fat Free	½ cup	90
Chocolate Caramel No Sugar Added	½ cup	110
Chocolate Chip	½ cup	160
Chocolate Chip Cookie Dough	½ cup	170
Chocolate Rainbow	½ cup	140
Coffee	½ cup	140
Cookies & Cream	½ cup	160
Creamsicle	½ cup	130
Deep Chocolate Fudge	½ cup	200
Dulce De Leche	½ cup	150
French Vanilla	½ cup	150
French Vanilla Light	½ cup	120
French Vanilla No Sugar Added	½ cup	110
Fresa Banana	½ cup	140
Heath English Toffee	½ cup	190
Hershey w/ Almonds	½ cup	170
Ice Cream Cake Oreo	1 slice	190
Ice Cream Cake Vanilla	1 slice	190
Klondike Sandwich	½ cup	160
Mint Chocolate Chip	½ cup	160
Mint Chocolate Chip Light	½ cup	130
Mint Oreo	½ cup	170
Mocha Almond Fudge	½ cup	170
Oreo	½ cup	160
Peach	½ cup	130
Peanut Butter & Fudge	½ cup	170
Reese's Peanut Butter Cups	½ cup	180
Rocky Road	½ cup	160
SpongeBob Cookie Dough	½ cup	160
Strawberry	½ cup	120

FOOD	PORTION	CALS
Strawberry Shortcake	½ cup	160
Turtle Sundae	½ cup	190
Vanilla	½ cup	140
Vanilla Calcium Rich	½ cup	130
Vanilla Caramel Brownie	½ cup	170
Vanilla Fudge Brownie	½ cup	180
Vanilla Fudge Twirl	½ cup	140
Vanilla Fudge Twirl No Sugar Added	½ cup	110
Vanilla Homemade	½ cup	140
Vanilla Lactose Free	½ cup	130
Vanilla Light	½ cup	110
Vanilla Light 2% Milk	½ cup	130
Vanilla No Sugar Added	½ cup	100
Wild Berry Swirl	½ cup	140
Butterfinger		
Bar	1 (1.9 oz)	210
Carnation		
Cup Chocolate	1 (3 oz)	140
Cup Chocolate Malt	1 (12 oz)	270
Cup Strawberry	1 (3 oz)	100
Cup Vanilla	1 (3 oz)	100
Cup Vanilla	1 (5 oz)	170
Cup Vanilla Malt	1 (12 oz)	260
Sundae Cup Strawberry	1 (5 oz)	200
Sunday Cup Chocolate	1 (5 oz)	210
Cool Creations		
Cookies & Cream Sandwich	1 (3.5 oz)	240
Mickey Mouse Bar	1 (2.5 oz)	120
Mini Sandwich	1 (2.3 oz)	110
Dippin' Dots		
Chocolate	⅜ cup (3 oz)	190
Dove		
Beyond Vanilla	½ cup	260
Cappuccino Chocolate Thrill	½ cup	300
Caramel Pecan Perfection	½ cup	310
Caramel Toffee Crunch	1 bar (2.8 oz)	270
Chocolate & Brownie Affair	½ cup	310
Give In To Mint	½ cup	310
Irresistably Raspberry	½ cup	240
Milk Chocolate w/ Almonds	1 bar (2.7 oz)	270

FOOD	PORTION	CALS
Milk Chocolate w/ Vanilla Ice Cream	1 bar (2.7 oz)	260
Original Dove w/ Vanilla Ice Cream	1 bar (2.7 oz)	260
Original Dove Miniatures	5 pieces (3.1 oz)	300
Toffe Caramel Almond	½ cup	320
Triple Chocolate	1 bar (2.8 oz)	200
Unconditional Chocolate	½ cup	300
Vanilla w/ A Chocolate Soul	½ cup	300
Drumstick		
Cone Chocolate	1 (4.6 oz)	320
Cone Chocolate Dipped	1 (4.6 oz)	320
Cone Vanilla	1 (4.6 oz)	340
Cone Vanilla Caramel	1 (4.6 oz)	360
Cone Vanilla Fudge	1 (4.6 oz)	360
Edy's		
Carb Benefit Butter Pecan	½ cup	170
Carb Benefit Chocolate	½ cup	150
Carb Benefit Chocolate Chip	½ cup	160
Carb Benefit Mint Chocolate Chip	½ cup	160
Carb Benefit Vanilla Bean	½ cup	140
Dips Chocolate	26 pieces	420
Dips Mint	26 pieces	420
Dips Vanilla	26 pieces	420
Grand Andes Cool Mint	½ cup	170
Grand Butter Pecan	½ cup	170
Grand Chocolate	½ cup	150
Grand Chocolate Caramel Swirl	½ cup	170
Grand Chocolate Chip	½ cup	160
Grand Chocolate Chips	½ cup	170
Grand Chocolate Fudge Mousse	½ cup	160
Grand Chocolate Fudge Sundae	½ cup	170
Grand Coffee	½ cup	140
Grand Cookie Dough	½ cup	180
Grand Cookies'N Cream	½ cup	160
Grand Double Fudge Brownie	½ cup	170
Grand Dulce De Leche	½ cup	150
Grand Espresso Chip	½ cup	150
Grand French Vanilla	½ cup	160
Grand Fudge Tracks	½ cup	180
Grand Ice Cream Sandwich	½ cup	150
Grand Mint Chocolate Chips	½ cup	170

FOOD	PORTION	CALS
Grand Peanut Butter Cup	½ cup	180
Grand Real Strawberry	½ cup	130
Grand Rocky Road	½ cup	170
Grand Spumoni	½ cup	150
Grand Toffee Bar Crunch	½ cup	170
Grand Toll House Cookie Swirl	½ cup	170
Grand Turtle Sundae	½ cup	160
Grand Utimate Caramel Cup	½ cup	170
Grand Vanilla	½ cup	140
Neapolitan	½ cup	140
Slow Churned Light Butter Pecan	½ cup	120
Slow Churned Light Caramel Delight	½ cup	120
Slow Churned Light Chocolate	½ cup	110
Slow Churned Light Chocolate Chip	½ cup	120
Slow Churned Light Chocolate Fudge Chunk	½ cup	120
Slow Churned Light Coffee	½ cup	105
Slow Churned Light Cookie Dough	½ cup	130
Slow Churned Light Cookies 'N Cream	½ cup	120
Slow Churned Light French Silk	½ cup	130
Slow Churned Light French Vanilla	½ cup	100
Slow Churned Light Fudge Tracks	½ cup	120
Slow Churned Light Mint Chocolate Chips	½ cup	120
Slow Churned Light Mocha Almond Fudge	½ cup	120
Slow Churned Light Neapolitan	½ cup	100
Slow Churned Light Rocky Road	½ cup	120
Slow Churned Light Strawberry	½ cup	110
Slow Churned Light Vanilla	½ cup	100
Slow Churned No Sugar Added Butter Pecan	½ cup	120
Slow Churned No Sugar Added Chocolate	½ cup	95
Slow Churned No Sugar Added Cookie Dough	½ cup	110
Slow Churned No Sugar Added Fat Free Chocolate Fudge	½ cup	100
Slow Churned No Sugar Added Fat Free Raspberry Vanilla Swirl	½ cup	90
Slow Churned No Sugar Added Fat Free Vanilla	½ cup	90
Slow Churned No Sugar Added Fat Free Vanilla Chocolate Swirl	½ cup	100
Slow Churned No Sugar Added Fudge Tracks	½ cup	110
Slow Churned No Sugar Added Mint Chocolate Chips	½ cup	110

FOOD	PORTION	CALS
Slow Churned No Sugar Added Neapolitan	½ cup	95
Slow Churned No Sugar Added Triple Chocolate	½ cup	110
Slow Churned No Sugar Added Vanilla	½ cup	90
Flintstones		
Cool Cream	1 (2.75 oz)	90
Push-Up Pebbles Treats	1 (2.75 oz)	120
Good Humor		
Bar Oreo	1 (4 oz)	250
Bar Reese's Peanut Butter	1 (4 oz)	310
Bar Toasted Almond	1 (3 oz)	180
Bar Vanilla Dark Chocolate	1 (3 oz)	190
Bar Vanilla Milk Chocolate	1 (3 oz)	180
Bar Candy Center Crunch	1 (4 oz)	310
Bar Strawberry Shortcake	1 (4 oz)	230
Chocolate Eclair Bar	1 (4 oz)	220
Cone Premium Sundae	1 (4.3 oz)	270
Cone Strawberry Shortcake	1 (4.3 oz)	230
Giant Sandwich Neapolitan	1 (6 oz)	250
Giant Sandwich Vanilla	1 (6 oz)	250
King Cone	1 (4.6 fl oz)	250
King Cone Giant	1 (8 oz)	190
Number 1 Bar	1 (4 oz)	200
Sandwich Chocolate Chip Cookie	1 (4.5 oz)	290
Sandwich Vanilla	1 (3.5 oz)	160
Sundae Twist Cup	1 (6 oz)	160
Haagen-Dazs		
Bars Chocolate & Almonds	1 (3.7 oz)	380
Bars Chocolate & Dark Chocolate	1 (3.6 oz)	350
Bars Chocolate Peanut Butter Swirl	1 (3 oz)	320
Bars Coffee & Almond Crunch	1 (3.7 oz)	370
Bars Cookies & Cream Crunch	1 (3.6 oz)	370
Bars Dulce De Leche Caramel	1 (3.7 oz)	370
Bars Tropical Coconut	1 (3.5 oz)	340
Bars Vanilla & Almonds	1 (3.7 oz)	380
Bars Vanilla & Dark Chocolate	1 (3.6 oz)	350
Bars Vanilla & Milk Chocolate	1 (3.5 oz)	340
Butter Pecan	½ cup	310
Cappuccino Commotion	½ cup	310
Cherry Vanilla	½ cup	240

FOOD	PORTION	CALS
Chocolate	½ cup	270
Chocolate Brownie w/ Walnuts	½ cup	290
Chocolate Chocolate Fudge	½ cup	290
Chocolate Chocolate Chip	½ cup	300
Chocolate Swiss Almond	½ cup	300
Cinnamon	½ cup	250
Coffee	½ cup	270
Coffee Mocha Chip	½ cup	290
Cookie Dough Chip	½ cup	310
Cookies & Cream	½ cup	270
Creme Caramel Pecan	½ cup	320
Dulce De Leche Caramel	½ cup	290
Low Fat Chocolate	½ cup	170
Low Fat Coffee Fudge	½ cup	170
Low Fat Strawberry	½ cup	150
Low Fat Vanilla	½ cup	170
Macadamia Brittle	½ cup	300
Mango	½ cup	250
Mint Chip	½ cup	300
Pineapple Coconut	½ cup	230
Pistachio	½ cup	290
Rum Raisin	½ cup	270
Strawberry	½ cup	250
Vanilla	½ cup	270
Vanilla Chocolate Chip	½ cup	310
Vanilla Fudge	½ cup	290
Vanilla Swiss Almond	½ cup	300
Healthy Choice		
Bar Sorbet & Cream	1	100
Brownie Bliss	½ cup	130
Butter Pecan Crunch	½ cup	100
Cappuccino Chocolate Chunk	½ cup	120
Caramel Fudge Brownie	½ cup	120
Cherry Chocolate Mambo	½ cup	130
Chocolate Chocolate Chunk	½ cup	120
Cookies 'N Cream	½ cup	120
Crazy Caramel	½ cup	120
Double Karma	½ cup	140
French Silk	½ cup	120
Happy Together	½ cup	150

FOOD	PORTION	CALS
Jumpin' Java	½ cup	130
Low Fat Bar Fudge	1	90
Low Fat Bar Mocha Fudge	1	90
Low Fat Bar Strawberry & Cream	1	90
Mint Chocolate Chip	½ cup	120
No Sugar Added Chocolate Fudge Brownie	½ cup	120
No Sugar Added Coffee Almond Fudge	½ cup	110
No Sugar Added Mint Chocolate Chip	½ cup	110
No Sugar Added Vanilla	½ cup	100
Peanut Butter Cup	½ cup	120
Praline & Caramel	½ cup	120
Rocky Road	½ cup	130
Sandwich Caramel	1	140
Sandwich Fudge Swirl	1	140
Sandwich Vanilla	1	130
Turtle Fudge Cake	½ cup	130
Vanilla	½ cup	110
Vanilla Bean	½ cup	120
Vanilla Caramel Fudge	½ cup	140
Hershey's		
Butter Pecan	½ cup	170
French Vanilla	½ cup	170
Vanilla Chocolate Strawberry	½ cup	160
Hood		
Ice Cream Sandwich	1	180
Klondike		
Bar Almond	1	300
Bar Cappuccino	1	280
Bar Caramel & Peanut	1	290
Bar Caramel Crunch	1	270
Bar Chocolate	1	280
Bar Dark Chocolate	1	280
Bar Heath	1	300
Bar Krunch	1	280
Bar Oreo	1	160
Bar Original	1	280
Bar Peppermint Patty	1	280
Bar Reese's	1	220
Big Bear Sandwich Neapolitan	1	300
Big Bear Sandwich Vanilla	1	300

FOOD	PORTION	CALS
Big Bear Cone Vanilla	1	330
Big Bear Cone Vanilla Caramel	1	360
Big Bear Cone Vanilla Fudge	1	380
CarbSmart Fudge Bar	1	60
CarbSmart Ice Cream Bar	1	130
Choco Taco	1	290
Cone Oreo	1	250
Cone Reese's	1	290
Cookie Sandwich Chips	1	470
Cookie Sandwich Oreo	1	230
Minis	2 pieces	170
Sandwich Double Decker	1	370
Slim-A-Bear 98% Fat Free Sandwich Vanilla	1	130
Slim-A-Bear No Sugar Added Cone Vanilla	1	270
Slim-A-Bear No Sugar Added Fudge Bar	1	90
Slim-A-Bear No Sugar Added Reduced Fat Bar Vanilla	1	160
Slim-A-Bear No Sugar Added Sandwich Vanilla	1	120
Sundae Cup	1	280
Nestle Crunch		
Chocolate	1 bar (3 oz)	200
Crunch King	1 (4 oz)	270
Nuggets	8 pieces	310
Reduced Fat	1 (2.5 oz)	130
Vanilla	1 bar (3 oz)	200
No Pudge!		
Giant Chocolate Eclair Low Fat	1 bar	110
Giant Cone Chocolate No Sugar Added	1	110
Giant Cone Cookies & Cream Low Fat	1	140
Giant Cone Fudgy Brownie Low Fat	1	140
Giant Cone Vanilla No Sugar Added	1	110
Giant Cookie & Cream Low Fat No Sugar Added	1 bar	100
Giant Fudgy Fat Free No Sugar Added	1 bar	60
Giant Sandwich Brownie Batter Low Fat	1	140
Giant Sandwich Brownie Chunk Low Fat	1	140
Giant Sandwich Vanilla & Chocolate No Sugar Added	1	130
Giant Strawberry Shortcake Low Fat	1 bar	110
NutraShake		
High Calorie High Protein All Flavors	1 serv (4 oz)	200

FOOD	PORTION	CALS
Popsicle		
Bar Snoopy	1 (3.5 oz)	150
Bar Sprinklers	1 (2.1 oz)	130
Cone Crispy	1 (2.5 oz)	150
Creamsicle Pop	1 (1.75 oz)	70
Cup Cookies & Cream	1 (10 oz)	310
Fruit Juicee Cups	1 (4 oz)	80
Ice Cream Bar Vanilla	1 (3 oz)	160
Ice Cream Pops Minis	2 (2.8 oz)	190
Sandwich Cookie Rugrats	1 (2.5 oz)	140
Sandwiches MInis	1 (2 oz)	100
Scribblers Ice Cream Pops	2 (2.4 oz)	130
Swirl Bar Bubble Gum	1 (2.6 oz)	60
WWE Bar	1 (3.6 oz)	180
X-Men Wolverine Bar	1 (4 oz)	100
Rice Dream		
Cappuccino	½ cup (3.2 oz)	150
Carob	½ cup (3.2 oz)	150
Carob Almond	½ cup (3.2 oz)	170
Cherry Vanilla	½ cup (3.2 oz)	150
Cocoa Marble Fudge	½ cup (3.2 oz)	150
Cookies N' Dream	½ cup (3.2 oz)	170
Mint Chocolate Chip	½ cup (3.2 oz)	170
Neapolitan	½ cup (3.2 oz)	150
Orange Vanilla Swirl	½ cup (3.2 oz)	250
Strawberry	½ cup (3.2 oz)	140
Vanilla Swiss Almond	½ cup (3.2 oz)	180
Rice Dream Supreme		
Cappuccino Almond Fudge	½ cup (3.2 oz)	170
Cherry Chocolate Chunk	½ cup (3.2 oz)	170
Chocolate Almond Chunk	½ cup (3.2 oz)	170
Chocolate Fudge Brownie	½ cup (3.2 oz)	170
Double Espresso Bean	½ cup (3.2 oz)	160
Mint Chocolate Cookie	½ cup (3.2 oz)	170
Peanut Butter Cup	½ cup (3.2 oz)	180
Pralines N' Dream	½ cup (3.2 oz)	180
Silhouette		
The Skinny Cow Low Fat Ice Cream Sandwich Vanilla	1	130

FOOD	PORTION	CALS
Slim-Fast		
Chocolate Fudge Bar	1 bar	110
Ice Cream Sandwich Chocolate	1	130
Ice Cream Sandwich Vanilla	1	130
Starbucks		
Caramel Cappuccino Swirl	½ cup	240
Classic Coffee	½ cup	230
Coffee Almond Fudge	½ cup	250
Frappuccino Bar Java Fudge	1 bar	130
Frappuccino Bar Mocha	1 bar	120
Java Chip	½ cup	250
Low Fat Latte	½ cup	170
Mud Pie	½ cup	240
White Chocolate Latte	½ cup	280
Tofutti		
Cuties Chocolate	1 (1.4 oz)	130
Cuties Vanilla	1 (1.4 oz)	120
Monkey Bars Peanut Butter	1 bar (2.5 oz)	220
Turkey Hill		
Black Cherry	½ cup	140
Black Raspberry	½ cup	140
Butter Pecan	½ cup	170
Carb IQ Vanilla Bean	½ cup	110
Chocolate Marshmallow	½ cup	160
Chocolate Mint Chip	½ cup	180
Chocolate Peanut Butter Cup	½ cup	180
Colombian Coffee	½ cup	140
Cookies 'N Cream	½ cup	160
Death By Chocolate	½ cup	160
Dutch Chocolate	½ cup	150
Egg Nog	½ cup	150
Fat Free No Sugar Added Caramel Fudge Decadence	½ cup	100
Fat Free No Sugar Added Cherry Vanilla Fudge	½ cup	90
Fat Free No Sugar Added Dutch Chocolate	½ cup	90
Fat Free No Sugar Added Vanilla Bean	½ cup	90
Fudge Ripple	½ cup	140
Light Butter Pecan	½ cup	130
Light Choco Mint Chip	½ cup	140

FOOD	PORTION	CALS
Light Tin Lissie Sundae	½ cup	140
Light Vanilla & Chocolate	½ cup	110
Light Vanilla Bean	½ cup	110
Neapolitan	½ cup	150
Orange Swirl	½ cup	140
Original Vanilla	½ cup	140
Peanut Butter Ripple	½ cup	170
Philadelphia Style Butter Almond	½ cup	180
Philadelphia Style Chocolate	½ cup	170
Philadelphia Style Mint Chocolate Chip	½ cup	180
Philadelphia Style Sweet Cherry Vanilla	½ cup	160
Philadelphia Style Vanilla Bean	½ cup	170
Rocky Road	½ cup	170
Rum Raisin	½ cup	150
Sandwich Choco Mint Chip	1	200
Sandwiches Vanilla	1	190
Strawberries 'N Cream	½ cup	140
Sundae Cones Rocky Road	1	340
Sundae Cones Tin Roof Sundae	1	290
Tin Roof Sundae	½ cup	160
Vanilla & Chocolate	½ cup	150
Vanilla Bean	½ cup	140
Weight Watchers		
Smart Ones Giant Sundae	1 serv (8 oz)	150
TAKE-OUT		
cone vanilla light soft serve	1 (4.6 oz)	164
gelato chocolate hazelnut	½ cup (5.3 oz)	370
gelato vanilla	½ cup (3 oz)	211
sundae caramel	1 (5.4 oz)	303
sundae hot fudge	1 (5.4 oz)	284
sundae strawberry	1 (5.4 oz)	269

ICE CREAM CONES AND CUPS

sugar cone	1	40
wafer cone	1	17
Dutch Mill		
Chocolate Covered Wafer Cups	1 (0.5 oz)	80
Frookie		
Chocolate Crunch	1 (0.4 oz)	50
Honey Crunch	1 (0.4 oz)	45

FOOD	PORTION	CALS
Keebler		
Chocolatey Cone	1 (0.4 oz)	50
Fudge Dipped Cup	1 (0.3 oz)	35
Ice Creme Cup	1 (0.2 oz)	15
Sugar Cone	1 (0.4 oz)	50
Waffle Bowl	1 (0.4 oz)	50
Waffle Cone	1 (0.4 oz)	50
ICE CREAM TOPPINGS		
butterscotch	2 tbsp (1.4 oz)	103
caramel	2 tbsp (1.4 oz)	103
marshmallow cream	1 oz	88
marshmallow cream	1 jar (7 oz)	615
pineapple	1 cup (11.5 oz)	861
pineapple	2 tbsp (1.5 oz)	106
strawberry	2 tbsp (1.5 oz)	107
strawberry	1 cup (11.5 oz)	863
walnuts in syrup	2 tbsp (1.4 oz)	167
Colac		
Passion Fruit	1 tbsp	31
Strawberry	1 tbsp	31
Hershey's		
Chocolate Shoppe Caramel	2 tbsp	100
Chocolate Shoppe Double Chocolate	1 tbsp	60
Chocolate Shoppe Hot Fudge	1 tbsp	70
Chocolate Shoppe Hot Fudge Fat Free	2 tbsp	100
Sprinkles Candy Coated Milk Chocolate	1 tbsp	70
Reese's		
Sprinkles Peanut Butter & Milk Chocolate	1 tbsp	70
Smucker's		
Butterscotch Caramel	2 tbsp	130
Dove Dark Chocolate	2 tbsp	140
Dove Milk Chocolate	2 tbsp	130
Dulce De Leche Milk Caramel Spread	2 tbsp	110
Hot Fudge	2 tbsp	140
Hot Fudge Sugar Free Fat Free	2 tbsp	90
Magic Shell Caramel	2 tbsp	220
Magic Shell Chocolate	2 tbsp	210
Magic Shell Chocolate Fudge	2 tbsp	120

FOOD	PORTION	CALS
Magic Shell Turtle Delight	2 tbsp	210
Magic Shell Twix	2 tbsp	210
Steel's		
Sugar Free Butterscotch	2 tbsp	60
Sugar Free Chocolate Fudge	2 tbsp	45
Sugar Free Hot Fudge	2 tbsp	65
Sugar Free Peanut Butter Fudge	2 tbsp	75
ICED TEA		
MIX		
Atkins		
Sugar Free Lemon not prep	2 tbsp	0
Carb Options		
Lemon as prep	1 serv	0
Nestea		
100% Tea	2 tsp (1 g)	0
100% Tea Decafe	2 tsp (1 g)	0
Ice Teasers Lemon	1 serv (0.5 oz)	5
Ice Teasers Orange	1 serv (0.5 oz)	5
Ice Teasers Wild Cherry	1 serv (0.5 oz)	5
Lemon	2 tsp (1 g)	5
Lemon & Sugar	2 tbsp (0.7 oz)	80
Lemonade Tea	2 tbsp (0.7 oz)	80
Sugar Free	2 tbsp (0.7 oz)	5
Sugar Free Decafe	1 tbsp (0.7 oz)	5
Sun Tea	1 tsp (1 g)	0
READY-TO-DRINK		
Apple & Eve		
Lemon Fruit	8 fl oz	100
Peach Fruit	8 fl oz	100
Raspberry Fruit	8 fl oz	100
Tangerine Fruit	8 fl oz	100
Arizona		
Green Tea w/ Ginseng & Honey	8 oz	70
Lemon	8 oz	90
Bolthouse Farms		
Perfectly Protein Vanilla Chai Tea	8 oz	160
Brazil Gourmet		
Nectar Tea All Flavors	8 oz	90
Nectar Tea Light Mango Passion	8 oz	60

FOOD	PORTION	CALS
Delta Blues		
Spearmint Tea Punch	8 oz	90
Fuze		
LemonAID	8 oz	70
Slender Energy All Flavors	8 oz	20
Vitamin Tea Diet Peach	8 oz	5
Vitamin Tea Green Tea w/ Ginseng	8 oz	60
Vitamin Tea Lemon	8 oz	70
White Tea	8 oz	60
White Tea No Carb Diet Pomegranate	8 oz	0
Glaceau Vitamin Water		
Vital-T	8 oz	50
Hansen's		
Chai	8 oz	150
China Black	8 oz	90
Green	8 oz	70
Green Diet Lemon	8 oz	0
Green Diet Peach	8 oz	0
Green Lemon	8 oz	70
Green Peach	8 oz	70
Oolong	8 oz	70
Spice	8 oz	90
Hawaiian		
Iced Tea	1 can	120
Honest Tea		
Assam	8 oz	17
Black Forest Berry	8 oz	25
Gold Rush	8 oz	9
Green Dragon	8 oz	30
Kashmiri Chai	8 oz	17
Lori's Lemon	8 oz	30
Moroccan Mint	8 oz	17
Peach Oo-La-Long	8 oz	30
Inko's		
White Tea All Flavors	1 bottle (16 oz)	56
White Tea Honeysuckle	1 bottle	0
Joe Tea		
All Flavors	8 oz	100
Kalahari		
Rooibos Red Tea All Flavors	8 oz	50

FOOD	PORTION	CALS
Mad River		
Red Tea w/ Guarana	8 oz	90
New Leaf		
All Flavors	8 oz	75
Republic Of Tea		
No Carb Unsweetened All Flavors	1 bottle (12 oz)	0
Snapple		
Diet Lemonade Ice Tea	8 oz	10
Diet Lime Green Tea	8 oz	0
Just Plain Tea	8 oz	0
Lemonade Ice Tea	8 oz	110
Lime Green Tea	8 oz	100
Mint	8 oz	110
Peach	8 oz	100
Raspberry	8 oz	100
Very Cherry	8 oz	100
SoBe		
Lean Diet Green Tea	8 oz	0
Lean Diet Peach Tea	8 oz	5
Lemon	8 oz	90
Soy20		
Lemon Green Tea	1 bottle (12 oz)	90
Sri Lankan		
Apple	8 oz	70
Lemon	8 oz	60
Sweet Leaf Tea		
Diet Sweet	8 oz	0
Hibiscus Herbal	8 oz	25
Lemon & Lime	8 oz	0
Mint & Honey Green	8 oz	60
Peach	8 oz	75
Raspberry & Tangerine	8 oz	75
Sweet Tea	8 oz	75
T42		
A Classic Earl Grey	8 oz	60
Herbal All Flavors	8 oz	70
Jamaican Ginger Green Tea	8 oz	70
Lemon And Honey Green Tea	8 oz	60
Wake-Up Blend English Breakfast	8 oz	45
With Lemon	8 oz	60

FOOD	PORTION	CALS
Tao Tea		
Grapefruit Green Tea	8 oz	71
Lemon Green Tea	8 oz	67
Tradewinds		
Diet Green Tea	8 oz	0
Diet Raspberry	8 oz	0
Mango Green Tea	8 oz	80
Turkey Hill		
Blueberry Oolong w/ Vitamins C & E	1 cup	100
Decaffeinated	1 cup	80
Decaffeinated Orange	1 cup	10
Diet	1 cup	0
Diet Decaffeinated	1 cup	0
Diet Green Tea w/ Ginseng & Honey	1 cup	5
Green Tea w/ Ginseng & Honey	1 cup	70
Lemon	1 cup	100
Mint Tea w/ Chamomile	1 cup	90
Oolong w/ Ginkgo Biloba & Ginseng	1 cup	100
Orange	1 cup	100
Peach	1 cup	110
Raspberry Tea	1 cup	110
Regular	1 cup	90
XS Energy		
Energy Tea Berry Typhoon	1 can (8.4 oz)	12

ICES AND ICE POPS

FOOD	PORTION	CALS
fruit & juice bar	1 (3 fl oz)	75
gelatin pop	1 (1.5 oz)	31
ice coconut pineapple	½ cup (4 fl oz)	109
ice fruit w/ Equal	1 bar (1.7 oz)	12
ice lime	½ cup (4 fl oz)	75
ice pop	1 (2 fl oz)	42
Breyers		
Fruit Bars No Sugar Added	1 (1.75 oz)	25
Juice Bar Strawberry	1 (3.75 oz)	120
Soft Frozen Cup Lemonade	1 pkg (12 oz)	290
Soft Frozen Cup Strawberry	1 pkg (12 oz)	260
Carnation		
Cup Orange Sherbet	1 (5 oz)	150
Cup Orange Sherbet	1 (3 oz)	90

FOOD	PORTION	CALS
Cold Fusion		
Protein Juice Bar All Flavors	1 bar (3.8 oz)	130
Cool Creations		
Ice Pop	1 pop (2 oz)	50
Mickey Mouse Bar	1 (4 oz)	170
Surprise Pops	1 (2 oz)	60
CoolFruits		
Fruite Juice Freezer Pops Grape & Cherry	3 pops (3 oz)	70
Dole		
Fruit'n Juice Coconut	1 bar (4 oz)	210
Fruit'n Juice Lemonade	1 bar (4 oz)	120
Fruit'n Juice Lime	1 bar (4 oz)	110
Fruit'n Juice Peach Passion	1 bar (2.5 oz)	70
Fruit'n Juice Pineapple Coconut	1 bar (4 oz)	150
Fruit'n Juice Pineapple Orange Banana	1 bar (4 oz)	110
Fruit'n Juice Pineapple Orange Banana	1 bar (2.5 oz)	70
Fruit'n Juice Raspberry	1 bar (2.5 oz)	70
Fruit'n Juice Strawberry	1 bar (2.5 oz)	70
Fruit'n Juice Strawberry	1 bar (4 oz)	110
Grape No Sugar Added	1 bar (1.75 oz)	25
Raspberry	1 bar (1.75 oz)	45
Raspberry No Sugar Added	1 bar (1.75 oz)	25
Strawberry	1 bar (1.75 oz)	45
Strawberry No Sugar Added	1 bar (1.75 oz)	25
Edy's		
Sherbet Berry Rainbow	½ cup	130
Sherbet Key Lime	½ cup	130
Sherbet Orange Cream	½ cup	120
Sherbet Raspberry	½ cup	130
Sherbet Swiss Orange	½ cup	150
Sherbet Tropical Rainbow	½ cup	130
Whole Fruit Creamy Coconut	1 bar	120
Whole Fruit Lemonade	1 bar	80
Whole Fruit Lime	1 bar	80
Whole Fruit Orange & Cream	1 bar	80
Whole Fruit Peach	½ cup	90
Whole Fruit Strawberry	1 bar	80
Whole Fruit Tangerine	1 bar	80
Whole Fruit Tropical	1 bar	100
Whole Fruit Wild Berry	1 bar	80

FOOD	PORTION	CALS
Flintstones		
Push-Up Sherbet Treats	1 (2.75 oz)	100
Good Humor		
Great White	1 (3 oz)	70
Hyper Stripe	1 (2.7 oz)	80
Haagen-Dazs		
Sorbet Bars Chocolate	1 (2.7 oz)	80
Sorbet Bars Orange	1 (2.5 oz)	120
Sorbet Bars Raspberry & Vanilla Yogurt	1 (2.5 oz)	90
Sorbet Bars Strawberry & Vanilla Ice Cream	1 (2.5 oz)	110
Sorbet Chocolate	½ cup	120
Sorbet Mango	½ cup	120
Sorbet Orange	½ cup	120
Sorbet Orchard Peach	½ cup	130
Sorbet Raspberry	½ cup	120
Sorbet Strawberry	½ cup	120
Sorbet Zesty Lemon	½ cup	120
Minute Maid		
Fruit And Cream Swirl	1 tube (3 oz)	90
Fruit Bars	1 bar	60
Natural Choice		
Organic Banana	½ cup (3.6 oz)	110
Organic Blueberry	½ cup (3.6 oz)	100
Organic Kiwi	½ cup (3.6 oz)	110
Organic Lemon	½ cup (3.6 oz)	110
Organic Mango	½ cup (3.6 oz)	110
Organic Strawberry	½ cup (3.6 oz)	110
Organic Strawberry Kiwi	½ cup (3.6 oz)	110
Popsicle		
All Natural Ice Pops	1 (1.75 oz)	50
Bar Bart Simpson	1 (4 oz)	110
Bar Dora The Explorer	1 (4 oz)	100
Bar Fruti Holanda Lemon Lime	1 (3 oz)	90
Bar Fruti Holanda Strawberry	1 (3 oz)	90
Bar Incredible Hulk	1 (4 oz)	100
Bar Jimmy Neutron	1 (4 oz)	100
Bar Mega Warheads	1 (4 oz)	110
Bar Power Ranger	1 (4 oz)	100
Bar Spider Man	1 (4 oz)	100
Bar SpongeBob	1 (4 oz)	100

FOOD	PORTION	CALS
Big Stick Pops Big Reds	1 (3.5 oz)	70
Big Stick Pops Cherry Pineapple	1 (3.5 oz)	50
Bubble Play	1 (4 oz)	100
Creamsicle Bar	1 (2.5 oz)	100
Creamsicle Sugar Free	2 (3.3 oz)	40
Creamsicle Pop No Sugar Added	1 (1.75 oz)	25
Cup Cherry	1 (12 oz)	240
Cup Frostee Fudge	1 (10 oz)	280
Cup Lemon	1 (12 oz)	230
Cup Screwball	1 (3.75 oz)	110
Firecracker	1 (1.6 oz)	35
Fruita Holanda Coconut Bar	1 (3 oz)	120
Fudgsicle Bar	1 (2.5 oz)	90
Fudgsicle Bar Fat Free	1 (1.75 oz)	60
Fudgsicle Pop	1 (1.75 oz)	60
Fudgsicle Pops No Sugar Added	2 (1.75 oz)	90
Minis Fudge Bar	2 (2.4 oz)	80
Pop Great White	1 (1.75 oz)	45
Pop Lick-A-Color	1 (2 oz)	50
Pop Sherbet Cyclone	1 (1.8 oz)	50
Pop Towering Tornado	1 (3.5 oz)	90
Pop Ups Orange Burst	1 (2.75 oz)	80
Pop Ups Reckless Rainbow	1 (2.75 oz)	90
Pop Ups SpongeBob	1 (2.75 oz)	90
Pops Tropical Sugar Free	1 (1.75 oz)	15
Pops Wild Bunch	2 (2.2 oz)	60
Rainbow Floats	1 (1.75 oz)	60
Rainbow Pops	1 (1.75 oz)	45
Scribblers Juice Pops	2 (2.4 oz)	60
Shots	1 serv (1.7 oz)	40
Snow Cone	1 (7 oz)	30
Sugar Free Pops Orange Cherry Grape	1 (1.75 oz)	15
Super Mario Bros Bar	1 (4 oz)	100
Swirl Bar Cotton Candy	1 (2.6 oz)	60
Tingle Twister Ice Pops	1 (1.75 oz)	45
Torpedo Pop Cherry	1 (1.75 oz)	35
Silhouette		
Fat Free Fudge Bars	1	90
Tropicana		
Fruit Juice Bar Orange	1	45

FOOD	PORTION	CALS
Fruit Juice Bar Raspberry	1	45
Strawberry	1	45
Wawona		
Peach	1 pop	78
Strawberry	1 pop	77

JACKFRUIT

fresh	3.5 oz	70

JALAPENO (see PEPPERS)

JAM/JELLY/PRESERVES

all flavors jam	1 tbsp (0.7 oz)	48
all flavors jam	1 pkg (0.5 oz)	34
all flavors jelly	1 tbsp (0.7 oz)	52
all flavors jelly	1 pkg (0.5 oz)	38
all flavors preserve	1 tbsp (0.7 oz)	48
all flavors preserve	1 pkg (0.5 oz)	34
apple butter	1 tbsp (0.6 oz)	33
orange marmalade	1 tbsp (0.7 oz)	49
orange marmalade	1 pkg (0.5 oz)	34
Colac		
Jelly All Flavors	1 tbsp	37
Eden		
Cherry Butter	1 tbsp	35
Organic Apple Butter	1 tbsp	20
El Angel		
Strawberry Marmelade	1 tbsp	25
Jok'n'Al		
Low Carb Fruit Spreads All Flavors	1 tbsp	10
Matouk's		
Guava Jam	1 tbsp	50
Mango Jam	1 tbsp	50
Polaner		
All Fruit Grape	1 tbsp	40
All Fruit Peach	1 tbsp	40
All Fruit Raspberry	1 tbsp	40
Sarabeth's		
Spreadable Fruit Orange Apricot	1 tbsp	30
Spreadable Fruit Peach Apricot	1 tbsp	40
Spreadable Fruit Strawberry Raspberry	1 tbsp	40

FOOD	PORTION	CALS
Smucker's		
Cider Apple Butter	1 tbsp	45
Jam Concord Grape	1 tbsp	50
Jam Red Plum	1 tbsp	50
Jam Seedless Red Raspberry	1 tbsp	50
Jam Seedless Strawberry	1 tbsp	50
Jelly Apple	2 tbsp	50
Jelly Concord Grape	1 tbsp	50
Jelly Currant	1 tbsp	50
Jelly Elderberry	1 tbsp	50
Jelly Guava	1 tbsp	50
Jelly Mixed Fruit	2 tbsp	50
Low Sugar All Flavors	1 tbsp	25
Preserves All Flavors	1 tbsp	50
Simply Fruit All Flavors	1 tbsp	40
Sugar Free All Flavors	1 tbsp	10
Welch's		
Grape Jam	1 tbsp	50
Wild Thyme Farms		
Fruit Spreads Blackberry Currant Ginger	1 tsp	8
Fruit Spreads Mango Apricot	1 tsp	7

JAPANESE FOOD (see ASIAN FOOD, SUSHI)

JAVA PLUM

fresh	3	5
fresh	1 cup	82

JELLY (see JAM/JELLY/PRESERVE)

JICAMA

cooked	¾ cup	38
Frieda's		
Jicama	¾ cup	35

JUTE

cooked	1 cup	32

KALE

chopped cooked	½ cup	21
frzn chopped cooked	½ cup	20
raw chopped	½ cup	21
scotch chopped cooked	½ cup	18

FOOD	PORTION	CALS
KANGAROO		
kangaroo	3 oz	120
KEFIR		
kefir	7 oz	132
KETCHUP		
banana	1 tsp	10
ketchup	1 tbsp	16
ketchup	1 pkg (0.2 oz)	6
low sodium	1 tbsp	16
Atkins		
Ketch-A-Tomato	1 tbsp	10
Del Monte		
Ketchup	1 tbsp	15
Estee		
No Sugar Added	1 tbsp	15
Healthy Choice		
Ketchup	1 tbsp (0.5 oz)	9
Heinz		
Ketchup	1 tbsp	15
No Salt	1 tbsp	20
One Carb	1 tbsp	5
Organic	1 tbsp	20
Hunt's		
Ketchup	1 tbsp	15
No Salt Added	1 tbsp	20
Squeeze	1 tbsp	15
Keto		
Ketchup	1 tbsp	4
Muir Glen		
Organic	1 tbsp (0.6 oz)	15
Steel's		
Sugar Free	1 tbsp	10
Stokelys		
Tomato	1 tbsp	15
Tree Of Life		
Ketchup	1 tbsp (0.5 oz)	10
Walden Farms		
Calorie Free	1 tbsp	0

FOOD	PORTION	CALS
KIDNEY		
beef simmered	3 oz	134
lamb braised	3 oz	117
pork cooked	3 oz	128
pork cooked	1 cup	211
veal braised	3 oz	139
KIDNEY BEANS		
canned	½ cup	105
dried cooked	½ cup	112
Bush's		
Light Red	½ cup	110
Eden		
Organic Cannellini	½ cup (4.6 oz)	100
Hunt's		
Kidney Beans	½ cup (4.5 oz)	94
Progresso		
Dark Red	½ cup (4.5 oz)	110
Red	½ cup	110
Rienzi		
Cannellini	½ cup	80
Red	½ cup	90
S&W		
Dark Red Premium	½ cup (4.6 oz)	100
Van Camp's		
Dark Red	½ cup (4.6 oz)	90
Light Red	½ cup (4.6 oz)	90
KIWIS		
fresh	1 med	46
Chiquita		
Fresh	2 med (5.2 oz)	100
KNISH		
Gabila's		
Potato	1 (4.5 oz)	170
TAKE-OUT		
cheese & blueberry	1 (7 oz)	378
cheese & cherry	1 (7 oz)	378
everything	1 (7 oz)	221
kashe	1 (7 oz)	270

FOOD	PORTION	CALS
potato	1 med (3.5 oz)	166
potato	1 lg (7 oz)	332
potato w/ broccoli & cheese	1 (7 oz)	312
potato w/ spinach & mushroom	1 (7 oz)	214
KOHLRABI		
raw sliced	½ cup	19
sliced cooked	½ cup	24
Frieda's		
Kohlrabi	⅔ cup	25
KRILL		
fresh	1 oz	22
KUMQUATS		
fresh	1	12
LAMB		
cubed lean only braised	3 oz	190
cubed lean only broiled	3 oz	158
ground broiled	3 oz	240
leg lean & fat Choice roasted	3 oz	219
loin chop w/ bone lean & fat Choice broiled	1 chop (2.3 oz)	201
loin chop w/ bone lean only Choice broiled	1 chop (1.6 oz)	100
new zealand lean & fat cooked	3 oz	259
new zealand lean only cooked	3 oz	175
rib chop lean & fat Choice broiled	3 oz	307
rib chop lean only Choice broiled	3 oz	200
shank lean & fat Choice braised	3 oz	206
shank lean & fat Choice roasted	3 oz	191
shoulder chop w/ bone lean & fat Choice braised	1 chop (2.5 oz)	244
shoulder chop w/ bone lean only Choice braised	1 chop (1.9 oz)	152
sirloin lean & fat Choice roasted	3 oz	248
LAMB DISHES		
TAKE-OUT		
couscous lamb	1 serv	275
lamb curry	1 cup	257
lamb fattoush salad	1 serv	606
lamb tagine casserole	1 serv	261

FOOD	PORTION	CALS
moroccan pilaf w/ bulgur	1 serv	327
moussaka	5.6 oz	312
sambousa lamb & vegetable pocket	1	645
stew	¾ cup	124

LAMBSQUARTERS
chopped cooked	½ cup	29

LEEKS
chopped cooked	¼ cup	8
cooked	1 (4.4 oz)	38
freeze dried	1 tbsp	1
raw	1 (4.4 oz)	76
raw chopped	¼ cup	16
Frieda's		
Fresh	1 cup	50

LEMON
fresh	1 med	22
lemon extract	½ tsp	12
peel	1 tbsp	0
wedge	1	5
Sunkist		
Fresh	1 (2 oz)	15

LEMON CURD
lemon curd made w/ egg	2 tsp	29
lemon curd made w/ starch	2 tsp	28

LEMON EXTRACT
True Lemon		
Crystallized Lemon	1 pkg (1 g)	0
Virginia Dare		
Extract	1 tsp	22

LEMON GRASS
fresh	1 tbsp (5 g)	5
fresh	1 cup (2.4 oz)	66

LEMON JUICE
bottled	1 tbsp	3
fresh	1 tbsp	4
frzn	1 tbsp	3

FOOD	PORTION	CALS
Adina		
Hibiscus Lemon Bissap	8 oz	80
Canarino		
Italian Hot Lemon Beverage	1 cup	0
Realemon		
Juice	1 tsp (5 ml)	0
LEMONADE		
FROZEN		
as prep w/ water	1 cup	100
not prep	1 can (6 oz)	397
MIX		
powder as prep w/ water	9 fl oz	113
powder w/ equal	1 pitcher (67 oz)	40
Keto		
Kooler Pink	½ tsp	0
Low Carb Creations		
Lemonade as prep	1 serv	10
Raspberry as prep	1 serv	10
Sipper Sweets		
Sugar Free Low Carb	1 serv	8
READY-TO-DRINK		
Bolthouse Farms		
Mango Lemonade	8 oz	120
Hansen's		
Sparkling	8 fl oz	100
Sparkling Pink	8 fl oz	120
Hi-C		
Blast Pink	8 oz	120
Honest Ade		
Cranberry	8 oz	50
Langers		
Raspberry Lemonade	8 oz	120
White Cranberry Lemonade	8 oz	120
Minute Maid		
Chilled	8 oz	100
Coolers Pink	1 pouch (7 oz)	90
Light	8 oz	15
Naked Juice		
Just Made	8 oz	110

FOOD	PORTION	CALS
Ocean Spray		
Spritzer	8 oz	160
Odwalla		
Pure Squeezed	8 fl oz	96
Strawberry Quencher	8 fl oz	110
Purity Organic		
Lemonade	8 oz	123
Santa Cruz		
Organic	1 can	160
Organic Raspberry	1 can	120
Snapple		
Lemonade	8 oz	110
Super Sour	8 oz	130
T42		
Lemonade	8 oz	90
Pink	8 oz	90
Three Drinks		
Sparkling	12 oz	12
Tropicana		
Sugar Free	1 can	10
Turkey Hill		
Lemonade	1 cup	120
Raspberry	1 cup	120
Strawberry Kiwi	1 cup	120
Zeigler's		
Old Fashioned	8 oz	120

LENTILS

FOOD	PORTION	CALS
dried cooked	1 cup	231
Natural Touch		
Lentil Rice Loaf	1 in slice (3.2 oz)	170
Near East		
Lentil Pilaf as prep	1 cup	200
Shiloh Farms		
Organic Green not prep	¼ cup (1.6 oz)	150
TastyBite		
Bengal Lentils	½ pkg (5 oz)	190
Jodhpur Lentils	½ pkg (5 oz)	190
Madras Lentils	½ pkg (5 oz)	130

FOOD	PORTION	CALS
TAKE-OUT		
indian sambar	1 serv	236
middle eastern lentil salad	1 serv (4.5 oz)	158
yemiser selatta ethiopian lentil salad	1 serv (3 oz)	115
LETTUCE (see also SALAD)		
bibb	1 head (6 oz)	21
boston	1 head (6 oz)	21
boston	2 leaves	2
cornsalad field salad	1 cup (1.9 oz)	7
iceberg	1 head (19 oz)	70
iceberg	1 leaf	3
looseleaf shredded	½ cup	5
romaine shredded	½ cup	4
Dole		
Iceberg	1 cup (3 oz)	15
Romaine	1½ cups (3 oz)	15
Shredded	1½ cups (3 oz)	15
Earthbound Farm		
Romaine Salad Organic	1½ cups (2.9 oz)	15
Frieda's		
Limestone	⅔ cup	10
Green Giant		
Hearts Of Romaine	6 leaves (3 oz)	14
Mann's		
Romaine Jumbo Hearts	3 oz	15
Ready Pac		
Baby Arugula	4 cups	20
Bella Romaine	1½ cups	15
River Ranch		
Hearts Of Romaine	1½ cups	12
Romaine Chopped	1½ cups	10
Romaine Hearts	1½ cups	10
LILY ROOT		
dried	1 oz	89
fresh	1 oz	32
LIMA BEANS		
CANNED		
large	1 cup	191
lima beans	½ cup	88

FOOD	PORTION	CALS
Del Monte		
Green	½ cup	80
Eden		
Organic Baby	½ cup (4.6 oz)	100
S&W		
Small Green	½ cup (4.4 oz)	80
Van Camp's		
Butter Beans	½ cup (4.6 oz)	110
Veg-All		
Baby Green	½ cup	90
DRIED		
baby cooked	1 cup	229
cooked	½ cup	104
large cooked	1 cup	217
FROZEN		
cooked	½ cup	94
fordhook cooked	½ cup	85
Birds Eye		
Baby	½ cup	130
Butter Beans Speckled	½ cup	100
Fordhook	½ cup	100
Fresh Like		
Baby	3.5 oz	138
LIME		
fresh	1	20
Sunkist		
Fresh	1 (2 oz)	20
LIME JUICE		
bottled	1 tbsp	3
fresh	1 tbsp	4
limeade frzn	1 can (6 oz)	408
Adina		
Lime Mint Mojita	8 oz	70
Honest Ade		
Limeade	8 oz	50
Minute Maid		
Light Limeade	8 oz	15
Odwalla		
Summertime Lime	8 fl oz	90

FOOD	PORTION	CALS
Realime		
Juice	1 tsp (5 ml)	0
LING		
blue raw	3.5 oz	83
fresh baked	3 oz	95
fresh fillet baked	5.3 oz	168
LINGCOD		
baked	3 oz	93
fillet baked	5.3 oz	164

LIQUOR/LIQUEUR *(see also* BEER AND ALE, CHAMPAGNE, MALT, WINE*)*

FOOD	PORTION	CALS
7&7	1 serv	178
alabama slammer	1 serv	103
amaretto sour	1 serv	295
angel's kiss	1 serv	85
anisette	1 oz	111
antifreeze	1 serv	177
apricot brandy	1 oz	96
apricot sour	1 serv	164
aquavit	1 oz	65
b 52	1 serv	247
b&b	1 serv	75
bahama breeze	1 serv	70
bahama mama	1 serv	153
bailey's & amaretto	1 serv	184
banana colada	1 serv	376
bay breeze	1 serv	173
bend me over	1 serv	242
benedictine	1 oz	104
betsy ross	1 serv	206
black devil	1 serv	220
black russian	1 serv	184
bloody mary	1 serv	150
blue whale	1 serv	222
bourbon & soda	1 serv (4 oz)	105
bourbon sour	1 serv	166
brandy	2 oz	255
brandy alexander	1 serv	266
brandy sour	1 serv	164

FOOD	PORTION	CALS
bushwacher	1 serv	286
campari	2 oz	245
cherry heering	2 oz	245
coffee liqueur	1 serv (1.5 oz)	175
cognac	1 oz	67
cosmopolitan martini	1 serv	126
creme de almonde	1 oz	102
creme de banana	1 oz	99
creme de cassis	1 oz	82
creme de menthe	1 serv (1.5 oz)	186
curacao liqueur	1 oz	81
daiquiri	1 serv (2 oz)	112
daiquiri banana	1 serv	277
dark & stormy	1 serv	64
doctor pepper	1 serv	95
drambuie	2 oz	225
frozen daiquiri	1 serv	393
frozen daiquiri pineapple	1 serv	186
frozen tequila screwdriver	1 serv	159
fuzzy navel	1 serv	247
gibson	1 serv (4 oz)	254
gimlet vodka	1 serv	150
gin	1 serv (1.5 oz)	110
gin & tonic	1 serv (7.5 oz)	171
gin ricky	1 serv	114
grasshopper	1 serv	275
happy hawaiian	1 serv	434
harvey wallbanger	1 serv	198
head banger	1 serv	165
hot buttered rum	1 serv	219
hot toddy	1 serv	188
hurricane	1 serv	205
kamikaze	1 serv	136
long island iced tea	1 serv	292
lynchburg lemonade	1 serv	465
mai tai	1 serv	165
manhattan	1 serv	171
margarita	1 serv	173
margarita strawberry	1 serv	106
martini	1 serv (3 oz)	206

FOOD	PORTION	CALS
martini apple	1 serv	147
martini rum	1 serv	131
mellow yellow	1 serv	95
mexican grasshopper	1 serv	638
mint julep	1 serv	136
mississippi mud	1 serv	496
mudslide	1 serv	566
narragansett	1 serv	168
nutcracker	1 serv	730
old fashioned	1 serv	223
orange crush	1 serv	461
pain killer	1 serv	277
peppermint pattie	1 serv	344
pina colada	1 serv (4.5 oz)	245
planter's cocktail	1 serv	105
planter's punch	1 serv	233
presbyterian	1 serv	170
purple passion	1 serv	215
rob roy	1 serv	171
rum	1 serv (1.5 oz)	97
rum boogie	1 serv	134
rum cola	1 serv	209
rum highball	1 serv	170
rum punch	1 serv	448
rusty nail	1 serv	159
sake	1 serv (1 oz)	39
salty dog	1 serv	210
scotch & soda	1 serv	104
screwdriver rum	1 serv	166
sea breeze	1 serv	207
sex on the beach	1 serv	190
singapore sling	1 serv (4 oz)	115
slippery nipple	1 serv	142
sloe gin fizz	1 serv (2.5 oz)	132
snake bite	1 serv	362
sour rum	1 serv	156
southern comfort	1 serv (1.5 oz)	184
swizzle rum	1 serv	187
tequila	1 serv (1.5 oz)	117
tequila gimlet	1 serv	150

FOOD	PORTION	CALS
tequila sour	1 serv	156
tequila stinger	1 serv	221
tequila sunrise	1 serv (6.8 oz)	232
tom collins	1 serv (7.5 oz)	121
vermouth cassis	1 serv	97
vodka	1 serv (1.5 oz)	97
vodka sour	1 serv	138
vodka stinger	1 serv	378
whiskey	1 serv (1.5 oz)	105
whiskey sour	1 serv (3.5 oz)	162
white russian	1 serv	290
zombie	1 serv	235

LITCHI JUICE
Ceres
Litchi	8 oz	120

LIVER (see also PATE)
beef pan-fried	3 oz	175
chicken stewed	1 cup (5 oz)	219
duck raw	1 (1.5 oz)	60
goose raw	1 (3.3 oz)	125
lamb braised	3 oz	187
lamb fried	3 oz	202
pork braised	3 oz	140
sheep raw	3.5 oz	131
turkey simmered	1 cup (5 oz)	237
veal braised	3 oz	140
veal fried	3 oz	208

LIVER SUBSTITUTES
Sabra
Vegetarian Liver	1 oz	70

LLAMA
llama	3 oz	120

LOBSTER
northern cooked	1 cup	142
northern cooked	3 oz	83
northern raw	3 oz	77
northern raw	1 lobster (5.3 oz)	136

FOOD	PORTION	CALS
spiny steamed	1 (5.7 oz)	233
spiny steamed	3 oz	122
Progresso		
Lobster Sauce	½ cup (4.3 oz)	100
TAKE-OUT		
newburg	1 cup	485

LOGANBERRIES
frzn	1 cup	80

LONGANS
fresh	1	2

LOQUATS
fresh	1	5

LOTUS
root raw sliced	10 slices	45
root sliced cooked	10 slices	59
seeds dried	1 oz	94
Eden		
Root	1 serv (0.3 oz)	35
Frieda's		
Lotus Root Fresh	1 cup	50

LOX (see SALMON)

LUPINES
dried cooked	1 cup	197

LYCHEES
fresh	1	6
Frieda's		
Fresh	6 to 8 (3.5 oz)	60

MACADAMIA NUTS
dry roasted w/ salt	10–12 nuts (1 oz)	200
oil roasted	1 oz	204
Hawaiian Host		
Chocolate Covered	1 piece (0.5 oz)	53
Keto		
Chocolately Covered	1 oz	171
Maranatha		
Macadamia Butter	2 tbsp	230

FOOD	PORTION	CALS
Mauna Loa		
Chocolate Trio	9 pieces	200
Dry Roasted Salted	¼ cup	200
Dry Roasted Unsalted	¼ cup	200
Honey Roasted	¼ cup	210
Kona Coffee Glazed	¼ cup	190
Maui Onion & Garlic	¼ cup	200
Milk Chocolate Coated	3 pieces	230
Milk Chocolate Toffee	7 pieces	210
MACE		
ground	1 tsp	8
MACKEREL		
CANNED		
jack	1 can (12.7 oz)	563
jack	1 cup	296
Brunswick		
Jack In Water	2 oz	100
Chicken Of The Sea		
Jack In Tomato Sauce	¼ cup	70
Jack In Water	⅓ cup	90
Orleans		
Jack	¼ cup	90
DRIED		
Eden		
Bonito Flakes	2 tbsp	4
FRESH		
atlantic cooked	3 oz	223
atlantic raw	3 oz	174
jack baked	3 oz	171
jack fillet baked	6.2 oz	354
king baked	3 oz	114
king fillet baked	5.4 oz	207
pacific baked	3 oz	171
pacific fillet baked	6.2 oz	354
spanish cooked	1 fillet (5.1 oz)	230
spanish cooked	3 oz	134
spanish raw	3 oz	118
SMOKED		
atlantic	3.5 oz	296

FOOD	PORTION	CALS
MALANGA		
Frieda's		
Malanga	⅔ cup	90
MALT		
malt liquor	1 bottle (12 oz)	148
nonalcoholic	1 bottle (12 oz)	133
Skyy		
Blue	1 bottle	235
Sport	1 bottle	160
MALTED MILK		
chocolate as prep w/ milk	1 cup	179
chocolate flavor powder	3 heaping tsp (0.7 oz)	79
natural flavor as prep w/ milk	1 cup	186
natural flavor powder	3 heaping tsp (0.7 oz)	87
MAMMY-APPLE		
fresh	1	431
MANGO		
fresh	1	135
Tomorrow's Tropicals		
Fresh	½ (3.6 oz)	70
MANGO JUICE		
Ceres		
Mango	8 oz	120
Fresh Samantha		
Mango Mama	1 cup (8 oz)	120
Guzzler		
Mango Passion	8 fl oz	140
Langers		
Mongo Mango	8 oz	120
Naked Juice		
Mighty Mango	8 oz	120
MARGARINE		
squeeze	1 tsp	34
stick corn	1 stick (4 oz)	815
stick corn	1 tsp	34
tub corn	1 tsp	34
tub diet	1 tsp	17

FOOD	PORTION	CALS
Benecol		
Single Serve Light	1 pkg (0.3 oz)	30
Tub Light	1 tbsp (0.5 oz)	45
Tub Regular	1 tbsp (0.5 oz)	80
Blue Bonnet		
Light Stick	1 tbsp	50
Soft Spread	1 tbsp	60
Soft Spread Light	1 tbsp	40
Stick	1 tbsp	80
Brummel & Brown		
Spread Made With Yogurt	1 tbsp	45
Fleischmann's		
Soft Spread Light	1 tbsp	40
Soft Spread Original	1 tbsp	70
Soft Spread Unsalted	1 tbsp	70
Soft Spread w/ Olive Oil	1 tbsp	70
I Can't Believe Its Not Butter		
Regular Stick	1 tbsp	90
Soft Fat Free	1 tbsp	5
Soft Light	1 tbsp	50
Soft Regular	1 tbsp	80
Soft w/ Calcium	1 tbsp	50
Spray	5 sprays	0
Squeeze	1 tbsp	60
Stick Light	1 tbsp	50
Parkay		
Light Spread	1 tbsp	50
Original Spread	1 tbsp	60
Original Stick	1 tbsp	90
Spray	5 sprays	0
Spread + Calcium	1 tbsp	45
Squeeze	1 tbsp	70
Stick Light	1 tbsp	50
Promise		
Buttery Spread	1 tbsp	80
Stick	1 tbsp	90
Smart Balance		
Buttery Spread No Trans Fat	1 tbsp	80
Spectrum		
Essential Omega	1 tbsp	80

FOOD	PORTION	CALS
Spread	1 tbsp	88
Take Control		
Light	1 tbsp	45
Spread	1 tbsp (0.5 oz)	80

MARINADE *(see SAUCE)*

MARJORAM
dried	1 tsp	2

MARLIN
raw	3 oz	110

MARSHMALLOW
marshmallow	1 reg (0.3 oz)	23
marshmallow	1 cup (1.6 oz)	146
Gol D Lite		
Sugar Free	⅓ pkg (0.9 oz)	51

MATZO
egg	1 (1 oz)	111
egg & onion	1 (1 oz)	111
matzo ball	1 med	80
plain	1 (1 oz)	112
whole wheat	1 (1 oz)	99
Eddyleon		
Dark Chocolate Coated Egg Matzo	1 oz	97
Milk Chocolate Coated Egg Matzo	1 oz	97
Manischewitz		
Dark Chocolate Coated Egg	½ (1.5 oz)	90
Egg	1 (1.2 oz)	120
Matzo Meal	¼ cup (1 oz)	130
Streit's		
Egg	1 (1.1 oz)	120
Egg & Onion	1 (1 oz)	100
Passover	1 (1 oz)	110

MAYONNAISE
mayonnaise	1 tbsp	99
mayonnaise	1 cup	1577
reduced calorie	1 cup	556
reduced calorie	1 tbsp	34
sandwich spread	1 tbsp	60

FOOD	PORTION	CALS
Blue Plate		
Squeeze	1 tbsp	100
Hellman's		
Mayonnaise	1 tbsp	90
Spectrum		
Canola Squeeze	1 tbsp	100
Canola Squeeze Light Eggless Vegan	1 tbsp	35
Organic Dijon	1 tbsp	90
Organic Olive Oil	1 tbsp	100
Organic Roasted Garlic	1 tbsp	100
Organic Squeeze	1 tbsp	100
Organic Wasabi	1 tbsp	100

MAYONNAISE TYPE SALAD DRESSING

mayonnaise type salad dressing	1 cup	916
mayonnaise type salad dressing	1 tbsp	57
reduced calorie w/o cholesterol	1 cup	1084
reduced calorie w/o cholesterol	1 tbsp	68
Carb Options		
Whipped Dressing	1 tbsp	50
Nasoya		
Fat Free Nayonaise	1 tbsp	10
Nayonaise	1 tbsp	35

MEAT STICKS

jerky beef	1 piece (0.7 oz)	82
smoked	1 (0.7 oz)	110
Big Ones		
BBQ	1 (1 oz)	130
Hot n'spicy	1 (1 oz)	130
Original	1 (1 oz)	130
Teriyaki	1 (1 oz)	130
Jack Link's		
Beef Jerky Teriyaki	1 oz	80
Lowrey's		
Smokehouse Tender Hickory Smoked	1 pkg (1 oz)	80
Smokehouse Tender Original	1 pkg (1 oz)	60
Smokehouse Tender Peppered	1 pkg (1 oz)	60
Oberto		
Beef Jerky	1 pkg (1.3 oz)	100

FOOD	PORTION	CALS
Pemmican		
Homestyle Tender All Flavors	1 oz	80
Kippered Beef Original	1 pkg (1 oz)	60
Kippered Beef Peppered	1 pkg (1 oz)	60
Kippered Beef Sweet & Hot	1 pkg (1 oz)	70
Kippered Beef Teriyaki	1 pkg (1 oz)	60
Long Lasting Hot & Spicy	1 oz	60
Long Lasting Original	1 oz	60
Long Lasting Peppered	1 oz	60
Long Lasting Teriyaki	1 oz	70
Premium Cut Beef Jerky	1 oz	80
Premium Cut Turkey Peppered	1 oz	70
Premium Cut Turkey Sweet Smoked	1 oz	70
Shredded Beef Jerky All Flavors	¼ cup	80
Steak Tips All Flavors	1 oz	70
Rustlers Roundup		
Beef Jerky	1 serv (5 g)	20
Flamin' Hot	1 serv (8 g)	40
Smoky Steak	1 serv (0.8 oz)	60
Spicy	1 serv (0.5 oz)	70

MEAT SUBSTITUTES *(see also* BACON SUBSTITUTES, CANADIAN BACON SUBSTITUTES, CHICKEN SUBSTITUTES, HAMBURGER SUBSTITUTES, SAUSAGE SUBSTITUTES, TURKEY SUBSTITUTES*)*

FOOD	PORTION	CALS
Ken & Robert's		
Veggie Pockets	1 (4.5 oz)	250
Veggie Pockets Bar B Que	1 (4.5 oz)	290
Veggie Pockets Broccoli & Cheddar	1 (4.5 oz)	250
Veggie Pockets Greek	1 (4.5 oz)	250
Veggie Pockets Indian	1 (4.5 oz)	260
Veggie Pockets Pizza	1 (4.5 oz)	270
Veggie Pockets Pot Pie	1 (4.5 oz)	250
Veggie Pockets Potato & Cheddar	1 (4.5 oz)	260
Veggie Pockets Santa Fe	1 (4.5 oz)	250
Veggie Pockets Tex Mex	1 (4.5 oz)	260
Lightlife		
Balogna	4 slices (2 oz)	60
Gimme Lean Ground Beef	1 serv (2 oz)	50
Smart BBQ	¼ cup	70
Smart Cutlet Salisbury Steak	1 (4.5 oz)	130

FOOD	PORTION	CALS
Smart Deli Country Ham	4 slices (2 oz)	90
Smart Deli Pastrami Style	4 slices (2 oz)	60
Smart Deli Pepperoni Style	13 slices (1 oz)	45
Smart Ground Original	⅓ cup (1.9 oz)	80
Smart Ground Taco Burrito	⅓ cup (2 oz)	70
Smart Menu Crumbles	⅓ cup	80
Smart Menu Meatless Meatballs	5	160
Smart Menu Steak Strips	1 serv (3 oz)	80
Smart Tex Mex	¼ cup	50
Loma Linda		
Dinner Cuts	2 slices (3.2 oz)	90
Nuteena	⅜ in slice (1.9 oz)	160
Sandwich Spread	¼ cup (1.9 oz)	80
Savory Dinner Loaf Mix not prep	⅓ cup (0.9 oz)	90
Swiss Stake	1 piece (3.2 oz)	120
Tender Bits	6 pieces (3 oz)	110
Tender Rounds	6 pieces (2.8 oz)	120
Vita Burger Chunks not prep	¼ cup (0.7 oz)	70
Vita Burger Granules	3 tbsp (0.7 oz)	70
Morningstar Farms		
Burger Style Recipe Crumbles	⅔ cup (1.9 oz)	80
Ground Meatless	½ cup (1.9 oz)	60
Harvest Burger Recipe Crumbles	½ cup (2 oz)	70
Quarter Prime	1 patty (3.4 oz)	140
Natural Touch		
Dinner Entree	1 patty (3 oz)	220
Loaf Mix not prep	4 tbsp (1 oz)	100
Stroganoff Mix not prep	4 tbsp (0.8 oz)	90
Taco Mix not prep	3 tbsp (0.6 oz)	60
Vegan Burger Crumbles	½ cup (1.9 oz)	60
Quorn		
Grounds	⅔ cup (3 oz)	80
Meatballs	4 (2.4 oz)	110
Soy7		
Burger Bits as prep	½ cup	60
Burger Mix as prep	1 serv (3.2 oz)	120
Recipe Strips as prep	¾ cup	70
Taco Mix as prep	¼ cup	70
Worthington		
Beef Style Meatless	⅜ in slice (1.9 oz)	110

FOOD	PORTION	CALS
Bolono	3 slices (2 oz)	80
Choplets	2 slices (3.2 oz)	90
Corned Beef Meatless	4 slices (2 oz)	140
Country Stew	1 cup (8.4 oz)	210
Dinner Roast	¼ in slice (3 oz)	180
FriPats	1 patty (2.2 oz)	130
Multigrain Cutlets	2 slices (3.2 oz)	100
Numete	⅜ in slice (1.9 oz)	130
Prime Stakes	1 piece (3.2 oz)	120
Prosage Roll	⅝ in slice (1.9 oz)	140
Protose	⅜ in slice (1.9 oz)	130
Yves		
Veggie Bologna	4 slices (2.2 oz)	70
Veggie Ground Italian	⅓ cup (2 oz)	60
Veggie Ground Round Italian	⅓ cup (1.9 oz)	60
Veggie Ground Round Original	2 oz	60
Veggie Pizza Pepperoni Slices	1 serv (1.7 oz)	70
Veggie Salami Deli Slices	1 serv (2.2 oz)	90

MELON
melon balls frzn	1 cup	55
Frieda's		
Camouflage	1 cup (5 oz)	50
SpriteMelon	1 (10.5 oz)	115
Temptation	⅒ melon (4.7 oz)	55

MEXICAN FOOD (see SALSA, SPANISH FOOD, TORTILLA)

MILK
CANNED
condensed sweetened	1 cup	982
condensed sweetened	1 oz	123
evaporated	½ cup	169
evaporated skim	½ cup	99
Carnation		
Evaporated	2 tbsp	40
Evaporated Fat Free	2 tbsp	25
Sweetened Condensed	⅓ cup	330
Meyenberg		
Evaporated Goat Milk	8 oz	145

FOOD	PORTION	CALS
Pet		
Evaporated	2 tbsp	40
DRIED		
buttermilk	1 tbsp	25
nonfat instantized	1 pkg (3.2 oz)	244
Carnation		
Nonfat	⅓ cup	80
Meyerberg		
Instant Goat Milk as prep	1 cup	142
Sanalac		
Powder	¼ cup (0.8 oz)	85
REFRIGERATED		
1%	1 cup	102
1%	1 qt	409
1% protein fortified	1 qt	477
1% protein fortified	1 cup	119
2%	1 cup	121
2%	1 qt	485
buffalo	7 oz	224
buttermilk	1 cup	99
buttermilk	1 qt	396
camel	7 oz	160
donkey	7 oz	86
goat	1 qt	672
goat	1 cup	168
human	1 cup	171
indian buffalo	1 cup	236
low sodium	1 cup	149
mare	7 oz	98
nonfat	1 cup	86
nonfat protein fortified	1 qt	400
sheep	1 cup	264
whole	1 cup	150
Borden		
Fat Free Skim	1 cup	80
Hood		
Carb Countdown	8 oz	138
Carb Countdown 2%	8 oz	100
Carb Countdown Fat Free	8 oz	78

FOOD	PORTION	CALS
Horizon Organic		
Fat Free	1 cup (8 oz)	80
Lactaid		
1% Lowfat	1 cup	110
2% Reduced Fat	1 cup	130
Calcium Fortified	1 cup	80
Fat Free	1 cup	90
Whole	1 cup	150
Land O Lakes		
1% Lowfat	1 carton (10 oz)	120
Fat Free	1 carton (10 oz)	100
Whole	1 carton (10 oz)	180
Meyenberg		
Goat Milk	8 oz	142
Goat Milk Low Fat	8 oz	89
NutraBalance		
LactaCare	1 pkg (8 oz)	500
Organic Valley		
Low Fat	1 cup	100
Nonfat	1 cup	80
Reduced Fat	1 cup	130
Whole	1 cup	150
Stonyfield Farm		
Organic Whole Milk	1 cup (8 oz)	180
Organic Whole Milk Vanilla	1 cup (8 oz)	230
Turkey Hill		
Cool Moos 2% Reduced Fat	1 cup	130
Cool Moos Whole Milk	1 cup	160
MILK DRINKS		
chocolate milk	1 cup	208
chocolate milk	1 qt	833
chocolate milk 1%	1 cup	158
chocolate milk 1%	1 qt	630
chocolate milk 2%	1 cup	179
Cal-C		
Orange Tangerine	8 oz	70
Peach Mango	8 oz	70
Strawberry Citrus	8 oz	70

FOOD	PORTION	CALS
Cocio		
Chocolate Milk	1 bottle	225
Garelick		
Colossal Coffee	1 cup	145
Ultimate Chocolate	1 cup	150
Hershey's		
Chocolate Milk Fat Free	1 bottle	160
Chocolate Milk Reduced Fat	1 bottle	200
Hood		
Carb Countdown Chocolate Milk	8 oz	100
Horizon Organic		
Lowfat Chocolate Milk	1 cup (8 oz)	160
Keto		
Chocolate Milk Mix	1 scoop	36
Land O Lakes		
Chocolate	1 cup (8.4 oz)	200
Nesquik		
Chocolate as prep w/ lowfat milk	1 cup	210
Chocolate No Sugar as prep w/ lowfat milk	1 cup	130
Double Chocolate as prep w/ lowfat milk	1 cup	210
Ready-To-Drink Banana	1 cup	200
Ready-To-Drink Chocolate	1 cup	200
Ready-To-Drink Double Chocolate	1 cup	200
Ready-To-Drink Fat Free Chocolate	1 cup	160
Ready-To-Drink Strawberry	1 cup	200
Ready-To-Drink Very Vanilla	1 cup	200
Strawberry as prep w/ lowfat milk	1 cup	210
Vanilla as prep w/ lowfat milk	1 cup	210
Organic Valley		
Chocolate Milk Reduced Fat	1 cup	180
Quaker		
Chocolate	8 oz	140
Strawberry	8 oz	130
Vanilla	8 oz	130
Quik		
Banana Lowfat	1 cup (8.4 oz)	200
Banana Powder	2 tbsp (0.8 oz)	90
Chocolate	1 cup (8.4 oz)	230
Chocolate Lowfat	1 carton (8.4 oz)	200
Cookies n Cream Powder	2 tbsp (0.8 oz)	100

FOOD	PORTION	CALS
Strawberry	1 cup (8.4 oz)	230
Strawberry Lowfat	1 carton (8.4 oz)	210
Strawberry Powder	2 tbsp (0.8 oz)	90
Rosa's Original		
Horchata All Flavors	8 oz	160
Turkey Hill		
Cool Moos Chocolate 1% Lowfat	1 cup	180
Cool Moos Orange Cream 1% Lowfat	1 cup	190
Cool Moos Strawberry 1% Lowfat	1 cup	160
Cool Moos Vanilla 1% Lowfat	1 cup	160

MILK SUBSTITUTES

FOOD	PORTION	CALS
imitation milk	1 qt	600
imitation milk	1 cup	150
8th Continent		
Soymilk Low Fat Chocolate	1 bottle (8 oz)	140
Soymilk Low Fat Original	1 bottle (8 oz)	80
Soymilk Low Fat Vanilla	1 bottle (8 oz)	90
Almond Breeze		
Chocolate	8 oz	115
Original	8 oz	57
Original Unsweetened	8 oz	40
Vanilla	8 oz	91
Better Than Milk		
Rice Original	2 tbsp (0.66 oz)	78
Rice Original Light	2 tbsp (0.66 oz)	66
Rice Vanilla	2 tbsp (0.66 oz)	78
Rice Vanilla Light	2 tbsp (0.66 oz)	66
Soy Carob	2 tbsp (1 oz)	90
Soy Chocolate	2 tbsp (1.1 oz)	112
Soy Light	2 tbsp (0.66 oz)	73
Soy Original	2 tbsp (0.8 oz)	100
Soy Vanilla	2 tbsp (0.7 oz)	77
EdenBlend		
Organic	8 oz	120
Edensoy		
Organic Light	8 oz	93
Organic Light Vanilla	8 oz	120
Galaxy		
Veggie Milk Chocolate	1 cup (8 oz)	150

FOOD	PORTION	CALS
Veggie Milk Original	1 cup (8 oz)	110
Hansen's		
Soy Smoothie Lemon Chiffon	8 oz	150
Soy Smoothie Orange Dream	8 oz	150
Harmony Farms		
Original Rice Beverage	1 cup (8 oz)	90
Harmony House		
Enriched Rice Beverage	1 cup (8 oz)	90
Enriched Soy Beverage	1 cup (8 oz)	90
Original Soy Beverage	1 cup (8 oz)	90
Keto		
Low Carb Mix	1 scoop	54
NutraBalance		
NuTaste	1 pkg (8 oz)	80
Pacific Foods		
Almond Low Fat Original	1 cup	70
Almond Low Fat Vanilla	1 cup	100
Multi Grain Low Fat Original	1 cup	160
Oat Organic Low Fat Original	1 cup	130
Oat Organic Low Fat Vanilla	1 cup	130
Rice Low Fat Plain	1 cup	130
Rice Low Fat Vanilla	1 cup	130
Soy Organic Unsweetened Original	1 cup	90
Soy Select Low Fat Plain	1 cup	70
Soy Select Low Fat Vanilla	1 cup	80
Soy Ultra	1 cup	130
Soy Ultra Plain	1 cup	120
Rice Dream		
Carob	1 box (8 oz)	150
Chocolate	1 box (8 oz)	170
Chocolate Enriched	1 box (8 oz)	170
Organic Original	1 box (8 oz)	120
Organic Original Enriched	1 box (8 oz)	120
Vanilla	1 box (8 oz)	130
Vanilla Enriched	1 box (8 oz)	130
Silk		
Chocolate	1 cup	140
Organic Plain	1 cup	100
Vanilla	1 bottle (11 oz)	140

FOOD	PORTION	CALS
Soy Dream		
Carob	8 oz	210
Chocolate Enriched	8 oz	210
Original	8 oz	140
Original Enriched	8 oz	140
Vanilla	8 oz	170
Vanilla Enriched	8 oz	140
Tree Of Life		
Original Rice Beverage	1 cup	90
Vitamite		
Non-Dairy	1 cup (8 oz)	110
Vitasoy		
Classic Original	8 oz	120
Complete Original	8 oz	70
Complete Vanille	8 oz	50
Creamy Original	8 oz	110
Green Tea Soymilk	8 oz	120
Light Original	8 oz	60
Light Chocolate	8 oz	100
Lite Vanilla	8 oz	70
Original Unsweetened	8 oz	80
Rich Chocolate	8 oz	160
Smooth Vanilla	8 oz	120
Vanilla Delight	8 oz	120
White Wave		
Mocha	1 cup	140
MILKFISH (AWA)		
baked	3 oz	162
MILKSHAKE		
chocolate	1 serv (10 oz)	393
malted milk shake	1 serv (10 oz)	402
vanilla	1 serv (10 oz)	379
Breyers		
Quick Vanilla	1 serv (10 oz)	320
Carb Options		
Chocolate Delite	1 can (11 oz)	190
Creamy Vanilla	1 can (11 oz)	190
Hershey's		
Chocolate	1 bottle	270

FOOD	PORTION	CALS
Cookies 'N' Cream	1 bottle	280
Strawberry	1 bottle	280
Vanilla Cream	1 bottle	320
Nesquik		
Ready-To-Drink	1 cup	170

MILLET
cooked	1 cup (6.1 oz)	207

MINERAL WATER (see WATER)

MISO
dried	1 oz	86
miso	½ cup	284
Eden		
Organic Genmai	1 tbsp	25
Tekka	1 tsp	5

MOLASSES
blackstrap	1 tbsp (0.7 oz)	47
blackstrap	1 cup (11.5 oz)	771
molasses	1 tbsp (0.7 oz)	53
molasses	1 cup (11.5 oz)	873
Brer Rabbit		
Dark	1 tbsp	60
Grandma's		
Robust	1 tbsp	60
Mott's		
Sulphured	1 tbsp	50
Unsulphured	1 tbsp	50

MONKFISH
baked	3 oz	82

MOOSE
roasted	3 oz	114

MOTH BEANS
dried cooked	1 cup	207

MOUSSE
FROZEN
Sara Lee
Chocolate	⅕ pkg (4.3 oz)	400

FOOD	PORTION	CALS
TAKE-OUT		
chocolate	½ cup (7.1 oz)	447
orange	½ cup	87
MUFFIN		
FROZEN		
Pepperidge Farm		
Blueberry	1 (2 oz)	180
Bran w/ Raisins	1 (2 oz)	180
Corn	1 (2 oz)	190
Orange Cranberry	1 (2 oz)	180
Sara Lee		
Blueberry	1 (2.2 oz)	220
Corn	1 (2.2 oz)	260
MIX		
blueberry	1 (1.75 oz)	149
corn	1 (1.75 oz)	160
wheat bran as prep	1 (1.75 oz)	138
Betty Crocker		
Apple Cinnamon as prep	1	170
Apple Streusel as prep	1	210
Banana Nut as prep	1	170
Cranberry Orange as prep	1	150
Double Chocolate as prep	1	220
Golden Corn as prep	1	160
Lemon Poppyseed as prep	1	180
Sunkist Lemon Poppyseed as prep	1	190
Twice The Blueberries as prep	1	140
Wild Blueberry as prep	1	170
Carbsense		
Honey Bran not prep	1 serv (1.3 oz)	120
Hodgson Mill		
Bran	¼ cup (1.3 oz)	130
Cornbread	¼ cup (1.3 oz)	130
Whole Wheat	¼ cup (1.3 oz)	130
Jiffy		
Apple Cinnamon as prep	1	190
Banana Nut as prep	1	180
Blueberry as prep	1	190
Bran w/ Dates as prep	1	170

FOOD	PORTION	CALS
Corn as prep	1	180
Raspberry as prep	1	180
Ketogenics		
Apple Cinnamon Bran as prep	1	190
Chocolate Chip as prep	1	215
Wild Blueberry as prep	1	190
MiniCarb		
Apple Cinnamon as prep	1	225
Sweet Corn as prep	1	225
Miracle Maize		
Country Style as prep	1	155
Sweet as prep	1	180
Sweet Rewards		
Low Fat Apple Cinnamon as prep	1	140
READY-TO-EAT		
blueberry	1 (2 oz)	158
oat bran wheat free	1 (2 oz)	154
toaster type blueberry	1	103
toaster type corn	1	114
toaster type wheat bran w/ raisins	1 (1.3 oz)	106
Atkins		
Blueberry	1 (3.5 oz)	210
Dolly Madison		
Blueberry	1 (1.75 oz)	170
Mega Banana Nut	1 (5.9 oz)	620
Mega Blueberry	1 (5.9 oz)	590
Mega Chocolate Chip	1 (5.9 oz)	620
Mega Cranberry Orange	1 (5.9 oz)	590
Mega Cream Cheese	1 (5.9 oz)	620
Dutch Mill		
Apple Oat Bran	1 (2 oz)	180
Banana Walnut	1 (2 oz)	220
Carrot	1 (2 oz)	190
Corn	1 (2 oz)	190
Cranberry Orange	1 (2 oz)	170
Raisin Bran	1 (2 oz)	230
Fred's Incredible Muffins		
All Flavors	1 (2.5 oz)	100
Hostess		
Banana Bran Low Fat	1 (2.7 oz)	240

FOOD	PORTION	CALS
Blueberry Low Fat	1 (2.7 oz)	230
Hearty Banana Nut	1 (5.9 oz)	620
Hearty Blueberry	1 (5.9 oz)	590
Hearty Chocolate Chip	1 (5.9 oz)	620
Hearty Cranberry Orange	1 (5.9 oz)	590
Hearty Cream Cheese	1 (5.9 oz)	620
Mini Banana Walnut	3 (1.2 oz)	160
Mini Blueberry	3 (1.2 oz)	150
Mini Chocolate Chip	3 (1.2 oz)	160
Mini Cinnamon Apple	3 (1.2 oz)	160
Mini Cinnamon Bites	3 (1.1 oz)	130
Mini Rocky Road	3 (1.2 oz)	160
Muffin Loaf Apple Spice	1 (3.7 oz)	430
Muffin Loaf Banana Nut	1 (3.8 oz)	460
Muffin Loaf Blueberry	1 (3.8 oz)	440
Muffin Loaf Chocolate Chocolate Chip	1 (3.8 oz)	400
Muffin Loaf Raspberry	1 (3.8 oz)	440
Oat Bran	1 (1.5 oz)	160
Natural Ovens		
Blueberry	1 (2.5 oz)	180
Carrot Nut	1 (2.5 oz)	170
Raisin Bran	1 (2.5 oz)	170
Otis Spunkmeyer		
Apple Cinnamon	1 (4 oz)	420
Cheese Streusel	½ muffin (2 oz)	220
Low Fat Wild Blueberry	1 (2.25 oz)	200
Mayport Almond Poppy Seed	½ muffin (2 oz)	210
Mayport Banana Nut	1 (2.25 oz)	270
Mayport Chocolate Chocolate Chip	1 (2.25 oz)	260
Mayport Chocolate Chip	½ muffin (2 oz)	240
Mayport Cinnamon Spice	½ muffin (2 oz)	230
Mayport Corn	½ muffin (2 oz)	230
Mayport Harvest Bran	1 (2.25 oz)	240
Mayport Lemon	½ muffin (2 oz)	230
Mayport Low Fat Apple Cinnamon	1 (4 oz)	380
Mayport Low Fat Banana Nut	1 (4 oz)	350
Mayport Low Fat Chocolate Chocolate Chip	1 (4 oz)	370
Mayport Orange	½ muffin (2 oz)	230
Mayport Pineapple	½ muffin (2 oz)	210
Mayport Wild Blueberry	1 (2.25 oz)	230

FOOD	PORTION	CALS
Uncle Wally's		
Chocolate Passion	1 (2 oz)	130
Cranberry Orange Supreme	1 (2 oz)	130
Fat Free Apple Cinnamon Delight	1 (2 oz)	110
Fat Free Wild Blueberry Bliss	1 (2 oz)	120
Golden Waves Of Corn	1 (2 oz)	120
Honey Raisin Bran	1 (2 oz)	130
No Nut Banana	1 (2 oz)	130
VitaMuffin		
Apple Berry Bran	1 (2 oz)	100
Blue Bran	1 (2 oz)	100
Cran Bran	1 (2 oz)	100
Deep Chocolate	1 (4 oz)	200
Multi Bran	1 (2 oz)	100
VitaTops Apple Berry Bran	1 (2 oz)	100
VitaTops Blue Bran	1 (2 oz)	100
VitaTops Cran Bran	1 (2 oz)	100
VitaTops Deep Chocolate	1 (2 oz)	100
VitaTops MultiBran	1 (2 oz)	100
TAKE-OUT		
corn	1 lg (2.5 oz)	214
raisin bran lowfat	1 (4 oz)	270
MULBERRIES		
fresh	1 cup	61
MULLET		
striped cooked	3 oz	127
striped raw	3 oz	99
MUNG BEANS		
dried cooked	1 cup	213
MUNGO BEANS		
dried cooked	1 cup	190
MUSHROOMS		
CANNED		
chanterelle	3.5 oz	12
pieces	½ cup	19
straw	1 cup (6.4 oz)	58
whole	1 (0.4 oz)	3

FOOD	PORTION	CALS
DRIED		
chanterelle	1 oz	25
cloud ear	1 (5 g)	13
cloud ears	1 cup (1 oz)	80
shiitake	4 (0.5 oz)	44
straw	1 piece (6 g)	2
tree ear	½ cup (0.4 oz)	36
wood ear mok yee	½ cup (0.4 oz)	25
Eden		
Shitake	6 (0.4 oz)	35
Frieda's		
Chanterelle	2 pieces (4 g)	15
Wood Ear	3 pieces (4 g)	15
FRESH		
chanterelle	3.5 oz	11
enoki raw	1 (4 in)	2
morel	3.5 oz	9
oyster raw	1 sm (0.5 oz)	6
oyster raw	1 lg (5.2 oz)	55
portabella	1 serv (2 oz)	14
raw	1 (0.5 oz)	5
raw sliced	½ cup	9
shitake cooked	4 (2.5 oz)	40
sliced cooked	½ cup	21
whole cooked	1 (0.4 oz)	3
Frieda's		
Enoki	¼ pkg (1 oz)	10
MUSKRAT		
roasted	3 oz	199
MUSSELS		
blue raw	3 oz	73
blue raw	1 cup	129
fresh blue cooked	3 oz	147
MUSTARD		
dry mustard	1 tsp	15
organic yellow	1 tsp	5
yellow ready-to-use	1 tsp	5

FOOD	PORTION	CALS
Boar's Head		
Delicatessen Style	1 tsp (5 g)	0
Honey	1 tsp (5 g)	10
Country Cupboard		
Smokey Garlic or Horseradish	1 tsp	10
Eden		
Organic Stone Ground	1 tsp	0
French's		
Classic Yellow	1 tsp	0
Gulden's		
Spicy Brown	1 tsp	5
Hebrew National		
Deli	1 tsp	4
Hunt's		
Mustard	1 tsp (5 g)	3
Kosciuszko		
Spicy Brown	1 tsp	5
Luzianne		
Creole Mustard	1 tbsp	10
Tree Of Life		
Dijon	1 tsp (5 g)	0
Dijon Imported	1 tsp (5 g)	5
Stone Ground	1 tsp (5 g)	0
Yellow	1 tsp (5 g)	0
Wild Thyme Farms		
Chili Pepper Garlic	1 tsp	5
Dill Horseradish	1 tsp	5
MUSTARD GREENS		
fresh chopped cooked	½ cup	11
fresh raw chopped	½ cup	7
frozen chopped cooked	½ cup	14
Birds Eye		
Chopped	1 cup	30
NATTO		
natto	½ cup	187
NAVY BEANS		
CANNED		
navy	1 cup	296

FOOD	PORTION	CALS
DRIED		
cooked	1 cup	259
NECTARINE		
fresh	1	67
Chiquita		
Fresh	1 med (4.9 oz)	70
NEUFCHATEL		
neufchatel	1 pkg (3 oz)	221
neufchatel	1 oz	74
Back To Nature		
Organic	⅛ pkg (1 oz)	70
Horizon Organic		
Neufchatel	2 tbsp	70
Organic Valley		
Neufchatel	1 oz	70
NOODLE DISHES (see PASTA DINNERS)		
NOODLES		
cellophane	1 cup	492
chow mein	1 cup (1.6 oz)	237
egg	1 cup (38 g)	145
egg cooked	1 cup (5.6 oz)	213
japanese soba cooked	1 cup (4 oz)	113
japanese somen cooked	1 cup (6.2 oz)	231
korean acorn noodles not prep	2 oz	195
rice cooked	1 cup (6.2 oz)	192
spinach/egg cooked	1 cup (5.6 oz)	211
A Taste Of Thai		
Rice Wide	2 oz	200
Annie Chun's		
Chow Mein	2 oz	200
Rice	2 oz	210
Rice Hunan	2 oz	210
Rice Pad Thai	2 oz	210
Rice Pad Thai Basil	2 oz	210
Azumaya		
Asian Style Thin Cut	1 cup	210
Catelli		
Egg	3 oz	317

FOOD	PORTION	CALS
Chun King		
Chow Mein	½ cup (1 oz)	137
Eden		
Kudzu	2 oz	200
Hodgson Mill		
Four Color Veggie Egg	2 oz	200
Whole Wheat Egg not prep	2 oz	190
La Choy		
Chow Mein	½ cup (1 oz)	137
Chow Mein Crispy Wide	½ cup (1 oz)	148
Rice	½ cup (1 oz)	121
Manischewitz		
Fine Yolk Free	1½ cups	210
Fine Egg	1½ cups	220
Wide Yolk Free	1¾ cups	210
Nasoya		
Chinese	1 cup	210
Japanese	1 cup	210
Spinach	1 cup	210
Pennsylvania Dutch		
Yolk Free Ribbons as prep	1½ cups	210
NOPALES		
cooked	1 cup (5.2 oz)	23
raw sliced	1 cup (3 oz)	14
NUTMEG		
ground	1 tsp	12

NUTRITION SUPPLEMENTS *(see also* CEREAL BARS, ENERGY BARS, ENERGY DRINKS*)*

FOOD	PORTION	CALS
Boost		
High Protein Powder Vanilla as prep w/ water	1 serv (8 oz)	200
DiabetiTrim		
Shake French Vanilla	1 pkg	90
Enlive!		
Drink All Flavors	1 box (8.1 oz)	300
Ensure		
Creamy Milk Chocolate Shake	1 can (8 oz)	350
Plus Vanilla Shake	1 bottle (8 oz)	350

FOOD	PORTION	CALS
GeniSoy		
Soy Natural Protein Powder	1 scoop (1 oz)	100
Glucerna		
Shakes All Flavors	1 can (8 oz)	220
Juven		
Grape w/ Arginine, Glutamine, HMB	1 pkg (0.8 oz)	90
Orange w/ HMB	1 pkg (0.8 oz)	90
Met-Rx		
Lite	1 pkg (1.6 oz)	170
Mass Action	1 scoop (0.9 oz)	60
Original	1 pkg (2.5 oz)	250
Protein Shake	1 can	200
Ultra	1 pkg (2.6 oz)	250
Nature Made		
CalBurst	1 piece	15
Nestle		
Additions	2⅓ tsp (0.7 oz)	100
NutraBalance		
EggPro	1 tbsp (7.5 g)	30
Nutribar		
Shake Chocolate Supreme as prep w/ 2% milk	1 serv (10 oz)	262
Shake Vanilla as prep w/ 2% milk	1 (10 oz)	259
PermaLean		
Protein Powder Bodacious Berry	1 scoop (1 oz)	104
Protein Powder Chocoholic Chocolate	1 scoop (1 oz)	104
Pounds Off		
All Flavors	1 bar (2.1 oz)	210
PowerBar		
Powergel All Flavors	1 pkg (1.4 oz)	120
Pria		
Complete Shake Creamy Milk Chocolate	1 pkg (11.6 oz)	170
Complete Shake French Vanilla	1 pkg (11.6 oz)	170
Resource		
Beneprotein Protein Powder	1 scoop	25
Optisource High Protein Drink	1 box (4 oz)	100
Slim-Fast		
Optima Ready-To-Drink All Flavors	1 can	180
Optima Shake Mix Chocolate Royale as prep with fat free milk	1 serv	190

FOOD	PORTION	CALS
Optima Shake Mix French Vanilla as prep w/ fat free milk	1 serv	200
Viactiv		
Calcium Chews	1	20
Chocolate	1	20
Vitasoy		
Weight Management Meal All Flavors	1 bottle (10 oz)	200
NUTS MIXED *(see also individual names)*		
dry roasted w/ peanuts	1 oz	169
dry roasted w/ peanuts salted	1 oz	169
mixed nuts chocolate covered	¼ cup (1.5 oz)	240
oil roasted w/ peanuts	1 oz	175
oil roasted w/ peanuts salted	1 oz	175
oil roasted w/o peanuts	1 oz	175
oil roasted w/o peanuts salted	1 oz	175
Estee		
Chocolate Covered Fruit & Nut Mix Fructose Sweetened	¼ cup	210
Here's Howe		
Royal Mixed Nuts	1 oz	180
Judy's		
Sugar Free Mixed Nut Brittle	¼ piece (1 oz)	120
Kind		
Nut Delight	1 bar (1.4 oz)	203
Maranatha		
Cashew Macadamia Butter	2 tbsp	210
Tamari Organic	¼ cup	160
Tamari Roasted	¼ cup	160
Mauna Loa		
Macadamia Mixed	¼ cup	190
Macadamias & Cashews	¼ cup	100
Organic Trails		
Tamari Roasted Nuts & Seeds	¼ cup	190
Planters		
NUT-rition Heart Healthy Mix	1 pkg (1.5 oz)	260
OCA		
Frieda's		
Oca	½ cup	70

FOOD	PORTION	CALS
OCTOPUS		
fresh steamed	3 oz	140
OHELOBERRIES		
fresh	1 cup	39
OIL		
almond	1 cup	1927
almond	1 tbsp	120
apricot kernel	1 tbsp	120
apricot kernel	1 cup	1927
avocado	1 cup	1927
avocado	1 tbsp	124
babassu palm	1 tbsp	120
butter oil	1 cup	1795
butter oil	1 tbsp	112
canola	1 cup	1927
canola	1 tbsp	124
coconut	1 tbsp	117
corn	1 tbsp	120
corn	1 cup	1927
cottonseed	1 tbsp	120
cottonseed	1 cup	1927
cupu assu	1 tbsp	120
garlic oil	1 tbsp	150
grapeseed	1 tbsp	120
hazelnut	1 cup	1927
hazelnut	1 tbsp	120
mustard	1 cup	1927
mustard	1 tbsp	124
oat	1 tbsp	120
olive	1 tbsp	119
olive	1 cup	1909
palm	1 cup	1927
palm	1 tbsp	120
palm kernel	1 cup	1879
palm kernel	1 tbsp	117
peanut	1 tbsp	119
peanut	1 cup	1909
peppermint	1 tsp	42
poppyseed	1 tbsp	120

FOOD	PORTION	CALS
pumpkin seed	1 oz	217
rice bran	1 tbsp	120
safflower	1 cup	1927
safflower	1 tbsp	120
sesame	1 tbsp	120
sheanut	1 tbsp	120
soybean	1 cup	1927
soybean	1 tbsp	120
soybean organic	1 tbsp	120
sunflower	1 tbsp	120
sunflower	1 cup	1927
teaseed	1 tbsp	120
tomatoseed	1 tbsp	120
vegetable	1 tbsp	120
vegetable	1 cup	1927
walnut	1 cup	1927
walnut	1 tbsp	120
wheat germ	1 tbsp	120
Alpha		
Hazelnut	1 oz	257
Consorzio		
Dipping Oil	1 tbsp	120
Olive Basil	1 tbsp	120
Olive Roasted Pepper	1 tbsp	120
Organic Extra Virgin Olive Meyer Lemon	1 tbsp	120
Eden		
Olive Spanish Extra Virgin	1 tbsp	120
Enova		
Oil	1 tbsp	120
Hollywood		
Safflower	1 tbsp	120
Loriva		
5 Pepper Hot	1 tbsp	120
Avocado	1 tbsp	120
Basil Flavored	1 tbsp	120
Canola	1 tbsp	120
Canolive	1 tbsp	120
Garlic Flavored	1 tbsp	120
Grapeseed	1 tbsp	120
Olive	1 tbsp	120

FOOD	PORTION	CALS
Olive Organic Extra Virgin	1 tbsp	120
Peanut	1 tbsp	120
Rice Bran	1 tbsp	120
Safflower	1 tbsp	120
Sesame	1 tbsp	120
Sunflower	1 tbsp	120
Toasted Sesame	1 tbsp	120
Walnut	1 tbsp	120
Mazola		
Corn	1 tbsp	120
No Stick Spray	⅓ sec spray	0
Pure Cooking Spray Canola All Flavors	¼ sec spray	0
Right Blend	1 tbsp	120
Vegetable	1 tbsp	120
Monini		
Olive Extra Virgin	1 tbsp	118
Nutiva		
Coconut Organic Extra Virgin	1 tbsp	120
Hemp Organic Cold Pressed	1 tbsp	120
Orville Redenbacher's		
Popping & Topping	1 tbsp	120
Pam		
Cooking Spray All Types	⅓ sec spray	0
Pompeian		
Olive	1 tbsp	130
Progresso		
Olive Extra Mild	1 tbsp (0.5 oz)	120
Olive Extra Virgin	1 tbsp (0.5 oz)	120
Olive Riviera Blend	1 tbsp (0.5 oz)	120
Spectrum		
Almond	1 tbsp	120
Apricot Kernel	1 tbsp	120
Avocado	1 tbsp	120
Canola Organic	1 tbsp	120
Coconut Organic	1 tbsp	120
Corn	1 tbsp	120
Grapeseed	1 tbsp	120
Grapeseed Oil Spray	⅓ sec spray	0
Hazelnut Toasted Organic	1 tbsp	120
Mediterranean Olive Organic	1 tbsp	120

FOOD	PORTION	CALS
Organic Extra Virgin Oil Spray	⅓ sec spray	0
Peanut	1 tbsp	120
Pumpkin Seed Organic	1 tbsp	120
Sesame Organic	1 tbsp	120
Sesame Toasted Organic	1 tbsp	120
Soy Organic	1 tbsp	120
Sunflower Organic	1 tbsp	120
Walnut	1 tbsp	120
Walnut Organic	1 tbsp	120
Tree Of Life		
Olive Extra Virgin Organic	1 tbsp (0.5 g)	130
Wesson		
Canola	1 tbsp	120

OKRA
FRESH

raw	8 pods	36
raw sliced	½ cup	19
sliced cooked	½ cup	25
sliced cooked	8 pods	27
FROZEN		
sliced cooked	1 pkg (10 oz)	94
sliced cooked	½ cup	34
Birds Eye		
Cut	¾ cup	25
Whole	9 pods	25
McKenzie's		
Breaded Okra	1 serv (2.8 oz)	90

OLIVES

green	4 med	15
green	3 extra lg	15
green olive tapenade	1 tbsp	25
ripe	1 sm	4
ripe	1 lg	5
ripe	1 colossal	12
ripe	1 jumbo	7
spanish stuffed	5 (0.5 oz)	15
Progresso		
Olive Salad (drained)	2 tbsp (0.8 oz)	25

FOOD	PORTION	CALS
Vlasic		
Ripe Colossal Pitted	2 (0.6 oz)	20
Ripe Jumbo Pitted	3 (0.6 oz)	25
Ripe Large Pitted	4 (0.5 oz)	25
Ripe Medium Pitted	5 (0.5 oz)	25
Ripe Sliced	¼ cup (0.5 oz)	25
Ripe Small Pitted	6 (0.5 oz)	25
ONION		
CANNED		
chopped	½ cup	21
whole	1 (2.2 oz)	12
Boar's Head		
Sweet Vidalia In Sauce	1 tbsp	10
DRIED		
flakes	1 tbsp	16
powder	1 tsp	7
shallots	1 tbsp	3
FRESH		
chopped cooked	½ cup	47
raw chopped	½ cup	30
raw chopped	1 tbsp	4
scallions raw chopped	1 tbsp	2
scallions raw sliced	½ cup	16
shallots raw chopped	1 tbsp	7
welsh raw	3½ oz	34
Antioch Farms		
Vidalia	1 med	60
Frieda's		
Cipolline	3 (3 oz)	30
Maui	⅓ cup (1.1 oz)	10
Pearl	⅔ cup (3 oz)	30
Nature's Harvest		
Onion	1 med (5.2 oz)	60
FROZEN		
chopped cooked	1 tbsp	4
chopped cooked	½ cup	30
rings	7 (2.5 oz)	285
rings cooked	2 (0.7 oz)	81
whole cooked	3½ oz	28

FOOD	PORTION	CALS
Birds Eye		
Diced	⅔ cup	30
Pearl Onions In Real Cream Sauce	½ cup	60
Small Whole	17	30
McKenzie's		
Onion Rounds	1 serv (3.2 oz)	220
TAKE-OUT		
fried	½ cup (7.5 oz)	176
rings breaded & fried	8 to 9	275

OPOSSUM
roasted	3 oz	188

ORANGE
CANNED

FOOD	PORTION	CALS
Del Monte		
SunFresh Mandarin	½ cup	80
Dole		
Fruit Bowls Mandarin Oranges	1 pkg	70
FRESH		
california navel	1	65
california valencia	1	59
florida	1	69
peel	1 tbsp	6
sections	1 cup	85
Frieda's		
Cara Cara	1 med (5 oz)	70
Mandarin Delite	1 cup (5 oz)	60
Mandarin Page	1 cup (5 oz)	60
Mandarin Pixie	1 cup (5 oz)	60
Mandarin Satsuma	1 (5 oz)	60
Melogold	½ (6 oz)	50
Seville	1 (3 oz)	40
Sunkist		
Cara Cara Navel	1 med	80
Minneola Tangelo	1 (3.8 oz)	70
Moro	1 (5.4 oz)	70
Orange	1 med	80
Satsuma Mandarin	1 (3.8 oz)	50

FOOD	PORTION	CALS
ORANGE EXTRACT		
Virginia Dare		
Extract	1 tsp	22
ORANGE JUICE		
canned	1 cup	104
chilled	1 cup	110
fresh	1 cup	111
frzn as prep	1 cup	112
frzn not prep	6 oz	339
mandarin orange	7 oz	94
orange drink	6 oz	94
Big Juicy		
Drink	8 oz	110
Bright & Early		
Orange Drink	8 oz	110
Dole		
100% Juice	8 oz	110
Fresh Samantha		
Juice	1 cup (8 oz)	100
Hi-C		
Blast Orange Drink	8 oz	120
Orange Lavaburst	1 box	90
Horizon Organic		
Juice Pulp Free	8 fl oz	110
Italian Volcano		
Blood Orange Organic	1 serv (6.75 oz)	84
Juicy Juice		
Punch	1 box (8.45 oz)	130
Punch	1 box (4.23 oz)	60
Minute Maid		
Country Style	8 oz	110
Heart Wise	8 oz	110
Kids+	8 oz	110
Light	8 oz	50
Original	8 oz	110
Plus Calcium	8 oz	110
W/ Extra Vitamin C & E Plus Zinc	8 oz	110
Mott's		
100% Juice	8 fl oz	130
100% Juice	1 box (8 oz)	130

FOOD	PORTION	CALS
Naked Juice		
Just OJ	8 oz	110
NutraShake		
Fortified	1 pkg (4 oz)	50
Ocean Spray		
100% Juice	8 oz	120
Odwalla		
Organic	8 fl oz	110
Simply Orange		
Pulp Free w/ Calcium	8 oz	110
Snapple		
Orangeade	8 oz	120
Tropicana		
Grovestand	8 oz	110
Healthy Heart	8 oz	110
Healthy Kids	8 oz	110
HomeStyle	8 oz	110
Immunity Defense	8 oz	110
Light'N Healthy	8 oz	50
Low Acid	8 oz	110
Original No Pulp	8 oz	110
Season's Best	8 oz	110
With Calcium + Vitamin D	8 oz	110
Turkey Hill		
Orangeade	1 cup	120
TAKE-OUT		
orange julius	1 serv (24 oz)	443
OREGANO		
ground	1 tsp	5

ORGAN MEATS *(see BRAINS, GIBLETS, GIZZARD, HEART, KIDNEY, LIVER, SWEETBREADS)*

OSTRICH		
cooked	3 oz	120
OYSTERS		
canned eastern	3 oz	58
canned eastern	1 cup	170
eastern cooked	3 oz	117
eastern cooked	6 med	58

FOOD	PORTION	CALS
eastern raw	6 med	58
eastern raw	1 cup	170
pacific raw	1 med	41
pacific raw	3 oz	69
steamed	3 oz	138
steamed	1 med	41
Brunswick		
Smoked	1 can (3 oz)	140
Bumble Bee		
Smoked	¼ cup	120
Whole	¼ cup	70
Chicken Of The Sea		
Smoked In Oil	1 can (3.75 oz)	140
Smoked In Water	1 can (3.75 oz)	120
Smoked Teriyaki	1 can (3.75 oz)	120
Whole	½ can (2 oz)	80
TAKE-OUT		
breaded & fried	6 (4.9 oz)	368
oysters rockefeller	3 oysters	66
stew	1 cup	278
PANCAKE/WAFFLE SYRUP		
lite	¼ cup	98
maple	1 tbsp	52
maple	1 cup (11.1 oz)	824
pancake syrup	¼ cup	209
pancake syrup	1 pkg (2 oz)	156
Atkins		
Sugar Free	¼ cup	0
Aunt Jemima		
Original	¼ cup	210
Country Cupboard		
Boysenberry	¼ cup	0
Maple Butter	¼ cup	0
Strawberry	¼ cup	0
Estee		
Maple	¼ cup	30
Karo		
Pancake Syrup	¼ cup	240

FOOD	PORTION	CALS
Keto		
Maple Butter	¼ cup	0
Ketogenics		
Zero Carb	¼ cup	0
Log Cabin		
Lite	¼ cup	100
Original	¼ cup	210
Mrs. Butter-worth's		
Lite	¼ cup	100
Original	¼ cup (2 oz)	230
Smucker's		
Breakfast Syrup Sugar Free	¼ cup	30
Stonewall Kitchen		
Maine Maple	¼ cup	210

PANCAKES

FOOD	PORTION	CALS
FROZEN		
buttermilk	1 (4 in diam)	83
plain	1 (4 in diam)	83
Golden		
Potato	1 (1.3 oz)	70
Inland Valley		
Potato	1 (2 oz)	120
MIX		
buckwheat	1 (4 in diam)	62
buttermilk	1 (4 in diam)	74
plain	1 (4 in diam)	74
sugar free low sodium	1 (3 in diam)	44
whole wheat	1 (4 in diam)	92
Atkins		
Quick Quisine Buttermilk not prep	⅓ cup	100
Quick Quisine Original not prep	¼ cup	80
Aunt Jemima		
Buttermilk Pancake & Waffle Mix not prep	⅓ cup	160
Pancake & Waffle Mix Whole Wheat as prep	3 pancakes	200
Aunt Paula's		
Pancake & Waffle Mix as prep	2	132
Betty Crocker		
Buttermilk as prep	3	200
Original as prep	3	200

FOOD	PORTION	CALS
Big Train		
Low Carb Pancake & Waffle Mix as prep	3	190
Bisquick		
Shake 'N Pour Blueberry as prep	3	210
Bruce		
Sweet Potato Pancakes	2	210
Carbolite		
Low Carb Mix not prep	⅓ cup	100
Carbsense		
Buckwheat not prep	½ cup	140
Buttermilk not prep	½ cup	140
Hodgson Mill		
Buckwheat	⅓ cup (1.8 oz)	160
Hungry Jack		
Buttermilk Pancake & Waffle as prep	3 (4 in) pancakes	150
Keto		
Banana not prep	⅓ cup	114
Original not prep	⅓ cup	114
Ketogenics		
Low Carb not prep	⅔ cup	185
MiniCarb		
Apple Cinnamon as prep	2	150
Robin Hood		
Buttermilk as prep	3	230
TAKE-OUT		
blueberry	1 (4 in diam)	84
plain	1 (4 in diam)	86
potato	1 (4 in diam)	78
w/ butter & syrup	2 (8.1 oz)	520

PANINI *(see SANDWICHES)*

PAPAYA

fresh	1	117
fresh cubed	1 cup	54
Del Monte		
In Extra Light Syrup w/ Passion Fruit Puree	½ cup	70
Frieda's		
Mexican	1 cup (5 oz)	50

FOOD	PORTION	CALS
PAPAYA JUICE		
nectar	1 cup	142
Ceres		
Papaya	8 oz	120
PAPRIKA		
paprika	1 tsp	6
PARSLEY		
dry	1 tsp	1
dry	1 tbsp	1
fresh chopped	½ cup	11
Frieda's		
Parsley Root	⅔ cup	10
PARSNIPS		
fresh cooked	1 (5.6 oz)	130
fresh sliced cooked	½ cup	63
raw sliced	½ cup	50
Frieda's		
Sliced	1 cup	100
PASSION FRUIT		
purple fresh	1	18
PASSION FRUIT JUICE		
purple	1 cup	126
yellow	1 cup	149
Ceres		
Passion Fruit	8 oz	120
PASTA (see also NOODLES, PASTA DINNERS, PASTA SALAD)		
DRY		
corn cooked	1 cup (4.9 oz)	176
corn spaghetti	2 oz	180
elbows	1 cup	389
elbows cooked	1 cup (4.9 oz)	197
shells small cooked	1 cup (4 oz)	162
spaghetti cooked	1 cup (4.9 oz)	197
spinach spaghetti cooked	1 cup (4.9 oz)	182
spirals cooked	1 cup (4.7 oz)	189
vegetable cooked	1 cup (4.7 oz)	172
whole wheat all shapes cooked	1 cup	174

FOOD	PORTION	CALS
Annie Chun's		
Soba Noodles	2 oz	200
Atkins		
All Shapes not prep	2 oz	230
Quick Quisine All Shapes as prep	¾ cup	210
Barilla		
Pastina	2 oz	210
Penne	1 cup (2 oz)	200
Plus Penne	2 oz	200
Tortelloni Porcini Mushroom	¾ cup	240
Tortelloni Ricotta & Asparagus	¾ cup	240
Tortelloni Ricotta & Spinach	¾ cup	240
Bella Vita		
Low Carb Penne Rigate	2 oz	190
Catelli		
All Shapes	3 oz	301
Bistro Cracked Black Pepper Fettucine	¼ pkg	320
Bistro Italian Herb Fettuccine	¼ pkg	310
Bistro Lemon Pepper Linguine	¼ pkg	320
Bistro Rainbows	3 oz	320
Bistro Spinach Lasagne	3 oz	320
Bistro Sun Dried Tomato & Basil Spaghettini	¼ pkg	320
Bistro Vegetable Fusilli	3 oz	320
Healthy Harvest Flax Omega-3	3 oz	290
Healthy Harvest Multigrain	3 oz	310
Healthy Harvest Organic Whole Wheat	3 oz	320
Healthy Harvest Whole Wheat All Shapes	3 oz	310
Darielle		
All Shapes not prep	2 oz	160
DaVinci		
Rotini	1 cup	210
Spaghetti	2 oz	210
Dreamfields		
All Shapes not prep	2 oz	190
Duc Amici		
Pasta Lite Low Carb Fusilli	2 oz	160
Eden		
Organic Extra Fine	2 oz	210
Organic Gemelli	2 oz	210
Organic Pesto Gemelli	2 oz	210

FOOD	PORTION	CALS
Organic Ribbons Saffron	2 oz	210
Organic Spaghetti Semolina	2 oz	200
Organic Spaghetti 50% Whole Grain	2 oz	210
Organic Spirals Kamut Vegetable	2 oz	210
Organic Spirals Sesame Rice	2 oz	200
Organic Spirals Mixed Grain	2 oz	210
Organic Spirals Spinach	2 oz	210
Organic Vegetable Alphabets	2 oz	200
Spirals Rye	2 oz	200
Food For Life		
Ezekiel 4:9	2 oz	210
Sprouted Grain		
Goya		
Coditos not prep	½ cup	230
Hodgson Mill		
Four Color Veggie Bows	2 oz	200
Four Color Veggie Rotini Spirals	2 oz	200
Pastamania! Durum Wheat Fettuccine	2 oz	200
Pastamania! Fettuccine Garlic & Parsley	2 oz	200
Pastamania! Fettuccine w/ Jerusalem Artichoke	2 oz	210
Pastamania! Fettucinne w/ Mushroom	2 oz	210
Pastamania! Fusilli Tre Colore w/ Tomato & Spinach	2 oz	200
Pastamania! Sea Shell Mix	2 oz	200
Pastamania! Spinach Fettuccine	2 oz	200
Pastamania! Thin Linguine	2 oz	200
Pastamania! Tomato Spinach & Durum Wheat	2 oz	210
Spaghetti Whole Wheat not prep	2 oz	190
Whole Wheat Lasagne not prep	2 oz	190
Whole Wheat Spinach Spaghetti not prep	2 oz	190
Keto		
Elbows not prep	1.6 oz	108
Spaghetti not prep	1.3 oz	130
LifeStream		
Organic All Shapes	2 oz	208
Lundberg		
Spaghetti Organic Brown Rice	2 oz	210
Notta Pasta		
Rice Pasta All Shapes	2 oz	200

FOOD	PORTION	CALS
Pastalia		
Heart Health Low Carb not prep	2 oz	176
Real Torino		
Tirali not prep	1 cup (2 oz)	210
Revival		
Soy Penne	⅙ box	200
Soy Thin Spaghetti	⅙ box	200
Ronzoni		
Elbows not prep	½ cup (2 oz)	210
Healthy Harvest Whole Wheat Blend Thin Spaghetti	⅐ pkg (2 oz)	180
Lasagne	2½ pieces (2 oz)	210
Tradizione D'Italia All Shapes	2 oz	210
San Giorgio		
Elbows not prep	½ cup	210
Soy7		
Pasta All Shapes	2 oz	200
Whey Cool		
High Protein Xtreme Rotini	1 serv (2 oz)	210
FRESH		
cooked	2 oz	75
spinach cooked	2 oz	74
REFRIGERATED		
Buitoni		
Angel Hair	1¼ cups	230
Fettuccine	1¼ cups	240
Fettuccine Spinach	1¼ cups	260
Linguine	1¼ cups	240
Ravioletti Three Cheese	1 cup	270
Ravioli Doublestuffed Mozzarella & Herb	1½ cups	340
Ravioli Four Cheese	1¼ cups	330
Ravioli Chicken & Roasted Garlic	1¼ cups	340
Ravioli Chicken Parmesan	1¼ cups	310
Ravioli Classic Beef	1¼ cups	340
Ravioli Garden Vegetable	1 cup	250
Ravioli Light Four Cheese	1¼ cups	230
Tortellini Herb Chicken	1 cup	340
Tortellini Mixed Cheese	1 cup	320

FOOD	PORTION	CALS
Tortellini Spinach Cheese	1 cup	330
Tortellini Three Cheese	1 cup	320
Tortelloni Cheese & Roasted Garlic	1 cup	270
Tortelloni Chicken & Prosciutto	1 cup	330
Tortelloni Mozzarella & Herb	1 cup	330
Tortelloni Mozzarella & Pepperoni	1 cup	330
Tortelloni Portabello Mushroom & Cheese	1 cup	270
Tortelloni Sun Dried Tomato	1 cup	310
Tortelloni Sweet Italian Sausage	1 cup	330

PASTA DINNERS *(see also PASTA SALAD)*
CANNED
Annie's Homegrown

Organic All Stars	1 cup	150
Organic BernieOs	1 cup	150
Organic Cheesy Ravioli	1 cup	180
Organic P'sghetti Loops	1 cup	190

Chef Boyardee

99% Fat Free Beef Ravioli	1 cup (8.6 oz)	210
99% Fat Free Cheese Ravioli	1 cup (8.8 oz)	210
Beef Ravioli	1 cup (8.6 oz)	230
Beefaroni	1 cup	260
Macaroni & Cheese	½ can (7.5 oz)	180
Mini Ravioli	1 cup (8.8 oz)	252
Spaghetti & Meat Balls	1 cup (8.4 oz)	240
Tortellini Cheese	½ can (7 oz)	230
Tortellini Meat	½ can (7 oz)	260

Franco-American

Beef Raviolios	1 can (7.7 oz)	250
Beefy Mac	1 can (7.5 oz)	228
Elbow Macaroni & Cheese	1 can (7.5 oz)	187
Spaghetti 'N Beef	1 can (7.5 oz)	226
Spaghetti w/ Meatballs	1 can (7.2 oz)	249

Hunt's

Noodles & Chicken	1 cup (8.7 oz)	176
Noodles & Beef	1 cup (8.7 oz)	151

Progresso

Beef Ravioli	1 cup (9.1 oz)	260
Cheese Ravioli	1 cup (9.1 oz)	220

FOOD	PORTION	CALS
FROZEN		
Amy's		
Bowl Stuffed Pasta Shells	1 pkg (10 oz)	300
Cannelloni w/ Vegetables	1 pkg (9 oz)	330
Lasagna Cheese	1 pkg (10.25 oz)	330
Lasagna Garden Vegetable	1 pkg (10.25 oz)	290
Macaroni & Cheese	1 pkg (9 oz)	410
Macaroni & Soy Cheese	1 pkg (9 oz)	370
Pasta & Vegetable Alfredo	1 cup	220
Pasta Primavera	1 pkg (9 oz)	300
Ravioli w/ Sauce	1 pkg (8 oz)	340
Rice Mac & Cheese	1 pkg (9 oz)	140
Skillet Meals	1 cup	250
Tofu Vegetable Lasagna	1 pkg (9.5 oz)	300
Vegetable Lasagna	1 pkg (9.5 oz)	280
Banquet		
Chicken Pasta Primavera	1 meal (9.5 oz)	320
Family Size Egg Noodles w/ Beef & Brown Gravy	1 serv	150
Family Size Lasagna w/ Meat Sauce	1 cup	270
Family Size Macaroni & Cheese	1 cup	230
Fettuccine Alfredo	1 meal (9.5 oz)	350
Homestyle Noodles & Chicken	1 meal (12 oz)	390
Lasagna w/ Meat Sauce	1 meal (9.5 oz)	260
Macaroni & Cheese	1 meal (12 oz)	420
Birds Eye		
Easy Recipe Creations Basil Herb Primavera	2¼ cups	260
Easy Recipe Creations Tortellini Parmigiana	2¼ cups	240
Pasta Secrets Italian Pesto	2⅓ cups	240
Pasta Secrets Primavera	2⅓ cups	230
Pasta Secrets Ranch	2⅓ cups	300
Pasta Secrets Three Cheese	2 cups	230
Pasta Secrets White Cheddar	2 cups	240
Pasta Secrets Zesty Garlic	2 cups	240
Golden Cuisine		
Cheese Manicotti	1 pkg	360
Spaghetti & Meatballs	1 pkg	490
Tuna Casserole	1 pkg	386
Healthy Choice		
Beef Macaroni	1 meal (8.5 oz)	220

FOOD	PORTION	CALS
Breaded Chicken Breast Stips w/ Macaroni & Cheese	1 meal (8 oz)	270
Breaded Chicken Breast w/ Mac & Cheese	1 pkg	290
Cheese Ravioli Parmigiana	1 meal (9 oz)	260
Fettuccine Alfredo	1 pkg	280
Fettuccini Alfredo Chicken	1 pkg	290
Lasagna Bake	1 pkg	270
Macaroni & Cheese	1 meal (9 oz)	240
Macaroni & Cheese	1 pkg	290
Manicotti	1 pkg	280
Manicotti w/ Three Cheeses	1 meal (11 oz)	300
Rigatoni w/ Broccoli & Chicken	1 pkg	270
Spaghetti & Sauce w/ Seasoned Beef	1 meal (10 oz)	260
Spaghetti w/ Meat Sauce	1 pkg	310
Stuffed Pasta Shells	1 pkg	290
Joseph's Pasta		
Grilled Chicken Ravioli w/ Roasted Red Pepper Sauce	1 pkg (14 oz)	540
Kid Cuisine		
Cheese Blaster Mac & Cheese	1 meal	380
Twist & Twirl Spaghetti w/ Mini Meatballs	1 meal	460
Lean Cuisine		
Cafe Classics Bow Tie Pasta & Chicken	1 pkg (9.5 oz)	240
Cafe Classics Bowl Three Cheese Stuffed Ragatoni	1 pkg (10 oz)	260
Cafe Classics Cheese Lasagna w/ Chicken Breast Scallopini	1 pkg (10 oz)	290
Cafe Classics Four Cheese Cannelloni	1 pkg (9.1 oz)	260
Cafe Classics Grilled Chicken & Penne Pasta	1 pkg (12 oz)	320
Cafe Classics Jumbo Rigatoni w/ Meatballs	1 pkg (15.4 oz)	400
Cafe Classics Lasagna w/ Meat Sauce	1 pkg (10.5 oz)	310
Cafe Classics Macaroni & Beef	1 pkg (9.5 oz)	270
Cafe Classics Macaroni & Cheese	1 pkg (10 oz)	300
Cafe Classics Penne Pasta w/ Tomato Basil Sauce	1 pkg (10 oz)	270
Cafe Classics Roasted Chicken w/ Lemon Pepper Fettuccini	1 pkg (8.1 oz)	250
Cafe Classics Shrimp & Angel Hair Pasta	1 pkg (10 oz)	240
Cafe Classics Spaghetti w/ Meat Sauce	1 pkg (11.5 oz)	280

FOOD	PORTION	CALS
Cafe Classics Spaghetti w/ Meatballs	1 pkg (9.5 oz)	270
Dinnertime Selects Chicken Fettuccini	1 pkg (12 oz)	360
One Dish Favorites Alfredo Pasta w/ Chicken & Broccoli	1 pkg (10 oz)	270
One Dish Favorites Angel Hair Pasta Marinara	1 pkg (10 oz)	260
One Dish Favorites Cheese Ravioli	1 pkg (8.5 oz)	250
One Dish Favorites Chicken Fettuccini	1 pkg (9.25 oz)	280
One Dish Favorites Lasagna Cheese Florentine Bake	1 pkg (10 oz)	270
One Dish Favorites Lasagna Chicken Florentine	1 pkg (10 oz)	270
One Dish Favorties Lasagna Classic Five Cheese	1 pkg (11.5 oz)	330
Skillet Chicken Alfredo	1 serv	180
Marie Callender's		
Cheese Ravioli In Marinara Sauce w/ Spirals & Garlic Bread	1 meal (16 oz)	750
Extra Cheese Lasagna	1 meal (15 oz)	590
Fettuccine Alfredo & Garlic Bread	1 meal (14 oz)	920
Fettuccine Alfredo Supreme	1 meal (13 oz)	450
Fettuccine Primavera w/ Tortellini	1 meal (14 oz)	750
Fettuccine w/ Broccoli & Chicken	1 meal (13 oz)	710
Lasagna w/ Meat Sauce	1 meal (15 oz)	630
Macaroni & Cheese	1 meal (12 oz)	540
Skillet Meal Chicken Alfredo	½ pkg	490
Skillet Meal Penne Pasta & Meatballs	½ pkg	600
Skillet Meal Rigatoni Vegetables In Cheese Sauce	1 cup	290
Spaghetti w/ Meat Sauce & Garlic Bread	1 meal (17 oz)	670
Stuffed Pasta Trio	1 meal (10.5 oz)	380
Michelina's		
Lasagna w/ Meat Sauce	1 pkg (9 oz)	280
Morton		
Macaroni & Cheese	1 serv (8 oz)	240
Spaghetti w/ Meat Sauce	1 meal (8.5 oz)	200
Savvy Faire		
Lasagna Florentine	1 pkg (9.2 oz)	300
Seeds Of Change		
Organic Lasagna Creamy Spinach	1 pkg (11 oz)	370
Slim-Fast		
Fettuccine Alfredo	1 pkg	240
Rotini w/ Tomato & Italian Herb	1 pkg	240

FOOD	PORTION	CALS
Shells & Creamy Cheese Sauce	1 pkg	240
South Beach Diet		
Penne & Chicken In Roasted Red Pepper Sauce	1 pkg	290
Stouffer's		
Lasagna w/ Meat Sauce	1 cup	250
Yves		
Veggie Lasagna	1 pkg (10.5 oz)	300
Veggie Macaroni	1 pkg (10.5 oz)	230
Veggie Penne	1 pkg (10.5 oz)	220
MIX		
A Taste Of Thai		
Coconut Ginger	1 cup	280
Pad Thai For Two	½ pkg	345
Peanut Noodles as prep	1 cup	330
Red Curry Noodles as prep	1 cup	280
Annie's Homegrown		
Gluten Free Rice Pasta & Cheddar as prep	1 cup	330
Organic Shells & Real Aged Wisconsin Cheddar as prep	1 cup	370
Organic Skillet Meals Beef Stroganoff as prep	1 cup	320
Organic Skillet Meals Cheddar & Herb Chicken as prep	1 cup	310
Organic Skillet Meals Cheese Lasagna as prep	1 cup	280
Organic Skillet Meals Cheeseburger Macaroni as prep	1 cup	350
Orangic Skillet Meals Chicken Fettucine as prep	1 cup	330
Organic Skillet Meals Creamy Tuna Spirals as prep	1 cup	260
Organic Whole Wheat Shells & Cheddar as prep	1 cup	360
Shells & Real Aged Wisconsin Cheddar as prep	1 cup	290
Shells & White Cheddar as prep	1 cup	290
Aramana		
Cheddar Cheeseburger as prep	1 cup	260
Creamy Chicken Alfredo as prep	1 cup	260
Mild Mexican as prep	1 cup	260
Atkins		
Quick Quisine Elbows & Cheese as prep	1 cup	250
Quick Quisine Fettuccine Alfredo as prep	1 cup	210
Quick Quisine Pesto Cream as prep	1 cup	240

FOOD	PORTION	CALS
Back To Nature		
Alfredo & Gemelli as prep	1 cup	340
Macaroni & Cheese as prep	1 cup	320
White Cheddar & Spirals as prep	1 cup	330
Hodgson Mill		
Macaroni & Cheese Whole Wheat	1 serv	250
Keto		
Macaroni & Cheese not prep	1 serv	112
Near East		
Angel Hair w/ Spicy Tomato as prep	1 cup	240
Radiatore Basil & Herb as prep	1 cup	240
Vermicelli Garlic & Oil as prep	1 cup	310
Whey Cool		
High Protein Macaroni & Cheese as prep	1 serv	260
REFRIGERATED		
Country Crock		
Elbow Macaroni & Cheese	1 cup	380
SHELF-STABLE		
It's Pasta Anytime		
Penne With Tomato Italian Sausage Sauce	1 pkg (15.25 oz)	540
Lunch Bucket		
Beef Ravioli In Tomato Sauce	1 pkg (7.5 oz)	180
Italian Pasta w/ Chicken	1 pkg (7.5 oz)	130
Lasagna 'n Meatsauce	1 pkg (7.5 oz)	160
Macaroni 'n Beef in Meatsauce	1 pkg (7.5 oz)	180
Macaroni'n Cheese	1 pkg (7.5 oz)	190
Pasta'n Chicken	1 pkg (7.5 oz)	150
Spaghetti'n Meatsauce	1 pkg (7.5 oz)	160
TAKE-OUT		
bami goreng indonesian noodle dish	1 cup	170
fettuccini alfredo	1 cup	715
lasagna	1 piece (2.5 in x 2.5 in)	374
lasagna vegetarian	2 cups	720
macaroni & cheese	1 cup	230
manicotti	¾ cup (6.4 oz)	273
noodle pudding	½ cup	132
ravioli cheese w/ tomato sauce	2 cups	530
rigatoni w/ sausage sauce	¾ cup	260
spaghetti w/ clam sauce	1 serv	395

FOOD	PORTION	CALS
spaghetti w/ marinara sauce	1 cup	260
spaghetti w/ meatballs & cheese	1 cup	407
tortellini cheese w/ tomato sauce	1 cup	470

PASTA SALAD
TAKE-OUT
elbow macaroni salad	3.5 oz	160
mustard macaroni salad	3.5 oz	190
pasta salad w/ crab vegetables mayonnaise	1 cup	317
pasta salad w/ vegetables	3.5 oz	140

PATE
chicken liver canned	1 tbsp (13 g)	109
duck pate	1 oz	96
fish pate	1 oz	76
goose liver smoked canned	1 tbsp (13 g)	60
liver canned	1 tbsp (13 g)	41
mushroom anchovy pate	1 can (2.25 oz)	130
pate foie gras	1 oz	127
pork pate	1 oz	107
pork pate en croute	1 oz	91
rabbit pate	1 oz	66
shrimp	1 can (2.25 oz)	140

PEACH
CANNED
halves in heavy syrup	1 half	60
halves in light syrup	1 half	44
halves juice pack	1 half	34
halves water pack	1 half	18
peachsauce	½ cup	120
spiced in heavy syrup	1 cup	180
spiced in heavy syrup	1 fruit	66
Del Monte		
Carb Clever Sliced	½ cup	30
Freestone Lite Slices	½ cup	60
Freestone Sliced	½ cup	100
Fruit Cup Diced Extra Light Syrup	1 pkg (4 oz)	50
Fruit Cup Diced In Heavy Syrup	1 serv (4 oz)	80
Fruit Naturals Chunks	½ cup	70
Fruit To Go Banana Berry Peaches	1 pkg (4 oz)	70

FOOD	PORTION	CALS
Halves In Heavy Syrup	½ cup	100
Orchard Select Sliced Cling	½ cup	80
Sliced In 100% Juice	½ cup	60
Dole		
All Natural Yellow Cling Sliced	½ cup	80
S&W		
Slices Lightly Sweetened Juice	½ cup	80
DRIED		
halves	10	311
halves	1 cup	383
halves cooked w/ sugar	½ cup	139
halves cooked w/o sugar	½ cup	99
Crispy Green		
Crispy Peaches	1 pkg (0.36 oz)	38
FRESH		
peach	1	37
sliced	1 cup	73
Chiquita		
Peach	1 med (3.4 oz)	40
FROZEN		
slices sweetened	1 cup	235

PEACH JUICE

nectar	1 cup	134
Ceres		
Peach	8 oz	120

PEANUT BUTTER

chunky	1 cup	1520
chunky	2 tbsp	188
chunky w/o salt	2 tbsp	188
chunky w/o salt	1 cup	1520
smooth	2 tbsp	188
smooth	1 cup	1517
smooth w/o salt	2 tbsp	188
smooth w/o salt	1 cup	1517
Carb Options		
Creamy	2 tbsp	190
Estee		
Creamy Low Sodium	2 tbsp	180

FOOD	PORTION	CALS
Jif		
Apple Cinnamon	2 tbsp (1.3 oz)	200
Berry Blend	2 tbsp (1.2 oz)	200
Chocolate Silk	2 tbsp (1.3 oz)	190
Creamy	2 tbsp	190
Extra Crunchy	2 tbsp (1.1 oz)	190
Reduced Fat Creamy	2 tbsp (1.3 oz)	190
Reduced Fat Crunchy	2 tbsp (1.3 oz)	190
Simply	2 tbsp (1.1 oz)	190
Maranatha		
Crunchy	2 tbsp	190
Salted	2 tbsp	190
P.B.		
Slices	1 slice (1 oz)	170
Peanut Butter & Co.		
Cinnamon Raisin Swirl	2 tbsp	143
Crunch Time	2 tbsp	200
Dark Chocolate Dreams	2 tbsp	175
Smooth Operator	2 tbsp	200
The Heat Is On	2 tbsp	164
White Chocolate Wonderful	1 tbsp	165
Peanut Wonder		
Low Sodium	2 tbsp	100
Regular	2 tbsp	100
Reese's		
Peanut Butter Chips	1 tbsp	80
Skippy		
Creamy	2 tbsp	190
Creamy w/ 2 slices white bread	1 sandwich	340
Reduced Fat Creamy	2 tbsp	190
Roasted Honey Nut	2 tbsp	190
Roasted Honey Nut Super Chunk	2 tbsp	190
Squeeze Stix	1 pkg	140
Squeeze Stix Chocolate	1 pkg	140
Squeez'It	2 tbsp	190
Super Chunk	2 tbsp	190
Super Chunk Reduced Fat	2 tbsp	190
Smucker's		
Goober All Flavors	3 tbsp	240
Natural Chunky	2 tbsp	210

FOOD	PORTION	CALS
Natural Creamy	2 tbsp	210
Natural Honey	2 tbsp	200
Natural No Salt Added Creamy	2 tbsp	210
Natural Reduced Fat Creamy	2 tbsp	200
Tropical Source		
Chips Dairy Free	13 pieces (1.5 oz)	80

PEANUTS

chocolate coated	10 (1.4 oz)	208
chocolate coated	1 cup (5.2 oz)	773
cooked	½ cup	102
dry roasted	1 cup	855
dry roasted w/ salt	30 nuts (1 oz)	170
A Taste Of Thai		
Spicy Peanut Bake	¼ pkg	45
At Last!		
Chocolate Covered	1 pkg (0.9 oz)	150
Brach's		
Double Dippers Chocolate Covered	15 pieces	210
Estee		
Chocolate Coated Fructose Sweetened	¼ cup	170
Frito Lay		
Salted	1 oz	160
Salted w/ Shells	½ cup	160
Judy's		
Sugar Free Coconut Peanut Brittle	¼ piece (1 oz)	90
Little Debbie		
Salted	¼ cup (1 oz)	160
Low Carb Creations		
Soft Peanut Brittle	2 pieces (1 oz)	140
Planters		
Honey Roasted	1 oz	160
Sweet Delight		
Peanut Roasters	⅓ pkg (1 oz)	160
Tom's		
Double Coated	1 pkg (1.35 oz)	220
Toasted	1 pkg (1.4 oz)	240

PEAR
CANNED

halves in heavy sirup	1 cup	188

FOOD	PORTION	CALS
halves in heavy syrup	1 half	68
halves in light syrup	1 half	45
halves juice pack	1 cup	123
halves water pack	1 half	22
Del Monte		
Carb Clever Sliced	½ cup	40
Fruit Cup Diced In Heavy Syrup	1 pkg (4 oz)	80
Fruit Cup Diced Extra Light Syrup	1 pkg (4 oz)	50
Fruit To Go Peachy Peaches	1 pkg (4 oz)	70
Halves In 100% Juice	½ cup	60
Halves In Light Syrup	½ cup	60
Orchard Select Sliced Bartlett	½ cup	80
S&W		
Halves In Lightly Sweetened Juice	½ cup	80
DRIED		
halves	10	459
halves	1 cup	472
halves cooked w/ sugar	½ cup	196
halves cooked w/o sugar	½ cup	163
FRESH		
asian	1 (4.3 oz)	51
pear	1	98
sliced w/ skin	1 cup	97
Chiquita		
Pear	1 med (5.8 oz)	100
PEAR JUICE		
nectar	1 cup	149
Ceres		
Pear	8 oz	120
PEAS		
CANNED		
green	½ cup	59
green low sodium	½ cup	59
Del Monte		
Sweet	½ cup	60
Sweet Very Young Small	½ cup	60
Green Giant		
Sweet	½ cup	60

FOOD	PORTION	CALS
Libby's		
No Salt No Sugar Added	½ cup	70
S&W		
Petite	½ cup (4.4 oz)	70
Small	½ cup (4.4 oz)	70
Veg-All		
Tender Sweet	½ cup	60
DRIED		
split cooked	1 cup	231
FRESH		
green cooked	½ cup	67
green raw	½ cup	58
snap peas cooked	½ cup	34
snap peas raw	½ cup	30
Frieda's		
Snow Peas	1 cup	35
Sugar Snap	⅔ cups (3 oz)	35
River Ranch		
Sugar Snap	1½ cups	35
FROZEN		
green cooked	½ cup	63
snap peas cooked	½ cup	42
Birds Eye		
Butter Peas	½ cup	110
Crowder	½ cup	120
Field Peas w/ Snaps	⅔ cup	130
Green	½ cup	70
Purple Hull Peas	½ cup	110
Sugar Snap	½ cup	40
Tiny Tender	¾ cup	40
Fresh Like		
Garden	3.5 oz	85
Green Giant		
Sweet	⅔ cup	70
La Choy		
Snow Pea Pods	½ pkg (3 oz)	35
Pictsweet		
Green Peas	⅔ cup	70
Tree Of Life		
Peas	⅔ cup (3.1 oz)	70

FOOD	PORTION	CALS
SHELF-STABLE		
TastyBite		
Agra Peas & Greens	½ pkg (5 oz)	260
TAKE-OUT		
pea & potato curry	1 serv (7 oz)	284
pea curry	1 serv (4.4 oz)	438
PECANS		
candied	1 oz	190
dry roasted	1 oz	187
dry roasted salted	1 oz	187
halves dry roasted w/ salt	20 (1 oz)	200
halves dried	1 cup	721
oil roasted	1 oz	195
oil roasted salted	1 oz	195
Keto		
Chocolately Covered	1 oz	207
Sweet Delights		
Pecan Roasters	⅓ pkg (1 oz)	210
PECTIN		
powder	1 pkg (1.75 oz)	163
powder	¼ pkg (0.4 oz)	39
Slim Set		
Packet	1 pkg	208
Powder	1 tbsp	3
Sure Jell		
For Lower Sugar Recipes	1 tsp (2.8 g)	20
Fruit Pectin	1 tsp (3.6 g)	20
PEPEAO		
dried	½ cup	36
raw sliced	1 cup	25
PEPPER		
black	1 tsp	5
cayenne	1 tsp	6
red	1 tsp	6
white	1 tsp	7
McCormick		
Lemon & Pepper Seasoning Salt	¼ tsp	0

FOOD	PORTION	CALS
PEPPERS		
CANNED		
chili green	1 cup (5.5 oz)	29
chili green hot chopped	½ cup	17
chili red hot	1 (2.6 oz)	18
chili red hot chopped	½ cup	17
green halves	½ cup	13
jalapeno chopped	½ cup	17
red halves	½ cup	13
Old El Paso		
Green Chiles Chopped	2 tbsp (1 oz)	5
Progresso		
Cherry Sliced & So Hot	2 tbsp (1 oz)	25
Hot Cherry	1 (1 oz)	10
Pepper Salad (drained)	2 tbsp (1 oz)	15
Roasted	1 piece (1 oz)	10
Sweet Fried w/ Onions	2 tbsp (0.9 oz)	20
Tuscan	3 (1 oz)	10
Rosarita		
Chilies Diced Green	2 tbsp (1 oz)	6
Chilies Green Strips	¼ cup (1.2 oz)	5
Chilies Whole Green	2 tbsp (1.2 oz)	5
Jalapeno Whole w/ Escabeche	¼ cup (1.2 oz)	8
Jalapenos Diced	2 tbsp (1 oz)	5
Jalapenos Nacho Sliced	2 tbsp (1 oz)	2
Vlasic		
Hot Sliced Cherry	1 oz	5
Jalapeno Sliced	1 oz	10
Mild Cherry	1 oz	5
Pepper Rings Hot	1 oz	5
Pepper Rings Mild	1 oz	5
DRIED		
ancho	1 (0.6 oz)	48
green	1 tbsp	1
pasilla	1 (7 g)	24
red	1 tbsp	1
FRESH		
banana	1 (4 in) (1.2 oz)	9
banana	1 cup (4.4 oz)	33
chili green hot	1	18

FOOD	PORTION	CALS
chili green hot chopped	½ cup	30
chili red chopped	½ cup	30
chili red hot	1 (1.6 oz)	18
green	1 (2.6 oz)	20
green chopped	½ cup	13
green chopped cooked	½ cup	19
green cooked	1 (2.6 oz)	20
habanero chile	1 tsp	9
hungarian	1 (0.9 oz)	8
jalapeno	1 (0.5 oz)	4
jalapeno sliced	1 cup (3.2 oz)	27
red	1 (2.6 oz)	20
red chopped	½ cup	13
red chopped cooked	½ cup	19
red cooked	1 (2.6 oz)	20
serrano	1 (6 g)	2
serrano chopped	1 cup (3.7 oz)	34
yellow	10 strips	14
yellow	1 (6.5 oz)	50
Chiquita		
Pepper	1 med (5.2 oz)	30
FROZEN		
green chopped	1 oz	6
red chopped	1 oz	6
Birds Eye		
Diced Green	¾ cup	20

PERCH
FRESH
cooked	3 oz	99
cooked	1 fillet (1.6 oz)	54
ocean perch atlantic cooked	1 fillet (1.8 oz)	60
ocean perch atlantic cooked	3 oz	103
ocean perch atlantic raw	3 oz	80
raw	3 oz	77
red raw	3.5 oz	114

PERSIMMONS
dried japanese	1	93
fresh	1	32
fresh japanese	1	118

FOOD	PORTION	CALS
Frieda's		
Dried Fuyu	⅓ cup (1.4 oz)	140
PHEASANT		
breast w/o skin raw	½ breast (6.4 oz)	243
leg w/o skin raw	1 (3.6 oz)	143
roasted	3.5 oz	215
w/ skin raw	½ pheasant (14 oz)	723
w/o skin raw	½ pheasant (12.4 oz)	470
PHYLLO		
phyllo dough	1 oz	85
sheet	1	57
Ekizian		
Sheets	¼ lb	433
Fillo Factory		
Fillo Dough Spelt Vegan	3 sheets (2 oz)	180
Fillo Dough Vegan	3 sheets (2 oz)	170
Fillo Dough Whole Wheat Vegan	3 sheets (2 oz)	190
Pastry Shells Vegan	3 (0.4 oz)	45
PICANTE *(see SALSA)*		
PICKLES		
dill	1 (2.3 oz)	12
dill low sodium	1 (2.3 oz)	12
dill low sodium sliced	1 slice	1
dill sliced	1 slice	1
gerkins	1 oz	6
kosher dill	1 (2.3 oz)	12
polish dill	1 (2.3 oz)	12
quick sour	1 (1.2 oz)	4
quick sour low sodium	1 (1.2 oz)	4
quick sour sliced	1 slice	1
sweet	1 (1.2 oz)	41
sweet gherkin	1 sm (½ oz)	20
sweet low sodium	1 (1.2 oz)	41
sweet sliced	1 slice	7
Claussen		
Bread 'N Butter Chips	4 slices (1 oz)	20
Deli Style Hearty Garlic Whole	½ (1 oz)	5
Kosher Dill Spears	1 spear (1.2 oz)	5

FOOD	PORTION	CALS
Kosher Dills Halves	1 half (1 oz)	5
Kosher Dills Mini	1 (0.8 oz)	5
Kosher Dills Whole	½ (1 oz)	5
New York Deli Style Half Sours Whole	½ (1 oz)	5
Sandwich Slices Bread 'N Butter	2 (1.2 oz)	25
Sandwich Slices Deli Style Hearty Garlic	2 (1.2 oz)	5
Sandwich Slices Kosher Dills	2 (1.2 oz)	5
Super Slices For Burgers	1 (0.8 oz)	5
Del Monte		
Dill Halves	1 piece (1 oz)	5
Hamburger Dill Chips	1 serv (1 oz)	0
Sweet	1 serv (1 oz)	40
Sweet Gerkins	1 serv (1 oz)	40
Tiny Kosher Dill	1 serv (1 oz)	5
Hebrew National		
Dill	1	23
Mt Olive		
Bread & Butter No Sugar Added	1 oz	0
Vlasic		
Hamburger Dill Chips	1 oz	5
Kosher Cross Cuts	1 oz	5
Kosher Spears	1 oz	5
Kosher Whole	1 oz	5
Sweet Butter Chips	1 oz	30
Sweet Gerkins	1 oz	35
Whole Dills	1 oz	5

PIE
FROZEN
Amy's

Apple	1 serv (4 oz)	240
Edwards		
Pie Slices Oreo Cream	1 slice (2.6 oz)	290
Mrs. Smith's		
Apple	1 slice (4.3 oz)	350
Blueberry	1 slice (4.6 oz)	330
Cappuccino	1 slice (4.2 oz)	300
Cherry	1 slice (4.3 oz)	320
Cherry Crumb	1 slice (4.2 oz)	320

FOOD	PORTION	CALS
Chocolate Cream	1 slice (4.6 oz)	340
Chocolate Mint Cream	1 slice (4.3 oz)	360
Coconut Custard	1 slice (4.4 oz)	260
Cookies 'N Cream	1 slice (4.3 oz)	360
Dutch Apple	1 slice (3.3 oz)	260
French Silk	1 slice (4.4 oz)	560
Key West Lime	1 slice (4.3 oz)	430
Lemon Cream	1 slice (5 oz)	440
Lemonade	1 slice (4.3 oz)	340
Mince	1 slice (4.6 oz)	380
Mixed Berry	1 slice (4.2 oz)	300
Peach	1 slice (4.6 oz)	320
Peach Lattice	1 slice (4.2 oz)	290
Peanut Butter Silk	1 slice (4.6 oz)	600
Pecan	1 slice (4.8 oz)	560
Pumpkin Custard	1 slice (4.6 oz)	270
Raspberry	1 slice (4.6 oz)	330
S'Mores Cream	1 slice (4.3 oz)	360
Strawberry Banana	1 slice (4.3 oz)	330
Sweet Potato Custard	1 slice (4.6 oz)	340
Sara Lee		
Apple 45% Reduced Fat	⅙ pie (4.5 oz)	290
Chocolate Silk	⅕ pie (4.8 oz)	500
Coconut Cream	⅕ pie (4.8 oz)	480
Homestyle Apple	⅛ pie (4.6 oz)	340
Homestyle Blueberry	⅛ pie (4.6 oz)	360
Homestyle Cherry	⅛ pie (4.6 oz)	320
Homestyle Dutch Apple	⅛ pie (4.6 oz)	350
Homestyle Mince	⅛ pie (4.6 oz)	390
Homestyle Peach	⅛ pie (4.6 oz)	320
Homestyle Pecan	⅛ pie (4.2 oz)	520
Homestyle Pumpkin	⅛ pie (4.6 oz)	260
Homestyle Raspberry	⅛ pie (4.6 oz)	380
Lemon Meringue	⅙ pie (5 oz)	350
SNACK		
Dolly Madison		
Apple	1 (4.5 oz)	480
Blueberry	1 (4.5 oz)	480
Cherry	1 (4.5 oz)	470
Chocolate Pudding	1 (4.5 oz)	530

FOOD	PORTION	CALS
Lemon	1 (4.5 oz)	500
Peach	1 (4.5 oz)	480
Pecan	1 (3 oz)	360
Pecan Fried	1 (4.5 oz)	530
Pineapple	1 (4.5 oz)	460
Hostess		
Apple	1 (4.5 oz)	480
Blackberry	1 (4.5 oz)	520
Blueberry	1 (4.5 oz)	480
Cherry	1 (4.5 oz)	470
French Apple	1 (4.5 oz)	480
Lemon	1 (4.5 oz)	500
Peach	1 (4.5 oz)	480
Pineapple	1 (4.5 oz)	460
Strawberry	1 (4.5 oz)	510
Tastykake		
Apple	1 (4 oz)	270
Blueberry	1 (4 oz)	300
Cherry	1 (4 oz)	290
Coconut Creme	1 (4 oz)	370
French Apple	1 (4.2 oz)	310
Lemon	1 (4 oz)	300
Peach	1 (4 oz)	280
Pineapple	1 (4 oz)	290
Pineapple Cheese	1 (4 oz)	320
Pumpkin	1 (4 oz)	340
Strawberry	1 (3.5 oz)	320
Tastyklair	1 (4 oz)	400
Tom's		
Apple	1 pkg (3 oz)	330
Banana Marshmallow	1 pkg (2.75 oz)	320
Cherry	1 pkg (3 oz)	320
Chocolate Marshmallow	1 pkg (2.75 oz)	320
TAKE-OUT		
apple	⅛ of 9 in (5.4 oz)	411
banana cream	⅛ of 9 in (5.2 oz)	398
blueberry	⅛ of 9 in (5.2 oz)	360
butterscotch	⅛ of 9 in (4.5 oz)	355
cherry	⅛ of 9 in (6.3 oz)	486
chocolate creme	1 slice (4 oz)	344

FOOD	PORTION	CALS
coconut creme	⅛ of 9 in (4.7 oz)	396
coconut custard	⅙ of 8 in (3.6 oz)	271
custard	⅛ of 9 in (4.5 oz)	262
key lime	⅙ (5 oz)	420
lemon meringue	1 slice (4.5 oz)	303
lemon meringue	⅛ of 9 in (4.5 oz)	362
mince	⅛ of 9 in (5.8 oz)	477
pecan	⅙ of 8 in (4 oz)	452
pumpkin	⅙ of 8 in (3.8 oz)	229
vanilla cream	⅛ of 9 in (4.4 oz)	350
PIE CRUST		
FROZEN		
baked	⅛ of 9 in (0.6 oz)	82
baked	9 in shell (4.4 oz)	647
puff pastry baked	1 shell (1.4 oz)	223
Pepperidge Farm		
Puff Pastry Sheets	⅙ sheet (1.4 oz)	170
Puff Pastry Shell	1 (1.6 oz)	190
Puff Pastry Squares	1 sq (2 oz)	240
Pet-Ritz		
Deep Dish	⅛ pie (0.7 oz)	90
Regular	⅛ pie (0.6 oz)	80
Tart Shells	1 (1 oz)	130
MIX		
as prep	9 in crust (5.6 oz)	801
as prep	⅛ of 9 in (0.7 oz)	100
Betty Crocker		
Pie Crust as prep	⅛ crust	110
Jiffy		
Pie Crust Mix	⅐ crust	180
MiniCarb		
Pie Crust Mix	1 slice	105
READY-TO-EAT		
chocolate cookie crumb	9 in crust (7.7 oz)	1130
chocolate cookie crumb	⅛ of 9 in pie (1 oz)	139
graham cracker	9 in crust (8.4 oz)	1181
graham cracker	⅛ of 9 in (1 oz)	148
vanilla wafer cracker crumbs	9 in crust (6.1 oz)	937
vanilla wafer cracker crumbs	⅛ of 9 in pie (0.8 oz)	119

FOOD	PORTION	CALS
Keebler		
Graham Single Serve	1 (0.8 oz)	120
Reduced Fat Graham	⅛ pie (0.7 oz)	90
REFRIGERATED		
All Ready		
Crust	⅛ pie (0.9 oz)	120
PIE FILLING		
apple	1 can (21 oz)	599
apple	⅛ can (2.6 oz)	74
cherry	1 can (21 oz)	683
cherry	⅛ can (2.6 oz)	85
pumpkin pie mix	1 cup	282
Colac		
All Flavors	1 tbsp	19
Comstock		
Light Cherry	⅓ cup	60
Red Ruby Cherry	⅓ cup (3.1 oz)	90
Libby's		
Pumpkin Pie Mix	⅓ cup	90
PIEROGI		
pierogi	¾ cup (4.4 oz)	307
Health Is Wealth		
Potato & Cheddar	2 (2.8 oz)	140
Potato & Onion	2 (2.8 oz)	140
Mrs. T's		
Broccoli & Cheddar	3 (4.2 oz)	200
Jalapeno & Cheddar	3 (4.2 oz)	190
Potato & American Cheese	3 (4.2 oz)	220
Potato & Roasted Garlic	3 (4.2 oz)	190
Potato & Cheddar	3 (4.2 oz)	180
Potato & Onion	3 (4.2 oz)	180
Rogies Cheddar & Bacon	7 (3 oz)	140
Rogies Jalapeno & Cheddar	7 (3 oz)	120
Rogies Potato & Cheddar	7 (3 oz)	130
PIGEON PEAS		
dried cooked	½ cup	102
dried cooked	1 cup	204

FOOD	PORTION	CALS

PIGNOLIA (see PINE NUTS)

PIG'S EARS AND FEET

ear simmered	1	184
feet pickled	1 lb	921
feet pickled	1 oz	58
feet simmered	3 oz	165

PIKE

northern cooked	3 oz	96
northern cooked	½ fillet (5.4 oz)	176
northern raw	3 oz	75
roe raw	1 oz	37
walleye baked	3 oz	101
walleye fillet baked	4.4 oz	147

PILLNUTS

canarytree dried	1 oz	204

PIMIENTOS

canned	1 slice	0
canned	1 tbsp	3
Dromedary		
Peeled	½ tsp (4 g)	0
Unpeeled	½ tsp (4 g)	0

PINE NUTS

pignolia dried	1 tbsp	51
pignolia dried	1 oz	146
pinyon dried	1 oz	161
Frieda's		
Pine Nuts	¼ cup	150
Progresso		
Pignoli	1 jar (1 oz)	170

PINEAPPLE

CANNED

chunks in heavy syrup	1 cup	199
chunks juice pack	1 cup	150
crushed in heavy syrup	1 cup	199
slices in heavy syrup	1 slice	45
slices in light syrup	1 slice	30
slices juice pack	1 slice	35

FOOD	PORTION	CALS
slices water pack	1 slice	19
tidbits in heavy syrup	1 cup	199
tidbits in juice	1 cup	150
tidbits in water	1 cup	79
Del Monte		
Chunks In Heavy Syrup	½ cup	90
Chunks In Its Own Juice	½ cup	70
Crushed In Heavy Syrup	½ cup	90
Crushed In Its Own Juice	½ cup	70
Fruit Cup Tidbits	1 pkg (4 oz)	50
Fruit Naturals Chunks	½ cup	70
Dole		
All Natural Chunks	½ cup	60
Chunks Juice Pack	½ cup	60
FRESH		
diced	1 cup	77
slice	1 slice	42
Bonita Hill		
Golden Extra Sweet	2 slices (3.9 oz)	60
Cala Fruit		
Golden Sliced	1 serv (3.5 oz)	50
Frieda's		
Zululand Queen	1 cup (5 oz)	70
Frosty Fresh		
Peeled & Cored	½ cup	60
FROZEN		
chunks sweetened	½ cup	104
PINEAPPLE JUICE		
canned	1 cup	139
frzn as prep	1 cup	129
frzn not prep	6 oz	387
Adina		
Pineapple Ginger Gin-Jah	8 oz	80
Ceres		
Pineapple	8 oz	120
Del Monte		
Juice	6 fl oz	80
Dole		
Chilled	8 oz	130

FOOD	PORTION	CALS
PINK BEANS		
dried cooked	1 cup	252
PINTO BEANS		
CANNED		
pinto	1 cup	186
Eden		
Organic Spicy	½ cup (4.6 oz)	125
Progresso		
Pinto Beans	½ cup (4.6 oz)	110
DRIED		
cooked	1 cup	235
FROZEN		
cooked	3 oz	152
PISTACHIOS		
dried	1 cup	739
dry roasted	1 oz	172
dry roasted salted	1 oz	172
dry roasted salted	1 cup	776
dry roasted w/ salt	47 nuts (1 oz)	160
dry roasted w/ shells unsalted	½ cup	180
American Almond		
Pistachio Paste	2 tbsp	160
Sweet Delights		
Pistachio Roasters	⅓ pkg (1 oz)	190
PITANGA		
fresh	1	2
fresh	1 cup	57
PIZZA *(see also PIZZA CRUST, PIZZA SAUCE)*		
Amy's		
Cheese	⅓ pie	300
Mushroom & Olive	⅓ pie	250
Pesto	⅓ pie	310
Pocket Sandwich Cheese Pizza	1 (4.5 oz)	300
Pocket Sandwich Vegetarian Pizza	1 (4.5 oz)	250
Roasted Vegetable	⅓ pie	260
Snacks Cheese	5–6 pieces	180
Soy Cheese	⅓ pie	290

FOOD	PORTION	CALS
Spinach	⅓ pie	300
Veggie Combo	⅓ pie	280
Appian Way		
Pizza Mix Thick Crust	⅓ pie (4.2 oz)	290
Pizza Mix Thin Crust	⅓ pie (4.1 oz)	250
Banquet		
Pepperoni	1 pie (6.75 oz)	490
Pizza Snack Cheese	6 pieces (7.5 oz)	200
Pizza Snack Pepperoni	6 pieces (7.5 oz)	230
Pizza Snack Pepperoni & Sausage	6 pieces (7.5 oz)	210
Celeste		
Cheese	1 (5.5 oz)	360
Freschetta		
Pepperoni	½ pie (5.8 oz)	470
Health Is Wealth		
Pizza Munchees	6 (3 oz)	190
Healthy Choice		
French Bread Cheese	1 pie	340
French Bread Cheese	1 piece (6 oz)	340
French Bread Pepperoni	1 pie	340
French Bread Pepperoni	1 piece (6 oz)	340
French Bread Sausage	1 piece (6 oz)	320
French Bread Supreme	1 pie	340
French Bread Supreme	1 piece (6.35 oz)	330
French Bread Vegetable	1 pie	320
Jeno's		
Crisp 'N Tasty Cheese	1 pie (6.8 oz)	460
Jiffy		
Crust Mix as prep	⅓ crust	180
Kid Cuisine		
Cheese Pizza Painter	1 meal	320
Dip & Dunk Cheese Pizza Strips	1 meal	510
Primo Pepperoni Pizza	1 meal	400
Lean Cuisine		
Casual Eating French Bread Cheese	1 serv (6 oz)	320
Casual Eating French Bread Pepperoni	1 pkg (5.25 oz)	300
Casual Eating Margherita	1 pkg (6 oz)	320
Casual Eating Pepperoni	1 pkg (6 oz)	380
Casual Eating Roasted Vegetable	1 pkg (6 oz)	330
Casual Eating Spinach & Mushroom	1 pkg (6.1 oz)	310

FOOD	PORTION	CALS
Casual Eating Three Meat	1 pkg (6.4 oz)	350
Causal Eating Deluxe	1 pkg (6 oz)	370
Causal Eating Four Cheese	1 pkg (6 oz)	400
Causal Eating French Bread Deluxe	1 pkg (6.1 oz)	310
Lean Pockets		
Pepperoni	1 (4.5 oz)	280
Sausage & Pepperoni	1 (4.5 oz)	280
Marie Callender's		
French Bread Cheese	1 (7.2 oz)	530
French Bread Pepperoni	1 (7.5 oz)	570
French Bread Supreme	1 (7.5 oz)	510
Pepperidge Farm		
Gourmet Crust Cheese	1 (4.4 oz)	390
Gourmet Crust Pepperoni	1 (4.5 oz)	420
Red Baron		
Deep Dish Single Pepperoni	1 pizza	460
South Beach Diet		
Deluxe	1 pie (6.8 oz)	280
Four Cheese	1 pie (6.3 oz)	290
Grilled Chicken & Vegetable	1 pie (6.8 oz)	280
Pepperoni	1 pie (6.3 oz)	290
Totino's		
Crisp Crust Cheese	½ pie	320
TAKE-OUT		
cheese	⅛ of 12 in pie	140
cheese	12 in pie	1121
cheese deep dish individual	1 (5.5 oz)	460
cheese meat & vegetables	⅛ of 12 in pie	184
cheese meat & vegetables	12 in pie	1472
pepperoni	12 in pie	1445
pepperoni	⅛ of 12 in pie	181
PIZZA CRUST		
crust	1 slice (1.7 oz)	130
whole wheat	⅛ crust	140
Alvarado Street Bakery		
Sprouted Wheat California Style	⅛ pie	190
Betty Crocker		
Italian Herb Crust Mix	¼ crust (1.6 oz)	180

FOOD	PORTION	CALS
Boboli		
Thin Crust	⅓ crust (2 oz)	160
Carbsense		
Garlic & Herb as prep	1 slice	100
Keto		
Dough Mix as prep	1 slice	79
MiniCarb		
Parmesan Herb Mix as prep	1 slice	130
Pillsbury		
Crust	⅓ crust (2 oz)	150

PIZZA SAUCE
Hunt's
Family Favorites	¼ cup	25
Muir Glen		
Organic	¼ cup (2.2 oz)	40
Progresso		
Pizza Sauce	¼ cup (2.1 oz)	20

PLANTAINS
cooked mashed	1 cup	232
sliced cooked	1 cup	179
Chester's		
Chips	1 oz	150
TAKE-OUT		
mofongo	1 serv	320
ripe fried	2.8 oz	214
sweet baked w/ ice cream	1 serv	285

PLUMS
CANNED
purple in heavy syrup	1 cup	320
purple in heavy syrup	3	119
purple in light syrup	3	83
purple in light syrup	1 cup	158
purple juice pack	1 cup	146
purple juice pack	3	55
purple water pack	3	39
purple water pack	1 cup	102
Eden		
Umeboshi Paste	1 tsp	5

FOOD	PORTION	CALS
Umeboshi Plums	1	5
FRESH		
plum	1	36
sliced	1 cup	91
Chiquita		
Purple	2 med (4.6 oz)	80
POI		
poi	½ cup	134
POKEBERRY SHOOTS		
cooked	½ cup	16
fresh	½ cup	18
POLENTA		
Frieda's		
Organic	2 slice (3.5 oz)	70
Original	4 oz	80
Melissa's		
Original	4 oz	80
POLLACK		
altantic fillet baked	5.3 oz	178
atlantic baked	3 oz	100
POMEGRANATE		
fresh	1	104
POMEGRANATE JUICE		
Cortas		
Concentrated Juice	1 tbsp (0.6 oz)	40
Naked Juice		
Pomegranate Passion	8 oz	150
POM		
100% Juice	8 oz	140
Pomegranate Blueberry	8 oz	140
Pomegranate Cherry	8 oz	140
Pomegranate Mango	8 oz	140
Pomegranate Tangerine	8 oz	150
POMPANO		
florida cooked	3 oz	179
florida raw	3 oz	140

FOOD	PORTION	CALS
POPCORN (see also POPCORN CAKES)		
air-popped	1 cup (0.3 oz)	31
caramel coated	1 cup (1.2 oz)	152
caramel coated w/ peanuts	⅔ cup (1 oz)	114
cheese	1 cup (0.4 oz)	58
oil popped	1 cup (0.4 oz)	55
Cape Cod		
White Cheddar	2⅓ cups	170
Chester's		
Caramel Craze	¾ cup	130
Microwave Butter	3 cups	170
Microwave Cheddar Cheese	3 cups	200
Cracker Jack		
Butter Toffee	¾ cup	140
Original	½ cup	120
Husman's		
Cheese Corn	2¼ cups (1 oz)	160
Jolly Time		
American's Best White	5 cups	100
American's Best Yellow	5 cups	100
America's Best 94% Fat Free	5 cups	100
Blast O Butter Light	4 cups	120
Butter Licious Light	5 cups	125
Crispy & White Light	5 cups	125
Healthy Pop 94% Fat Free	5 cups	100
Healthy Pop Caramel Apple	5 cups	100
Healthy Pop Kettle	4 cups	100
White	5 cups	100
Yellow	5 cups	100
Judy's		
Sugar Free Popcorn Nut Brittle	¼ piece (1 oz)	100
Mauna Loa		
Macadamia Nut Butter Corn Crunch	1 oz	150
Orville Redenbacher's		
Gourmet Original	3 cups	92
Hot Air	1 cup	15
Kernel Original	1 cup	15
Microwave Butter Light	1 cup	20
Microwave Kettle Korn Sweet	1 cup	35
Microwave Movie Theater Butter Light	1 cup	20

FOOD	PORTION	CALS
Microwave Movie Theater Extra Butter	1 cup	35
Microwave Natural Light	1 cup	20
Microwave Pour Over Butter	1 cup	40
Microwave Pour Over Cheddar	1 cup	50
Microwave Regular Butter	1 cup	35
Microwave Regular Corn On The Cob	1 cup	35
Microwave Regular Natural	1 cup	15
Microwave Regular Old Fashioned Butter	1 cup	35
Microwave Regular Tender White	1 cup	40
Microwave Smart Pop Butter	1 cup	15
Microwave Smart Pop Kettle Korn	1 cup	20
Microwave Smart Pop Movie Theater Butter	1 cup	20
Microwave Sweet Cinnabon	1 cup	50
Microwave Sweet Honey Butter	1 cup	35
Microwave Sweet 'N Buttery	1 cup	40
Microwave Ultimate Butter	1 cup	30
Microwave Sweet Caramel	1 cup	90
White	1 cup	15
Poppycock		
The Original	½ cup	160
Smart Balance		
No Trans Fat Low Sodium Low Fat	1 cup	20
Smartfood		
Low Fat Toffee Crunch	¾ cup	110
Reduced Fat White Cheddar	3 cups	140
White Cheddar	2 cups	190
White Cheddar	1 pkg	160
Snyder's Of Hanover		
Butter	⅝ oz	110
Tom's		
Caramel Corn	1 pkg (1.6 oz)	180
Utz		
Au Natural	3 cups (1 oz)	120
Butter	2 cups (1 oz)	170
Cheese	2 cups (1 oz)	150
Hulless Puff'N Corn	2 cups (1 oz)	180
Hulless Puff'N Corn Cheese	2 cups (1 oz)	170
Hulless Puff'N Corn Hot Cheese	1 pkg (1.75 oz)	290
White Cheddar	2 cups (1 oz)	150

FOOD	PORTION	CALS
POPCORN CAKES		
Orville Redenbacher's		
Butter	2	60
Caramel	1	40
Chocolate	1	45
Mini Butter	8	60
Mini Caramel	7	50
Mini Peanut Caramel Crunch	6	60
Mini Peanut Crunch	6	60
Mini Sour Cream & Onion	8	60
White Cheddar	2	60
POPOVER		
home recipe as prep w/ 2% milk	1 (1.4 oz)	87
home recipe as prep w/ whole milk	1 (1.4 oz)	90
mix as prep	1 (1.2 oz)	67
POPPY SEEDS		
poppy seeds	1 tsp	15
American Almond		
Baker's Style Poppy Seed Filling	2 tbsp	120
PORGY		
fresh	3 oz	77
PORK (see also HAM, PORK DISHES)		
FRESH		
boston blade roast lean & fat cooked	3 oz	229
boston blade steak lean & fat cooked	3 oz	220
center loin roast lean bone in cooked	3 oz	169
center loin chop lean bone in cooked	3 oz	172
center rib chop lean & fat bone in cooked	3 oz	213
center rib roast lean & fat bone in cooked	3 oz	217
fresh ham rump lean roasted	3 oz	175
fresh ham rump lean & fat roasted	3 oz	214
fresh ham shank lean roasted	3 oz	183
fresh ham shank lean & fat roasted	3 oz	246
fresh ham whole lean roasted	3 oz	179
fresh ham whole lean roasted diced	1 cup	285
fresh ham whole lean & fat roasted	3 oz	232
fresh ham whole lean & fat roasted diced	1 cup	369
ground 97% fat free	4 oz	130

FOOD	PORTION	CALS
ground cooked	3 oz	252
leg loin & shoulder lean only roasted	3 oz	198
loin chop lean bone in braised	3 oz	191
loin chop lean bone in broiled	3 oz	199
loin roast lean bone in roasted	3 oz	210
loin whole lean & fat braised	3 oz	203
loin whole lean & fat broiled	3 oz	206
loin whole lean & fat roasted	3 oz	211
lungs braised	3 oz	84
pancreas cooked	3 oz	186
ribs country style lean & fat braised	3 oz	252
shoulder arm picnic lean & fat roasted	3 oz	269
shoulder whole lean & fat roasted	3 oz	248
shoulder whole lean & fat roasted diced	1 cup	394
shoulder whole lean roasted	3 oz	196
shoulder whole lean roasted diced	1 cup	311
sirloin chop lean & fat bone in braised	3 oz	208
sirloin roast lean & fat bone in cooked	3 oz	222
spareribs braised	3 oz	338
spleen braised	3 oz	127
tail simmered	3 oz	336
tenderloin lean roasted	3 oz	139
top loin chop boneless lean & fat cooked	3 oz	198
top loin roast boneless lean & fat cooked	3 oz	192
Freirich		
Porkette	4 oz	220
TAKE-OUT		
chicharrones pork cracklings fried	1 cup	844

PORK DISHES
Hormel

Center Cut Loin Lemon Garlic	1 serv (4 oz)	130
Extra Lean Apple Burbon	1 serv (4 oz)	140
Extra Lean Teriyaki	4 oz	140
Pork Roast Au Jus	1 serv (5 oz)	180
Morton's Of Omaha		
Tender Pork Roast w/ Gravy & Vegetables	1 serv (5 oz)	210
Smithfield		
Pulled Pork w/ Barbecue Sauce	2 oz	90
Tenderloin Garlic & Herb	3 oz	100
Tenderloin Hickory Sweet	4 oz	110

FOOD	PORTION	CALS
Tyson		
Lemon Pepper Pork Roast	1 serv (3 oz)	110
TAKE-OUT		
chinese spareribs	1 serv	776
pork roast	2 oz	70
pork vandaloo curry	1 serv	620
tourtiere	1 piece (4.9 oz)	451

PORK RINDS (see SNACKS)

POT PIE
Amy's		
Broccoli	1 (7.5 oz)	430
Country Vegetable	1 (7.5 oz)	370
Shepard's	1 (8 oz)	160
Vegetable	1 (7.5 oz)	420
Vegetable Non-Dairy	1 (7.5 oz)	320
Banquet		
Beef	1 (7 oz)	400
Cheesy Potato & Broccoli w/ Ham	1 (7 oz)	410
Chicken	1 (7 oz)	380
Family Size Hearty Chicken	1 cup	460
Macaroni & Cheese	1 pkg (6.5 oz)	210
Turkey	1 (7 oz)	370
Vegetable Cheese	1 (7 oz)	340
Marie Callender's		
Beef	1 (9.5 oz)	680
Chicken	1 (9.5 oz)	680
Chicken & Broccoli	1 (9.5 oz)	670
Chicken Au Gratin	1 (9.5 oz)	690
Turkey	1 (9.5 oz)	680
Morton		
Macaroni & Cheese	1 (6.5 oz)	210
Vegetable w/ Beef	1 (7 oz)	340
Vegetable w/ Chicken	1 (7 oz)	320
Vegetable w/ Turkey	1 (7 oz)	310
Swanson		
Beef	1 (7 oz)	376
Chicken	1 (7 oz)	416
Turkey	1 (7 oz)	440

FOOD	PORTION	CALS
TAKE-OUT		
beef	⅓ of 9 in pie (7.4 oz)	515
beef	1 serv (6.9 oz)	449
chicken	⅓ of 9 in pie (8.1 oz)	545
POTATO (see also CHIPS, KNISH, PANCAKES)		
CANNED		
potatoes	½ cup	54
Del Monte		
New Whole	2 med (5.5 oz)	60
Savory Sides Au Gratin	½ cup	80
S&W		
Whole Small	2 (5.5 oz)	60
FRESH		
baked skin only	1 skin (2 oz)	115
baked w/ skin	1 (6.5 oz)	220
baked w/o skin	½ cup	57
baked w/o skin	1 (5 oz)	145
boiled	½ cup	68
microwaved	1 (7 oz)	212
microwaved w/o skin	½ cup	78
raw w/o skin	1 (3.9 oz)	88
Arrowfarms		
Yukon Gold	1 med (5 oz)	100
Dole		
Idaho	1 (5.3 oz)	100
Frieda's		
Fingerling	4 (5 oz)	100
Green Giant		
Red Potatoes	1 med (5 oz)	100
Lucinda's		
Red "C"	1 med (5.2 oz)	100
SunLite		
SunLite	1 (5 oz)	87
FROZEN		
french fries	10 strips	111
french fries thick cut	10 strips	109
hashed brown	½ cup	170
potato puffs	½ cup	138
potato puffs as prep	1	16

FOOD	PORTION	CALS
Birds Eye		
Baby Gourmet	7 (4 oz)	100
Whole	3	50
Fillo Factory		
Petite Fillo Puffs Potato & Herb	7 (4.6 oz)	280
Healthy Choice		
Cheddar Broccoli Potatoes	1 pkg	270
Inland Valley		
Crinkle Cuts	15 pieces (3 oz)	150
Crisscut Fries	13 pieces (3 oz)	160
Curly QQQ's	1⅓ cups (3 oz)	180
Fajita Fries	17 pieces (3 oz)	170
French Fries	15 pieces (3 oz)	130
Hash Browns	⅔ cup	70
Home Browns	1 patty (2.2 oz)	130
Mashed Homestyle	⅔ cup	160
Simply Shreds	1 cup	70
Stix	5 pieces (3 oz)	170
Stuffed Spudz w/ Cheese	5 pieces	210
Tater Babies	8 pieces (3 oz)	130
Tater Puffs	10 pieces	160
Twice Baked	1 (5.2 oz)	230
Twice Baked Sour Cream Bacon & Chives	1 (5.2 oz)	240
Twice Baked Triple Cheese	1 (5.2 oz)	250
Lean Cuisine		
One Dish Favorites Deluxe Cheddar	1 pkg (10.4 oz)	260
Oh Boy!		
Stuffed With Cheddar Cheese	1 (5 oz)	130
Tree Of Life		
Organic French Fries	20 pieces (3 oz)	110
MIX		
au gratin as prep	½ cup	160
instant mashed flakes as prep w/ whole milk & butter	½ cup	118
instant mashed flakes not prep	½ cup	78
instant mashed granules as prep w/ whole milk & butter	½ cup	114
instant mashed granules not prep	½ cup	372
scalloped	½ cup	105

FOOD	PORTION	CALS
Betty Crocker		
Mashed Butter & Herb	½ cup	160
Mashed Chicken & Herb	½ cup	120
Reduced Fat Recipe		
Hungry Jack		
Mashed Potato Flakes as prep	½ cup	160
Idahoan		
AuGratin as prep	½ cup	150
Hash Browns as prep	½ cup	160
Hash Browns Cheesy not prep	½ cup	120
Mashed Baked as prep	½ cup	110
Mashed Butter & Herb as prep	½ cup	110
Mashed Buttery Homestyle as prep	½ cup	110
Mashed Four Cheese as prep	½ cup	100
Mashed Southwest as prep	½ cup	110
Roasted Garlic as prep	½ cup	600
Scalloped as prep	½ cup	150
REFRIGERATED		
Country Crock		
Garlic Mashed	⅔ cup	170
Homestyle Mashed	⅔ cup	190
PurelyIdaho		
Cheddar Crusted	¾ cup	120
Oven Roasts	1 serv (3 oz)	70
SHELF-STABLE		
Lunch Bucket		
Scalloped w/ Ham Chunks	1 pkg (7.5 oz)	170
TastyBite		
Bombay Potatoes	½ pkg (5 oz)	190
Mumbai Pav Bhaji	½ pkg (5 oz)	229
Simla Potatoes	½ pkg (5 oz)	180
TAKE-OUT		
au gratin w/ cheese	½ cup	178
baked topped w/ cheese sauce	1	475
baked topped w/ cheese sauce & bacon	1	451
baked topped w/ cheese sauce & broccoli	1	402
baked topped w/ cheese sauce & chili	1	481
baked topped w/ sour cream & chives	1	394
cheese fries w/ ranch dressing	1 serv	3010
curry	1 serv (6 oz)	292

FOOD	PORTION	CALS
french fries	1 reg	235
hash brown	½ cup (2.5 oz)	151
indian yogurt potatoes	1 serv	315
mashed	½ cup	111
mustard potato salad	3.5 oz	120
o'brien	1 cup	157
potato dumpling	3.5 oz	334
potato pancakes	1 (1.3 oz)	101
potato salad	½ cup	179
potato salad w/ vegetables	3.5 oz	120
red new boiled	5 sm (5 oz)	120
scalloped	½ cup	127
twice backed w/ cheese	1 half (10 oz)	392

POTATO STARCH

potato starch	1 oz	96

POUT

ocean baked	3 oz	86
ocean fillet baked	4.8 oz	139

PRETZELS

chocolate covered	1 oz	130
dutch twist	4 (2.1 oz)	229
milk chocolate covered twists	4 (1 oz)	140
pretzels	1 oz	108
rods	4 (2 oz)	229
sticks	10	10
sticks	120 (2 oz)	229
twists	10 (2.1 oz)	229
whole wheat	2 sm (1 oz)	103
whole wheat	2 med (2 oz)	205
Aramana		
Soy Pretzels	15 (1 oz)	100
Bachman		
Thin'n Right	12 (1 oz)	120
Cape Cod		
Pretzls	25	130
Gardetto's		
Mustard	1 pkg (0.5 oz)	50

FOOD	PORTION	CALS
Landies Candies		
Sugar Free Chocolate	4 (1.5 oz)	220
Little Debbie		
Mini Twists	1 pkg (1.2 oz)	140
Rold Gold		
Braided Twists	8	110
Braided Twists Honey Wheat	8	110
Checkers	20	110
Rods	3	110
Sourdough Hard	1	100
Sourdough Specials	5	110
Sticks	48	100
Thins	9 pieces	110
Tiny Twists	18 pieces	110
Tiny Twists Cheddar	20	110
Tiny Twists Honey Mustard	13	110
Snyder's Of Hanover		
Dips White Fudge	1 oz	130
Hard Sourdough	1 oz	100
Hard Sourdough Unsalted	1 oz	100
Logs	1 oz	110
Mini	1 oz	120
Mini Unsalted	1 oz	110
Nibblers	1 oz	120
Nibblers Honey Mustard & Onions	1 oz	130
Nibblers Oat Bran	1 oz	130
Nibblers Unsalted	1 oz	120
Oat Bran	1 oz	100
Old Fashioned Dipping Stix	1 oz	100
Old Tyme Unsalted	1 oz	120
Olde Tyme	1 oz	120
Olde Tyme Stix	1 oz	120
Pieces Buttermilk Ranch	1 oz	130
Pieces Cheddar Cheese	1 oz	190
Pieces Honey Mustard & Onions	1 oz	140
Pieces Peppered Pizza	1 oz	150
Rods	1 oz	120
Snaps	24 (1 oz)	110

FOOD	PORTION	CALS
Thin	1 oz	130
Whole Wheat Honey	1 oz	120
Spinzels		
Braided	1 pkg (0.5 oz)	55
Utz		
Country Store Stix	5 (1 oz)	110
Fat Free Hard	1 (0.8 oz)	90
Fat Free Hard No Salt Added	1 (0.8 oz)	90
Fat Free Sour Dough Nuggets	10 (1 oz)	100
Fat Free Stix	14 (1 oz)	100
Fat Free Thin	10 (1 oz)	100
Honey Mustard & Onion	⅓ cup (1 oz)	130
Rods	3 (1 oz)	120
Specials	5 (1 oz)	110
Specials Extra Dark	5 (1 oz)	110
Specials Unsalted	5 (1 oz)	110
Wheels	20 (1 oz)	100
Wege		
Honey Wheat	1 (0.8 oz)	120
PRUNE JUICE		
jarred	1 cup	182
Ocean Spray		
100% Juice	8 oz	180
PRUNES		
canned heavy syrup	¼ cup	61
dried	6	121
dried	½ cup	158
cooked w/o sugar		
American Almond		
Baker's Style Ledvar	2 tbsp	90
St Dalfour		
French Prunes	3	100
Sunsweet		
Dried Plums	5	100
PUDDING		
MIX		
Betty Crocker		
Rice as prep	1 serv	200

FOOD	PORTION	CALS
Jell-O		
Vanilla as prep w/ 2% milk	½ cup (5.1 oz)	150
Keto		
Banana not prep	½ scoop	62
Chocolate not prep	½ scoop	66
French Vanilla not prep	½ scoop	62
Louisiana Purchase		
Bread	1 serv (1.3 oz)	150
Lundberg		
Elegant Rice Cinnamon Raisin	½ cup (3.9 oz)	70
Elegant Rice Coconut	½ cup (3.9 oz)	70
Elegant Rice Honey Almond	½ cup (3.9 oz)	70
Uncle Ben's		
Rice Pudding Cinnamon & Raisins as prep	½ cup (1.5 oz)	160
READY-TO-EAT		
Boost		
Vanilla	1 pkg (5 oz)	240
Healthy Choice		
Low Fat Chocolate Raspberry	½ cup (3.5 oz)	102
Low Fat Chocolate Almond	½ cup (3.5 oz)	109
Low Fat Double Chocolate Fudge	½ cup (3.5 oz)	101
Low Fat French Vanilla	½ cup (3.5 oz)	98
Low Fat Tapioca	½ cup (3.5 oz)	101
Hunt's		
Dessert Favorites Banana Cream Pie	1 serv (3.5 oz)	140
Dessert Favorites Chocolate Brownie	1 serv (3.5 oz)	190
Dessert Favorites Chocolate Mud Pie	1 serv (3.5 oz)	170
Dessert Favorites Chocolate Peanut Butter Pie	1 serv (3.5 oz)	190
Dessert Favorites Dulce De Leche Caramel Cream	1 serv (3.5 oz)	140
Dessert Favorites Lemon Merinque Pie	1 serv (3.5 oz)	130
Snack Pack Butterscotch	1 serv (3.5 oz)	130
Snack Pack Chocolate	1 serv (3.5 oz)	104
Snack Pack Chocolate Fudge	1 serv (3.5 oz)	150
Snack Pack Chocolate Marshmallow	1 serv (3.5 oz)	130
Snack Pack Fat Free Chocolate	1 serv (3.5 oz)	90
Snack Pack Fat Free Tapioca	1 serv (3.5 oz)	80
Snack Pack Fat Free Vanilla	1 serv (3.5 oz)	80
Snack Pack Lemon	1 serv (3.5 oz)	120
Snack Pack Swirl Chocolate Caramel	1 serv (3.5 oz)	140
Snack Pack Swirl S'mores	1 serv (3.5 oz)	140

FOOD	PORTION	CALS
Snack Pack Tapioca	1 serv (3.5 oz)	130
Snack Pack Vanilla	1 serv (3.5 oz)	130
Imagine		
Banana	1 pkg (4 oz)	150
Butterscotch	1 pkg (4 oz)	150
Chocolate	1 pkg (4 oz)	170
Lemon	1 pkg (4 oz)	150
Jell-O		
Fat Free Chocolate Vanilla Swirl	1 serv (4 oz)	100
Fat Free Chocolate Fudge & Caramel	1 serv (4 oz)	100
Fat Free Tapioca	1 serv (4 oz)	100
Fat Free Vanilla Caramel	1 serv (4 oz)	100
Tapioca	1 serv (4 oz)	110
Kozy Shack		
Banana	1 pkg (4 oz)	132
Chocolate	1 pkg (4 oz)	139
Chocolate No Sugar Added	1 pkg (4 oz)	93
Rice	1 pkg (4 oz)	135
Tapioca	1 pkg (4 oz)	134
Tapioca No Sugar Added	1 pkg	90
Vanilla	1 pkg (4 oz)	130
Vanilla No Sugar Added	1 pkg (4 oz)	90
NutraBalance		
Low Lactose All Flavors	1 serv (4 oz)	225
Swiss Miss		
Butterscotch	1 pkg (4 oz)	156
Chocolate	1 pkg (4 oz)	166
Chocolate Fudge	1 pkg (4 oz)	175
Fat Free Chocolate	1 pkg (4 oz)	98
Fat Free Chocolate Fudge	1 pkg (4 oz)	101
Fat Free Vanilla	1 pkg (4 oz)	93
Fat Free Parfait Vanilla Chocolate	1 pkg (4 oz)	96
Lemon Meringue Pie	1 pkg (4 oz)	150
Low Fat Tapioca	1 pkg (4 oz)	130
Low Fat Vanilla	1 serv (4 oz)	120
Milk Chocolate	1 pkg (4 oz)	166
Parfait Vanilla Chocolate	1 pkg (4 oz)	164
Swirl Chocolate Caramel	1 pkg (4 oz)	169
Swirl Chocolate Vanilla	1 pkg (4 oz)	169
Swirl Chocolate Vanilla Chocolate	1 pkg (4 oz)	169

FOOD	PORTION	CALS
Tapioca	1 pkg (4 oz)	138
Vanilla	1 pkg (4 oz)	156
TAKE-OUT		
blancmange	1 serv (4.7 oz)	154
bread pudding	½ cup (4.4 oz)	212
bread w/ raisins	½ cup	180
chocolate	½ cup (5.5 oz)	221
corn	⅔ cup	181
queen of puddings	1 serv (4.4 oz)	266
rice pudding	1 serv (6 oz)	220
rice w/ raisins	½ cup	246
tapioca	½ cup (5.3 oz)	189
vanilla	½ cup (4.3 oz)	130
yorkshire	1 serv (3 oz)	177
PUFFERFISH		
raw	3 oz	72
PUMMELO		
fresh	1	228
sections	1 cup	71
Sunkist		
Fresh	¼	90
PUMPKIN		
butter	1 tbsp	32
canned	½ cup	41
cooked mashed	½ cup	24
flowers cooked	½ cup	10
flowers raw	1	0
leaves cooked	½ cup	7
leaves raw	½ cup	4
raw cubed	½ cup	15
Libby's		
Puree	½ cup	40
PUMPKIN SEEDS		
dried	1 oz	154
roasted	¼ cup	296
salted & roasted	¼ cup	296
whole roasted	¼ cup	71
whole roasted	1 oz	127

FOOD	PORTION	CALS
whole salted	¼ cup	71
roasted		
David		
All Natural	¼ cup	160
PURSLANE		
cooked	1 cup	21
fresh	1 cup	7
QUAIL		
breast w/o skin raw	1 (2 oz)	69
w/ skin raw	1 quail (3.8 oz)	210
w/o skin raw	1 quail (3.2 oz)	123
QUICHE		
Atkins		
Crustless Bacon & Onion	1 serv	320
Crustless Four Cheese	1 serv	290
Crustless Smoked Ham & Cheese	1 serv	290
TAKE-OUT		
cheese	⅛ 9-inch pie	566
lorraine	⅛ 9-inch pie	568
mushroom	1 slice (3 oz)	256
spinach	⅛ 9-inch pie	342
QUINCE		
fresh	1	53
QUINOA		
quinoa not prep	1 cup (6 oz)	636
RABBIT		
domestic w/o bone roasted	3 oz	167
wild w/o bone stewed	3 oz	147
RACCOON		
roasted	3 oz	217
RADICCHIO		
raw shredded	½ cup	5
RADISHES		
chinese dried	½ cup	157
chinese raw	1 (12 oz)	62

FOOD	PORTION	CALS
chinese raw sliced	½ cup	8
chinese sliced cooked	½ cup	13
daikon dried	½ cup	157
daikon raw	1 (12 oz)	62
daikon raw sliced	½ cup	8
daikon sliced cooked	½ cup	13
red raw	10	7
red sliced	½ cup	10
white icicle raw	1 (0.5 oz)	2
white icicle raw sliced	½ cup	7
Eden		
Daikon Dried Shredded	2 tbsp	45
Daikon Pickled	2 slices	5
Frieda's		
Black	¾ cup	15
Chinese Lo Bok	⅔ cup	25
Daikon	½ cup	15
Korean Moo	⅔ cup	15
TAKE-OUT		
korean kimchee	½ cup	31
moo namul saengche korean salad	1 serv (3.7 oz)	34

RAISINS

FOOD	PORTION	CALS
chocolate coated	10 (0.4 oz)	39
chocolate coated	1 cup (6.7 oz)	741
golden seedless	1 cup	437
jumbo golden	¼ cup	130
seedless	1 cup	434
seedless	1 tbsp	27
sultanas	1 oz	88
Brach's		
California Chocolate Covered	35 pieces	170
Dole		
CinnaRaisins	1 pkg (1 oz)	95
Estee		
Chocolate Covered Fructose Sweetened	¼ cup	180
Mariana		
Fruitn Yogurt Milk Chocolate Covered Raisins	32 pieces (1 oz)	130
Nestle		
Chocolate Covered	1⅓ tbsp	70

FOOD	PORTION	CALS
Sun-Maid		
California Golden	¼ cup	130
California Seedless	1 box (1.5 oz)	130
Tree Of Life		
Organic	¼ cup (1.4 oz)	130
RASPBERRIES		
canned in heavy syrup	½ cup	117
fresh	1 cup	61
fresh	1 pint	154
frozen sweetened	1 pkg (10 oz)	291
frozen sweetened	1 cup	256
frzn unsweetened	¾ cup	130
Birds Eye		
Red	5 oz	90
Frieda's		
Dried	⅓ cup (1.4 oz)	145
RASPBERRY JUICE		
Dole		
Country Raspberry	8 fl oz	140
Fresh Samantha		
Raspberry Dream	1 cup (8 oz)	120
Naked Juice		
Raspberry Ade	8 oz	90
Nantucket Nectars		
Organic Very Raspberry	8 oz	120
RED BEANS		
CANNED		
Hunt's		
Small	½ cup (4.5 oz)	89
Van Camp's		
Red Beans	½ cup (4.6 oz)	90
MIX		
Bean Cuisine		
Pasta & Beans Barcelona Red With Radiatore	1 serv	210
RELISH		
cranberry orange	½ cup	246
hamburger	1 tbsp	19

FOOD	PORTION	CALS
hamburger	½ cup	158
hot dog	1 tbsp	14
hot dog	½ cup	111
piccalilli	1.4 oz	13
sweet	½ cup	159
sweet	1 tbsp	19
Claussen		
Sweet Pickle	1 tbsp (0.5 oz)	15
Del Monte		
Hamburger	1 tbsp	20
Hot Dog	1 tbsp	15
Sweet Pickle	1 tbsp	20
Frieda's		
Kim Chee	¼ cup	15
Matouk's		
Hot Chow	2 tbsp	20
Kuchela	1 tsp	9
Vlasic		
Fancy Sweet	1 tbsp	15
RENNIN		
tablet	1 (0.9 g)	1
RHUBARB		
fresh	½ cup	13
frozen	½ cup	60
frzn as prep w/ sugar	½ cup	139
RICE *(see also* RICE CAKES, WILD RICE*)*		
arborio	½ cup	100
brown long grain cooked	1 cup (6.8 oz)	216
brown medium grain cooked	1 cup (6.8 oz)	218
glutinous cooked	1 cup (6.1 oz)	169
starch	1 oz	98
white long grain cooked	1 cup (5.5 oz)	205
white long grain instant cooked	1 cup (5.8 oz)	162
white medium grain cooked	1 cup (6.5 oz)	242
white short grain cooked	1 cup (6.5 oz)	242
A Taste Of Thai		
Coconut Garlic Basil as prep	¾ cup	160
Coconut Ginger as prep	¾ cup	190
Jasmine not prep	¼ cup	160

FOOD	PORTION	CALS
Yellow Curry as prep	¾ cup	180
Amy's		
Bowls Brown Rice & Vegetables	1 pkg (10 oz)	240
Birds Eye		
Rice & Broccoli In Cheese Sauce	1 pkg	290
White & Wild w/ Green Beans	1 cup (6.6 oz)	180
Buitoni		
Risotto Garden Vegetable	1 serv	210
Risotto Portobello Mushrooms	1 serv	210
Risotto Rosemary & Potatoes	1 serv	210
Risotto Tomato Basil	1 serv	210
Carolina		
Black Beans & Rice Mix as prep	1 serv	200
Gold as prep	1 cup	160
Spanish Rice Mix as prep	1 serv	180
Chun King		
Fried Rice Mix	½ cup (1.4 oz)	126
Country Crock		
Chicken Rice w/ Herbs	1 cup	210
Gourmet House		
Brown & White not prep	¼ cup	160
La Choy		
Fried Rice	1 cup (4.9 oz)	236
Lundberg		
One-Step Curry	1 cup (7.4 oz)	160
Quick Brown Rice Savory Vegetarian Chicken	1 cup (2.5 oz)	260
Risotto Tomato Basil	1 serv	140
Mahatma		
Jambalaya as prep	1 cup	190
Nacho Cheese Mix as prep	1 serv	250
Thai Jasmine as prep	¾ cup	160
Minute		
Instant Brown as prep	⅔ cup	170
Near East		
Creative Grains Chicken & Herb as prep	1 cup	270
Creative Grains Creamy Parmesan as prep	1 cup	280
Creative Grains Roasted Garlic as prep	1 cup	220
Creative Grains Roasted Pecan as prep	1 cup	240
Long Grain & Wild Rice Roasted Vegetable & Chicken as prep	1 cup	220

FOOD	PORTION	CALS
Long Grain & Wild Rice Garlic & Herb as prep	1 cup	220
Pilaf Brown Rice as prep	1 cup	210
Pilaf Chicken as prep	1 cup	220
Pilaf Mix Curry as pre	1 cup	220
Pilaf Mix Garlic & Herb as prep	1 cup	220
Pilaf Mix Long Grain & Wild as prep	1 cup	220
Pilaf Mix Rice as prep	1 cup	220
Pilaf Mix Roasted Chicken & Garlic as prep	1 cup	220
Pilaf Mix Spanish Rice as prep	1 cup	310
Pilaf Mix Toasted Almond as prep	1 cup	230
Pilaf Mix Wild Mushroom & Herb as prep	1 cup	220
Nueva Cocina		
Arroz A La Mexicana	1 cup	190
Arroz Con Pollo	1 cup	150
Gallo Pinto	⅓ pkg	220
Moros Y Cristianos	⅓ pkg	220
Paella	⅓ pkg	160
Pacific Foods		
Ready-To-Serve Lemon & Herb	½ pkg	240
Ready-To-Serve Roasted Chicken	½ pkg	240
Ready-To-Serve Spanish Style	½ pkg	230
Ready-To-Serve Wild Rice & Mushroom	½ pkg	230
Rice Expressions		
Indian Basmati	1 cup	180
Organic Brown	1 cup	160
Organic Long Grain	1 cup	180
Organic Rice Pilaf	1 cup	170
Organic Tex Mex	1 cup	190
River Rice		
Brown Long Grain not prep	¼ cup	150
S&W		
Arborio as prep	¾ cup	150
Basmati Mix as prep	¾ cup	160
Brown Long Grain not prep	¼ cup	150
Long Grain Organic not prep	¼ cup	150
Success		
Beef Mix as prep	1 cup	240
Broccoli & Cheese	½ cup	130
Brown	1 cup	150

FOOD	PORTION	CALS
Brown & Wild Mix	½ cup	120
Classic Chicken	½ cup	90
Grilled Chicken & Broccoli Mix as prep	1 cup	240
Long Grain & Wild	½ cup	120
Pilaf	½ cup	120
Red Beans & Rice Mix as prep	1 cup	300
Spanish	½ cup	120
White as prep	1 cup	190
Yellow Mix as pre	1 cup	170
TastyBite		
Pilaf Curried Vegetable	½ pkg (4.5 oz)	180
Pilaf Green Peas	½ pkg (4.5 oz)	208
Pilaf Vegetable Kofta	½ pkg (4.5 oz)	229
Uncle Ben's		
Original Brown as prep	1 cup	170
Ready Rice Whole Grain	½ pkg	190
White Converted as prep	1 cup	170
Van Camp's		
Spanish	½ cup (4.5 oz)	90
Water Maid		
White Medium Grain not prep	¼ cup	160
Zatarain's		
Dirty Rice Mix as prep w/o meat and oil	½ cup	130
Red Beans & Rice as prep w/o oil	½ cup	100
TAKE-OUT		
coconut rice	1 serv	500
congee	½ cup (4.1 oz)	44
nasi goreng (fried rice)	1 serv	206
nasi goreng indonesian rice & vegetables	1 cup (4.9 oz)	130
paella	1 serv (7 oz)	308
pilaf	½ cup	84
risotto	1 serv (6.6 oz)	426
spanish	¾ cup	363

RICE CAKES (see also POPCORN CAKES)
Lundberg

FOOD	PORTION	CALS
Nutra Farmed Brown Rice	1 (0.7 oz)	70
Nutra Farmed Sesame Tamari	1 (0.7 oz)	70
Organic Koku Sesame	1 (0.7 oz)	80

FOOD	PORTION	CALS
Tastemorr		
Rice Crisps Caramel	7	55
ROCKFISH		
pacific cooked	3 oz	103
pacific cooked	1 fillet (5.2 oz)	180
pacific raw	3 oz	80
ROE (*see also* INDIVIDUAL FISH NAMES)		
fish	1 oz	11
fresh baked	1 oz	58
ROLL		
FROZEN		
Pillsbury		
Dinner Rolls Crusty French	1	110
Sara Lee		
Deluxe Cinnamon Rolls w/o Icing	1 (2.7 oz)	370
READY-TO-EAT		
bialy	1 (2.2 oz)	138
brioche sweet roll	1 (3.5 oz)	410
brown & serve	1 (1 oz)	85
cheese	1 (2.3 oz)	238
cinnamon raisin	1 (2¾ in)	223
dinner	1 (1 oz)	85
egg	1 (2½ in)	107
french	1 (1.3 oz)	105
hamburger	1 (1.5 oz)	123
hamburger multi-grain	1 (1.5 oz)	113
hamburger reduced calorie	1 (1.5 oz)	84
hard	1 (3½ in)	167
hot cross bun	1	202
hotdog	1 (1.5 oz)	123
hotdog reduced calorie	1 (1.5 oz)	84
hotdog whole wheat	1 (1.5 oz)	110
kaiser	1 (3½ in)	167
oat bran	1 (1.2 oz)	78
rye	1 (1 oz)	81
submarine	1 (4.7 oz)	155
wheat	1 (1 oz)	77
whole wheat	1 (1 oz)	75

FOOD	PORTION	CALS
Alvarado Street Bakery		
Sprouted Wheat Burger Bun	1 (2.2 oz)	140
Bread Du Jour		
Cracked Wheat	1 (1.2 oz)	100
Italian	1 (1.2 oz)	90
Sourdough	1 (1.2 oz)	90
Country Kitchen		
Wheat Light	1	80
Natural Ovens		
Best Burger Bun	1	178
Better Wheat Buns	1	140
Gourmet Dinner	1	70
Pepperidge Farm		
Brown & Serve Club	1 (1.6 oz)	120
Dinner Rolls Finger Poppy	1 (0.9 oz)	80
Kaiser Soft 100% Whole Wheat	1	200
Stroehmann		
Hamburger	1 (1.4 oz)	100
Hamburger Potato	1 (1.9 oz)	140
Hot Dog	1 (1.4 oz)	100
Hot Dog Potato	1 (1.9 oz)	140
Super Bakery		
Daily Donut Reduced Fat	1 (2.2 oz)	200
Organic Sandwich Bun	1 (3.6 oz)	250
Sub Roll	1 (3.6 oz)	250
Wonder		
Brown & Serve	1 (1 oz)	80
Brown & Serve Sourdough	1 (1 oz)	70
Brown & Serve Wheat	1 (1 oz)	80
Bun	1 (3 oz)	220
Club French	1 (1.6 oz)	120
Club Grain	1 (1.6 oz)	120
Club Sourdough	1 (1.6 oz)	120
Dinner	2 (1.6 oz)	130
Dinner Honey Rich	1 (1.3 oz)	100
Dinner Wheat	2 (1.6 oz)	140
Hamburger	1 (2.5 oz)	180
Hamburger	1 (2 oz)	150
Hamburger	1 (1.5 oz)	110
Hamburger Wheat	1 (1.5 oz)	120

FOOD	PORTION	CALS
Hamburger Wheat	1 (1.9 oz)	140
Hoagie French	1 (3 oz)	220
Hoagie Grain	1 (3 oz)	220
Hoagie Sourdough	1 (3 oz)	220
Hot Dog	1 (2 oz)	160
Kaiser	1 (2.2 oz)	180
Kaiser Hoagie	1 (3 oz)	220
Multigrain	1 (1.8 oz)	140
Potato Bun	1 (1.5 oz)	110
Steak	1 (2.5 oz)	190
REFRIGERATED		
cinnamon w/ frosting	1	109
crescent	1 (1 oz)	98
Pillsbury		
Apple Cinnamon	1 (1.5 oz)	150
Caramel	1 (1.7 oz)	170
Cinnamon w/ Icing	1 (1.5 oz)	150
Cinnamon w/ Icing Reduced Fat	1 (1.5 oz)	140
Cinnamon Raisin w/ Icing	1 (1.7 oz)	170
Cornbread Twists	1 (1.4 oz)	140
Crecents Reduced Fat	1 (1 oz)	100
Crescent	1 (1.7 oz)	170
Dinner	1 (1.4 oz)	110
Dinner Wheat	1 (1.4 oz)	110
Orange Sweet Roll w/ Icing	1 (1.7 oz)	150

ROSE APPLE

fresh	3.5 oz	32

ROSE HIP

fresh	1 oz	26

ROSELLE

fresh	1 cup	28

ROSEMARY

dried	1 tsp	4

ROUGHY

orange baked	3 oz	75

RUBS (see HERBS/SPICES)

FOOD	PORTION	CALS
RUTABAGA		
cooked mashed	½ cup	41
raw cubed	½ cup	25
SABLEFISH		
baked	3 oz	213
fillet baked	5.3 oz	378
smoked	3 oz	218
smoked	1 oz	72
SAFFLOWER		
seeds dried	1 oz	147
SAFFRON		
saffron	1 tsp	2
SAGE		
ground	1 tsp	2
SALAD		
MIX		
Dole		
All American Toss	2 cups (3.5 oz)	50
American Blend	1½ cups (3 oz)	15
Classic	1½ cups (3 oz)	15
Classic Romaine Blend	1½ cups (3 oz)	15
Coleslaw	1½ cups (3 oz)	25
European Special Blend	2 cups (3 oz)	15
Garlic Caesar Complete w/ Dressing	1½ cups (3.5 oz)	180
Greek Marinade	1½ cups (3.5 oz)	100
Greener Selection	1½ cups (3 oz)	15
Light Caesar Complete w/ Dressing	1½ cups (3.5 oz)	60
Light Herb Ranch Complete w/ Dressing	1½ cups (3.5 oz)	50
Light Roasted Garlic Caesar Complete w/ Dressing	1½ cups (3.5 oz)	60
Light Zesty Italian Complete w/ Dressing	1½ cups (3.5 oz)	50
Mediterranean Marinade	2 cups (3.5 oz)	90
Oriental Complete w/ Dressing	1½ cups (3.5 oz)	120
Romano Complete w/ Dressing	1½ cups (3.5 oz)	150
Sunflower Ranch Complete w/ Dressing	1½ cups (3.5 oz)	160
Tomato & Mozzarella Medley	2 cups (3.5 oz)	60
Triple Cheese Toss	2 cups (3.5 oz)	80

FOOD	PORTION	CALS
Earthbound Farm		
Baby Caesar Mix	1 pkg (5 oz)	25
Baby Greens w/ Low Fat Honey Dijon Vinaigrette & Tomato Croutons	1 serv (3.5 oz)	90
Caesar w/ Garlic Croutons	1 serv (3.5 oz)	170
Italian Salad Organic	1⅔ cups (2.9 oz)	15
Mixed Baby Greens Organic	1 pkg (4 oz)	30
Organic Baby Greens w/ Vinaigrette & Garlic Croutons	1 serv (3.5 oz)	230
Organic Baby Spinach w/ Sesame Soy Vinaigrette & Peanuts	1 serv (3.5 oz)	150
Organic Italian Salad w/ Blue Cheese Dressing & Walnuts	1 serv (3.5 oz)	190
Romaine Blend Organic	1⅔ cups (2.9 oz)	15
Fresh Express		
Baby Spinach Trio	4 cups (3 oz)	20
Fancy Field Greens	1½ cups (3 oz)	15
Original Iceberg Garden w/ Zip	1½ cups (3 oz)	15
Veggie Lover's	1½ cups (3 oz)	20
Krakus		
Bordeaux	1 pkg (5 oz)	35
Ready Pac		
All American	2.5 cups	15
Bowl Salad Chef	1 pkg	350
Bowl Salad Chicken Caesar	1 pkg	380
Bowl Salad Greek	1 pkg	400
Bowl Salad Spinach Bacon	1 pkg	300
Bowl Salad Spring Mix Veggie	1 pkg	330
Caesar Romaine	1½ cups	15
Classic Crisp Salad	2¼ cups	10
Continental	3 cups	20
Costa Brava	3 cups	15
Hearty Green Salad	2½ cups	10
Lafayette	3 cups	10
Milano	3 cups	15
Organic Caesar Romaine	2¼ cups	15
Organic Mesclun Blend	1 pkg (4.5 oz)	35
Organic Monterey	3 cups	15
Parisian	2 cups	20
Portofino	1 pkg (5 oz)	25

FOOD	PORTION	CALS
Santa Barbara	3½ cups	15
Spring Mix	1 pkg (5 oz)	35
River Ranch		
American Bland	1½ cups	15
Caesar Kit	1½ cups	110
European Blend	1¾ cups	10
Garden	1½ cups	15
Garden Supreme	1½ cups	15
Italian Blend	1¾ cups	15
Raspberry Vinaigrette Kit	1¾ cups	130
Riviera Blend	1½ cups	10
TAKE-OUT		
caesar	2 cups	337
chef w/o dressing	1½ cups	386
cobb w/ dressing	4 cups	635
greek w/ dressing	2 cups	210
tossed 7-layer	2 cups	557
tossed w/o dressing	1½ cups	32
tossed w/o dressing w/ cheese & egg	1½ cups	102
tossed w/o dressing w/ chicken	1½ cups	105
tossed w/o dressing w/ pasta & seafood	1½ cups	380
tossed w/o dressing w/ shrimp	1½ cups	107
waldorf	1 cup	242

SALAD DRESSING
MIX
A Taste Of Thai
Peanut Dressing as prep	2 tbsp	40
Et Tu		
Caesar Salad Kit	1 serv	140
Good Seasons		
Italian as prep	2 tbsp	130
Italian not prep	⅛ pkg (3 g)	5
McCormick		
Mediterrenean Potato Salad	1 tbsp	25
Pasta Salad Vinagarette	1 tsp (5 g)	15
READY-TO-EAT		
blue cheese	1 tbsp	77
french	1 tbsp	67
french reduced calorie	1 tbsp	22

FOOD	PORTION	CALS
italian	1 tbsp	69
italian reduced calorie	1 tbsp	16
russian	1 tbsp	76
russian reduced calorie	1 tbsp	23
sesame seed	1 tbsp	68
thousand island	1 tbsp	59
thousand island reduced calorie	1 tbsp	24
Annie Chun's		
Lemongrass	2 tbsp	60
Sesame Cilantro	1 tbsp	4
Carb Options		
Italian	2 tbsp	70
Ranch	2 tbsp	150
Consorzio		
Balsamic Vinaigrette	2 tbsp	60
Caesar Parmesan & Romano	2 tbsp	120
Honey Mustard	2 tbsp	100
Italian	2 tbsp	60
Mango	1 tbsp	15
Raspberry & Balsamic	1 tbsp	15
Strawberry Balsamic	1 tbsp	10
Drew's		
Low Carb Garlic Italian	1 tbsp	80
Low Carb Lemon Tahini Goddess	1 tbsp	80
Low Carb Sesame Orange	1 tbsp	80
Hellmann's		
Citrus Splash Ruby Red Ginger	2 tbsp (1 oz)	90
Kraft		
Free Thousand Island	2 tbsp	45
LaMartinique		
Blue Cheese Vinaigrette	2 tbsp	160
Poppy Seed	2 tbsp	170
Nasoya		
Creamy Dill	1 tbsp	30
Creamy Italian	2 tbsp	70
Garden Herb	2 tbsp	60
Sesame Garlic	2 tbsp	60
Old Dutch		
Sweet & Sour	2 tbsp	50

FOOD	PORTION	CALS
Paul's		
No-Fat Raspberry & Balsamic	2 tbsp	20
No-Oil Orange & Basil	2 tbsp	15
Spectrum		
Honey Dijon	2 tbsp	35
Organic Creamy Dill	2 tbsp	25
Organic Creamy Garlic	2 tbsp	20
Organic Greek Goddess	2 tbsp	110
Organic Omega 3 Balsamic Vinaigrette	2 tbsp	80
Organic Omega 3 Ginger Garlic Vinaigrette	2 tbsp	80
Organic Omega 3 Raspberry Vinaigrette	2 tbsp	80
Organic Porcini Mushroom Vinaigrette	2 tbsp	70
Organic Rocky Mountain Ranch	2 tbsp	130
Organic Sweet Onion & Garlic	2 tbsp	15
Organic Toasted Sesame	2 tbsp	15
Provencal Garlic Lover's	2 tbsp	50
Zesty Italian	2 tbsp	30
Steel's		
Honey Mustard	1 tbsp	90
Sweet Ginger Lime	1 tbsp	68
Wishbone		
Italian	2 tbsp	80
Just 2 Good! Creamy Caesar	2 tbsp	45
Thousand Island	2 tbsp	130
TAKE-OUT		
vinegar & oil	1 tbsp	72
SALMON		
CANNED		
chum w/ bone	1 can (13.9 oz)	521
chum w/ bone	3 oz	120
pink w/ bone	1 can (15.9 oz)	631
pink w/ bone	3 oz	118
sockeye w/ bone	3 oz	130
sockeye w/ bone	1 can (12.9 oz)	566
Bumble Bee		
Blueback	¼ cup	110
Keta	¼ cup	90
Pink	¼ cup	90
Red	¼ cup	110

FOOD	PORTION	CALS
Skinless & Boneless	¼ cup	50
Smoked Fillets In Oil	⅓ cup	150
Chicken Of The Sea		
Pink	1 pkg (3 oz)	90
Pink Skinless Boneless	¼ cup	60
Red	¼ cup	110
Smoked Pacific	1 pkg (3 oz)	120
Libby's		
Alaskan Sockeye Red	¼ cup	110
Pink Skinless Boneless	¼ cup	50
Red	¼ cup	110
FRESH		
atlantic baked	3 oz	155
chinook baked	3 oz	196
chum baked	3 oz	131
coho cooked	½ fillet (5.4 oz)	286
coho cooked	3 oz	157
coho raw	3 oz	124
pink baked	3 oz	127
roe raw	1 oz	59
sockeye cooked	3 oz	183
sockeye cooked	½ fillet (5.4 oz)	334
sockeye raw	3 oz	143
SMOKED		
chinook	1 oz	33
Lascco		
Nova Sliced	2 oz	60
TAKE-OUT		
roulette w/ spinach stuffing	1 serv (4 oz)	160
salmon cake	1 (3 oz)	241
SALSA		
black bean & corn	2 tbsp	15
cirtus	2 tbsp (1 oz)	10
peach	2 tbsp	15
tomato-less corn & chile	2 tbsp	45
Cape Cod		
Medium & Mild	2 tbsp	15
Del Salsa		
Fire Roasted All Flavors	2 tbsp	8

FOOD	PORTION	CALS
Gringo Billy's		
Salsa Mix	1 tsp	5
Guiltless Gourmet		
Roasted Red Pepper	2 tbsp	10
Southwestern Grill	2 tbsp	15
Hunt's		
Alfresco All Varieties	2 tbsp (1.1 oz)	10
Hot	2 tbsp (1.1 oz)	27
Medium	2 tbsp (1.1 oz)	27
Mild	2 tbsp (1.1 oz)	27
Picante All Varieties	2 tbsp (1.1 oz)	11
Squeeze Mild & Medium	2 tbsp (1.1 oz)	27
Muir Glen		
Black Bean & Corn Medium	2 tbsp (1.1 oz)	15
Chipotle Medium	2 tbsp (1.1 oz)	10
Fire Roasted Tomato Medium	2 tbsp (1.1 oz)	10
Garlic Cilantro Medium	2 tbsp (1.1 oz)	10
Habanero Hot	2 tbsp (1.1 oz)	10
Organic Medium	2 tbsp (1.1 oz)	10
Organic Mild	2 tbsp (1.1 oz)	10
Roasted Garlic Medium	2 tbsp (1.1 oz)	10
Pace		
Picante Mild or Medium	2 tbsp	10
Thick & Chunky Mild or Medium	2 tbsp	10
Rosarita		
Extra Chunky Medium	2 tbsp (1 oz)	7
Green Tomatillo Medium	2 tbsp (1 oz)	8
Picante Zesty Jalapeno Hot	2 tbsp (1 oz)	8
Picante Zesty Jalapeno Medium	2 tbsp (1 oz)	9
Picante Zesty Jalapeno Mild	2 tbsp (1 oz)	8
Roasted Mild	2 tbsp (1 oz)	10
Traditional Medium	2 tbsp (1 oz)	7
Traditional Mild	2 tbsp (1 oz)	7
Snyder's Of Hanover		
Mild	2 tbsp	10
Tostitos		
All Natural	2 tbsp	15
Con Queso	2 tbsp	40
Monterey Jack Queso	2 tbsp	40
Restaurant Style	2 tbsp	15

FOOD	PORTION	CALS
Tree Of Life		
Medium	2 tbsp (1 oz)	10
Mild	2 tbsp (1 oz)	10
Utz		
Chunky	2 tbsp (1 fl oz)	60
SALSIFY		
fresh sliced cooked	½ cup	46
Frieda's		
Salsify	¾ cup	70
SALT SUBSTITUTES		
Eden		
Shiso Leaf Powder	1 tsp	0
Halsosalt		
All Flavors	¼ tsp (7 g)	1
Molly McButter		
Lite Sodium	1 tsp	5
Morton		
Salt Substitute	¼ tsp (1.2 g)	tr
Mrs. Dash		
Onion & Herb	¼ tsp	0
SALT/SEASONED SALT		
salt	1 tsp (6 g)	0
salt	1 tbsp (18 g)	0
Eden		
Atlantic Sea Salt	¼ tsp	0
Brittany Sea Salt	¼ tsp	0
McCormick		
Celery Salt	¼ tsp	0
Morton		
Garlic	1 tsp	3
Iodized	1 tsp	tr
Kosher	1 tsp	0
Lite	¼ tsp (1.4 g)	tr
Nature's Season Seasoning Blend	1 tsp	3
Non-Iodized	1 tsp	0
Seasoned	1 tsp	4

FOOD	PORTION	CALS
SANDWICHES		
Amy's		
Pocket Sandwich Broccoli & Cheese	1 (4.5 oz)	270
Pocket Sandwich Roasted Vegetables	1 (4.5 oz)	220
Pocket Sandwich Spinach Feta	1 (4.5 oz)	250
Pocket Sandwich Tofu Scramble	1 (4 oz)	160
Pocket Sandwich Vegetable Pie	1 (5 oz)	300
Toaster Pops Grilled Cheese	1	180
Lean Pockets		
Bacon Egg & Cheese	1 (4.5 oz)	150
Barbecue Sauce w/ Beef	1 (4.5 oz)	290
Chicken Cheddar & Broccoli	1 (4.5 oz)	260
Chicken Fajita	1 (4.5 oz)	260
Chicken Parmesan	1 (4.5 oz)	280
Ham & Cheese	1 (4.5 oz)	280
Meatballs & Mozzarella	1 (4.5 oz)	290
Philly Steak & Cheese	1 (4.5 oz)	280
Sausage Egg & Cheese	1 (4.5 oz)	140
Steak Fajita	1 (4.5 oz)	260
Three Cheese & Chicken Quesadilla	1 (4.5 oz)	280
Turkey & Ham w/ Cheddar	1 (4.5 oz)	280
Turkey Broccoli & Cheese	1 (4.5 oz)	270
Madalena's Masterpiece		
Calzone Artichoke Parmesan	1 (10 oz)	570
Calzone Grilled Chicken	1 (10 oz)	520
Calzone Sausage Pepperoni	1 (10 oz)	640
Panini Garlic Chicken	1 (8 oz)	450
Panini Honey Ham	1 (8 oz)	520
Panini Turkey Pesto	1 (8 oz)	500
Panini Veggie	1 (8 oz)	480
Quesabake Mexican Sausage	1 (7 oz)	510
Quesabake Roasted Veggie	1 (7 oz)	460
Smucker's		
Uncrustables Grilled Cheese	1 (1.8 oz)	150
Uncrustables Peanut Butter & Grape Jelly	1 (2 oz)	210
Uncrustables Peanut Butter & Strawberry Jam	1 (2 oz)	210
South Beach Diet		
Wrap Kit Deli Ham & Turkey	1 pkg	220
Wrap Kit Grilled Chicken Caesar	1 pkg	230
Wrap Kit Southwestern Style Chicken	1 pkg	240

FOOD	PORTION	CALS
Wrap Kits Turkey & Bacon Club	1 pkg	250
TAKE-OUT		
calzone beef & cheese	1	330
calzone cheese	1 (12 oz)	1020
calzone pepperoni	1	450
chicken fillet plain	1	515
chicken fillet w/ cheese lettuce mayonnaise & tomato	1	632
crab cake w/ bun	1	308
croque monsieur	1 (12.4 oz)	765
fish fillet w/ tartar sauce	1	431
fish fillet w/ tartar sauce & cheese	1	524
fried egg	1	226
fried egg w/ cheese	1	340
fried egg w/ cheese & ham	1	348
gyro	1 (13.7 oz)	604
ham w/ cheese	1	353
roast beef submarine sandwich w/ tomato lettuce & mayonnaise	1	411
roast beef w/ cheese	1	402
roast beef plain	1	346
steak w/ tomato lettuce salt & mayonnaise	1	459
submarine w/ salami ham cheese lettuce tomato onion & oil	1	456
tuna salad submarine sandwich w/ lettuce & oil	1	584
SAPODILLA		
fresh	1	140
fresh cut up	1 cup	199
SAPOTES		
fresh	1	301
SARDINES		
CANNED		
atlantic in oil w/ bone	2	50
atlantic in oil w/ bone	1 can (3.2 oz)	192
pacific in tomato sauce w/ bone	1	68
pacific in tomato sauce w/ bone	1 can (13 oz)	658

FOOD	PORTION	CALS
Beach Cliff		
In Louisiana Hot Sauce	1 can (3.7 oz)	150
In Mustard Sauce	1 can (3.7 oz)	150
In Olive Oil	1 can (3.7 oz)	200
In Tomato Sauce	1 can (3.7 oz)	140
In Water	1 can (3.7 oz)	150
Small In Soybean Oil	1 can (3.7 oz)	200
W/ Hot Green Chilies	1 can (3.7 oz)	180
Brunswick		
In Louisiana Hot Sauce	1 can (3.7 oz)	150
In Mustard Sauce	1 can (3.7 oz)	150
In Soybean Oil	1 can (3.7 oz)	110
In Spring Water	1 can (3.7 oz)	150
In Tomato Sauce	1 can (3.7 oz)	150
W/ Hot Tabasco Peppers	1 can (3.7 oz)	110
Bumble Bee		
In Hot Sauce	¼ cup	90
In Mustard	¼ cup	70
In Oil	1 can (3.7 oz)	130
In Water	1 can (3.7 oz)	120
Chicken Of The Sea		
In Hot Sauce	1 can (3.75 oz)	130
In Mustard Sauce	1 can (3.75 oz)	150
In Oil	1 can (3.75 oz)	190
In Tomato Sauce	1 can (3.75 oz)	130
In Water	1 can (3.75 oz)	100
Goya		
In Tomato Sauce	2 pieces (2.2 oz)	50
King Oscar		
In Olive Oil	1 can (3.75 oz)	150
Skinless Boneless In Soya Oil	3 pieces (1.9 oz)	120
Season		
Brisling In Water	1 can (3.75 oz)	145
FRESH		
raw	3.5 oz	135

SAUCE *(see also BARBECUE SAUCE, GRAVY, PIZZA SAUCE, SPAGHETTI SAUCE)*

JARRED		
fish sauce chinese	1 tbsp	9
fish sauce vietnamese nuoc mam	1 tbsp	6

FOOD	PORTION	CALS
hoisin	1 tbsp	35
morroccan tagine	½ cup (4 oz)	70
oyster	1 tbsp	8
teriyaki	1 tbsp	15
teriyaki	1 oz	30
A Taste Of Thai		
Chili Sauce Garlic Pepper	1 tsp	10
Chili Sauce Sweet Red	1 tsp	10
Fish Sauce	1 tbsp	15
Peanut Satay	2 tbsp	80
A1		
Bold Steak Sauce	1 tbsp	20
Annie Chun's		
Shiitake Mushroom	1 tbsp	15
Thai Peanut	2 tbsp	120
Armour		
Chili Hot Dog	¼ cup (2.2 oz)	120
Meatless Sloppy Joe Sauce	¼ cup (2.2 oz)	30
Asian Gourmet		
Duck Sauce Peking Style	2 tbsp	40
Atkins		
Steak Sauce	1 tbsp	5
Teriyaki	1 tbsp	10
Boar's Head		
Ham Glaze Brown Sugar & Spice	2 tbsp (1.4 oz)	120
Carb Options		
Alfredo	¼ cup	110
Asian Teriyaki Marinade	1 tbsp	5
Cheese	¼ cup	90
Garden Style	½ cup	80
Steak Sauce	1 tbsp	5
Chun King		
Sweet And Sour	2 tbsp (1.2 oz)	58
Teriyaki	1 tbsp (0.6 oz)	17
Teriyaki Hot	1 tbsp (0.6 oz)	17
Consorzio		
Marinade Baja Lime	1 tbsp	60
Marinade California Teriyaki	1 tbsp	40
Marinade Dijon Peppercorn	1 tbsp	15

FOOD	PORTION	CALS
Marinade Jamaican Jerk	1 tbsp	10
Marinade Lemon Pepper	1 tbsp	60
Marinade Roasted Garlic	1 tbsp	35
Marinade Sesame Ginger	1 tbsp	25
Marinade Southwestern Chipotle	1 tbsp	30
Marinade Tropical Grill	1 tbsp	40
Del Monte		
Seafood Cocktail	¼ cup	100
Sloppy Joe Hickory Flavor	¼ cup	60
Sloppy Joe Original	¼ cup	50
Fage		
Tzatziki	2 tbsp	30
Gebhardt		
Enchilada Sauce	¼ cup (2.2 oz)	35
Hot Dog Chili Sauce	¼ cup (2.2 oz)	60
Hot Sauce	1 tsp (5 g)	1
Gringo Billy's		
Chipotle Dipping & Grilling Sauce	1 tsp	5
Jok'n'Al		
Cocktail	¼ cup	29
Plum	1 tbsp	10
Just Rite		
Hot Dog	¼ cup (2.2 oz)	50
Kikkoman		
Teriyaki	1 tbsp	15
La Choy		
Duck Sauce Sweet & Sour	2 tbsp (1.3 oz)	61
Sweet & Sour	2 tbsp (1.2 oz)	58
Teriyaki	1 tbsp (0.6 oz)	17
Lea & Perrins		
Worcestershire	1 tsp	5
Lee Kum Kee		
Plum Sauce	2 tbsp	100
Manwich		
Bold	¼ cup (2.2 oz)	62
Mexican	¼ cup (2.2 oz)	27
Original	¼ cup (2.2 oz)	32
Taco Season	¼ cup (2.2 oz)	27
Thick & Chunky	¼ cup (2.3 oz)	44

FOOD	PORTION	CALS
Matouk's		
Calypso	1 tsp	0
Flambeau Sauce	1 tsp	0
McCormick		
Flavor Medleys Garlic & Herb	2 tbsp	50
Flavor Medleys Italian Herb	2 tbsp	50
Flavor Medleys Lemon Pepper	2 tbsp	50
Flavor Medleys Tomato & Basil	2 tbsp	50
Nando's		
Curry Coconut	¼ cup	71
Fresh Lemon	¼ cup	61
Marinade Lime & Cilantro	1 tbsp	27
Marinade Sundried Tomato	1 tbsp	15
Peri-Peri Pepper Extra Hot	1 oz	17
Peri-Peri Pepper Garlic	1 oz	12
Peri-Peri Pepper Hot	1 oz	16
Peri-Peri Pepper Wild Herb	1 oz	14
Roasted Red	¼ cup	70
Sweet Apricot	¼ cup	51
Old El Paso		
Enchilada Mild	¼ cup	25
Open Range		
Hot Dog Chili	¼ cup (2.2 oz)	61
Pace		
Enchilada Sauce	¼ cup	36
Taco Sauce	¼ cup	32
Progresso		
Alfredo	½ cup (4.4 oz)	200
Sauce Arturo		
Original	¼ cup (2.2 fl oz)	50
Steel's		
Sugar Free Cocktail w/ Dill & Lemon	¼ cup	36
Sugar Free Hoisin	2 tbsp	15
Sugar Free Mango Curry	1 tbsp	13
Sugar Free Peanut Sauce	1 tbsp	34
Sugar Free Sweet & Sour	2 tbsp	10
Tostitos		
Beef Fiesta Nacho	2.4 oz	120
Chicken Quesadilla Topping	2.5 oz	90

FOOD	PORTION	CALS
Ty Ling		
Duck	2 tbsp	70
Walden Farms		
Calorie Free Seafood Sauce	1 tbsp	0
Scampi Sauce Calorie Free	2 tbsp	0
Wild Thyme Farms		
Chili Ginger Honey	1 tbsp	30
MIX		
cheese as prep w/ milk	1 cup	307
curry as prep	1 cup	120
curry as prep w/ milk	1 cup	270
mushroom as prep w/ milk	1 cup	228
sour cream as prep w/ milk	1 cup	509
stroganoff as prep	1 cup	271
sweet & sour as prep	1 cup	294
teriyaki as prep	1 cup	131
white as prep w/ milk	1 cup	241
A Taste Of Thai		
Pad Thai Sauce	2 tbsp	90
Peanut Sauce	¼ pkg	45
Durkee		
A La King as prep	1 cup	60
Cheese as prep	¼ cup	25
Hollandaise as prep	2 tbsp	10
White as prep	¼ cup	20
French's		
Cheese as prep	¼ cup	25
Hollandaise as prep	2 tbsp	10
Manwich		
Mix	¼ oz	22
McCormick		
Bernaise Blend	1 tsp (3 g)	10
Chicken Dijon Blend	1⅔ tbsp (10 g)	40
Green Peppercorn Blend as prep	¼ cup	20
Grill Mates Mesquite Marinade as prep	1 tbsp	15
Grill Mates Southwest Marinade	2 tsp (5 g)	15
Hollandaise Blend	2 tsp (4 g)	15
Hunter Blend as prep	¼ cup	25
Meat Marinade	1 tsp (4 g)	15

FOOD	PORTION	CALS
Pepper Medley Blend as prep	¼ cup	30
White Blend	2 tsp (6 g)	20
TAKE-OUT		
adobo fresco	2 tbsp	81
bearnaise	1 oz	177
cucumber yogurt sauce	1.5 tbsp	20

SAUERKRAUT

FOOD	PORTION	CALS
canned	½ cup	22
B&G		
Sauerkraut	2 tbsp (1 oz)	6
Boar's Head		
Sauerkraut	2 tbsp (1 oz)	5
Claussen		
Sauerkraut	¼ cup (1.1 oz)	5
Del Monte		
Bavarian Style	2 tbsp	15
Sauerkraut	2 tbsp	0
Eden		
Organic	½ cup	25
Hebrew National		
Sauerkraut	2 tbsp	5
S&W		
Canned	2 tbsp (1 oz)	5
Red Cabbage	2 tbsp (1 oz)	15
Silver Floss		
Sauerkraut	½ cup	20

SAUSAGE

FOOD	PORTION	CALS
beef & pork	1 link (2.3 oz)	196
beef & pork w/ cheddar cheese	1 link (2.7 oz)	228
bierschinken	3.5 oz	174
bierwurst	3.5 oz	258
blutwurst uncooked	3.5 oz	424
bockwurst	3.5 oz	276
bratwurst pork cooked	1 link (2.5 oz)	226
brotwurst pork & beef	1 link (2.5 oz)	226
chipolata	3.5 oz	342
chorizo	1 link (2.1 oz)	273
fleischwurst	3.5 oz	305
free range chicken breakfast	2 links (2.7 oz)	110

FOOD	PORTION	CALS
gelbwurst uncooked	3.5 oz	363
italian pork cooked	1 (2.4 oz)	230
jagdwurst	3.5 oz	211
knockwurst pork & beef	1 (2.5 oz)	221
mettwurst uncooked	3.5 oz	483
plockwurst uncooked	3.5 oz	312
polish kielbasa	2 oz	127
pork cooked	2 links (1.7 oz)	163
regensburger uncooked	3.5 oz	354
vienna canned	1 can (4 oz)	260
vienna canned	1 link (0.5 oz)	37
weisswurst uncooked	3.5 oz	305
zungenwurst (tongue)	3.5 oz	285
Armour		
Brown 'N Serve Lite Original	3	120
Brown 'N Serve Turkey	3 links	120
Vienna Sausage 25% Less Fat	3 (1.9 oz)	130
Vienna Sausage 50% Less Fat	3 (1.9 oz)	90
Vienna Sausage Chicken & Beef	3 (1.9 oz)	120
Vienna Sausage Hot 'n Spicy	3 (2.1 oz)	150
Vienna Sausage In BBQ Sauce	3 (2.1 oz)	150
Vienna Sausage In Beef Stock	3 (1.9 oz)	150
Vienna Sausage Jalapeno In Beef Stock	3 (1.9 oz)	170
Banner		
Sausage Stomachs	2 oz	90
Sausage Tripe	2 oz	90
Bilinski's		
Chicken Bratworst With Wild Rice	1 (2 oz)	70
Chicken Cajun-Style Andouille	2 oz	80
Chicken Italian With Peppers	1 (2 oz)	70
Chicken With Apples & Chardonnay	2 oz	70
Chicken With Cilantro	2 oz	70
Chicken With Jalapenos	2 oz	70
Chicken With Pesto	2 oz	90
Chicken With Spinach	2 oz	70
Chicken With Sun-Dried Tomato	2 oz	70
Boar's Head		
Bratwurst	1 (4 oz)	300
Hot Smoked	1 (3.2 oz)	280

FOOD	PORTION	CALS
Kielbasa	2 oz	120
Knockwurst	1 (4 oz)	310
Hebrew National		
Knockwurst Beef	1 (3 oz)	260
Jennie-O		
Italian Hot	1 (3.9 oz)	160
Turkey Italian Sweet	1 link (3.9 oz)	160
Jones		
Light 50% Less Fat	2 (1.6 oz)	100
Little Pork	3	190
Murray's		
Chicken Hot Italian	3 oz	130
Chicken Spinach & Garlic	3 oz	100
Chicken Sun Dried Tomato	3 oz	110
Chicken Sweet Italian	3 oz	130
Perdue		
Hot Italian Turkey Cooked	1 link (2.4 oz)	150
Sweet Italian Turkey Cooked	1 link (2.4 oz)	150
Shady Brook		
Turkey Sweet Italian	1 (2.5 oz)	110
Soy Lean		
Pork Breakfast Patty	1 (2 oz)	75
Turkey Store		
Breakfast	2 links (2 oz)	140
Breakfast Sausage Patties Mild	2 patties (2.3 oz)	160
Wampler		
Breakfast Turkey	2 (2.4 oz)	110
Italian Turkey	1 (2.7 oz)	120

SAUSAGE DISHES
TAKE-OUT

italian sausage w/ peppers & onions	1 cup	210
sausage roll	1 (2.3 oz)	311

SAUSAGE SUBSTITUTES

meatless	1 patty (1.3 oz)	98
meatless	1 link (0.9 oz)	64
Boca Burgers		
Breakfast Patties	1 (1.3 oz)	70
Lightlife		
Gimme Lean	2 oz	50

FOOD	PORTION	CALS
Smart Brats	1 (2 oz)	120
Smart Links Breakfast	2 (2 oz)	100
Smart Links Italian	1 (2 oz)	120
Smart Menu Breakfast Patty	1	45
Loma Linda		
Linketts	1 (1.2 oz)	70
Little Links	2 (1.6 oz)	90
Morningstar Farms		
Breakfast Links	2	60
Breakfast Patties	1 (1.3 oz)	80
Grillers	1 patty (2.2 oz)	140
Sausage Style Recipe Crumbles	⅔ cup (1.9 oz)	90
Natural Touch		
Vegan Sausage Crumbles	½ cup (1.9 oz)	60
Quron		
Links	2 (1.6 oz)	70
Worthington		
Leanies	1 link (1.4 oz)	100
Prosage Links	2 (1.6 oz)	60
Yves		
Veggie Breakfast Links	1 (1.6 oz)	60
Veggie Breakfast Patties	1 (2 oz)	70

SAVORY

| ground | 1 tsp | 4 |

SCALLOP

raw	3 oz	75
TAKE-OUT		
breaded & fried	2 lg	67

SCONE

Finnegan's		
Irish Raisin	1 (2 oz)	170
King Arthur		
Cranberry Orange as prep	1	248
TAKE-OUT		
apricot	1	232
blueberry	1 (3 oz)	270
cheese	1 (3.5 oz)	364
orange poppy	1 (3 oz)	260

FOOD	PORTION	CALS
plain	1 (3.5 oz)	362
raisin	1 (3 oz)	270

SCUP
fresh baked	3 oz	115

SEA BASS (see BASS)

SEA CUCUMBER
dried	1 oz	74
fresh	1 oz	20

SEA TROUT (see TROUT)

SEA URCHIN
canned	1 oz	39
fresh	1 oz	36
roe paste	1 tbsp	19

SEAWEED
agar dried	1 oz	87
agar fresh	1 oz	tr
hijiki dried	1 tbsp	9
irishmoss fresh	1 oz	14
kelp fresh	1 oz	12
kombu fresh	1 oz	12
laver fresh	1 oz	10
nori fresh	1 oz	10
nori sheet dried	1 (8 x 8 in)	5
seahair dried	1 tbsp	13
spirulina dried	1 oz	83
spirulina fresh	1 oz	7
tangle fresh	1 oz	12
wakame fresh	1 oz	13

SEITAN (see WHEAT)

SEMOLINA
dry	1 cup (5.9 oz)	601

SESAME
seeds	1 tsp	16
sesame butter	1 tbsp	95
sesame crunch candy	20 pieces (1.2 oz)	181

FOOD	PORTION	CALS
sesame crunch candy	1 oz	146
tahini from roasted & toasted kernels	1 tbsp	89
tahini from stone ground kernels	1 tbsp	86
tahini from unroasted kernels	1 tbsp	85
Eden		
Organic Seaweed Gomasio	1 serv (1.5 oz)	10
Organic Gomasio	½ tsp	10
Organic Gomasio Garlic	½ tsp	10
Maranatha		
Raw Tahini	2 tbsp	190
Roasted Tahini	2 tbsp	210
SESBANIA		
flower	1	1
flowers	1 cup	5
flowers cooked	1 cup	23
SHAD		
american baked	3 oz	214
roe baked w/ butter & lemon	1 oz	36
roe raw	1 oz	37
SHALLOTS		
Christopher Ranch		
Fresh	1 (1 oz)	20
Frieda's		
Fresh	1 tbsp (1 oz)	20
SHARK		
fin dried	1 oz	32
raw	3 oz	111
TAKE-OUT		
batter-dipped & fried	3 oz	194
SHEEPSHEAD FISH		
cooked	1 fillet (6.5 oz)	234
cooked	3 oz	107
raw	3 oz	92

SHELLFISH (see individual names, SHELLFISH SUBSTITUTES)

SHELLFISH SUBSTITUTES

crab imitation	1 cup (4.4 oz)	144

FOOD	PORTION	CALS
scallop imitation	3 oz	84
shrimp imitation	3 oz	86
surimi	1 oz	28
surimi	3 oz	84
Chicken Of The Sea		
Imitation Crab	1 pkg (2.5 oz)	40
Louis Kemp		
Crab Delights	½ cup (3 oz)	80
Crab Delights Chunk Style	½ cup (3 oz)	80
Crab Delights Easy Shred	½ cup (3 oz)	80
Crab Delights Leg Style	½ cup (3 oz)	80
Lobster Delights Chunk or Salad Style	½ cup (3 oz)	80
Scallop Delights Bay Style	½ cup (3 oz)	80
TAKE-OUT		
crab salad	1 cup	395

SHELLIE BEANS

FOOD	PORTION	CALS
canned	½ cup	37

SHERBET

FOOD	PORTION	CALS
orange	½ gal	2158
orange	½ cup (4 fl oz)	132
orange	1 bar (2.75 fl oz)	91
Breyers		
Orange	½ cup	120
Rainbow	½ cup	120
Turkey Hill		
Fruit Rainbow	½ cup	120
Orange Grove	½ cup	120

SHRIMP
CANNED

FOOD	PORTION	CALS
chinese shrimp paste	1 tbsp	15
Bumble Bee		
Broken Shrimp	¼ cup	40
Medium Or Large Or Jumbo	¼ cup	40
Small	¼ cup	40
Tiny	¼ cup	40
Chicken Of The Sea		
Tiny Small or Medium	½ can (2 oz)	45

FOOD	PORTION	CALS
FRESH		
cooked	4 large	22
FROZEN		
Chicken Of The Sea		
Cooked Large Peeled Deveined Tail On	3 oz	80
Large Raw Cleaned Tail Off	4 oz	120
Gorton's		
Popcorn Garlic & Herb	22 pieces (3.6 oz)	270
Popcorn Original	20 pieces (3.2 oz)	240
Margaritaville		
Calypso Coconut + Sauce	5 pieces	350
Island Lime	6 pieces	130
Jammin' Jerk	7 pieces	140
Paradise Cocktail + Sauce	5 pieces	85
Sunset Scampi	1 serv (½ pkg)	270
Surfside Skewers + Sauce	2 skewers	105
TAKE-OUT		
breaded & fried	3 oz	206
gingered	4	80
jambalaya	¾ cup	188
scampi	2 cups	438
shrimp newburg	1 serv (6.4 oz)	456
shrimp w/ crab stuffing	5	158
SMELT		
rainbow cooked	3 oz	106
rainbow raw	3 oz	83
SMOOTHIE (see also FRUIT DRINKS, YOGURT DRINKS)		
Bolthouse Farms		
Strawberry Banana Fruit	8 oz	124
Hansen's		
Apricot Nectar	1 can	170
Cranberry Twist	1 can	180
Energy Island Blast	1 can	170
Guava Strawberry	1 can	170
Lite Cranberry Raspberry	1 can	50
Mango Pineapple	1 can	170
Peach Berry	1 can	170
Pineapple Coconut	1 can	180
Strawberry Banana	1 can	180

FOOD	PORTION	CALS
Tropical Passion	1 can	170
Whipped Orange	1 can	180
Jammin' Juice		
Mambo Mango	6 oz	92
Jammin' Nectars		
C-Beta Carrot	6 oz	96
Ginger Party	6 oz	6
Guanabana Limbo	6 oz	78
Pure Passion	6 oz	78
Razz-Ade	6 oz	89
Naked Juice		
Chocolate Karma	8 oz	190
Vanilla Chai	8 oz	170
Odwalla		
Blackberry Fruit Shake	8 fl oz	140
Orange Pina	8 fl oz	140
Sambazon		
Acai Energy Mango Banana	8 oz	190
Acai Soy Energy	8 oz	210
Amazon Cherry	8 oz	156
Soy Blendz		
Mango Orange Dream	1 bottle (10 oz)	220
Mixed Berry Medley	1 bottle (10 oz)	210
Orange Citrus Splash	1 bottle (10 oz)	220
Strawberry Banana Blast	1 bottle (10 oz)	230
Tree Of Life		
Organic Smoothie Banana Raspberry Strawberry	⅔ cup (5 oz)	90
Organic Smoothie Mango Strawberry Raspberry	⅔ cup (5 oz)	70
Organic Smoothie Strawberry Banana	⅔ cup (5 oz)	90
Organic Smoothie Strawberry Blueberry Banana	⅔ cup (5 oz)	90
WholeSoy & Co.		
Organic Soy Peach	8 oz	210
Organic Soy Raspberry	8 oz	210
Organic Soy Strawberry	8 oz	210

FOOD	PORTION	CALS
SNACKS		
cheese puffs	1 oz	157
corn puffs cheese	1 bag (8 oz)	1256
corn twists cheese	1 oz	157
corn twists cheese	1 bag (8 oz)	1256
oriental mix	1 oz	155
pork skins	1 oz	154
pork skins barbecue	1 oz	152
trail mix	1 oz	131
trail mix	1 cup (5.3 oz)	693
trail mix tropical	1 oz	115
trail mix w/ chocolate chips	1 oz	137
trail mix w/ chocolate chips	1 cup (5.1 oz)	707
Baken-ets		
Fried Pork Skins	9 pieces	80
Fried Pork Skins Hot'n Spicy	9 pieces	80
Fried Pork Skins Sweet & Tangy BBQ	9 pieces	80
Pork Cracklins	8 pieces	90
Pork Cracklins Hot'n Spicy	8 pieces	80
Barbara's Bakery		
Cheese Puffs Bakes	1½ cups (1 oz)	160
Cheese Puffs Jalapeno	¾ cup (1 oz)	150
Cheese Puffs Original	¾ cup (1 oz)	150
Bowlby's		
Bits Almond	½ cup	100
Bits Pecan	½ cup	200
Bits Ranch	½ cup	170
Bits Salsa	½ cup	170
Bits Sour Cream Onion & Dill	½ cup	170
Bits'N'Pops	¾ cup	130
Mix-Ups Country Mix	½ cup	170
Mix-Ups Nuttyest-Of-All	½ cup	160
Mix-Ups Trail Mix	½ cup	165
Bugles		
Baked Original	1⅓ cups	130
Chile Con Queso	1⅓ cups	160
Nacho	1½ cups	160
Original	1½ cups	160
Smokin'BBQ	1⅓ cups	150

FOOD	PORTION	CALS
Cheetos		
Asteriods Go Snack	¾ cup (1 oz)	160
Baked Crunchy	34 pieces (1 oz)	130
Crunchy	21 pieces (1 oz)	160
Natural White Cheddar	32 pieces (1 oz)	150
Puffs	13 pieces (1 oz)	160
Twisted	7 pieces (1 oz)	160
Chester's		
Puffcorn Butter	3 cups	160
Puffcorn Cheese	3 cups	160
Chex Mix		
Cheddar	⅔ cup	140
Hot'N Spicy	⅔ cup	130
Nacho Fiesta	⅔ cup	120
Party Blend Bold	⅔ cup	140
Peanut Lovers	⅔ cup	140
Traditional	⅔ cup	130
Dakota Gourmet		
Amazing Corn Classic	1 pkg (1 oz)	360
Amazing Corn Cool Ranch	1 pkg (1 oz)	367
Amazing Corn Mesquite BBQ	1 pkg (1 oz)	369
Heart Smart Toasted Corn	⅓ cup (1 oz)	110
Heart Smart Toasted Corn	1 pkg (1.75 oz)	177
Trail Mix Heart Smart	1 pkg (1.75 oz)	172
Eden		
Rice Puffs Five Flavor Arare	1 oz	110
Frito Lay		
Funyuns	13 (1 oz)	140
Munchos	16 (1 oz)	160
Munchos BBQ	14 (1 oz)	160
Funyuns		
Mini Onion Rings Go Snacks	1 pkg	260
Onion Rings	13 pieces	140
Glenny's		
Slim Carb Curls Cheddar Cheese	1 pkg (1 oz)	121
Gram's Gourmet		
Crunchies Pork Rinds	⅛ pkg (0.5 oz)	70
_J&J_		
Microwave Pork Rinds All Flavors	1 oz	130

FOOD	PORTION	CALS
Kangaroo		
Pita Snackers Crispy Cinnamon	10 pieces (1 oz)	90
Pita Snackers Sea Salt	10 pieces (1 oz)	90
Maranatha		
High Energy Mix	¼ cup	120
Organic Harvest Mix	¼ cup	150
Organic Nature Mix	¼ cup	150
Snack Attack Mix	¼ cup	140
Trail Mix Deluxe	¼ cup	150
Trail Mix Navajo	¼ cup	140
Trail Mix Olympic w/ Chocolate	¼ cup	140
Trail Mix Organic Delight	¼ cup	150
Trail Mix Organic Raw	¼ cup	140
Mauna Loa		
Tropical Nut & Fruit	¼ cup	180
Munchies		
Snack Mix Flamin' Hot	1 oz	140
Snack Mix Kids	1 oz	130
Old Dutch Foods		
Baked Cheese Curls	2 cups (1.1 oz)	180
Cheese Puffcorn Curls	2 cups (1.1 oz)	170
Organic Trails		
Trail Mix Summit Blend	¼ cup	150
Planters		
Cheez Mania Original	42 pieces (1 oz)	150
Pumpkorn		
Caramel	⅓ cup	150
Chili	⅓ cup	150
Curry	⅓ cup	150
Maple Vanilla	⅓ cup	150
Mesquite	⅓ cup	150
Original	⅓ cup	150
Robert's American Gourmet		
Pirate's Booty Puffed Rice & Corn w/ Cheddar	1 oz	120
Sabritones		
Chile & Lime	23 pieces	150
Snyder's Of Hanover		
Cheese Twists	1 oz	230
Fried Pork Skins	1 oz	80
Fried Pork Skins Barbecue	1 oz	80

FOOD	PORTION	CALS
Kruncheez	1.25 oz	200
Onion Toasters	1 oz	188
Utz		
Caramel Corn Clusters	1⅛ cups (1 oz)	120
Cheese Balls	50 (1 oz)	150
Cheese Curls	18 (1 oz)	150
Cheese Curls Crunchy	30 (1 oz)	160
Cheese Curls Reduced Fat	32 (1 oz)	140
Onion Rings	41 (1 oz)	140
Party Mix	¾ cup (1 oz)	140
Pork Cracklins	0.5 oz	90
Pork Cracklins Hot & Spicy	0.5 oz	80
Pork Rinds	0.5 oz	80
Pork Rinds BBQ	0.5 oz	80
SNAIL		
cooked	3 oz	233
raw	3 oz	117
TAKE-OUT		
escargot cooked	5	25
SNAKE		
fresh	3 oz	78
SNAP BEANS		
FRESH		
Frieda's		
Purple Wax	⅔ cup	25
SNAPPER		
cooked	1 fillet (6 oz)	217
cooked	3 oz	109
raw	3 oz	85
SODA		
club	12 oz	0
cola	12 oz	151
cream	12 oz	191
diet cola	12 oz	2
diet cola w/ equal	12 oz	2
diet cola w/ saccharin	12 oz	2

FOOD	PORTION	CALS
ginger ale	12 oz can	124
grape	12 oz	161
lemon lime	12 oz	149
orange	12 oz	177
pepper type	12 oz	151
quinine	12 oz	125
root beer	12 oz	152
shirley temple	1 serv	159
tonic water	12 oz	125
7 Up		
Diet	8 oz	0
Original	8 oz	100
Plus	1 can (12 oz)	10
A & W		
Root Beer	1 can (12 oz)	170
AJ Stephans		
Birch Beer	1 bottle	170
Black Cherry	1 bottle	180
Cream	1 bottle	170
Jamaican Style Ginger Beer	1 bottle	170
Lemon & Lime	1 bottle	190
Olde Style Root Beer	1 bottle	170
Barq's		
Diet French Vanilla Creme	8 oz	1
Diet Red Creme	8 oz	4
Diet Root Beer	8 oz	1
Floatz	8 oz	127
French Vanilla Creme	8 oz	112
Red Creme	8 oz	113
Root Beer	8 oz	111
Barritts		
Ginger Beer	1 bottle (12 oz)	200
Best Health		
Root Beer	1 bottle (12 oz)	165
Vanilla Cream	1 bottle (12 oz)	170
Big Red		
Vanilla Float	1 can	180
Blumers		
Black Cherry	1 bottle (12 oz)	138
Blueberry Cream	1 bottle (12 oz)	190

FOOD	PORTION	CALS
Cream	1 bottle (12 oz)	181
Orange Cream	1 bottle (12 oz)	187
Root Beer	1 bottle (12 oz)	190
Bong Water		
Chronic Tonic	12 oz	144
Cottonmouth Quencher	12 oz	165
Green Dreams	12 oz	165
Purple Haze	12 oz	165
Briar's		
Black Cherry	1 bottle (12 oz)	180
Cream	1 bottle (12 oz)	180
Diet Root Beer	8 oz	4
Orange Cream	8 oz	120
Red Birch	8 oz	104
Root Beer	1 bottle (12 oz)	168
Canada Dry		
Ginger Ale	1 can (12 oz)	140
Tonic Water	8 fl oz	90
Capt'n Eli's		
Root Beer	8 oz	165
Carver's		
Ginger Ale	8 oz	94
Celsius		
All Flavors	1 bottle (12 oz)	5
Chronic 187		
Orange	1 bottle (12 oz)	300
Coca-Cola		
C2	8 oz	45
Classic	1 can (12 oz)	140
W/ Lime	8 oz	98
Zero	8 oz	0
Coke		
Cherry	8 oz	104
Diet	8 oz	1
Diet Cherry	8 oz	1
Diet Vanilla	8 oz	1
Diet w/ Lime	8 oz	2
Vanilla	8 oz	100

FOOD	PORTION	CALS
Dr Pepper		
Diet	1 oz	tr
Original	1 can (12 oz)	150
Fanta		
Apple	8 oz	121
Black Cherry	8 oz	110
Cherry	8 oz	117
Citrus	8 oz	91
Grape	8 oz	122
Lemon	8 oz	112
Orange	8 oz	111
Peach	8 oz	29
Pineapple	8 oz	120
Pink Grapefruit	8 oz	113
Strawberry	8 oz	120
Firefighter		
Backdraft Root Beer	8 oz	90
Courageous Cola	8 oz	90
Flashover Orange	8 oz	20
Incendiary Citrus	8 oz	90
Rolling Code Black Cherry	8 oz	90
Fresca		
Soda	8 oz	3
Frostie		
Diet Cherry Limeade	1 bottle (12 oz)	0
Diet Root Beer	1 bottle (12 oz)	0
Vanilla Root Beer	1 bottle (12 oz)	180
Hansen's		
Black Cherry	8 fl oz	110
Diet All Flavors	1 can	0
Ginger Beer	8 fl oz	100
Natural Black Cherry	1 can	160
Natural Cherry Vanilla	1 can	140
Natural Creamy Rootbeer	1 can	160
Natural Ginger Ale	1 can	140
Natural Grapefruit	1 can	130
Natural Key Lime	1 can	130
Natural Kiwi Strawberry	1 can	130
Natural Mandarin Lime	1 can	130

FOOD	PORTION	CALS
Natural Orange Mango	1 can	170
Natural Raspberry	1 can	130
Natural Tangerine	1 can	160
Natural Tropical Passion	1 can	160
Natural Vanilla Cola	1 can	140
Orange Creme	8 fl oz	110
Sangria	8 fl oz	110
Sarsaparilla	8 fl oz	110
Sparkling Orangeade	8 fl oz	100
Vanilla Creme	8 fl oz	110
Hiball		
Club	1 bottle (10 oz)	5
Tonic Water	1 bottle (10 oz)	120
IBC		
Cream	1 bottle (12 oz)	180
Root Beer	1 can	160
Inca Kola		
Diet	8 oz	1
Soda	8 oz	96
Jolt		
Blue	8 oz	120
Cherry Bomb	8 oz	90
Cola	8 oz	100
Red	8 oz	120
Ultra	8 oz	0
Jones Soda		
Sugar Free All Flavors	1 bottle (12 oz)	0
Kutztown		
Birch Beer	1 bottle (12 oz)	160
Red Cream	1 bottle (12 oz)	150
Sarsaparilla	1 bottle (12 oz)	150
Like		
Cola	1 oz	13
Lucozade		
Soda	7 oz	136
Maine Root		
All Flavors	1 bottle (12 oz)	165
Manzana Mia		
Soda	8 oz	99

FOOD	PORTION	CALS
Mello Yellow		
Cherry	8 oz	118
Diet	8 oz	3
Melon	8 oz	119
Soda	8 oz	118
Mountain Dew		
Pitch Black	8 oz	110
Mr. Pibb		
Diet	8 oz	1
Northern Neck		
Diet Ginger Ale	8 oz	4
Ginger Ale	8 oz	94
Nuky		
Rose Soda	8 oz	120
Olde Brooklyn		
Coney Island Cream	8 oz	130
Flatbush Orange	8 oz	130
Williamsburg Root Beer	8 oz	120
Olde Philadelphia		
Black Cherry	1 bottle (12 oz)	180
Cream	1 bottle (12 oz)	190
Cream Diet	1 bottle (12 oz)	0
Grape	1 bottle (12 oz)	180
Orange Cream	1 bottle (12 oz)	190
Pineapple	1 bottle	190
Root Beer	1 bottle (12 oz)	180
Orangina		
Sparkling Citrus	8 oz	90
Pennsylvania Dutch		
Birch Beer	8 fl oz	110
Pepsi		
Blue Berry Cola Fusion	8 fl oz	100
Diet	1 can (12 oz)	0
Edge	1 can (12 oz)	70
Regular	1 can (12 oz)	150
Vanilla	1 can	160
Vanilla Diet	1 can	0
Prism		
Green Tea Soda Cola	8 oz	105
Lemon Lime	8 oz	117

FOOD	PORTION	CALS
Qibla		
Cola	1 bottle (18 oz)	185
Diet Cola	1 bottle (18 oz)	1
Red Flash		
Soda	8 oz	105
Santa Cruz		
Organic Cherry	1 can	140
Organic Concord Grape	1 can	150
Organic Ginger Ale	1 can	150
Organic Lemon Lime	1 can	130
Organic Orange Mango	1 can	130
Organic Root Beer	1 can	150
Organic Vanilla Creme	1 can	160
Saranac		
Diet Root Beer	1 bottle (12 oz)	35
Ginger Beer	1 bottle (12 oz)	160
Root Beer	1 bottle (12 oz)	180
Schweppes		
Ginger Ale	8 oz	120
Seagram's		
Ginger Ale	1 can (12 oz)	130
Sex Cola		
All Flavors	1 bottle (12 oz)	0
Sierra Mist		
Lemon Lime	1 can (12 oz)	140
Ski		
Citrus	1 bottle (10 oz)	150
Snow		
Sparkling Mint	8 oz	75
Souix City		
Cream	1 bottle (12 oz)	180
Orange Cream	1 bottle (12 oz)	200
Root Beer	1 bottle (12 oz)	170
Sarsaparilla	1 bottle (12 oz)	170
Sprite		
Diet Zero	8 oz	0
ReMix Aruba Jam	8 oz	97
ReMix Berryclear	8 oz	97
Soda	8 oz	96

FOOD	PORTION	CALS
Steap		
Green Tea Soda Orange	8 oz	90
Green Tea Soda Root Beer	8 oz	90
Organic Green Tea Soda Raspberry	8 oz	90
Stewart's		
Cream	1 bottle (12 oz)	180
Diet Cream	1 bottle (12 oz)	0
Root Beer	1 bottle (12 oz)	160
Strawberries N' Cream	1 bottle	200
Wishniak Black Cherry	1 bottle	180
Stirrings		
Club	1 bottle (6.3 oz)	0
Ginger Ale	1 bottle (6.3 oz)	100
Tonic Water	1 bottle (6.3 oz)	85
Sunkist		
Diet Orange	8 oz	0
Orange	8 oz	130
Tab		
Soda	8 oz	1
Thomas Kemper		
Black Cherry	1 bottle	177
Old Fashion Birch	1 bottle	170
Orange Cream	1 bottle	180
Pure Draft Honey Cola	1 bottle	140
Pure Draft Root Beer	1 bottle	160
Vanilla Cream	1 bottle	170
Three Drinks		
Citrus	12 oz	12
Tommyknocker		
Almond Creme	1 bottle (12 oz)	150
Key Lime Creme	1 bottle (12 oz)	180
Orange Creme	1 bottle (12 oz)	180
Root Beer	1 bottle (12 oz)	150
Root Beer Float	1 bottle (12 oz)	110
Strawberry Creme	1 bottle (12 oz)	150
Uno Mas		
All Flavors	1 can (12 oz)	130
Vermont Sweetwater		
Country Apple Jack	1 bottle	180
Kickin' Cow Cola	1 bottle	129

FOOD	PORTION	CALS
Mango Moonshine	1 bottle	180
Maple	1 bottle	101
Raspberry Rhubarb Ramble	1 bottle	180
Tangerine Cream Twister	1 bottle	180
Vermont Maple Seltzer	1 bottle	53
Virgil's		
Micro Brewed Root Beer	1 bottle (12 oz)	160
White Rock		
Organics Raspberry Creme	1 can (12.4 oz)	120
Organics Red Peach	1 can (12.4 oz)	120
White T		
All Flavors	1 bottle (12 oz)	128
Diet All Flavors	1 bottle (12 oz)	0
Windy City		
Root Beer	1 bottle (12 oz)	170
Yoo-Hoo		
Original	9 fl oz	150
Z Cola		
No Artificial Sweeteners	8 oz	0
SOLE		
cooked	1 fillet (4.5 oz)	148
cooked	3 oz	99
lemon raw	3.5 oz	85
raw	3.5 oz	90
TAKE-OUT		
breaded & fried	3.2 oz	211
SORGHUM		
sorghum	1 cup (6.7 oz)	651
SOUFFLE		
lemon chilled	1 cup	176
raspberry chilled	1 cup	173
spinach	1 cup	218
Atkins		
Broccoli Cheddar & Bacon	1 serv	200
SOUP		
CANNED		
clam chowder new england as prep w/ milk	1 cup	163

FOOD	PORTION	CALS
Amy's		
Organic Barley	1 cup	50
Organic Black Bean Vegetable	1 cup	110
Organic Cream Of Mushroom	1 cup	120
Organic Cream Of Tomato	1 cup	100
Organic Lentil	1 cup	130
Organic Minestrone	1 cup	90
Organic No Chicken Noodle Soup	1 cup	90
Organic Vegetable	1 cup	35
Boston Market		
Chicken Broth Reduced Sodium	1 cup	15
Butterball		
Chicken Broth Reduced Sodium 99% Fat Free	1 cup	10
Campbell's		
98% Fat Free Cream Of Chicken as prep	1 cup	70
Cheddar Cheese	1 cup	110
Cheddar Cheese as prep	1 cup	134
Chicken Broth	½ cup	20
Chicken Gumbo as prep	1 cup	55
Chicken Vegetable as prep	1 cup	74
Chunky Beef Barley	1 cup	160
Chunky Chicken & Dumplings	1 cup	190
Chunky Chicken Corn Chowder	1 cup	230
Chunky Chili Roadhouse Beef & Bean	1 cup	220
Chunky New England Clam Chowder	1 cup	240
Chunky Old Fashioned Vegetable Beef	1 cup	130
Chunky Sirloin Burger w/ Country Vegetables	1 cup	180
Chunky Vegetable	1 cup	130
Clam Chowder New England as prep	1 cup	89
Classics Beef Noodle	1 cup	70
Classics Chicken Rice	1 cup (8.4 oz)	80
Classics Minestrone	1 cup	90
Classics Old Fashioned Vegetable	1 cup	90
Classics Vegetarian Vegetable as prep	1 cup	90
Consomme as prep	1 cup	24
Cream Of Asparagus as prep	1 cup	72
Cream Of Celery as prep	1 cup	107
Cream Of Chicken as prep	1 cup	120
Cream Of Chicken w/ Herbs	1 cup	90
Cream Of Mushroom as prep	1 cup	108

FOOD	PORTION	CALS
Double Noodle	1 cup	90
Fiesta Tomato as prep	1 cup	72
Garden Vegetable as prep	1 cup	69
Green Pea as prep	1 cup	173
Healthy Request Chicken Noodle as prep	1 cup	70
Healthy Request Chicken Rice as prep	1 cup	60
Healthy Request Cream Of Chicken as prep	1 cup	80
Healthy Request Cream Of Chicken & Broccoli as prep	1 cup	78
Healthy Request Cream Of Mushroom as prep	1 cup	66
Healthy Request Hearty Pasta w/ Vegetables	1 cup	87
Healthy Request Tomato as prep	1 cup	91
Healthy Request Vegetable as prep	1 cup	84
Home Cookin' Chicken Vegetable	1 cup (8.4 oz)	130
Italian Tomato as prep	1 cup	105
Kitchen Classics Bean With Bacon	1 cup	180
Kitchen Classics Chicken Noodle	1 cup	180
Kitchen Classics Chicken w/ White & Wild Rice	1 cup	100
Kitchen Classics Lentil	1 cup	120
Low Sodium Chicken W/ Noodles	1 can (10.75 oz)	162
Low Sodium Chunky Vegetable Beef	1 can (10.75 oz)	159
Low Sodium Cream of Mushroom	1 can (10.75 oz)	200
Low Sodium Green Pea	1 can (10.75 oz)	235
Low Sodium Tomato w/ Pieces	1 can (10.75 oz)	170
Ready To Serve Bean w/ Bacon 'N Ham	1 can (10.5 oz)	274
Ready To Serve Chicken Noodle	1 cup	80
Ready To Serve Chicken w/ Rice	1 can (10.5 oz)	122
Ready To Serve Vegetable Beef	1 can (10.5 oz)	143
Savory Tomato & Dill as prep	1 cup	99
Select Chicken & Pasta With Roasted Garlic	1 cup (8.4 oz)	100
Select Chicken Rice	1 cup	100
Select Chicken With Egg Noodles	1 cup	90
Select Creamy Potato w/ Roasted Garlic	1 cup	180
Select Fiesta Vegetable	1 cup (8.4 oz)	120
Select Herbed Chicken w/ Roasted Vegetables	1 cup	90
Select Italian Style Wedding	1 cup	110
Select Mexican Chicken Tortilla	1 cup	150
Select Roasted Chicken w/ Long Grain & Wild Rice	1 cup	130
Select Roasted Chicken w/ Rotini & Penne Pasta	1 cup	90

FOOD	PORTION	CALS
Select Rosemary Chicken w/ Roasted Potatoes	1 cup	110
Select Tuscany-Style Minestrone	1 cup (8.4 oz)	190
Soup At Hand Chicken & Stars	1 pkg	70
Soup At Hand Chicken w/ Mini Noodles	1 pkg (10.75 oz)	80
Soup At Hand Cream of Broccoli	1 pkg (10.75 oz)	160
Soup At Hand Creamy Chicken	1 pkg (10.75 oz)	150
Soup At Hand Creamy Tomato	1 pkg	180
Soup At Hand Vegetable Medley	1 pkg (10.75 oz)	110
Soup At Hand Velvety Potato	1 pkg (10.75 oz)	160
Vegetable Beef as prep	1 cup	68
College Inn		
Beef Broth 99% Fat Free	1 cup	20
Beef Broth Fat Free Lower Sodium	1 cup	15
Chicken Broth Light & Fat Free	1 cup	5
Gold's		
Borscht Low Calorie	1 cup	20
Borscht Unsalted	1 cup	70
Hungarian Cabbage	6 oz	70
Healthy Choice		
Bean & Ham	1 cup	170
Beef & Potato	1 cup	110
Broccoli Cheddar	1 cup (8.4 oz)	116
Chicken & Dumplings	1 cup	130
Chicken & Pasta	1 cup	110
Chicken Corn Chowder	1 cup	140
Chicken Fiesta	1 cup	100
Chicken w/ Roasted Garlic	1 cup	120
Chicken w/ Rice	1 cup	90
Chili Beef	1 cup	170
Clam Chowder	1 cup	110
Country Vegetable	1 cup	100
Cream Of Chicken Vegetable	1 cup (8.9 oz)	127
Cream Of Mushroom	1 cup (8.8 oz)	77
Creamy Tomato	1 cup	100
Garden Vegetable	1 cup	120
Hearty Chicken	1 cup	120
Italian Bean & Pasta	1 cup	100
Old Fashioned Chicken Noodle	1 cup	110
Roasted Italian Style Chicken	1 cup	120
Split Pea w/ Ham	1 cup	170

FOOD	PORTION	CALS
Turkey w/ Rice	1 cup	90
Vegetable Beef	1 cup	130
Vegetable Clam Chowder	1 cup	230
Zesty Gumbo	1 cup	100
Imagine		
Creamy Broccoli	1 serv (8 oz)	70
Creamy Butternut Squash	1 serv (8 oz)	120
Creamy Mushroom	1 serv (8 oz)	80
Creamy Potato Leek	1 serv (8 oz)	90
Creamy Sweet Corn	1 serv (8 oz)	100
Creamy Tomato	1 serv (8 oz)	90
No-Chicken Broth	1 serv (8 oz)	35
Vegetable Broth	1 serv (8 oz)	45
Zesty Gazpacho	1 serv (8 oz)	80
Manischewitz		
Clear Chicken Condensed	½ cup	15
Natural Choice		
Organic Vegan Classic Mushroom	1 cup	50
Organic Vegan Classic Tomato	1 cup	100
Organic Vegan Country Corn	1 cup	100
Organic Vegan Kabocha Squash	1 cup	60
Organic Vegan Southern Greens	1 cup	80
Organic Vegan Split Pea	1 cup	120
Organic Vegan Vegetable Curry	1 cup	110
Pacific Foods		
Beef Broth	1 cup	20
Creamy Butternut Squash	1 cup	90
Creamy Roasted Carrot	1 cup	100
Creamy Roasted Red Pepper & Tomato	1 cup	100
Hearty Beef Barley	1 cup	110
Hearty Chicken Noodle	1 cup	80
Hearty Chicken Tortilla	1 cup	130
Hearty Roasted Red Pepper & Corn Chowder	1 cup	210
Organic Creamy Tomato	1 cup	100
Organic Free Range Chicken Broth	1 cup	10
Organic French Onion	1 cup	35
Organic Low Sodium Chicken Broth	1 cup	10
Organic Mushroom Broth	1 cup	5
Organic Vegetarian Broth	1 cup	15

FOOD	PORTION	CALS
Progresso		
99% Fat Free Beef Barley	1 cup	130
99% Fat Free Beef Vegetable	1 cup (8.5 oz)	160
99% Fat Free Chicken Rice w/ Vegetables	1 cup (8.4 oz)	110
99% Fat Free Lentil	1 cup (8.5 oz)	130
99% Fat Free Minestrone	1 cup (8.5 oz)	130
99% Fat Free Split Pea	1 cup (8.9 oz)	170
99% Fat Free Tomato Garden Vegetable	1 cup (8.6 oz)	100
99% Fat Free Vegetable	1 cup (8.4 oz)	70
99% Fat Free White Cheddar Potato	1 cup (8.6 oz)	140
Bean & Ham	1 cup (8.4 oz)	160
Beef & Vegetable	1 cup	130
Beef Minestrone	1 cup (8.5 oz)	140
Beef Noodle	1 cup (8.5 oz)	140
Carb Monitor Chicken Vegetable	1 cup	70
Cheese & Herb Tortellini Tomato	1 cup (8.6 oz)	140
Chickarina	1 cup (8.3 oz)	130
Chicken Minestrone	1 cup (8.4 oz)	110
Chicken Vegetable	1 cup (8.4 oz)	90
Chicken & Wild Rice	1 cup (8.4 oz)	100
Chicken Barley	1 cup (8.5 oz)	110
Chicken Broth	1 cup (8.2 oz)	20
Chicken Rice w/ Vegetable	1 cup	100
Clam & Rotini Chowder	1 cup (8.8 oz)	190
Escarole In Chicken Broth	1 cup (8.1 oz)	25
Hearty Black Bean	1 cup (8.5 oz)	170
Hearty Penne In Chicken Broth	1 cup (8.4 oz)	80
Herb Rotini Vegetable	1 cup (9.1 oz)	120
Italian Herb Shells Minestrone	1 cup (9.1 oz)	120
Macaroni & Bean	1 cup (8.6 oz)	160
Manhattan Clam Chowder	1 cup (8.4 oz)	110
Meatballs & Pasta Pearls	1 cup (8.3 oz)	140
Minestrone Parmesan	1 cup (8.3 oz)	100
New England Clam Chowder	1 cup (8.4 oz)	190
Oregano Penne Italian Style Vegetable	1 cup (8.7 oz)	90
Peppercorn Penne Vegetable	1 cup (9.1 oz)	100
Potato Broccoli & Cheese	1 cup (8.8 oz)	160
Potato Ham & Cheese	1 cup (8.6 oz)	170
Rich & Hearty Beef Pot Roast	1 cup	130
Rich & Hearty Chicken & Homestyle Noodles	1 cup	110

FOOD	PORTION	CALS
Roasted Garlic Pasta Lentil	1 cup (9.3 oz)	120
Rotisserie Seasoned Chicken	1 cup (8.5 oz)	100
Spicy Chicken & Penne	1 cup (8.5 oz)	110
Split Pea w/ Ham	1 cup (8.4 oz)	150
Tomato	1 cup (8.5 oz)	100
Tomato Basil	1 cup (8.8 oz)	100
Tomato Vegetable	1 cup (8.5 oz)	90
Tortellini In Chicken Broth	1 cup (8.3 oz)	70
Traditional Beef Barley	1 cup	150
Traditional Chicken & Herb Dumplings	1 cup	110
Traditional Chicken Noodle	1 cup	100
Traditional Hearty Chicken & Rotini	1 cup	100
Turkey Noodle	1 cup	90
Turkey Rice w/ Vegetables	1 cup (8.5 oz)	110
Vegetable Classics French Onion	1 cup	50
Vegetable Classics Green Split Pea	1 cup	170
Vegetable Classics Hearty Tomato	1 cup	110
Vegetable Classics Lentil	1 cup	180
Vegetable Classics Minestrone	1 cup	110
Vegetable Classics Tomato Rotini	1 cup	140
Vegetable Classics Vegetable	1 cup	80
Rienzi		
Chicken & Rice	1 cup	110
Snow's		
Clam Chowder	1 cup	200
Streit's		
Hearty Vegetarian Vegetable	1 cup	90
Mushroom Barley	1 cup	100
Swanson		
Beef Broth 100% Fat Free Lower Sodium	1 cup	15
Beef Broth 99% Fat Free	1 cup	10
Beef Broth Onion Seasoned	1 cup (8.4 oz)	20
Chicken Broth 100% Fat Free 33% Less Sodium	1 cup	15
Chicken Broth 99% Fat Free	1 cup	15
Vegetable Broth	1 cup	19
Walnut Acres		
Organic Country Corn Chowder	1 cup (8.8 oz)	150
Wolfgang Puck		
Chicken Parmesan w/ Pasta	1 cup	300
Hearty Lentil & Vegetable	1 cup	170

FOOD	PORTION	CALS
FROZEN		
Birds Eye		
Hearty Spoonfuls Pasta & Chicken	1 bowl (11.2 oz)	140
Nature's Entree		
Chowder	1 pkg (12 oz)	230
Tortellini Minestone	1 pkg (12 oz)	360
MIX		
beef broth cube	1 cube (3.6 g)	6
chicken broth cube	1 cube (4.8 g)	9
A Taste Of Thai		
Coconut Ginger	2 tsp	15
Alpine Aire		
Low Carb Bay Shrimp Bisque	1 pkg	150
Low Carb Beefy Vegetable	1 pkg	100
Low Carb Broccoli Cheddar	1 pkg	140
Low Carb Mushroom & Chicken w/ Roasted Garlic	1 pkg	130
Armour		
Bouillon Cubes Beef	1 (4 g)	5
Bouillon Cubes Chicken	1 (4 g)	5
Azumaya		
Asian Style Thin Noodle	1 cup	120
Asian Style Wide Noodle	1 cup	120
Bean Cuisine		
13 Bean Bouillabasse	1 cup	220
Island Black Bean	1 cup	210
Lots of Lentil	1 cup	230
Mesa Maize	1 cup	160
White Bean Provencal	1 cup	250
Fantastic		
Noodle Bowls Mandarin Broccoli	1 pkg (2.2 oz)	220
Hodgson Mill		
Choice Bean not prep	¼ cup (1.5 oz)	150
MiniCarb		
Miso w/ Tofu & Shitake	1 pkg	33
Szechuan Beef	1 pkg	24
Thai Coconut Cream	1 pkg	100
Miso-Cup		
Golden Vegetable as prep	1 cup	30
Miso Reduced Sodium as prep	1 cup	25

FOOD	PORTION	CALS
Organic Miso as prep	1 cup	35
Savory Seaweed as prep	1 cup	30
Nueva Cocina		
Frijoles Negros Con Chipotle Chile	1 cup	140
Sopa De Calabaza	1 cup	180
Sopa De Frijoles Colorados	1 cup	140
Sopa De Frijoles Negros	1 cup	140
Sopa De Maiz	1 cup	150
Sopa De Tortilla	1 cup	140
Ramen Noodle		
Beef as prep	1 pkg (2.2 oz)	280
Beef Low Fat as prep	1 pkg (2.2 oz)	216
Chicken as prep	1 pkg (2.2 oz)	279
Chicken Low Fat as prep	1 pkg (2.2 oz)	216
Oriental Low Fat as prep	1 pkg (2.2 oz)	217
Shrimp as prep	1 pkg (2.2 oz)	294
Shrimp Low Fat as prep	1 pkg (2.2 oz)	218
Tomato as prep	1 pkg (2.2 oz)	295
Rapunzel		
Cubes Vegetable Bouillon No Salt Added	½ cube	25
Cubes Vegetable Bouillon w/ Sea Salt	½ cube	15
Cubes Vegetable Bouillon w/ Sea Salt & Herbs	½ cube	15
Simply Asia		
Soy Noodle Bowl	1 pkg	70
Slim-Fast		
Creamy Broccoli	1 pkg	210
Creamy Chicken	1 pkg	220
Creamy Potato Cheddar & Chive	1 pkg	220
Steero		
Beef Bouillon Cube	1 (3.5 g)	5
Beef Bouillon Cube Reduced Sodium	1 cube (3.5 oz)	5
Beef Bouillon Instant	1 tsp (3.5 oz)	5
Beef Bouillon Instant Reduced Sodium	1 tsp (3.5 oz)	5
Chicken Bouillon Cube	1 (3.5 g)	5
Chicken Bouillon Cube Reduced Sodium	1 (3.5 g)	5
Chicken Bouillon Instant	1 tsp (3.5 g)	5
Chicken Bouillon Instant Reduced Sodium	1 tsp (3.5 g)	5
Thai Kitchen		
Instant Rice Noodle Bangkok Curry	1 pkg	192

FOOD	PORTION	CALS
Rice Noodle Bowl Roasted Garlic	1 bowl	170
Rice Noodle Bowl Spring Onion	1 bowl	170
Wyler's		
Beef Bouillon Cube	1 (3.5 g)	5
Beef Bouillon Cube Reduced Sodium	1 (3.5 g)	5
Beef Bouillon Instant	1 tsp (3.5 g)	5
Beef Bouillon Instant Reduced Sodium	1 tsp (3.5 g)	5
Chicken Bouillon Cube	1 (3.5 g)	5
Chicken Bouillon Cube Reduced Sodium	1 (3.5 g)	5
Chicken Bouillon Instant	1 tsp (3.5)	5
Chicken Bouillon Instant Reduced Sodium	1 tsp (3.5 g)	5
SHELF-STABLE		
Annie Chun's		
Ginger Chicken	1 cup	30
Shiitake Mushroom	1 cup	25
Traditional Miso	1 cup	35
Campbell's		
Chunky Classic Chicken Noodle	1 pkg (15.25 oz)	110
Lunch Bucket		
Chicken Noodle	1 pkg (7.25 oz)	80
Country Vegetable	1 pkg (7.25 oz)	60
TastyBite		
Tom Yum	½ pkg (5.3 oz)	92
TAKE-OUT		
albondigas meatball soup	1 bowl	318
beef stew soup	1 cup (8.8 oz)	221
black bean turtle soup	1 cup	241
broccoli cheese	1 cup	165
brunswick stew soup	1 cup (8.5 oz)	232
caldo de res beef soup	1 bowl	327
chinese velvet corn	1¼ cups	135
corn & cheese chowder	¾ cup	215
egg drop	1 cup	73
gazpacho	1 cup	46
greek lemon	¾ cup	63
hot & sour	1 serv (14 oz)	173
matzo ball soup	1 cup	118
middle eastern chilled fruit	1 cup	99
middle eastern chilled yogurt & cucumber	1 bowl	85
minestrone	1 cup	154

FOOD	PORTION	CALS
miso w/ tofu	1 bowl	36
onion soup gratinee	1 serv	492
oxtail	5 oz	64
pasta e fagioll	1 cup (8.8 oz)	194
ratatouille	1 cup (7.5 oz)	266
sopa de feijao portuguese bean & sausage	1 cup	220
thai lemon grass	1 bowl	100
vietnamese pho beef noodle	1 serv (7.8 oz)	480
wonton soup	1 cup	205
zupa koprowa polish dill soup	1 bowl	54
zuppa toscana	1 bowl	543

SOUR CREAM

FOOD	PORTION	CALS
sour cream	1 cup (8 oz)	493
sour cream	1 tbsp (0.4 oz)	26
Breakstone's		
Sour Cream	2 tbsp (1 oz)	60
Cabot		
Light	2 tbsp	35
No Fat	2 tbsp	20
Sour Cream	2 tbsp	50
Crowley		
Sour Cream	2 tbsp	60
Land O Lakes		
Fat Free	2 tbsp (1.1 oz)	25
Light	2 tbsp (1 oz)	40
Sour Cream	2 tbsp (1 oz)	60

SOUR CREAM SUBSTITUTES

FOOD	PORTION	CALS
nondairy	1 oz	59
nondairy	1 cup	479

SOURSOP

FOOD	PORTION	CALS
fresh	1	416
fresh cut up	1 cup	150

SOY (see also CHEESE SUBSTITUTES, ICE CREAM AND FROZEN DESSERTS, MILK SUBSTITUTES, MISO, SOY SAUCE, SOYBEANS, TEMPEH, TOFU, YOGURT FROZEN)

FOOD	PORTION	CALS
lecithin	1 tbsp	104
soy milk	1 cup	79
soya cheese	1.4 oz	128

FOOD	PORTION	CALS
Bob's Red Mill		
Flour	⅓ cup	130
Dakota Gourmet		
Soy Nuts	1 oz	129
Fearn		
Granules	¼ cup	110
Powder	¼ cup	100
GeniSoy		
Soy Nuts Deep Sea Salted	1 oz	120
Soy Nuts Old Hickory Smoked	1 oz	120
Soy Nuts Praline	55 pieces (1 oz)	120
Soy Nuts Unsalted	1 oz	120
Soy Nuts Zesty Barbeque	1 oz	120
Health Trip		
Soynut Butter Honey Sweet	2 tbsp	170
Soynut Butter Original	2 tbsp	180
Soynut Butter Unsalted	2 tbsp	180
I.M. Healthy		
SoyNut Butter Chocolate	2 tbsp (1.1 oz)	190
SoyNut Butter Honey Creamy	2 tbsp (1.1 oz)	170
SoyNut Butter Original Creamy	2 tbsp (1.1 oz)	170
SoyNut Butter Unsweetened Chunky	2 tbsp (1.1 oz)	160
SoyNut Butter Unsweetened Creamy	2 tbsp (1.1 oz)	160
Loma Linda		
Soyagen All Purpose	¼ cup (1 oz)	130
Soyagen Carob	¼ cup (1 oz)	130
Soyagen No Sucrose	¼ cup (1 oz)	130
Natural Touch		
Roasted Soy Butter	2 tbsp (1.1 oz)	170
Revival		
Shake Chocolate Daydream Frustose	1 pkg	240
Shake Strawberry Smile Unsweetened	1 pkg	130
Shake Strawberry Smile Fructose	1 pkg	225
Shake Strawberry Smile Splenda	1 pkg	130
Soy Shake Plain	1 pkg	110
Soy Shake Vanilla Pleasure	1 pkg	220
Soy Shake Vanilla Pleasure Splenda	1 pkg	120
Soy Shake Vanilla Pleasure Unsweetened	1 pkg	120
Soynuts Chocolate Covered	⅙ cup	70
Soynuts Hot Jalapeno & Cheddar	⅙ cup	78

FOOD	PORTION	CALS
Soynuts Unsalted	⅙ cup	78
Soynuts Yogurt Covered	⅙ cup	720
Soy Juicy		
All Flavors	8 oz	160
Soy Wonder		
Creamy	2 tbsp	170
Crunchy	2 tbsp	170
SOY SAUCE		
shoyu	1 tbsp	9
soy sauce	1 tbsp	7
tamari	1 tbsp	11
Chun King		
Lite	1 tbsp (0.5 oz)	15
Soy Sauce	1 tbsp (0.6 oz)	11
Eden		
Organic Shoyu Reduced Sodium	1 tbsp	10
Organic Tamari	1 tbsp	15
Ponzu Sauce	1 tbsp	5
Shoyu	1 tbsp	15
Just Rite		
Soy Sauce	1 tbsp (0.5 oz)	11
Kikkoman		
Lite	1 tbsp (0.5 oz)	10
Soy Sauce	1 tbsp (0.5 oz)	10
La Choy		
Lite	1 tbsp (0.5 oz)	15
Soy Sauce	1 tbsp (0.6 oz)	11
Tree Of Life		
Shoyu	1 tbsp (0.5 oz)	15
Tamari Wheat Free	1 tbsp (0.5 oz)	15
SOYBEANS		
dried cooked	1 cup	298
dry roasted	½ cup	387
green cooked	½ cup	127
roasted	½ cup	405
roasted & toasted	1 cup	490
roasted & toasted salted	1 cup	490
sprouts raw	½ cup	43

FOOD	PORTION	CALS
sprouts steamed	½ cup	38
sprouts stir fried	1 cup	125
Arrowhead		
Organic not prep	¼ cup	180
Eden		
Organic Black	½ cup (4.6 oz)	120
Frieda's		
Edamame	½ cup (2.6 oz)	100
Seapoint Farms		
Edamame Organic	½ cup (2.6 oz)	100
Edamame In Pods frzn	½ cup (2.6 oz)	100
Edamame Rice Bowl Kung Pao Vegetable	1 pkg (12 oz)	420
Edamame Rice Bowl Szechwan Vegetable	1 pkg (12 oz)	420
Edamame Rice Bowl Teriyaki Vegetable	1 pkg (12 oz)	430
Edamame Rice Bowl Vegetable Fried Rice	1 pkg (11 oz)	220
Edamame Shelled	½ cup (2.6 oz)	100

SPAGHETTI *(see PASTA, PASTA DINNERS, PASTA SALAD, SPAGHETTI SAUCE)*

SPAGHETTI SAUCE
JARRED

FOOD	PORTION	CALS
marinara sauce	1 cup	171
spaghetti sauce	1 cup	272
Amy's		
Family Marinara	½ cup	50
Garlic Mushroom	½ cup	120
Puttanesca	½ cup	40
Tomato Basil	½ cup	80
Wild Mushroom	½ cup	60
Barilla		
Boscaiola Mushrooms & Garlic	½ cup	90
Restaurant Creations Cheese & Tomatoes	¼ cup	110
Restaurant Creations Garlic Herbs & Tomatoes	¼ cup	100
Restaurant Creations Pesto & Tomatoes	¼ cup	150
Catelli		
Garden Select Country Mushroom	½ cup	80
Garden Select Diced Tomatoes & Basil	½ cup	80
Garden Select Fine Herbs	½ cup	80
Garden Select Garlic & Onion	½ cup	80

FOOD	PORTION	CALS
Garden Select Parmesan & Romano	½ cup	80
Garden Select Zucchini Primavera	½ cup	80
Classico		
Italian Sausage	½ cup	90
Tomato & Basil	½ cup	60
Colavita		
Garden Style	½ cup (4.4 oz)	60
Del Monte		
Chunky Garlic & Herb	½ cup	60
Chunky Italian Herb	½ cup	60
Tomato & Basil	½ cup	70
W/ Four Cheese	½ cup	70
With Garlic & Onion	½ cup	80
With Green Peppers & Mushrooms	½ cup	80
With Meat	½ cup	60
With Mushrooms	½ cup	60
Eden		
Organic Lightly Seasoned	½ cup (4.4 oz)	80
Francesco Rinaldi		
Alfredo	¼ cup (2.1 oz)	70
Chunky Garden Mushroom & Onion	½ cup (4.4 oz)	80
Chunky Garden Tomato Garlic & Onion	½ cup (4.4 oz)	70
Dolce Sweet & Tasty Tomato	½ cup (4.4 oz)	110
Dolce Three Cheese	½ cup (4.4 oz)	90
Dulce Super Mushroom	½ cup (4.4 oz)	110
Hearty Diavolo	½ cup (4.4 oz)	70
Hearty Mushroom Pepper & Onion	½ cup (4.4 oz)	80
Hearty Tomato & Basil	½ cup (4.4 oz)	80
Puttanesca	½ cup (4.3 oz)	70
Tomato Alfredo	¼ cup (2.1 oz)	60
Traditional Meat Flavored	½ cup (4.4 oz)	90
Traditional Mushroom	½ cup (4.4 oz)	90
Traditional No Salt Added	½ cup (4.4 oz)	70
Traditional Original	½ cup (4.4 oz)	90
Vodka Sauce	¼ cup (2.1 oz)	60
Healthy Choice		
Chunky Italian Vegetable	½ cup (4.4 oz)	40
Chunky Mushroom	½ cup (4.4 oz)	42
Garlic & Herbs	½ cup (4.4 oz)	49

FOOD	PORTION	CALS
Garlic Lovers Garlic & Mushroom	½ cup (4.4 oz)	44
Garlic Lovers Roasted Garlic	½ cup (4.4 oz)	52
Garlic Lovers Roasted Garlic & Sun Dried Tomato	½ cup (4.4 oz)	52
Super Chunky Mushroom & Sweet Peppers	½ cup (4.4 oz)	43
Super Chunky Tomato Mushroom & Garlic	½ cup (4.4 oz)	45
Super Chunky Vegetable Primavera	½ cup (4.4 oz)	43
Traditional	½ cup (4.4 oz)	48
With Mushrooms	½ cup (4.4 oz)	48
Hunt's		
Basil Garlic & Oregano	¼ cup	15
Cheese & Garlic	½ cup	50
Chunky Vegetable	½ cup	50
Diced In Tomato Sauce	½ cup	30
Family Favorites Lasagna	¼ cup	30
Four Cheese	½ cup	50
Italian Sausage	½ cup	60
Light	½ cup	45
Meat	½ cup	68
No Added Sugar	½ cup	45
Roasted Garlic & Onion	½ cup	50
Traditional	½ cup	50
With Mushrooms	½ cup	50
Muir Glen		
Organic Balsamic Roasted Onion	½ cup (4.4 oz)	50
Organic Cabernet Marinara	½ cup (4.4 oz)	50
Organic Chunky Herb	½ cup (4.4 oz)	50
Organic Garden Vegetable	½ cup (4.4 oz)	50
Organic Garlic & Onion	½ cup (4.4 oz)	55
Organic Garlic Roasted Garlic	½ cup (4.4 oz)	50
Organic Green Olive	½ cup (4.4 oz)	60
Organic Italian Herb	½ cup (4.4 oz)	55
Organic Mushroom Marinara	½ cup (4.4 oz)	45
Organic Portabello Mushroom	½ cup (4.4 oz)	50
Organic Sun Dried Tomato	½ cup (4.4 oz)	55
Organic Tomato Basil	½ cup (4.4 oz)	50
Newman's Own		
Sockarooni	½ cup	60

FOOD	PORTION	CALS
Prego		
Pasta Bake Sauce Tomato Garlic & Basil	1 serv (3.4 oz)	80
Traditional	½ cup (4.2 oz)	140
Progresso		
Marinara	½ cup (4.3 oz)	80
Meat Flavored	½ cup (4.4 oz)	100
Sauce	½ cup (4.4 oz)	100
Ragu		
Chunky Garden Style Tomato Garlic & Onion	½ cup (4.5 oz)	110
Sara Lee		
Chunky Garden Mushroom & Peppers	½ cup (4.4 oz)	80
Tree Of Life		
Pasta Sauce	½ cup (4 oz)	50
Pasta Sauce Fat Free Classic	½ cup (3.9 oz)	40
Pasta Sauce Fat Free Mushroom & Basil	½ cup (3.9 oz)	30
Pasta Sauce Fat Free Onion & Garlic	½ cup (3.9 oz)	30
Pasta Sauce Fat Free Sweet Pepper	½ cup (3.9 oz)	30
Pasta Sauce No Salt Added	½ cup (3.9 oz)	50
Tuttorosso		
Pasta Sauce Meat	½ cup	90
Walden Farms		
Alfredo Sauce Calorie Free	¼ cup	0
Marinara Calorie Free	⅓ cup	0
MIX		
Durkee		
Spaghetti Sauce as prep	½ cup	15
With Mushrooms as prep	½ cup	15
French's		
Italian as prep	½ cup	16
Mushroom as prep	½ cup	20
Thick as prep	½ cup	10
McCormick		
Alfredo Pasta Blend as prep	½ cup	60
Pasta Rosa Blend	1 tbsp (10 g)	40
Pesto Pasta Sauce as prep	2 tsp (4 g)	10
Primavera Pasta Blend	1 tbsp (7 g)	30
Spaghetti Sauce	1 tbsp (8 g)	25
REFRIGERATED		
Buitoni		
Alfredo	¼ cup	140

FOOD	PORTION	CALS
Alfredo Portabello Mushroom	¼ cup	100
Alfredo Light	¼ cup	80
Marinara	½ cup	80
Marinara Roasted Garlic	½ cup	60
Pesto	¼ cup	330
Pesto w/ Basil	¼ cup	300
Pesto w/ Basil Reduced Fat	¼ cup	230
Pesto w/ Sun Dried Tomatoes	¼ cup	210
Tomato Herb Parmesan	½ cup	120
TAKE-OUT		
bolognese	5 oz	195

SPANISH FOOD
CANNED
Derby
Tamales	3 (6.5 oz)	253

Gebhardt
Enchiladas	2 (5.7 oz)	258
Tamales	2 (5.7 oz)	268
Tamales Jumbo	2 (6.9 oz)	332

Rosarita
Enchilada Sauce Mild	¼ cup (2.1 oz)	23

Van Camp's
Tamales	2 (5 oz)	210

FROZEN
Amy's
Black Bean Vegetable Enchilada	1 (4.75 oz)	130
Bowls Santa Fe Enchilada	1 pkg (10 oz)	340
Burrito Bean & Cheese	1 (6 oz)	280
Burrito Bean & Rice Non-Dairy	1 (6 oz)	270
Burrito Black Bean Vegetable	1 (6 oz)	320
Burrito Breakfast	1 (6 oz)	210
Burrito Especial	1 (6 oz)	260
Cheese Enchilada	1 (4.75 oz)	210
Mexican Tamale Pie	1 (8 oz)	150

Banquet
Chimichanga Meal	1 meal (9.5 oz)	500
Enchilada Beef	1 pkg (11 oz)	370
Enchilada Cheese	1 pkg (11 oz)	360
Enchilada Chicken	1 pkg (11 oz)	350

FOOD	PORTION	CALS
Enchilada Beef & Tamale Combo	1 pkg (11 oz)	450
Mexican Style Enchilada Combo	1 meal (11 oz)	360
Health Is Wealth		
Burrito Munchees	10 (5 oz)	310
Mexican Munchees	2 (1 oz)	49
Healthy Choice		
Chicken Enchiladas	1 pkg	360
Enchilada Chicken	1 pkg	300
Jose Ole		
Burrito Chicken	1 (5 oz)	260
Lean Cuisine		
One Dish Favorites Chicken Enchilada	1 pkg (9 oz)	280
Patio		
Beef & Cheese Enchiladas Chili 'N Beans	1 meal (15.5 oz)	670
Beef Enchiladas Chili 'N Beans	1 meal (15.5 oz)	540
Burrito Bean & Cheese	1 (5 oz)	300
Burrito Beef & Bean Hot	1 (5 oz)	320
Burrito Beef & Bean Mild	1 (5 oz)	330
Burrito Beef & Bean Medium	1 (5 oz)	310
Burrito Beef & Bean Red Chili Pepper Red Hot	1 (5 oz)	320
Burrito Chicken	1 (5 oz)	290
Enchilada Beef	1 meal (12 oz)	320
Enchilada Cheese	1 meal (12 oz)	370
Enchilada Chicken	1 meal (12 oz)	400
Fiesta	1 meal (12 oz)	350
Mexican Style	1 meal (13.25 oz)	470
MIX		
Gebhardt		
Menudo Mix	¼ tsp (0.4 g)	1
McCormick		
Burrito Seasoning	1 tbsp (8 g)	25
Fajitas Marinade Mix	2 tsp (4 g)	15
Taco Seasoning Hot	2 tsp (6 g)	20
Taco Seasoning Mild	2 tsp (7 g)	20
READY-TO-EAT		
taco shell baked	1 med (0.5 oz)	61
taco shell baked w/o salt	1 med (0.5 oz)	61
Gebhardt		
Taco Shells	3 (1.1 oz)	155

FOOD	PORTION	CALS
La Mexicana		
Flour Burritos	1 (1.6 oz)	160
Rosarita		
Taco Shells	3 (1.1 oz)	155
Tostada Shells	2 (1 oz)	125
TAKE-OUT		
burrito w/ apple	1 sm (2.6 oz)	231
burrito w/ apple	1 lg (5.4 oz)	484
burrito w/ beans	2 (7.6 oz)	448
burrito w/ beans & cheese	2 (6.5 oz)	377
burrito w/ beans & chili peppers	2 (7.2 oz)	413
burrito w/ beans & meat	2 (8.1 oz)	508
burrito w/ beans cheese & beef	2 (7.1 oz)	331
burrito w/ beans cheese & chili peppers	2 (11.8 oz)	663
burrito w/ beef -	2 (7.7 oz)	523
burrito w/ beef & chili peppers	2 (7.1 oz)	426
burrito w/ beef cheese & chili peppers	2 (10.7 oz)	634
burrito w/ cherry	1 sm (2.6 oz)	231
burrito w/ cherry	1 lg (5.4 oz)	484
chimichanga w/ beef	1 (6.1 oz)	425
chimichanga w/ beef & cheese	1 (6.4 oz)	443
chimichanga w/ beef & red chili peppers	1 (6.7 oz)	424
chimichanga w/ beef cheese & red chili peppers	1 (6.3 oz	364
enchilada eggplant	1	142
enchilada w/ cheese	1 (5.7 oz)	320
enchilada w/ cheese & beef	1 (6.7 oz)	324
enchirito w/ cheese beef & beans	1 (6.8 oz)	344
frijoles w/ cheese	1 cup (5.9 oz)	226
nachos w/ cheese	6 to 8 (4 oz)	345
nachos w/ cheese & jalapeno peppers	6 to 8 (7.2 oz)	607
nachos w/ cheese beans ground beef & peppers	6 to 8 (8.9 oz)	568
nachos w/ cinnamon & sugar	6 to 8 (3.8 oz)	592
quesadilla	1	290
taco	1 sm (6 oz)	370
taco salad	1½ cups	279
taco salad w/ chili con carne	1½ cups	288
tostada w/ beans & cheese	1 (5.1 oz)	223
tostada w/ beans beef & cheese	1 (7.9 oz)	334

FOOD	PORTION	CALS
tostada w/ beef & cheese	1 (5.7 oz)	315
tostada w/ guacamole	2 (9.2 oz)	360

SPICES *(see individual names,* HERBS/SPICES*)*

SPINACH
CANNED
spinach	½ cup	25
Del Monte		
Whole Leaf	½ cup	30
S&W		
Spinach	½ cup (4.5 oz)	30
FRESH		
baby raw	2 cups	20
cooked	½ cup	21
malabar cooked	1 cup (1.5 oz)	10
mustard chopped cooked	½ cup	14
mustard raw chopped	½ cup	17
new zealand chopped cooked	½ cup	11
new zealand raw	½ cup	4
raw chopped	1 pkg (10 oz)	46
raw chopped	½ cup	6
Dole		
Baby Spinach	3½ cups (3 oz)	35
Fresh Express		
Baby Spinach	3 cups	20
Spicy Spinach	3 cups (3 oz)	10
Ready Pac		
Baby	2 cups	20
Microwave Spinach as prep	½ cup	20
FROZEN		
cooked	½ cup	27
Amy's Organic		
Snacks Spinach Feta	5–6 pieces	170
Birds Eye		
Chopped	⅓ cup	20
Creamed	½ cup	100
Cut Leaf	1 cup	20
Fresh Like		
Cut Leaf	3.5 oz	21

FOOD	PORTION	CALS
Green Giant		
Creamed Low Fat Sauce	½ cup	80
Health Is Wealth		
Spinach Munchees	2 (1 oz)	60
Spinach Feta Munchees	2 (1 oz)	70
Tree Of Life		
Organic	1 cup (3 oz)	20
SHELF-STABLE		
TastyBite		
Kashmir Spinach	½ pkg (5 oz)	170
TAKE-OUT		
indian saag	1 serv	28
spanakopita spinach pie	1 cup (6 oz)	196

SPINACH JUICE
juice	7 oz	14

SPORTS DRINKS (see ENERGY DRINKS)

SPOT
baked	3 oz	134

SPROUTS
kidney bean	½ cup	27
lentil sprouts	½ cup	40
mung bean	½ cup	16
mung bean canned	½ cup	8
mung bean cooked	½ cup	13
pea	½ cup	77
radish	½ cup	8
Brassica		
Broccoli Sprouts	½ cup (1 oz)	16
Chun King		
Bean Sprouts	1 cup (3 oz)	11
Fresh Alternatives		
Deli Blend	½ cup (1 oz)	10
Salad Blend	½ cup (1 oz)	10
Sandwich Blend	½ cup (1 oz)	5
La Choy		
Bean Sprouts	1 cup (2.9 oz)	11

FOOD	PORTION	CALS
TAKE-OUT		
mung bean stir fried	½ cup	31
SQUAB		
boneless baked	3.5 oz	175
breast w/o skin raw	1 (3.5 oz)	135
w/o skin raw	1 squab (5.9 oz)	239
SQUASH (see also SQUASH SEEDS, ZUCCHINI)		
CANNED		
crookneck sliced	½ cup	14
FRESH		
acorn cooked mashed	½ cup	41
acorn cubed baked	½ cup	57
butternut baked	½ cup	41
crookneck sliced cooked	½ cup	18
hubbard baked	½ cup	51
hubbard cooked mashed	½ cup	35
scallop sliced cooked	½ cup	14
spaghetti cooked	½ cup	23
Frieda's		
Acorn	¾ cup (3 oz)	35
Baby Crookneck	⅔ cup (3 oz)	15
Baby Scallop	⅔ cup (3 oz)	15
Eight Ball	2 (4.4 oz)	18
Hubbard	¾ cup (3 oz)	35
Mini Pumpkin	¾ cup (3 oz)	20
Spaghetti	¾ cup (3 oz)	30
Star Spangled	⅔ cup (3 oz)	20
Turban	¾ cup (3 oz)	30
Martin Farms		
Butternut Fresh Cut	½ cup	40
FROZEN		
butternut cooked mashed	½ cup	47
crookneck sliced cooked	½ cup	24
Birds Eye		
Cooked Squash	½ cup	50
Sliced Yellow	⅔ cup	15

FOOD	PORTION	CALS
SQUASH SEEDS		
roasted	1 oz	148
salted & roasted	1 oz	148
seeds dried	1 oz	154
seeds whole roasted	1 oz	127
SQUIB		
pigeon w/ skin & bone	3.5 oz	169
SQUID		
fried	3 oz	149
raw	3 oz	78
Margaritaville		
Captain's Calamari Strips + Sauce	⅓ pkg	330
TAKE-OUT		
calamari deep fried	1 serv	451
SQUIRREL		
roasted	3 oz	147
STARFRUIT		
fresh	1	42
Frieda's		
Dried	⅓ cup (1.4 oz)	120
STRAWBERRIES		
CANNED		
in heavy syrup	½ cup	117
DRIED		
Frieda's		
Dried	½ cup (1.4 oz)	150
FRESH		
strawberries	1 cup	45
strawberries	1 pint	97
FROZEN		
sweetened sliced	1 pkg (10 oz)	273
sweetened sliced	1 cup	245
unsweetened	1 cup	52
whole sweetened	1 pkg (10 oz)	223
whole sweetened	1 cup	200
Birds Eye		
In Syrup	½ cup	120

FOOD	PORTION	CALS
Lite Syrup	1 pkg (10 oz)	120
Whole	½ cup	100
Tree Of Life		
Organic	¾ cup (5 oz)	50

STRAWBERRY JUICE
Adina
California Kiss Hibiscus Strawberry	8 oz	80

Ceres
Strawberry	8 oz	115

Giant Berry Farms
Just Strawberries	1 bottle (12 oz)	140

Hi-C
Blast	8 oz	120

Squeezit
Strawberry	1 bottle (7 oz)	110

STUFFING/DRESSING
Pepperidge Farm
Corn Bread	¾ cup (1.5 oz)	170
Herb Seasoned	¾ cup (1.5 oz)	170
Herb Seasoned Cubed	¾ cup (1.3 oz)	140
One Step Chicken	½ cup (1.2 oz)	140
One Step Southwestern Corn Bread	½ cup (1.2 oz)	150
One Step Turkey	½ cup (1.2 oz)	150

TAKE-OUT
bread	1 cup	352
cornbread	½ cup	179
sausage	½ cup	292

STURGEON
cooked	3 oz	115
raw	3 oz	90
roe raw	1 oz	59
smoked	1 oz	48
smoked	3 oz	147

SUCKER
white baked	3 oz	101

SUGAR
brown packed	1 cup (7.7 oz)	828

FOOD	PORTION	CALS
brown unpacked	1 cup (5.1 oz)	547
brown organic	1 tsp	17
cinnamon sugar	1 tsp	16
maple	1 piece (1 oz)	99
powdered	1 tbsp (0.3 oz)	31
powdered unsifted	1 cup (4.2 oz)	467
raw	1 pkg (5 g)	19
sugarcane stem	3 oz	54
white	1 packet (3 g)	12
white	1 cup (7 oz)	773
white	1 tsp (4 g)	15
Billington's		
Muscovado Light Brown	1 tsp	15
Domino		
Dark Brown	1 tsp	15
Light Brown	1 tsp	15
White	1 tsp	15
Gluco Burst		
Artic Cherry	1 pkg (1.3 oz)	70
Maui Brand		
Raw Sugar	1 tsp	15
Princess Of Yum		
Citrus Lemon	2.5 tsp	40
French Vanilla	2.5 tsp	40

SUGAR SUBSTITUTES
Equal
Flavor Sticks	1 pkg	0
Packet	1 pkg	0
Spoonful	1 tsp	0
Sugar Lite	1 tsp	8
Fran Gare's		
Miracle Sweet	1 tsp	10
Keto		
Sweet	½ tsp	0
Lo Han		
Sweet	2 scoops	2
SomerSweet		
Sweetener	¼ tsp	0

FOOD	PORTION	CALS
Splenda		
Sugar Blend For Baking	½ tsp	10
Sweetener	1 pkg	0
Steel's		
Brown	1 tsp	10
Sugar Substitute	1 tsp	10
Stevita		
Spoonable	⅓ tsp	0
Sugar Twin		
Packets	1	0
Spoonable Brown	1 tsp	0
Spoonable White	1 tsp	0
SweetLeaf		
SteviaPlus	1 pkg	0
Whey Low		
Gold	1 tsp	4
Granular	1 tsp	4
Powder	1 tsp	4
SUGAR-APPLE		
fresh	1	146
fresh cut up	1 cup	236
SUNCHOKE		
fresh raw sliced	½ cup	57
Frieda's		
Sunchoke	½ cup (3 oz)	70
SUNFISH		
pumpkinseed baked	3 oz	97
SUNFLOWER		
seeds dried	1 cup	821
seeds dried	1 oz	162
seeds dry roasted	1 oz	165
seeds dry roasted	1 cup	745
seeds dry roasted salted	1 cup	745
seeds dry roasted salted	1 oz	165
seeds oil roasted	1 cup	830
seeds oil roasted salted	1 oz	175
seeds oil roasted salted	1 cup	830
seeds toasted	1 oz	176

FOOD	PORTION	CALS
seeds toasted	1 cup	826
seeds toasted salted	1 cup	826
seeds toasted salted	1 oz	176
sunflower butter	1 tbsp	93
sunflower butter w/o salt	1 tbsp	93
Dakota Gourmet		
Honey Roasted Kernels	1 pkg (1 oz)	158
Lightly Salted Kernels	1 pkg (1 oz)	168
David		
Kernals Original	¼ cup	200
Seeds BBQ	¼ cup	190
Seeds BBQ Sizzlin	¼ cup	190
Seeds Jalapeno	¼ cup	190
Seeds Nacho Cheese	¼ cup	180
Seeds Original	¼ cup	190
Seeds Ranch	¼ cup	190
Seeds Reduced Sodium	¼ cup	190
Frito Lay		
Seeds	3 tbsp	180
Maranatha		
Tamari Seeds	¼ cup	160
SunGold		
SunButter	2 tbsp	200

SUSHI
TAKE-OUT

FOOD	PORTION	CALS
california roll	1 piece (0.8 oz)	28
fresh salmon rolls	4 pieces	250
sashimi	1 serv (6 oz)	198
tuna roll	1 piece (0.7 oz)	23
vegetable roll	1 piece (1.2 oz)	27
vinegared ginger	⅓ cup (1.6 oz)	48
wasabi	2 tsp (0.3 oz)	5
yellowtail roll	1 piece (0.6 oz)	25

SWAMP CABBAGE

FOOD	PORTION	CALS
chopped cooked	½ cup	10
raw chopped	1 cup	11

FOOD	PORTION	CALS
SWEET POTATO *(see also* YAM*)*		
baked w/ skin	1 (3.5 oz)	118
canned in syrup	½ cup	106
canned pieces	1 cup	183
frzn cooked	½ cup	88
leaves cooked	½ cup	11
mashed	½ cup	172
Princella		
In Light Syrup	⅔ cup	160
Royal Prince		
Orange Pineapple	½ cup	160
TAKE-OUT		
candied	3.5 oz	144
SWEETBREAD (PANCREAS)		
beef braised	3 oz	230
lamb braised	3 oz	199
veal braised	3 oz	218
SWISS CHARD		
cooked	½ cup	18
raw chopped	½ cup	3
Frieda's		
Bright Lights	1 cup (3 oz)	15
SWORDFISH		
cooked	3 oz	132
raw	3 oz	103
SYRUP		
corn dark & light	¼ cup	240
date syrup	1 tbsp	63
maple	1 tbsp	52
maple	1 cup (11.1 oz)	824
raspberry	1 oz	76
rose hip	1 oz	9
sorghum	1 tbsp (0.7 oz)	61
sorghum	1 cup (11.6 oz)	957
sugar syrup	¼ cup	76
DaVinci Gourmet		
Sugar Free All Flavors	1 tbsp	0

FOOD	PORTION	CALS
Eden		
Organic Barley Malt	1 tbsp	60
Estee		
Blueberry	¼ cup	30
Hershey's		
Strawberry	2 tbsp	100
Karo		
Corn Syrup Dark	1 tbsp	120
Corn Syrup Light	2 tbsp	120
Nesquik		
Strawberry Calcium Fortified	2 tbsp	100
Quik		
Strawberry	2 tbsp (1.5 oz)	110
Smucker's		
Blackberry	¼ cup	210
Blueberry	¼ cup	210
Boysenberry	¼ cup	210
Red Raspberry	¼ cup	210
Strawberry	¼ cup	210
Sundae Syrup 3 Musketeers	2 tbsp	110
Sundae Syrup Butterscotch	2 tbsp	100
Sundae Syrup Caramel	2 tbsp	100
Sundae Syrup Strawberry	2 tbsp	110
Spectrum		
Balsamic Organic	1 tbsp	35

TAHINI *(see SESAME)*

TAMARILLOS
Frieda's

Gold Or Red	2 (4.2 oz)	40

TAMARIND

fresh	1	5
fresh cut up	1 cup	287

TAMARIND JUICE
Teptip

Drink	1 can (11.2 oz)	210

FOOD	PORTION	CALS
TANGERINE		
CANNED		
in light syrup	½ cup	76
juice pack	½ cup	46
FRESH		
sections	1 cup	86
tangerine	1	37
Chiquita		
Tangerine	1 med (3.5 oz)	50
Sunkist		
Fresh	1 (3.8 oz)	50
TANGERINE JUICE		
canned sweetened	1 cup	125
fresh	1 cup	106
frzn sweetened as prep	1 cup	110
frzn sweetened not prep	6 oz	344
Fresh Samantha		
Fresh Juice	1 cup (8 oz)	110
Italian Volcano		
Organic	1 serv (6.75 oz)	94
Naked Juice		
Tangerine Scream	8 oz	110
Odwalla		
Juice	8 fl oz	110
TAPIOCA		
pearl dry	½ cup (2.7 oz)	272
starch	1 oz	98
TARO		
chips	10 (0.8 oz)	115
leaves cooked	½ cup	18
raw sliced	½ cup	56
shoots sliced cooked	½ cup	10
sliced cooked	½ cup (2.3 oz)	94
tahitian sliced cooked	½ cup	30
Frieda's		
Taro Root	⅔ cup (3 oz)	90
TARPON		
fresh	3 oz	87

FOOD	PORTION	CALS
TARRAGON		
ground	1 tsp	5
TEA/HERBAL TEA (*see also* ICED TEA)		
HERBAL		
chamomile brewed	1 cup	2
Celestial Seasonings		
Mandarin Orange Spice	1 tea bag	0
Eden		
Organic Genmaicha Tea	1 cup	0
Organic Kukicha Tea	1 cup	0
Guayaki		
Yerba Mate Magical Mint	1 tea bag	5
Yerba Mate Organic Chai Spice	1 tea bag	5
Yerba Mate Organic Chocolatte	1 tea bag	5
Yerba Mate Organic Orange Blossom	1 tea bag	5
Yerba Mate Organic Rooiboost	1 tea bag	5
Yerba Mate Organic Traditional	1 tea bag	5
Lipton		
Bedtime Story	1 tea bag	0
Cinnamon Apple	1 tea bag	0
Ginger Twist	1 tea bag	0
Lemon	1 tea bag	0
Orange	1 tea bag	0
Peppermint	1 tea bag	0
Quietly Chamomile	1 tea bag	0
Silk		
Chai	1 cup	140
Tetley		
Chamomile	1 cup	0
Orange & Peach	1 cup	0
Peppermint	1 cup	0
REGULAR		
brewed tea	6 oz	2
Activitea		
Green Tea	1 cup	36
Celestial Seasonings		
Green Tea Blueberry Breeze	1 cup	0
Green Tea Honey Lemon Ginseng	1 cup	0
Green Tea Raspberry Garden as prep	1 cup	0

FOOD	PORTION	CALS
Honey Darjeeling as prep	1 cup	0
Teahouse Chai Original India Spice	1 cup	0
DaVinci Gourmet		
Sugar Free Tea Concentrate Green	2 tbsp	0
Sugar Free Tea Concentrate Lemon	2 tbsp	0
Sugar Free Tea Concentrate Spiced Chai	1.5 tbsp	0
Guayaki		
Yerba Mate Organic Greener Green Tea	1 tea bag	5
Lipton		
100% Natural	1 teabag	0
Brisk Tea as prep	1 teabag	0
Decaffeinated Brisk Tea as prep	1 serv	0
Green Tea	1 tea bag	0
Low Carb Creations		
Chai as prep	1 cup	25
Oregon		
Chai Latte Cider	½ cup	110
Chai Latte Java	½ cup	42
Chai Latte Kashmir Green Tea	½ cup	81
Chai Latte Nog	½ cup	90
Chai Latte The Original	½ cup	78
Pacific Chai		
All Flavors as prep	1 serv	93
Paradise		
Tropical Tea	8 fl oz	1
Tropical Tea Decafe	8 fl oz	1
Tropical Tea Passion Fruit	8 fl oz	1
Red Rose		
Decaffeinated	1 cup	0
Salada		
Green Tea	1 cup	0
Green Tea Decaffeinated	1 tea bag	0
Original Blend Black Tea	1 tea bag	0
Tea Tech		
Instant Green Tea All Flavors	1 tube	0
XtraGreen Tea Mix All Flavors	1 tube	0
Tetley		
British Blend Round Teabags	1 cup	0
Chai Black Tea	1 cup	0
Decaffeinated Tea Bag as prep	1	0

FOOD	PORTION	CALS
Earl Grey	1 cup	0
English Breakfast	1 cup	0
Honey Lemon Green Tea	1 cup	0
TAKE-OUT		
chai spiced latte decaf	1 cup	130

TEMPEH

tempeh	½ cup	165
Lightlife		
Garden Veggie	1 serv (4 oz)	230
Organic Flax	1 serv (4 oz)	230
Organic Grilles Lemon	1 patty (2.7 oz)	140
Organic Grilles Tamari	1 patty (2.7 oz)	130
Organic Soy	1 serv (4 oz)	210
Organic Three Grain	1 serv (4 oz)	240
Organic Wild Rice	1 serv (4 oz)	280
Turtle Island		
Five Grain	3 oz	190
Low Fat Millet	3 oz	130
Soy	3 oz	160
Wild Rice Rhapsody	3 oz	160
White Wave		
Five Grain	⅓ block	140
Organic Original Soy	⅓ block	150
Organic Sea Veggie	⅓ block	120
Soy Rice	⅓ block	140

THYME

ground	1 tsp	4

TILAPIA

Beacon Light

Farm Raised Fillets	3 oz	85

TILEFISH

cooked	½ fillet (5.3 oz)	220
cooked	3 oz	125
raw	3 oz	81

TOFU

firm	¼ block (3 oz)	118
firm	½ cup	183

FOOD	PORTION	CALS
fresh fried	1 piece (0.5 oz)	35
fuyu salted & fermented	1 block (⅓ oz)	13
koyadofu dried frozen	1 piece (½ oz)	82
okara	½ cup	47
regular	¼ block (4 oz)	88
regular	½ cup	94
Azumaya		
Extra Firm	1 serv (2.8 oz)	70
Firm	1 serv (2.8 oz)	70
Lite Silken	1 serv (3.2 oz)	40
Lite Extra Firm	1 serv (2.8 oz)	60
Seasoned Oriental Spice	1 serv (3 oz)	90
Seasoned Zesty Garlic & Onion	1 serv (3 oz)	90
Silken	1 serv (3.2 oz)	40
Eden		
Dried	1 serv (0.4 oz)	50
Galaxy		
Slices Hickory Smoked	1 slice (1 oz)	50
Slices Italian Garlic Herb	1 slice (1 oz)	50
Slices Original	1 slice (1 oz)	50
Slices Savory	1 slice (1 oz)	50
Hinoichi		
Firm	1 inch slice (3 oz)	60
Nasoya		
Chinese Spice	¼ pkg (3 oz)	90
Extra Firm	⅕ pkg (2.8 oz)	80
Firm	⅕ pkg (2.8 oz)	70
Garlic & Onion	¼ pkg (3 oz)	90
Lite Firm	⅕ pkg (2.8 oz)	40
Lite Silken	⅕ pkg (3.2 oz)	30
Seasoned Ginger Sesame	½ pkg (5.5 oz)	210
Seasoned Sweet & Sour	½ pkg (5.5 oz)	190
Seasoned Teriyaki	½ pkg (5.5 oz)	190
Seasoned Thai Peanut	½ pkg (5.5 oz)	240
Silken	⅕ pkg (3.2 oz)	45
Soft	⅕ pkg (2.8 oz)	60
TofuMate Breakfast Scramble	¼ pkg	15
TofuMate Eggless Salad	¼ pkg	15
TofuMate Mandarin Stirfry	¼ pkg	25
TofuMate Mediterranean Herb	¼ pkg	15

FOOD	PORTION	CALS
TofuMate Szechwan StirFry	¼ pkg	25
TofuMate Texas Taco	¼ pkg	15
Pete's Tofu		
Dessert Peach Mango	1 serv (6 oz)	120
Dessert Very Berry	1 serv (6 oz)	120
Medium Firm	3 oz	70
Soft	3 oz	56
Super Firm	3 oz	130
Super Firm Italian Herb	3 oz	120
Tofu 2 Go Lemon Pepper	2 pieces + sauce	160
Tofu 2 Go Santa Fe	2 pieces + sauce	150
Tofu 2 Go Sesame Ginger	2 pieces + sauce	160
Tofu 2 Go Thai Tango	2 pieces + sauce	165
Tree Of Life		
30% Reduced Fat Firm	⅕ block (3.2 oz)	90
Easymeal Pasta Primavera as prep	1 serv	460
Easymeal Southwest Medley as prep	1 serv	380
Easymeal Teriyaki Stir Fry as prep	1 serv	270
Easymeal Thai Stir Fry as prep	1 serv	270
Organic Baked	⅓ block (2.7 oz)	150
Organic Baked Island Spice	⅓ pkg (2.7 oz)	130
Organic Baked Oriental	⅓ pkg (2.7 oz)	130
Organic Baked Savory	⅓ block (2.7 oz)	140
Organic Firm	⅕ block (3.2 oz)	100
Raw Firm	⅕ block (3.2 oz)	100
White Wave		
Baked Garlic Herb Italian	1 piece	120
Baked Hickory Smoke BBQ	1 piece	75
Baked Roma Italian Basil	1 piece	100
Baked Teriyaki Oriental	1 piece	120
Baked Thai Style	1 piece	120
Baked Zesty Lemon Pepper	1 piece	120
Extra Firm	¼ block	80
Organic Extra Firm	⅕ block	90
Organic Soft	⅕ block	90
Reduced Fat	⅕ block	90
TAKE-OUT		
soy sauce marinated & grilled	1 serv (4 oz)	181

FOOD	PORTION	CALS
TOMATILLO		
fresh	1 (1.2 oz)	11
fresh chopped	½ cup	21
TOMATO		
CANNED		
paste	½ cup	110
puree	1 cup	102
puree w/o salt	1 cup	102
red whole	½ cup	24
sauce	½ cup	37
sauce spanish style	½ cup	40
sauce w/ mushrooms	½ cup	42
sauce w/ onion	½ cup	52
stewed	½ cup	34
w/ green chiles	½ cup	18
wedges in tomato juice	½ cup	34
Big R		
Cajun Stewed	½ cup (4.2 oz)	25
Diced w/ Chilies	½ cup (4.2 oz)	25
Mexican Stewed	½ cups (4.2 oz)	25
Stewed	½ cup (4.2 oz)	25
Whole	½ cup (4.2 oz)	25
Cento		
Paste	2 tbsp	30
Puree	¼ cup	25
Claussen		
Halves	1 serv (1 oz)	5
Contadina		
Crushed w/ Italian Herbs	¼ cup	20
Italian Paste	2 tbsp	35
Italian Paste Roasted Garlic	2 tbsp	35
Paste	2 tbsp (1.2 oz)	30
Puree	¼ cup (2.2 oz)	20
Recipe Ready Diced Roasted Garlic	½ cup (4.3 oz)	45
Stewed	½ cup	35
Stewed w/ Celery & Green Peppers	½ cup	35
Del Monte		
Chunky Pasta Style	½ cup	45
Diced	½ cup	25

FOOD	PORTION	CALS
Diced No Salt Added	½ cup	25
Diced w/ Basil Garlic & Oregano	½ cup	50
Diced w/ Garlic & Onion	½ cup	40
Diced w/ Green Pepper & Onion	½ cup	40
Diced Zesty Chili Style	½ cup	30
Diced Zesty w/ Mild Green Chilies	½ cup	30
Petite Cut	½ cup	25
Petite Cut Garlic & Olive Oil	½ cup	45
Sauce	¼ cup	20
Stewed Cajun Recipe	½ cup	35
Stewed Italian Recipe	½ cup	30
Stewed Mexican Recipe	½ cup	35
Stewed No Salt Added	½ cup	35
Stewed Original	½ cup	35
Wedges	½ cup	35
Eden		
Organic Diced	½ cup	30
Organic Diced w/ Green Chilies	½ cup	30
Hunt's		
Crushed	½ cup	30
Diced Original	½ cup	20
Diced w/ Basil Garlic & Oregano	½ cup	25
Diced w/ Green Pepper Celery & Onions	½ cup	45
Diced w/ Mild Green Chilies	½ cup	30
Diced w/ Roasted Garlic	½ cup	30
Diced w/ Sweet Onion	½ cup	45
Family Favorites Meatloaf	¼ cup	30
Paste	2 tbsp	25
Paste No Salt Added	2 tbsp	30
Paste w/ Basil Garlic & Oregano	2 tbsp	25
Petite Diced	½ cup	20
Petite Diced w/ Mushrooms	½ cup	40
Puree	½ cup	30
Sauce	¼ cup	15
Sauce Garlic & Herb	½ cup	40
Sauce No Salt Added	2 tbsp	30
Sauce Roasted Garlic	¼ cup	15
Stewed	½ cup	35
Stewed No Salt Added	½ cup	40
Whole No Salt Added	¼ cup	20

FOOD	PORTION	CALS
Whole No Salt Added	4 oz	20
Muir Glen		
Diced Fire Roasted	¼ cup	30
Diced w/ Green Chilies	½ cup (4.5 oz)	25
Organic Chunky Sauce	¼ cup (2.3 oz)	20
Organic Crushed Fire Roasted	¼ cup	20
Organic Diced	½ cup (4.5 oz)	25
Organic Diced No Salt Added	½ cup (4.5 oz)	25
Organic Diced w/ Basil & Garlic	½ cup (4.5 oz)	25
Organic Diced w/ Italian Herbs	½ cup (4.4 oz)	25
Organic Ground Peeled	¼ cup (2.3 oz)	10
Organic Paste	2 tbsp (1.2 oz)	30
Organic Puree	¼ cup (2.2 oz)	20
Organic Sauce	¼ cup (2.2 oz)	20
Organic Sauce No Salt Added	¼ cup (2.2 oz)	20
Organic Stewed	½ cup (4.5 oz)	30
Organic Whole Peeled	½ cup (4.6 oz)	30
Whole Peeled w/ Basil	½ cup (4.6 oz)	30
Progresso		
Crushed w/ Added Puree	¼ cup (2.1 oz)	20
Italian Style Peeled	½ cup (4.2 oz)	20
Paste	2 tbsp (1.2 oz)	30
Puree	¼ cup (2.2 oz)	25
Puree Thick Style	¼ cup (2.2 oz)	20
Sauce	¼ cup (2.1 oz)	20
Whole Peeled	½ cup (4.2 oz)	25
Redpack		
Chunky Style In Puree	½ cup	30
Crushed In Puree	¼ cup	20
Paste	2 tbsp	0
Puree	¼ cup (2.2 oz)	25
Rienzi		
Paste	2 tbsp	25
Ro-Tel		
Diced In Sauce	½ cup	40
Mexican Festival	½ cup	30
Original	½ cup	20
Tuttorosso		
Puree	¼ cup	20

FOOD	PORTION	CALS
DRIED		
sun dried	1 cup	140
sun dried	1 piece	5
sun dried in oil	1 cup (4 oz)	235
sun dried in oil	1 piece (3 g)	6
Frieda's		
Red Chopped	⅓ cup (1.1 oz)	100
FRESH		
bruschetta	¼ cup	50
cooked	½ cup	32
grape tomatoes	20	30
green	1	30
red	1 (4.5 oz)	26
red chopped	1 cup	35
Chiquita		
Tomato	1 med (5.2 oz)	35
Eurofresh		
Tomatoes On The Vine	1 med (5.2 oz)	35
Frieda's		
Baby Roma	⅔ cup (3 oz)	120
Tear Drop	⅔ cup (3 oz)	20
TAKE-OUT		
bruschetta on toasted italian bread	1 slice	106
stewed	1 cup	80
TOMATO JUICE		
beef broth & tomato	1 can (5.5 oz)	62
clam & tomato	1 can (5½ oz)	77
tomato juice	6 oz	32
tomato juice	½ cup	21
Campbell's		
Juice	8 oz	50
Del Monte		
Juice	8 oz	50
Dole		
Juice	1 bottle (12 oz)	85
Hunt's		
Juice	1 can (6 oz)	22
No Salt Added	8 fl oz	34

FOOD	PORTION	CALS
Luvli Juices		
Smashing Tomato	1 bottle (10 oz)	125
Spicy Tomato	1 bottle (10 oz)	125
Mott's		
Tomato Juice	8 fl oz	40
Muir Glen		
Organic	5.5 oz	40
TONGUE		
beef simmered	3 oz	241
lamb braised	3 oz	234
pork braised	3 oz	230
TORTILLA		
corn	1 (6 in diam)	56
corn w/o salt	1 (6 in diam) .9 oz	56
flour w/o salt	1 (8 in diam) 1.2 oz	114
Alvarado Street Bakery		
Sprouted Wheat Burrito Size	1 (2.2 oz)	170
CarbOle		
Low-Carb	1 (2 oz)	100
Food For Life		
Sprouted Corn	2 (1.7 oz)	120
La Mexicana		
Corn	1 (0.8 oz)	50
Flour	1 (0.8 oz)	80
Tortillas de Trigo	1 (1 oz)	140
La Tortilla Factory		
Low Carb Whole Wheat	1 lg	100
Low Carb Whole Wheat	1 reg	60
Manny's		
Burrito Tortilla	1 (2.1 oz)	180
Fajita Tortilla	1 (2 oz)	170
Fat Free	1 (1 oz)	65
Low Carb	1 (1.7 oz)	140
Soft Taco Tortilla	1 (1 oz)	80
Tortilla Wrap Tomato Basil	1 (1.4 oz)	100
White Corn Gluten Free	1 (2 oz)	60
Whole Wheat	1 (2 oz)	170
Mariachi		
Tortilla	1	112

FOOD	PORTION	CALS
Old El Paso		
Flour	1 (1.4 oz)	130
Super Bakery		
Organic	1 (2.5 oz)	210
Tumaro's		
Low In Carb Garden Vegetable	1 (8 inch)	100
Low In Carb Green Onion	1 (8 inch)	100
Low In Carb Multi-grain	1 (8 inch)	100
Low In Carb Sour Cream & Salsa	1 (8 inch)	100

TORTILLA CHIPS (see CHIPS)

TRAIL MIX (see SNACKS)

TREE FERN

chopped cooked	½ cup	28

TRITICALE

dry	½ cup (3.4 oz)	323

TROUT

baked	3 oz	162
rainbow cooked	3 oz	129
seatrout baked	3 oz	113

TRUFFLES

fresh	0.5 oz	4

TUNA
CANNED

light in oil	3 oz	169
light in oil	1 can (6 oz)	399
light in water	3 oz	99
light in water	1 can (5.8 oz)	192
white in oil	1 can (6.2 oz)	331
white in oil	3 oz	158
white in water	1 can (6 oz)	234
white in water	3 oz	116
Bumble Bee		
Chunk Light In Water	2 oz	60
Chunk Light Touch Of Lemon In Water	¼ cup	60
Chunk Light In Oil	¼ cup	110
Chunk White In Water	¼ cup	60

FOOD	PORTION	CALS
Chunk White In Oil	¼ cup	100
Chunk White In Water Very Low Sodium	¼ cup	70
Light In Oil	¼ cup	110
Solid White In Oil	¼ cup	90
Solid White In Water	2 oz	70
Tonno In Olive Oil	¼ cup	120
Chicken Of The Sea		
Albacore In Spring Water	2 oz	80
Chunk Light In Water	¼ cup (2 oz)	60
Chunk Light In Oil	2 oz	110
Chunk White Low Sodium In Spring Water	1 can (3 oz)	80
Chunk White In Spring Water	½ can	60
Premium Albacore Pouch	2 oz	60
Coral		
Light In Water	¼ cup	60
Progresso		
In Olive Oil drained	¼ cup (2 oz)	160
StarKist		
Chunk Light In Water	¼ cup (2 oz)	60
Chunk Light No Drain Package	¼ cup (2 oz)	60
Low Sodium Chunk White In Water	2 oz	60
Solid White Albacore In Water	¼ cup	70
Tuna Fillet In Spring Water	¼ cup (2 oz)	60
FRESH		
bluefin cooked	3 oz	157
bluefin raw	3 oz	122
skipjack baked	3 oz	112
yellowfin baked	3 oz	118
MIX		
Chicken Of The Sea		
Salad Kit	1 serv (3.5 oz)	380
SHELF-STABLE		
Bumble Bee		
Steak Entrees Ginger & Soy	1 pkg (4 oz)	170
Steak Entrees Lemon & Cracked Pepper	1 pkg (4 oz)	160
Steak Entrees Mesquite Grilled	1 pkg (4 oz)	150

FOOD	PORTION	CALS
TUNA DISHES		
MIX		
Chicken Of The Sea		
Tuna Salad Kit Single Mayo & Onion	1 pkg	380
READY-TO-EAT		
StarKist		
Lunch To-Go	1 pkg	310
Ready-Mixed Tuna Salad Kit	1 pkg (3.5 oz)	190
Tuna Salad Lunch Kit	1 pkg (4.3 oz)	230
Wampler		
Salad	⅓ cup	180
Salad Chunky	⅓ cup	180
TAKE-OUT		
tuna salad	1 cup	383
tuna salad	3 oz	159
TURBOT		
european baked	3 oz	104
TURKEY (*see also* TURKEY DISHES, TURKEY SUBSTITUTES)		
CANNED		
w/ broth	1 can (5 oz)	231
w/ broth	½ can (2.5 oz)	116
FRESH		
back w/ skin roasted	½ back (9 oz)	637
breast w/ skin roasted	4 oz	212
dark meat w/ skin roasted	3.6 oz	230
dark meat w/o skin roasted	1 cup (5 oz)	262
dark meat w/o skin roasted	3 oz	170
ground cooked	3 oz	188
leg w/ skin roasted	2.5 oz	147
leg w/ skin roasted	1 (1.2 lbs)	1133
light meat w/ skin roasted	from ½ turkey (2.3 lbs)	2069
light meat w/ skin roasted	4.7 oz	268
light meat w/o skin roasted	4 oz	183
neck simmered	1 (5.3 oz)	274
skin roasted	from ½ turkey (9 oz)	1096
skin roasted	1 oz	141
w/ skin roasted	8.4 oz	498
w/ skin roasted	½ turkey (4 lbs)	3857

FOOD	PORTION	CALS
w/ skin neck & giblets roasted	½ turkey (8.8 lbs)	4123
w/o skin roasted	1 cup (5 oz)	238
w/o skin roasted	7.3 oz	354
wing w/ skin roasted	1 (6.5 oz)	426
Jennie-O		
Ground	4 oz	160
Perdue		
Breast Tenderloins Butter Garlic	3 oz	100
Burger Cooked	1 (4 oz)	160
Dark Cooked	3 oz	180
Drumsticks Cooked	1 (2.2 oz)	110
Ground Cooked	3 oz	160
Tenderloins Black Pepper Cooked	3 oz	90
Thighs Cooked	1 (3.2 oz)	240
White Cooked	3 oz	150
Shady Brook		
Cutlets	4 oz	110
Ground	4 oz	160
Ground Breast	4 oz	120
Tenderloin Rotisserie	4 oz	130
Turkey Store		
Lean Ground Italian Style	4 oz	190
Wampler		
Boneless Breast Roast	4 oz	160
Breast Half	4 oz	160
Breast Steaks	4 oz	120
Drumsticks	4 oz	180
Ground	4 oz	210
Ground Breast	4 oz	130
Ground Lean	4 oz	160
Thighs	4 oz	170
Wings	4 oz	220
Woodfire Grill Burger	1 (3 oz)	180
FROZEN		
roast boneless seasoned light & dark meat roasted	1 pkg (1.7 lbs)	1213
Wampler		
Burger BBQ	1 (4 oz)	240
Burgers Cracked Peppercorn & Garlic	1 (3 oz)	170

FOOD	PORTION	CALS
READY-TO-EAT		
bologna	1 slice (1 oz)	59
breast	1 slice (0.75 oz)	23
diced light & dark seasoned	1 oz	39
diced light & dark seasoned	½ lb	313
ham thigh meat	2 oz	73
ham thigh meat	1 pkg (8 oz)	291
pastrami	2 oz	80
pastrami	1 pkg (8 oz)	320
patties battered & fried	1 (3.3 oz)	266
patties breaded & fried	1 (2.3 oz)	181
prebasted breast w/ skin roasted	1 breast (3.8 lbs)	2175
prebasted breast w/ skin roasted	½ breast (1.9 lbs)	1087
prebasted thigh w/ skin roasted	1 thigh (11 oz)	494
roll light & dark meat	1 oz	42
roll light meat	1 oz	42
salami cooked beef	1 slice (0.9 oz)	67
turkey loaf breast meat	2 slices (1.5 oz)	47
turkey loaf breast meat	1 pkg (6 oz)	187
turkey salad sandwich spread	¼ cup	104
turkey sticks breaded & fried	1 stick (2.3 oz)	178
Alpine Lace		
Breast Fat Free	2 oz	45
Boar's Head		
Breast Cracked Pepper Smoked	2 oz	60
Breast Golden Skin On	2 oz	60
Breast Golden Skinless	2 oz	60
Breast Hickory Smoked	2 oz	70
Breast Low Sodium Skinless	2 oz	60
Breast Lower Sodium Skin On	2 oz	60
Breast Maple Glazed Honey Coat	2 oz	70
Breast Ovengold Skin On	2 oz	60
Breast Ovengold Skinless	2 oz	60
Breast Roasted Mesquite Smoked Skinless	2 oz	60
Breast Roasted Salsalito	2 oz	60
Pastrami Seasoned	2 oz	60

FOOD	PORTION	CALS
Carl Buddig		
Honey Roasted Turkey Breast	1 pkg (2.5 oz)	120
Lean Slices Honey Roasted Breast	1 pkg (2.5 oz)	70
Lean Slices Oven Roasted Breast	1 pkg (2.5 oz)	70
Lean Slices Smoked Breast	1 pkg (2.5 oz)	70
Oven Roasted Breast	1 pkg (2.5 oz)	110
Smoked Breast	1 pkg (2.5 oz)	110
Turkey Ham	1 pkg (2.5 oz)	100
Healthy Choice		
Smoked Breast	4 slices (1.8 oz)	60
Hebrew National		
98% Fat Free Oven Roasted	5 slices (2 oz)	50
98% Fat Free Smoked Breast	5 slices (2 oz)	60
Jennie-O		
Turkey Breast Golden Roast	3 oz	100
Jordan's		
Fat Free Turkey Breast	1 slice (1 oz)	25
Oscar Mayer		
Lunchables Turkey Bagels	1 pkg	420
Smoked Turkey Breast	2 oz	60
Smoked White	3 slices (3 oz)	90
Turkey Bologna	3 slices (3 oz)	160
Turkey Cotto Salami	3 slices (3 oz)	130
Perdue		
Breast Sliced Cajun Style	2 oz	50
Breast Sliced Honey Smoked	2 oz	50
Breast Sliced Pan Roasted	2 oz	70
Ham Hickory Smoked	2 oz	60
Healthsense Breast Sliced Oven Roasted	2 oz	60
Pastrami Hickory Smoked	2 oz	70
Shady Brook		
Meatballs Italian Style	3 (3 oz)	130
Wampler		
Bologna	2 oz	130
Dark Cured	2 oz	80
Deli Roast Breast	2 oz	50
Deli Roast Classic Spiced Breast	2 oz	70
Deli Roast Pan Roasted Breast	2 oz	70
Deli Roast Pan Roasted Skinless Breast	2 oz	50
Deli Roast Peppered Breast	2 oz	40

FOOD	PORTION	CALS
Deli Roast Rotisserie Breast	2 oz	50
Pastrami	2 oz	90
Salami	2 oz	90
Turkey Ham	2 oz	60

TURKEY DISHES
FROZEN

gravy & turkey	1 cup (8.4 oz)	160
gravy & turkey	1 pkg (5 oz)	95

Banquet

Homestyle Gravy & Sliced Turkey	2 slices + gravy	130
Sandwich Toppers Gravy & Sliced Turkey	1 pkg (5 oz)	160

READY-TO-EAT
Jennie-O

Stuffed Breast Cheddar Cheese & Broccoli	1 serv (6 oz)	240
Stuffed Turkey Breast Pepper Cheese & Rice	1 piece (6 oz)	250
Turkey Breast Roast In Homestyle Gravy	1 serv (5 oz)	110

Mosey's

Turkey Breast w/ Gravy	1 serv (5 oz)	140

Wampler

Turkey Ham Salad	⅓ cup	150

TAKE-OUT

boneless breast w/ cranberry apple stuffing	1 serv (5 oz)	260

TURKEY SUBSTITUTES
Lightlife

Smart Deli Roast Turkey	4 slices (2 oz)	80

Quorn

Roast	⅕ roast (3.2 oz)	90

Tofurkey

Deli Slices Hickory	1.5 oz	120
Deli Slices Original	1.5 oz	120
Deli Slices Peppered	1.5 oz	120
Drummettes	1 (3 oz)	105
Giblet Gravy	1 serv (3.5 oz)	42
Stuffed Tofu Roast	1 serv (4 oz)	193

Yves

Veggie Turkey Deli Slices	1 serv (2.2 oz)	85

FOOD	PORTION	CALS
TURMERIC		
ground	1 tsp	8
TURNIPS		
canned greens	½ cup	17
cooked mashed	½ cup (4.2 oz)	47
cubed cooked	½ cup (3 oz)	33
frzn greens cooked	½ cup	24
greens chopped cooked	½ cup	15
greens raw chopped	½ cup	7
raw cubed	½ cup (2.4 oz)	25
Birds Eye		
Greens w/ Diced Turnip	1 cup	25
TURTLE		
raw	3.5 oz	85
TUSK FISH		
raw	3.5 oz	79
VANILLA		
vanilla extract	1 tsp	17
Steel's		
Sugar Free	1 tbsp	24
Virginia Dare		
Extract	1 tsp	10
VEAL *(see also VEAL DISHES)*		
cutlet lean only braised	3 oz	172
cutlet lean only fried	3 oz	156
ground broiled	3 oz	146
loin chop w/ bone lean & fat braised	1 chop (2.8 oz)	227
loin chop w/ bone lean only braised	1 chop (2.4 oz)	155
shoulder w/ bone lean only braised	3 oz	169
sirloin w/ bone lean & fat roasted	3 oz	171
sirloin w/ bone lean only roasted	3 oz	143
VEAL DISHES		
TAKE-OUT		
parmigiana	4.2 oz	279
scallopini	1 serv (8 oz)	608

FOOD	PORTION	CALS
VEGETABLE JUICE		
vegetable juice cocktail	6 fl oz	34
vegetable juice cocktail	½ cup	22
Dole		
Vegetable Blend	1 bottle (12 oz)	90
Hunt's		
Cocktail	1 can (6 oz)	20
Muir Glen		
Organic	5.5 oz	50
V8		
Lemon Twist	1 bottle (12 oz)	70
Lightly Tangy	8 oz	58
Low Sodium	8 oz	53
Original	8 oz	51
Picante Vegetable	8 oz	51
Spicy Hot	8 oz	49
VEGETABLES MIXED		
CANNED		
mixed vegetables	½ cup	39
peas & carrots	½ cup	48
peas & carrots low sodium	½ cup	48
peas & onions	½ cup	30
succotash	½ cup	102
Chun King		
Chow Mein Vegetables	⅔ cup (3 oz)	14
Del Monte		
Mixed	½ cup	40
Mixed Vegetables w/ Potatoes	½ cup	45
Peas And Carrots	½ cup	60
Savory Sides Homestyle Vegetable Medley	½ cup	70
Savory Sides Rio Grande Vegetables	½ cup	70
La Choy		
Chop Suey Vegetables	½ cup (2.2 oz)	10
S&W		
Mixed	½ cup (4.4 oz)	35
Peas & Carrots	½ cup (4.5 oz)	60
Peas & Onions	½ cup (4.3 oz)	40
Veg-All		
Cajun Mixed	½ cup	50

FOOD	PORTION	CALS
FRESH		
River Ranch		
Broccoli & Carrots	1 cup	25
Broccoli & Cauliflower	1 cup	25
Stir Fry Blend	1 cup	30
Vegetable Medley	1 cup	25
FROZEN		
mixed vegetables cooked	½ cup	54
peas & carrots cooked	½ cup	38
peas & onions cooked	½ cup	40
succotash cooked	½ cup	79
Birds Eye		
Baby Pea & Vegetable Blend	¾ cup	40
Baby Sweet Peas & Pearl Onions	⅔ cup	60
Broccoli Cauliflower & Carrots	½ cup	25
Broccoli Cauliflower & Carrots In Cheese Sauce	½ cup	70
Broccoli Cauliflower & Red Peppers	½ cup	20
Broccoli & Cauliflower	½ cup	20
Broccoli Carrots & Water Chestnuts	½ cup	30
Broccoli Corn & Red Peppers	½ cup	50
Broccoli Red Peppers Onions & Mushrooms	½ cup	25
Brussels Sprouts Cauliflower & Carrots	½ cup	30
California Style Vegetables	½ cup	100
Cauliflower Nuggets Corn Carrots & Snow Pea Pods	½ cup	30
Gumbo Blend	¾ cup	40
Italian Style Vegetables & Bow Tie Pasta	1 cup	150
Mixed Vegetables	⅓ cup	50
New England Style Vegetables & Pasta Shells	1 pkg (9 oz)	260
Oriental Style Vegetables	½ cup	60
Peas & Pearl Onions	⅔ cup	90
Peas & Potatoes In Real Cream Sauce	½ cup	90
Radiatore Pasta & Vegetables	1 cup	200
Roasted Potatoes & Broccoli	⅔ cup (3.9 oz)	100
Roletti Pasta & Vegetables	1 cup (4.4 oz)	190
Simply Grillin' Garden Herb	1 cup	140
Stir Fry Asparagus	2 cups	90
Stir Fry Broccoli	1 cup	30
Stir Fry Pepper	1 cup	25
Stir Fry Sugar Snap	¾ cup	35

FOOD	PORTION	CALS
Stir Fry Whole Green Bean	1¾ cup	100
Szechuan Vegetables In A Sesame Sauce	1 cup	60
Vegetables For Soup	⅔ cup	45
Vegetables For Stew	⅔ cup	40
Voila! Italian Pesto Chicken	2 cups	240
Voila! Three Cheese Chicken	1¾ cups	220
Fresh Like		
California Blend	3.5 oz	31
Midwestern Blend	3.5 oz	42
Mixed	3.5 oz	69
Oriental Blend	3.5 oz	26
Winter Blend	3.5 oz	26
Green Giant		
Alfredo Vegetables	¾ cup	70
Cheese Sauce Broccoli Cauliflower Carrots	1 cup (4.1 oz)	60
Seasoned Broccoli & Carrots w/ Garlic & Herbs	½ cup	45
Health Is Wealth		
Veggie Munchees	2 (1 oz)	50
La Choy		
Fancy Chinese Mixed Vegetables	½ cup (2.9 oz)	9
Lean Cuisine		
Cafe Classics Roasted Potatoes w/ Broccoli & Cheddar Cheese Sauce	1 pkg (10.25 oz)	230
McKenzie's		
Gumbo Mixture	1 serv (2.9 oz)	35
Pictsweet		
Peas & Carrots	⅔ cup	50
Tree Of Life		
Mixed	½ cup (3 oz)	65
SHELF-STABLE		
TastyBite		
Curry Bangkok Red	½ pkg (5.3 oz)	88
Curry Patong Yellow	½ pkg (5.3 oz)	118
Curry Siam Green	½ pkg (5.3 oz)	63
Jaipur Vegetables	½ pkg (5 oz)	220
Malabar Mixed	½ pkg (5 oz)	67
TAKE-OUT		
buddha's delight	1 serv (16 oz)	174
caponata	¼ cup	28
curry	1 serv (7.7 oz)	398

FOOD	PORTION	CALS
gyoza potstickers vegetable	8 (4.9 oz)	210
pakoras	1 (2 oz)	108
ratatouille	1 serv (3.5 oz)	96
samosa	2 (4 oz)	170
succotash	½ cup	111
tapenade grilled vegetables	¼ cup	40

VENISON
roasted	4 oz	215

VINEGAR
balsamic of modena	1 tbsp (0.5 oz)	10
cider	1 tbsp	tr
Eden		
Organic Brown Rice	1 tbsp	2
Ume Plum	1 tsp	2
Heinz		
White	2 tbsp	2
Progresso		
Balsamic	2 tbsp (0.5 oz)	10
Regina		
Red Wine	1 tbsp	0
Spectrum		
Apple Cider Organic	1 tbsp	7
Balsamic Organic	1 tbsp	6
Brown Rice Organic	1 tbsp	10
Golden Balsamic Organic	1 tbsp	6
Red Wine Organic	1 tbsp	0
White Organic	1 tbsp	2
White Wine Organic	1 tbsp	0
Wild Thyme Farms		
Balsamic Red Raspberry	1 tbsp	13

WAFFLES
FROZEN
buttermilk	1 4 in sq (1.2 oz)	88
plain	1 4 in sq (1.2 oz)	88
EnviroKidz		
Organic Gorilla Banana	2 (2.7 oz)	230
Kid Cuisine		
Wave Rider Waffle Sticks	1 meal (6.6 oz)	380

FOOD	PORTION	CALS
MIX		
plain as prep	1 7 in diam (2.6 oz)	218
READY-TO-EAT		
Gol D Lite		
Low Carb Belgian	1 (0.9 oz)	100
Low Carb Belgian Chocolate Covered	1 (l.1 oz)	130
Kashi		
GoLean Blueberry	2	170
GoLean Original	2	170
Thomas'		
Buttermilk	1 (1.6 oz)	130
Homestyle	1 (1.6 oz)	140
TAKE-OUT		
plain	1 (7 in diam)	218
WALNUTS		
black dried chopped	1 cup	759
english dried	1 oz	182
english dried chopped	1 cup	770
halves	14 (1 oz)	190
Sweet Delights		
Walnut Roasters	⅓ pkg (1 oz)	210
WASABI (see HORSERADISH)		
WATER		
ice cubes	3	0
tap water	8 oz	0
Absopure		
Natural Spring	8 fl oz	0
Aquafina		
Essentials B-Power Wild Berry	8 fl oz	40
Essentials Calcium + Tangerine Pineapple	8 fl oz	40
Essentials Daily C Citrus	8 fl oz	40
Essentials Multi-V Watermelon	8 fl oz	40
Water	8 fl oz	0
Aquess		
Purified Water w/ Soluble Fiber	1 bottle (18 oz)	30
Base Energy + Water		
All Flavors	8 oz	28

FOOD	PORTION	CALS
Blu Italy		
Sparkling Lemon	8 oz	0
Calabria		
Mineral	8 oz	0
Castellina		
Sparkling Spring	8 fl oz	0
Clearly Canadian		
Sparkling All Flavors	8 oz	45
Crystal Geyser		
Spring Water	8 fl oz	0
Dasani		
Purfied Water	8 oz	0
w/ Lemon	8 oz	2
w/ Raspberry	8 oz	1
Evamor		
Artesian Water	8 fl oz	0
Evian		
Spring Water	1 bottle (11.5 oz)	0
Ferrarelle		
Sparkling	8 fl oz	0
Fiji		
Natural Artesian	1 bottle (16.9 oz)	0
FlavH20		
All Flavors	1 can (12.3 oz)	80
Gerolsteiner		
Sparkling Mineral	8 fl oz	0
Glaceau Vitamin Water		
Balance Cran Grapefruit	8 oz	50
Defense	8 oz	50
Endurance Peach Mango	8 oz	50
Energy Tropical Citrus	8 oz	40
Essential Orange Orange	8 oz	40
Focus Kiwi Strawberry	8 oz	40
Formula 50	8 oz	50
Multi-V Lemonade	8 oz	40
Perform Lemon Lime	8 oz	50
Power-C Dragonfruit	8 oz	40
Rescue Green Tea	8 oz	40
Revive Fruit Punch	8 oz	50
Stress-B Lemon Lime	8 oz	40

FOOD	PORTION	CALS
Hansen's		
Energy Water Lemon	8 oz	10
Hint		
Flavored Water All Flavors	1 bottle (15 oz)	0
Iceland Spring		
Spring Water	1 liter	0
Meridian		
Clear All Flavors	8 oz	100
Metromint		
Peppermint Water	8 oz	0
Multi Vitamin Enhanced Water		
All Flavors	8 oz	50
No Carb All Flavors	8 oz	0
O Waters		
All Flavors	8 oz	0
Paradiso		
Slightly Sparkling	8 oz	0
Pellegrino		
Mineral Water	8 oz	0
Pink2O		
Fortified	1 bottle (20 oz)	0
Propel		
Fitness Water All Flavors	8 oz	10
Rapid		
Hydra-Cell Water	1 bottle (16.9 oz)	0
Reebok		
Fitness Water Berry	1 bottle (24 oz)	30
Fitness Water Natural	1 bottle (24 oz)	0
Replenish		
Elements Enhanced Water Orange	8 oz	40
San Benedetto		
Natural Mineral Water	1 liter	0
Sanfaustino		
Mineral	8 oz	0
Saratoga		
Spring	8 oz	0
Spa		
Mineral Water Reine	1 bottle (17.5 oz)	0
Speedo Sportswater		
All Flavors	8 oz	10

FOOD	PORTION	CALS
Stacker 2		
Protein Water All Flavors	1 bottle (19.44 oz)	80
Sulinka		
Sparkling Mineral	8 oz	0
Tao Tea		
Lychee Water	8 oz	67
Thorpedo		
Ultra Low GI Energy Water	8 oz	45
Trinity		
Energize	8 oz	50
Multi-Esstential	8 oz	50
Revive	8 oz	50
Strength	8 oz	50
Think	8 oz	50
Ty Nant		
Mineral Water	1 liter	0
Vasa		
Natural Spring	8 oz	0
Veryfine		
Fruit 2 O Lemon	8 oz	0
Fruit 2 O Lemon Lime	8 oz	0
Fruit 2 O Orange	8 oz	0
Fruit 2 O Raspberry	8 oz	0
VitaZest		
All Flavors	8 oz	0
Vittel		
Mineral Water	1 bottle (18 oz)	0
Volvic		
Spring Water	8 oz	0
Voss		
Artesian	8 oz	0
W20 For Women		
All Flavors	8 oz	40
Water+		
Energy Fruit Punch	8 oz	45
Fitness + Lemon	8 oz	45
Focus Mixed Berry	8 oz	45
Lean Peach	8 oz	40
Recovery Strawberry Kiwi	8 oz	45
Ultra C Orange	8 oz	45

FOOD	PORTION	CALS
WATER CHESTNUTS		
chinese sliced canned	½ cup	35
fresh sliced	½ cup	66
Chun King		
Sliced	2 tbsp (0.8 oz)	11
Whole	2 (0.7 oz)	10
La Choy		
Chopped	2 tbsp (0.6 oz)	9
Sliced	2 tbsp (0.8 oz)	11
Whole	2 (0.7 oz)	10
WATERCRESS		
fresh chopped	½ cup	2
garden fresh	½ cup	8
garden fresh cooked	½ cup	16
Frieda's		
Watercress	1 cup	10
WATERMELON		
cut up	1 cup	50
seeds dried	1 cup	602
seeds dried	1 oz	158
wedge	1/16	152
Dulcinea		
Fresh Mini Seedless	2 cups	88
Frieda's		
Yellow Seedless	½ cup (3 oz)	25
Sundia		
Fresh	2 cups	80
WATERMELON JUICE		
Snapple		
What-A-Melon	8 oz	90
Squeezit		
Watermelon	1 bottle (7 oz)	110
Sundia		
100% Natural	8 oz	110
WAX BEANS		
CANNED		
Del Monte		
Wax Beans	½ cup	20

FOOD	PORTION	CALS
S&W		
Cut	½ cup (4.2 oz)	20
WHALE		
raw	3.5 oz	134
WHEAT		
sprouted	1 cup (3.8 oz)	214
starch	3.5 oz	348
Bob's Red Mill		
Vital Wheat Gluten	¼ cup	120
Near East		
Pilaf Mix Wheat as prep	1 cup	220
Taboule Salad Mix as prep	⅔ cup	110
NOW		
Wheat Gluten Flour	¼ cup	125
WHEAT GERM		
plain toasted	¼ cup (1 oz)	108
plain toasted	1 cup	431
w/ brown sugar & honey toasted	1 cup	426
w/ brown sugar & honey toasted	1 oz	107
Hodgson Mill		
Untoasted	2 tbsp	55
Kretschmer		
Original Toasted	2 tbsp (0.5 oz)	50
Mother's		
Toasted	2 tbsp	50
WHEY		
acid dry	1 tbsp (3 g)	10
acid fluid	1 cup (8 fl oz)	59
sweet dry	1 tbsp (8 g)	26
sweet fluid	1 cup (8 fl oz)	66
whey cheese	1 oz	126
WHIPPED TOPPINGS		
cream pressurized	1 tbsp (3 g)	8
cream pressurized	1 cup (2.1 oz)	154
nondairy frzn	1 tbsp	13
nondairy powdered as prep w/ whole milk	1 cup	151
nondairy powdered as prep w/ whole milk	1 tbsp (4 g)	8

FOOD	PORTION	CALS
nondairy pressurized	1 tbsp (4 g)	11
nondairy pressurized	1 cup	184
Cabot		
Whipped Cream	2 tbsp	30
Estee		
Whipped Topping as prep	1 serv	10
Reddiwip		
Chocolate	2 tbsp	15
Extra Creamy	2 tbsp	15
Fat Free	2 tbsp	5
Original	2 tbsp	15
WHITE BEANS		
canned	1 cup	306
dried regular cooked	1 cup	249
dried small cooked	1 cup	253
Progresso		
Cannellini	½ cup (4.6 oz)	100
WHITEFISH		
baked	3 oz	146
smoked	3 oz	92
smoked	1 oz	39
WHITING		
cooked	3 oz	98
hake raw	3.5 oz	84
raw	3 oz	77
WILD RICE		
cooked	1 cup (5.7 oz)	166
Gourmet House		
Cracked not prep	¼ cup	170
Hand Harvested not prep	¼ cup	170
Quick Cooking not prep	½ cup	170
White & Wild not prep	¼ cup	170
Wild & Rice Garden Blend no prep	¼ cup	190
WINE		
beaujolais	4 oz	95
bordeaux red	4 oz	95
chianti	4 oz	101

FOOD	PORTION	CALS
cooking	1 oz	15
dessert dry	1 glass (4 oz)	179
haiku	1 serv	93
japanese plum	3 oz	139
japanese sake	1 oz	33
kir	1 serv	78
liebfraumilch	4 oz	86
madeira	3.5 oz	169
marsala	4 oz	80
merlot	4 oz	95
muscatel	4 oz	160
port	3.5 oz	156
red	1 glass (4 oz)	85
rose	1 glass (4 oz)	84
sake screwdriver	1 serv	175
sangria	1 serv	88
sangria blanco	1 serv	155
sherry	2 oz	84
sweet dessert	1 glass (4 oz)	189
vermouth dry	3.5 oz	105
vermouth sweet	3.5 oz	167
wassail wine	1 serv	142
white	1 glass (4 oz)	80
wine cooler	1 serv	218
wine spritzer	1 serv	60
Boone's		
Country Kwencher	4 fl oz	96
Delicious Apple	4 fl oz	84
Sangria	4 fl oz	88
Snow Creek Berry	4 fl oz	72
Strawberry Hill	4 fl oz	88
Sun Peak Peach	4 fl oz	72
Wild Island	4 fl oz	72
Carlo Rossi		
Blush	4 fl oz	84
Burgundy	4 fl oz	88
Chablis	4 fl oz	84
Paisano	4 fl oz	92
Red Sangria	4 fl oz	92
Rhine	4 fl oz	84

FOOD	PORTION	CALS
Vin Rosé	4 fl oz	84
White Grenache	4 fl oz	80
Eden		
Mirin Rice Cooking Wine	1 tbsp	25
Fairbanks		
Port	4 fl oz	176
Sherry	4 fl oz	136
White Port	4 fl oz	136
Gallo		
Blush Chablis	4 fl oz	88
Burgundy	4 fl oz	88
Cabernet Sauvignon	4 fl oz	88
Chablis Blanc	4 fl oz	80
Chardonnay	4 fl oz	92
Classic Burgundy	4 fl oz	84
French Colombard	4 fl oz	84
Hearty Burgundy	4 fl oz	88
Pink Chablis	4 fl oz	80
Red Rosé	4 fl oz	92
Rhine	4 fl oz	88
Sheffield Cellars		
Sherry	4 fl oz	136
Tawny Port	4 fl oz	180
Vermouth Extra Dry	1 fl oz	28
Vermouth Sweet	1 fl oz	43
Very Dry Sherry	4 fl oz	128

WINGED BEANS
dried cooked	1 cup	252

WRAPS (see BREAD)

XANTHAN GUM
Bob's Red Mill
Xanthan Gum	1 tbsp	8

YAM (see also SWEET POTATO)
CANNED
Bruce
In Syrup	⅔ cup	150

S&W
Candied	½ cup (4.9 oz)	170

FOOD	PORTION	CALS
FRESH		
mountain yam hawaii cooked	½ cup	59
yam cubed cooked	½ cup	79
Frieda's		
Name	¾ cup	100
YARDLONG BEANS		
dried cooked	1 cup	202
YAUTIA *(see MALANGA)*		
YEAST		
baker's compressed	1 cake (0.6 oz)	18
baker's dry	1 pkg (¼ oz)	21
baker's dry	1 tbsp	35
brewer's dry	1 tbsp	25
Fleischmann's		
Active Dry	1 pkg (7 g)	23
Bread Machine	1 pkg (7 g)	26
RapidRise	1 pkg (7 g)	26
Hodgson Mill		
Fast Rise	1 tsp (9 g)	25
YELLOW BEANS		
canned low sodium	½ cup	14
dried cooked w/o salt	½ cup	127
fresh cooked w/o salt	½ cup	22
fresh raw	½ cup	17
frozen cooked	½ cup	20
snap canned	½ cup	1813
YELLOWTAIL		
baked	3 oz	159
YOGURT *(see also YOGURT DRINKS, YOGURT FROZEN)*		
coffee lowfat	8 oz	194
fruit lowfat	8 oz	225
fruit lowfat	4 oz	113
plain	8 oz	139
plain lowfat	8 oz	144
plain no fat	8 oz	127
vanilla lowfat	8 oz	194

FOOD	PORTION	CALS
Axelrod		
Fat Free Lemon	1 pkg (6 oz)	90
Fat Free Raspberry	6 oz	90
Fat Free Vanilla	1 pkg (6 oz)	90
Breyers		
Vanilla 98% Fat Free	½ cup	90
Cabot		
Non Fat	8 oz	100
Non Fat Berry Banana	8 oz	130
Non Fat Blueberry	8 oz	130
Non Fat French Vanilla	8 oz	130
Non Fat Lemon	8 oz	130
Non Fat Raspberry	8 oz	130
Non Fat Very Berry	8 oz	130
Colombo		
Fat Free Plain	8 oz	100
Fat Free Vanilla	8 oz	160
French Vanilla	8 oz	180
Fruit On The Bottom Strawberry Banana	8 oz	230
Lowfat Plain	8 oz	130
Multipack Blended All Flavors	4 oz	110
Strawberry	8 oz	190
Dannon		
Chunky Fruit Nonfat Apple Cinnamon	6 oz	160
Chunky Fruit Nonfat Blueberry	6 oz	160
Chunky Fruit Nonfat Cherry Vanilla	6 oz	160
Chunky Fruit Nonfat Peach	6 oz	160
Chunky Fruit Nonfat Strawberry	6 oz	160
Chunky Fruit Nonfat Strawberry Banana	6 oz	160
Creamy Fruit Blends Raspberry	6 oz	170
Danimals Lowfat Blueberry	4.4 oz	130
Danimals Lowfat Grape Lemonade	4.4 oz	120
Danimals Lowfat Lemon Ice	4.4 oz	120
Danimals Lowfat Orange Banana	4.4 oz	130
Danimals Lowfat Strawberry	4.4 oz	130
Danimals Lowfat Tropical Punch	4.4 oz	130
Danimals Lowfat Vanilla	4.4 oz	120
Danimals Lowfat Wild Raspberry	4.4 oz	120
Double Delights Banana Creme Strawberry	6 oz	160
Double Delights Bavarian Creme Raspberry	6 oz	170

FOOD	PORTION	CALS
Double Delights Cheesecake Cherry	6 oz	170
Double Delights Cheesecake Strawberry	6 oz	170
Double Delights Chocolate Cheesecake	6 oz	220
Double Delights Chocolate Dipped Strawberry	6 oz	210
Double Delights Chocolate Eclair	6 oz	220
Double Delights Vanilla Strawberry	6 oz	170
Double Delights Vanilla Peach & Apricot	6 oz	170
Fruit On The Bottom Lowfat Apple Cinnamon	8 oz	240
Fruit On The Bottom Lowfat Blueberry	8 oz	240
Fruit On The Bottom Lowfat Boysenberry	8 oz	240
Fruit On The Bottom Lowfat Cherry	8 oz	240
Fruit On The Bottom Lowfat Minipack Mixed Berry	4.4 oz	130
Fruit On The Bottom Lowfat Minipack Strawberry	4.4 oz	130
Fruit On The Bottom Lowfat Mixed Berries	8 oz	240
Fruit On The Bottom Lowfat Orange	8 oz	240
Fruit On The Bottom Lowfat Peach	8 oz	240
Fruit On The Bottom Lowfat Strawberry	8 oz	240
Fruit On The Bottom Lowfat Strawberry Banana	8 oz	240
La Creme Strawberry	1 pkg (4 oz)	140
La Creme Vanilla	1 pkg (4 oz)	140
Light Duets Cherry Cheesecake	6 oz	90
Light Duets Raspberry Royale	6 oz	90
Light Duets Strawberry Cheesecake	6 oz	90
Light 'N Crunchy Mint Chocolate Chip	8 oz	140
Light 'N Crunchy Nonfat Caramel Apple Crunch	8 oz	140
Light 'N Crunchy Nonfat Lemon Blueberry Cobbler	8 oz	140
Light 'N Crunchy Nonfat Mocha Cappuccino	8 oz	140
Light 'N Crunchy Nonfat Raspberry w/ Granola	8 oz	140
Light 'N Crunchy Nonfat Vanilla Chocolate Crunch	8 oz	130
Light 'N Fit Vanilla	6 oz	90
Light Nonfat Banana Cream Pie	8 oz	100
Light Nonfat Blueberry	8 oz	100
Light Nonfat Cappuccino	8 oz	100

FOOD	PORTION	CALS
Light Nonfat Cherry Vanilla	8 oz	100
Light Nonfat Coconut Cream Pie	8 oz	100
Light Nonfat Creme Caramel	8 oz	100
Light Nonfat Lemon Chiffon	8 oz	100
Light Nonfat Mint Chocolate Cream Pie	8 oz	100
Light Nonfat Peach	8 oz	100
Light Nonfat Raspberry	8 oz	100
Light Nonfat Strawberry	8 oz	100
Light Nonfat Strawberry Banana	8 oz	100
Light Nonfat Strawberry Kiwi	8 oz	100
Light Nonfat Tangerine Chiffon	8 oz	100
Light 'N Fit w/ Fiber Blueberry	4 oz	70
Lowfat Coffee	8 oz	210
Lowfat Cranberry Raspberry	8 oz	210
Lowfat Lemon	8 oz	210
Lowfat Vanilla	8 oz	210
Minipack Blended Nonfat Blueberry	4.4 oz	120
Minipack Blended Nonfat Cherry	4.4 oz	110
Minipack Blended Nonfat Peach	4.4 oz	120
Minipack Blended Nonfat Raspberry	4.4 oz	120
Minipack Blended Nonfat Strawberry	4.4 oz	120
Minipack Blended Nonfat Strawberry Banana	4.4 oz	120
Sprinkl'ins Cherry Vanilla	1 (4.1 oz)	130
Sprinkl'ins Strawberry	1 (4.1 oz)	130
Sprinkl'ins Strawberry Banana	1 (4.1 oz)	130
Sprinkl'ins Vanilla w/ Cherry Crystals	1 (4.1 oz)	110
Sprinkl'ins Vanilla w/ Orange Crystals	1 (4.1 oz)	110
Fage		
Sheep & Goat's Milk	1 pkg (7 oz)	190
Horizon Organic		
Fat Free Apricot Mango	¾ cup (6 oz)	120
Fat Free Honey	1 cup (8 oz)	160
LeCarb		
YoCarb Plain	1 pkg (4 oz)	50
Oberweis		
Peach	1 pkg (8 oz)	210
Pascual		
Nonfat Cherries & Berries	1 pkg (4.4 oz)	100
Nonfat Peach	1 pkg (4.4 oz)	100

FOOD	PORTION	CALS
Silk		
Organic Soy Strawberry	1 pkg (6 oz)	160
Soy Apricot Mango	1 pkg	160
Soy Banana Strawberry	1 pkg	160
Soy Black Cherry	1 pkg	160
Soy Blueberry	1 pkg	160
Soy Key Lime	1 pkg	170
Soy Lemon	1 pkg	160
Soy Lemon Kiwi	1 pkg	150
Soy Peach	1 pkg	170
Soy Plain	8 oz	120
Soy Raspberry	1 pkg	160
Soy Vanilla	1 pkg (8 oz)	120
Spega		
La Natura Low Fat	1 pkg (5.2 oz)	80
Stonyfield Farm		
Kids' Lowfat BaNilla	1 pkg (4 oz)	110
Light Black Cherry	1 pkg (6 oz)	100
Light Blueberry	1 pkg (4 oz)	100
Light Peach	1 pkg (6 oz)	100
Light Strawberry	1 pkg (4 oz)	100
Nonfat French Vanilla	1 pkg	90
Nonfat Strawberry	1 pkg	140
O'Soy Chocolate	1 pkg (6 oz)	160
O'Soy Peach	1 pkg (4 oz)	100
Squeezers Lowfat Strawberry	1 tube (2 oz)	60
Whole Milk French Vanilla	1 pkg (6 oz)	190
Total		
Greek Yogurt 0% Fat	1 pkg (5.3 oz)	80
Greek Yogurt 2% Fat	1 pkg (7 oz)	130
Greek Yogurt Classic	1 pkg (7 oz)	180
Greek Yogurt Light	1 pkg (5.3 oz)	130
Honey	1 pkg (3.5 oz)	250
WholeSoy & Co.		
Organic Soy Apricot Mango	1 pkg (6 oz)	160
Organic Soy Lemon	1 pkg (6 oz)	160
Organic Soy Plain	1 pkg (6 oz)	150
Organic Soy Raspberry	1 pkg (6 oz)	170
Organic Soy Vanilla	1 pkg (6 oz)	150

FOOD	PORTION	CALS
Yoplait		
Healthy Heart All Flavors	1 pkg (6 oz)	180
Whips! Orange Creme	1 pkg (4 oz)	140

YOGURT DRINKS (see also SMOOTHIES)

FOOD	PORTION	CALS
Dannon		
DanActive	1 bottle (3.5 oz)	90
Frusion Smoothie Peach Passion Fruit	1 bottle (10 oz)	270
Frusion Smoothie Tropical Fruit	1 bottle (10 oz)	270
Stonyfield		
Smoothie Lowfat Strawberry	1 bottle (10 oz)	250
Stonyfield Farm		
Kids' Juice Smoothie Orange Strawberry Banana Wave	1 bottle (6 oz)	160
Smoothie Light Strawberry	1 bottle (10 oz)	130
Yo-Goat		
Blueberry	8 oz	150
Yoplait		
Nouriche All Flavors	1 bottle (11 oz)	290

YOGURT FROZEN

FOOD	PORTION	CALS
chocolate soft serve	½ cup (4 fl oz)	115
vanilla soft serve	½ cup (4 fl oz)	114
Breyers		
Chocolate	½ cup	150
Vanilla	½ cup	140
Vanilla No Sugar Added	½ cup	100
Dannon		
Light'N Fit w/ Fiber Strawberry	4 oz	70
Edy's		
Black Cherry Vanilla Swirl	½ cup	90
Caramel Praline Crunch	½ cup	100
Chocolate	½ cup	90
Strawberry	½ cup	100
Vanilla	½ cup	90
Vanilla Chocolate Swirl	½ cup	90
Haagen-Dazs		
Lowfat Dulce De Leche	½ cup	190
Nonfat Chocolate	½ cup	140
Nonfat Coffee	½ cup	140
Nonfat Strawberry	½ cup	140

FOOD	PORTION	CALS
Nonfat Vanilla	½ cup	140
Nonfat Vanilla Raspberry Swirl	½ cup	130
Nonfat Vanilla Fudge	½ cup	160
Turkey Hill		
Black Raspberry	½ cup	110
Caramel Cashew Crunch	½ cup	160
Chocolate Chip Cookie Dough	½ cup	140
Clark Bar	½ cup	140
Fat Free Chocolate Cherry Cordial	½ cup	100
Fat Free Chocolate Marshmallow	½ cup	130
Fat Free Mint Cookie 'N Cream	½ cup	110
Fat Free Neapolitan	½ cup	100
Fat Free Orange Swirl	½ cup	100
Fat Free Vanilla Fudge	½ cup	110
Peach Raspberry	½ cup	110
Tin Roof Sundae	½ cup	140
Vanilla & Chocolate	½ cup	110
Vanilla Bean	½ cup	110
WholeSoy & Co.		
Organic All Flavors	½ cup	120
ZUCCHINI		
baby raw	1 (0.5 oz)	3
canned italian style	½ cup	33
frzn cooked	½ cup	19
raw sliced	½ cup	9
sliced cooked	½ cup	14
Frieda's		
Baby	⅔ cup (3 oz)	20
Progresso		
Italian Style	½ cup (4.2 oz)	50
TAKE-OUT		
indian paalkora	1 serv	46

PART TWO

Restaurant Chains

> *The larger the portion size you are served, and the more variety you are offered, the more likely you are to over-eat. Go easy on super-sizes and choose wisely at buffets.*

FOOD	PORTION	CALS
A&W		
BEVERAGES		
Coke	1 sm (11 oz)	145
Diet Coke	1 sm (11 oz)	0
Diet Root Beer	1 sm (15 oz)	0
Diet Root Beer Float	1 sm (14.4 oz)	170
Root Beer Float	1 sm (14.4 oz)	330
Root Beer	1 sm (15 oz)	220
MAIN MENU SELECTIONS		
Cheese Curds	1 serv	570
Cheese Dog	1	320
Cheeseburger	1	470
Cheeseburger Deluxe	1	510
Cheeseburger Deluxe Bacon	1	570
Cheeseburger Deluxe Bacon Double	1	800
Cheeseburger Deluxe Double	1	720
Coney Chili Dog	1	310
Coney Chili Dog Cheese	1	350
Fries	1 lg	430
Fries Cheese	1 serv	380
Fries Chili	1 serv	370
Fries Chili & Cheese	1 serv	400
Fries Kids	1 serv	310
Hamburger	1	430
Hamburger Deluxe	1	460
Hot Dog Plain	1	280
Onion Rings	1 serv	350
Sandwich Crispy Chicken	1	580
Sandwich Grilled Chicken	1	430
Sauce BBQ	1 serv (1 oz)	40
Sauce Honey Mustard	1 serv (1 oz)	100
Sauce Ranch	1 serv (1 oz)	160
Sauce Sweet & Sour	1 serv (1 oz)	45
APPLEBEE'S		
DESSERTS		
Apple Betty Cobbler Ala Mode	1 serv	598
Berry Lemon Cheesecake	1 slice	230
Chocolate Raspberry Cake	1 slice	230
Fudge Brownie Sundae	1 serv	739

FOOD	PORTION	CALS
Low Fat Bikini Banana Strawberry Shortcake	1 serv	248
Low Fat Brownie Sundae	1 serv	415
Low Fat Marble Cheesecake	1 serv	261
MAIN MENU SELECTIONS		
Applebee's Burger w/ Fries	1 serv	1274
Baja Chicken Rollup	1 serv	490
Basic Hamburger w/ Fries	1 serv	980
Beef Fajita Quesadilla	1 serv	1205
Bourbon Street Steak w/ Fried New Potatoes	1 serv	1115
Grilled Citrus Chicken Salad	1 serv	240
Grilled Talapia w/ Mango Salsa	1 serv	340
Low Fat Asian Chicken Salad	1 serv (5 oz)	623
Low Fat Asian Chicken Salad	1 med serv (2.5 oz)	370
Low Fat Blacked Chicken Salad	1 serv (5 oz)	411
Low Fat Blacked Chicken Salad	1 med serv (2.5 oz)	287
Low Fat Garlic Chicken Pasta	1 serv	587
Low Fat Lemon Chicken Pasta	1 serv	528
Low Fat Quesadilla Chicken Fajita	1 serv	518
Low Fat Quesadilla Veggie	1 serv	344
Mesquite Chicken Salad	1 serv	200
Mozzarella Stix	8 pieces	963
Onion Soup Au Gratin	1 serv	150
Quesadillas	1 serv	684
Riblet Basket w/ Fries	1 serv	1317
Salad Dinner w/o Dressing	1 serv	303
Salad Santa Fe Chicken	1 med	724
Sandwich Bacon Cheese Chicken Grill w/o Fries	1	746
Sandwich Gyro	1	880
Sizzling Chicken Skillet	1 serv	360
Stir Fry Chicken	1 serv	566
Teriyaki Shrimp Skewers	1 serv	260
Tortilla Chicken Melt	1 serv	480
ARBY'S		
BEVERAGES		
Chocolate Shake	1 (14 oz)	480
Hot Chocolate	1 serv (8.6 oz)	110
Jamocha Shake	1 (14 oz)	470
Milk	1 serv (8 oz)	120
Orange Juice	1 serv (10 oz)	140

FOOD	PORTION	CALS
Strawberry Shake	1 (14 oz)	500
Vanilla Shake	1 (14 oz)	470
BREAKFAST SELECTIONS		
Add Egg	1 serv (2 oz)	110
Add Swiss Cheese Slice	1 slice (0.5 oz)	45
Biscuit w/ Bacon	1 (3.2 oz)	320
Biscuit w/ Butter	1 (2.9 oz)	280
Biscuit w/ Ham	1 (4.3 oz)	330
Biscuit w/ Sausage	1 (4.2)	460
Croissant w/ Bacon	1 (2.5 oz)	300
Croissant w/ Ham	1 (3.7 oz)	310
Croissant w/ Sausage	1 (3.6 oz)	420
French Toast Syrup	1 serv (0.5 oz)	130
Sourdough w/ Bacon	1 (5 oz)	380
Sourdough w/ Ham	1 (4 oz)	220
Sourdough w/ Sausage	1 (4 oz)	330
Toastix w/o Syrup	1 serv (4.4 oz)	370
DESSERTS		
Apple Turnover Iced	1 (4.5 oz)	420
Cherry Turnover Iced	1 (4.5 oz)	410
MAIN MENU SELECTIONS		
Arby's Sauce	1 serv (0.5 oz)	15
Au Jus Sauce	1 serv (3 oz)	5
Baked Potato Broccoli'N Cheddar	1 (14 oz)	540
Baked Potato Deluxe	1 (13 oz)	650
Baked Potato w/ Butter & Sour Cream	1 (11.2 oz)	500
BBQ Dipping Sauce	1 serv (1 oz)	40
Bronco Berry Sauce	1 serv (1.5 oz)	90
Chicken Finger 4-Pak	1 serv (6.77 oz)	640
Chicken Finger Snack w/ Curly Fries	1 serv (6.4 oz)	580
Curly Fries	1 lg (7 oz)	620
Curly Fries	1 med (4.5 oz)	400
Curly Fries	1 sm (3.8 oz)	310
Curly Fries Cheddar	1 serv (6 oz)	460
German Mustard	1 pkg (0.25 oz)	5
Homestyle Fries	1 lg (7.5 oz)	560
Homestyle Fries	1 med (5 oz)	370
Homestyle Fries	1 sm (4 oz)	300
Homestyle Fries Child-Size	1 serv (3 oz)	220
Honey Mustard	1 serv (1 oz)	130

FOOD	PORTION	CALS
Horsey Sauce	1 pkg (0.5 oz)	60
Jalapeno Bites	1 serv (4 oz)	330
Ketchup	1 pkg (0.3 oz)	10
Marinara Sauce	1 serv (1.5 oz)	35
Mayonnaise	1 pkg (0.4 oz)	90
Mayonnaise Light Cholesterol Free	1 pkg (0.4 oz)	20
Mozzarella Sticks	4 (4.8 oz)	470
Onion Petals	1 serv (4 oz)	410
Potato Cakes	2 (3.5 oz)	250
Sandwich Chicken Bacon'N Swiss	1 (7.4 oz)	610
Sandwich Chicken Breast Fillet	1 (7.2 oz)	540
Sandwich Chicken Cordon Bleu	1 (8.4 oz)	630
Sandwich Grilled Chicken Deluxe	1 (8.7 oz)	450
Sandwich Hot Ham 'N Swiss	1 (5.9 oz)	340
Sandwich Market Fresh Roast Beef & Swiss	1 (12.5 oz)	810
Sandwich Market Fresh Roast Beef Ranch & Bacon	1 (13.5 oz)	880
Sandwich Market Fresh Roast Chicken Caesar	1 (12.7 oz)	820
Sandwich Market Fresh Roast Ham & Swiss	1 (12.5 oz)	730
Sandwich Market Fresh Roast Turkey & Swiss	1 (12.5 oz)	760
Sandwich Market Fresh Ultimate BLT	1 (10.5 oz)	820
Sandwich Roast Beef Arby-Q	1 (6.4 oz)	360
Sandwich Roast Beef Beef'N Cheddar	1 (6.9 oz)	480
Sandwich Roast Beef Big Montana	1 (11 oz)	630
Sandwich Roast Beef Giant	1 (7.9 oz)	480
Sandwich Roast Beef Junior	1 (4.4 oz)	310
Sandwich Roast Beef Melt w/ Cheddar	1 (5.2 oz)	340
Sandwich Roast Beef Regular	1 (5.4 oz)	350
Sandwich Roast Beef Super	1 (8.5 oz)	470
Sandwich Roast Chicken Club	1 (8.4 oz)	520
Sub Sandwich French Dip	1 (10 oz)	440
Sub Sandwich Hot Ham'N Swiss	1 (9.7 oz)	530
Sub Sandwich Italian	1 (11 oz)	780
Sub Sandwich Philly Beef'N Swiss	1 (10.8 oz)	700
Sub Sandwich Roast Beef	1 (11.6 oz)	760
Sub Sandwich Turkey	1 (10.6 oz)	630
Tangy Southwest Sauce	1 serv (1.5 oz)	250
SALAD DRESSINGS		
Bleu Cheese	1 serv (2 oz)	300

FOOD	PORTION	CALS
Buttermilk Ranch	1 serv (2 oz)	290
Buttermilk Ranch Light	1 serv (2 oz)	100
Caesar	1 serv (2 oz)	310
Honey French	1 serv (2 oz)	290
Italian Reduced Calorie	1 serv (2 oz)	25
Italian Parmesan	1 serv (2 oz)	240
Thousand Island	1 serv (2 oz)	290
SALADS		
Caesar Side Salad	1 (5 oz)	45
Caesar Salad w/o Dressing	1 serv (8 oz)	90
Chicken Finger w/o Dressing	1 serv (13 oz)	570
Croutons Seasoned	1 serv (0.25 oz)	30
Croutons Cheese & Garlic	1 serv (0.63 oz)	100
Garden Salad	1 (12.3 oz)	70
Grilled Chicken	1 serv (16.3 oz)	210
Grilled Chicken Caesar w/o Dressing	1 serv (12 oz)	230
Roast Chicken	1 serv (14.8 oz)	160
Side Salad	1 (5.7 oz)	25
Turkey Club Salad w/o Dressing	1 serv (12 oz)	350
AU BON PAIN		
BAKED SELECTIONS		
Bagel Cinnamon Crisp	1 (6 oz)	540
Baguette	1 loaf (10.6 oz)	680
Bread Stick	1 (2.3 oz)	200
Cinnamon Roll	1 (4 oz)	300
Cookie Chocolate Chip	1 (2 oz)	230
Cookie Chocolate Chunk Macadamia	1 (2 oz)	250
Cookie Gingerbread Man w/ Raisins & Icing	1 (2.7 oz)	280
Cookie Oatmeal Raisin	1 (2 oz)	210
Cookie Peanut Butter	1 (2 oz)	240
Cookie Shortbread	1 (2.3 oz)	240
Cookie Walnut Raisin	1 (2 oz)	250
Cookie English Toffee	1 (2 oz)	230
Creme De Fleur	1 serv (5.55 oz)	470
Croissant Almond	1 (4.7 oz)	480
Croissant Apple	1 (3.5 oz)	200
Croissant Chocolate	1 (3.1 oz)	330
Croissant Cinnamon Raisin	1 (3.8 oz)	300
Croissant Raspberry Cheese	1 (3.6 oz)	290

FOOD	PORTION	CALS
Croissant Sweet Cheese	1 (3.6 oz)	320
Danish Cranberry	1 (4.5 oz)	350
Danish Lemon	1 (4.3 oz)	340
Danish Sweet Cheese	1 (4.2 oz)	390
Focaccia	1 piece (5.4 oz)	430
Four Grain Bread	1 serv (4.7 oz)	400
French Roll	1 (4.2 oz)	260
French Roll Roast Beef	1 (11 oz)	540
Hearth Roll	1 (3 oz)	210
Holiday Cookie w/ Icing & Sprinkles	1 (1.6 oz)	150
Loaf Multigrain	1 slice (1.8 oz)	130
Muffin Banana Walnut	1 (5.4 oz)	430
Muffin Blueberry	1 (5.6 oz)	470
Muffin Bran Raisin	1 (5.5 oz)	400
Muffin Carrot	1 (5.8 oz)	520
Muffin Corn	1 (5.7 oz)	390
Muffin Cranberry Walnut	1 (5.4 oz)	500
Muffin Low Fat 3 Berry	1 (4.4 oz)	270
Muffin Low Fat Chocolate Cake	1 (4.2 oz)	470
Muffin Milk Chocolate Chunk	1 (5.3 oz)	530
Muffin Pumpkin	1 (6 oz)	510
Parisienne Loaf	1 loaf (19 oz)	1210
Petit Pain	1 (2.9 oz)	180
Roll Braided w/ Topping	1 (10 oz)	430
Roll Pecan	1 (6 oz)	620
Sandwich Loaf Country White	1 serv (1.75 oz)	110
Sandwich Loaf Tomato Herb	1 serv (1.75 oz)	120
Scone Chocolate Walnut	1 (4 oz)	420
Scone Cranberry Orange Almond	1 (4 oz)	400
Scone Maple Oat Pecan Date	1 (4 oz)	410
Scone Orange	1 (4.2 oz)	370
Shortbread Heart ½ Chocolate	1 (2.7 oz)	290
Shortbread Heart w/ Red Sugar	1 (2.5 oz)	270
Sourdough Bagel Asiago Cheese	1 (4.8 oz)	340
Sourdough Bagel Cheddar Scallion	1 (4.1 oz)	310
Sourdough Bagel Cinnamon Crisp	1 (4.6 oz)	360
Sourdough Bagel Cinnamon Raisin	1 (4.5 oz)	300
Sourdough Bagel Cranberry Nut	1 (4.7 oz)	400
Sourdough Bagel Double Cheddar Jalpeno	1 serv (4.1 oz)	320

FOOD	PORTION	CALS
Sourdough Bagel Dutch Apple	1 (4.7 oz)	380
Sourdough Bagel Everything	1 (4.4 oz)	330
Sourdough Bagel Focaccia	1 (4.1 oz)	320
Sourdough Bagel Honey 9 Grain	1 (4.8 oz)	310
Sourdough Bagel Onion	1 (4.4 oz)	320
Sourdough Bagel Plain	1 (4 oz)	300
Sourdough Bagel Poppy Seed	1 (4.4 oz)	330
Sourdough Bagel Sesame	1 (4.4 oz)	340
Sourdough Bagel Wild Blueberry	1 (4.1 oz)	280
Streudal Cherry	1 serv (4 oz)	380
Streudel Apple	1 serv (4.35 oz)	400
SALADS		
Caesar w/o Dressing	1 serv (7.8 oz)	240
Chef's	1 serv (10.3 oz)	290
Chicken Caesar	1 serv (10.2 oz)	380
Chicken Oriental	1 serv (8.6 oz)	220
Chicken Pesto Salad	1 serv (8 oz)	400
Garden	1 serv (9.3 oz)	160
Garden Side	1 serv (5.1 oz)	90
Gorgonzola & Walnut	1 serv (5 oz)	330
Mozzarella & Red Pepper Salad	1 serv (10.5 oz)	360
Tuna	1 serv (13.2 oz)	440
SANDWICHES AND FILLINGS		
Club Hot Roasted Turkey	1 (11.7 oz)	630
Cream Cheese Plain	1 serv (2 oz)	190
Cream Cheese Reduced Fat Honey Walnut	1 serv (2 oz)	150
Cream Cheese Reduced Fat Sundried Tomato	1 serv (2 oz)	140
Cream Cheese Reduced Fat Veggie	1 serv (2 oz)	140
Croissant Spinach & Cheese	1 (3.6 oz)	220
Croque Madame	1 (11 oz)	570
Croque Monsieur	1 (11 oz)	590
Egg On A Bagel	1 serv (7.1 oz)	500
Egg On A Bagel w/ Bacon	1 serv (7.6 oz)	580
Egg On A Bagel w/ Cheese	1 serv (7.85 oz)	590
Egg On A Bagel w/ Cheese & Bacon	1 serv (8.35 oz)	670
Focaccia Chicken & Mozzarella	1 serv (13.75 oz)	800
Focaccia Chicken Tarragon w/ Field Greens	1 (12.5 oz)	870
Focaccia Garden Vegetable Goat Cheese w/ Artichoke Spread	1 (14.25 oz)	570
Focaccia Hickory Smoked Ham & Brie	1 (13.3 oz)	620

FOOD	PORTION	CALS
Focaccia Smoked Turkey & Swiss w/ Cilantro	1 (13.25 oz)	810
Fo-Ca-Cha-Cha Chicken	1 serv (11.15 oz)	730
French Roll Ham	1 (11 oz)	390
French Roll Hot Grilled Chicken	1 (11 oz)	620
French Roll Hot Roast Turkey	1 (11 oz)	500
French Roll Tuna	1 (10.6 oz)	550
Hot Croissant Spinach & Cheese	1 (4 oz)	290
Pane Bagniate	1 (12 oz)	670
Sandwich Arizona Chicken	1 (12 oz)	600
Sandwich Cheese	1 (7.2 oz)	590
Sandwich Fresh Mozzarella Tomato & Pesto	1 (11 oz)	790
Sandwich Honey Dijon Chicken	1 (13.6 oz)	750
Sandwich Thai Chicken	1 (11.4 oz)	550
Wrap Chicken Caesar	1 (10.5 oz)	640
Wrap Fields & Feta	1 (13.5 oz)	620
Wrap Honey Smoked Turkey	1 (15 oz)	520
Wrap Roast Beef & Brie	1 (14 oz)	570
SOUPS		
Autumn Pumpkin	1 serv (8 oz)	170
Black Bean	1 serv (8 oz)	180
Chicken Florentine	1 serv (8 oz)	140
Chicken Noodle	1 serv (8 oz)	100
Clam Chowder	1 serv (8 oz)	220
Corn & Green Chili Bisque	1 serv (8 oz)	200
Corn Chowder	1 serv (8 oz)	270
Curried Rice & Lentil	1 serv (8 oz)	140
French Moroccan Tomato Lentil	1 serv (8 oz)	130
Garden Vegetable	1 serv (8 oz)	50
Low Sodium Mediterranean Pepper	1 serv (12 oz)	280
Low Sodium Southwest Vegetable	1 serv (12 oz)	220
Old Fashioned Tomato	1 serv (8 oz)	140
Pasta E Fagioli	1 serv (8 oz)	240
Potato Cheese	1 serv (8 oz)	190
Potato Leek	1 serv (8 oz)	200
Red Beans & Rice	1 serv (8 oz)	200
Soup Bread Bowl	1 (9.25 oz)	600
Southern Black Eyed Pea	1 serv (8 oz)	320
Split Pea	1 serv (8 oz)	160
Tomato Florentine	1 serv (8 oz)	120
Tuscan Vegetable	1 serv (8 oz)	140

FOOD	PORTION	CALS
Vegetable Beef Barley	1 serv (8 oz)	110
Vegetarian Lentil	1 serv (8 oz)	120
Vegetarian Chili	1 serv (8 oz)	170
Wild Mushroom Bisque	1 serv (8 oz)	140

AUNTIE ANNE'S
BEVERAGES

FOOD	PORTION	CALS
Dutch Ice Blue Raspberry	1 (14 oz)	165
Dutch Ice Grape	1 (14 oz)	180
Dutch Ice Kiwi Banana	1 (14 oz)	190
Dutch Ice Lemonade	1 (14 oz)	315
Dutch Ice Mocha	1 (14 oz)	400
Dutch Ice Orange Creme	1 (14 oz)	280
Dutch Ice Pina Colada	1 (14 oz)	220
Dutch Ice Strawberry	1 (14 oz)	220
Dutch Ice Wild Cherry	1 (14 oz)	210
Dutch Shake Chocolate	1 (14 oz)	580
Dutch Shake Coffee	1 (14 oz)	590
Dutch Shake Strawberry	1 (14 oz)	610
Dutch Shake Vanilla	1 (14 oz)	510
Dutch Smoothie Blue Raspberry	1 (14 oz)	230
Dutch Smoothie Grape	1 (14 oz)	230
Dutch Smoothie Kiwi Banana	1 (14 oz)	240
Dutch Smoothie Lemonade	1 (14 oz)	300
Dutch Smoothie Mocha	1 (14 oz)	330
Dutch Smoothie Orange Creme	1 (14 oz)	280
Dutch Smoothie Pina Colada	1 (14 oz)	260
Dutch Smoothie Strawberry	1 (14 oz)	250
Dutch Smoothie Wild Cherry	1 (14 oz)	250
Lemonade	1 (22 oz)	180
Lemonade Strawberry	1 (22 oz)	190

DIPPING SAUCES

FOOD	PORTION	CALS
Caramel Dip	1 serv (1.5 oz)	135
Cheese Sauce	1 serv (1.25 oz)	100
Chocolate Dip	1 serv (1.25 oz)	130
Cream Cheese Light	1 serv (1.25 oz)	70
Cream Cheese Strawberry	1 serv (1.25 oz)	110
Hot Salsa Cheese	1 serv (1.25 oz)	100
Marinara Sauce	1 serv (1.25 oz)	10
Sweet Mustard	1 serv (1.25 oz)	60

FOOD	PORTION	CALS
PRETZELS		
Almond	1	400
Almond w/o Butter	1	350
Cinnamon Raisin w/o Butter	1	350
Cinnamon Sugar	1	450
Garlic	1	350
Garlic w/o Butter	1	320
Glazin' Raisin	1	510
Glazin' Raisin w/o Butter	1	470
Jalapeno	1	310
Jalapeno w/o Butter	1	270
Maple Crumb	1	550
Maple Crumb w/o Butter	1	520
Original	1	370
Original w/o Butter	1	340
Parmesan Herb	1	440
Parmesan Herb w/o Butter	1	390
Sesame	1	410
Sesame w/o Butter	1	350
Sour Cream & Onion	1	340
Sour Cream & Onion w/o Butter	1	310
Stixs	4	247
Stixs w/o Butter	4	227
Whole Wheat	1	370
Whole Wheat w/o Butter	1	350
BAJA FRESH		
MAIN MENU SELECTIONS		
Baja Burrito Chicken	1 serv	820
Baja Burrito Steak	1 serv	920
Black Beans	1 serv	360
Burrito Bean & Cheese Chicken	1 serv	1000
Burrito Bean & Cheese Steak	1 serv	1100
Burrito Bean & Cheese Vegetarian	1 serv	870
Burrito Dos Manos Chicken	1 full serv	1480
Burrito Dos Manos Steak	1 full serv	1580
Burrito Mexicano Chicken	1 serv	830
Burrito Mexicano Steak	1 serv	920
Burrito Ultimo Chicken	1 serv	860
Burrito Ultimo Steak	1 serv	950

FOOD	PORTION	CALS
Cebollitas	1 serv	40
Chips & Salsa Baja	1 serv	1100
Enchiladas Cheese	1 serv	850
Enchiladas Chicken	1 serv	780
Enchiladas Steak	1 serv	890
Enchiladas Verde Cheese	1 serv	840
Enchiladas Verde Chicken	1 serv	770
Enchiladas Verde Vegetarian	1 serv	720
Fajitas Chicken Corn Tortillas	1 serv	1200
Fajitas Chicken Flour Tortillas	1 serv	1360
Fajitas Steak Corn Tortillas	1 serv	1360
Fajitas Steak Flour Tortillas	1 serv	1530
Grilled Vegetarian	1 serv	770
Mini Quesa-Dita Cheese	1 serv	620
Mini Quesa-Dita Chicken	1 serv	670
Mini Quesa-Dita Steak	1 serv	700
Mini Tosta-Dita Chicken	1 serv	570
Mini Tosta-Dita Steak	1 serv	630
Nachos Cheese	1 serv	1880
Nachos Chicken	1 serv	2010
Nachos Steak	1 serv	2100
Pinto Beans	1 serv	320
Quesadilla	1 serv	1180
Quesadilla Cheese	1 serv	1130
Quesadilla Chicken	1 serv	1260
Quesadilla Steak	1 serv	1350
Rice	1 serv	280
Taco Baja Style Chicken	1 serv	190
Taco Baja Style Steak	1 serv	220
Taco Baja Style Wild Gulf Shrimp	1 serv	190
Taco Chilio Chicken	1 serv	320
Taco Chilito Steak	1 serv	340
Taco Fish	1 serv	270
Taco Mahi Mahi	1 serv	260
Taquitos Chicken w/ Beans	1 serv	750
Taquitos Chicken w/ Rice	1 serv	710
Taquitos Steak w/ Beans	1 serv	820
Taquitos Steak w/ Rice	1 serv	790
Tostada Chicken	1 serv	1140
Tostada Steak	1 serv	1230

FOOD	PORTION	CALS
Tostada Vegetarian	1 serv	1010
SALAD DRESSINGS		
Fat Free Salsa Verde	1 serv (2.6 oz)	15
Guacamole	2 oz	70
Olive Oil Vinaigrette	1 serv (2.6 oz)	230
Pico De Gallo	1 serv	50
Pronto Guacamole	1 serv	550
Ranch	1 serv (2.6 oz)	220
Salsa Baja	1 serv	70
Salsa Roja	1 serv	70
Salsa Verde	1 serv	50
Sour Cream	1 oz	60
SALADS		
Baja Ensalada Chicken	1 serv	310
Baja Ensalada Fish	1 serv	360
Baja Ensalada Steak	1 serv	460
Side Salad	1 serv	70

BASKIN-ROBBINS
FROZEN YOGURT

FOOD	PORTION	CALS
Cafe Mocha Truly Free Soft Serve	1 reg	140
Chocolate Nonfat Soft Serve	1 reg	190
Lowfat Maui Brownie Madness	1 reg	250
ICE CREAM		
Cappuccino Blast w/ Whipped Cream	1 reg	340
Chocolate	1 reg	270
Chocolate Chip	1 reg	270
Espresso'n Cream Lowfat	1 reg	180
Jamoca Almond Fudge	1 reg	280
Peach Crumb Pie No Sugar Added	1 reg	180
Pralines'n Cream	1 reg	280
Shake Chocolate	16 oz	750
Shake Vanilla	16 oz	630
Smoothie Very Strawberry w/ Soft Serve Ice Cream	1 reg	320
Thin Mint No Sugar Added	1 reg	160
Vanilla	1 reg	270
ICES		
Daiquiri Ice	1 reg	130

FOOD	PORTION	CALS
Sherbet Rainbow	1 reg	160
Sorbet Peachy Keen	1 reg	110

BEAR ROCK CAFE
BAKED SELECTIONS

Almond French Horn	1	491
Bear Claw	1	260
Cinnamon Roll w/ Cream Cheese Icing	1	540
English Muffin	1	120
Pecan Sticky Bun	1	555

SALAD DRESSINGS

Balsamic Vinaigrette	1 serv (1.5 oz)	156
Blue Cheese	1 serv (1.5 oz)	230
Caesar	1 serv (1.5 oz)	198
Creamy Italian	1 serv (1.5 oz)	180
Fat Free Ranch	1 serv (1.5 oz)	40
Fat Free Vidalia Onion	1 serv (1.5 oz)	56
Honey Mustard	1 serv (1.5 oz)	184
Oil & Vinegar	1 serv (1.5 oz)	250
Ranch	1 serv (1.5 oz)	213
Red Wine Vinaigrette	1 serv (1.5 oz)	198
Sesame Oriental	1 serv (1.5 oz)	128
Sweet Vidalia Onion	1 serv (1.5 oz)	170
Thousand Island	1 serv (1.5 oz)	184

SALADS

Almond Citrus Chicken w/o Dressing	1 serv	443
BLT Chicken w/o Dressing	1 serv	394
BLT w/o Dressing	1 lg	285
BLT w/o Dressing	1 sm	146
Caesar Chicken w/ Dressing	1 serv	580
Caesar w/ Dressing	1 lg	451
Caesar w/ Dressing	1 sm	236
Dusk Mountain Blackened Chicken w/o Dressing	1 serv	304
Fruit Salad	1 serv (4 oz)	61
Lodge	1 sm	55
Lodge w/o Dressing	1 lg	82
Low Carb BLT	1 serv	721
Low Carb Side Salad w/ Dressing	1 serv	316
Low Carb w/ Chicken w/ Dressing	1 serv	567

FOOD	PORTION	CALS
Low Fat Grilled Chicken w/o Dressing	1 serv	151
Mount Fuji w/ Dressing	1 serv	554
SANDWICHES		
Bagel & Cream Cheese	1	378
Bear Cristo	1	310
BLT	1	585
Coop's Chicken Salad Croissant	1	439
Fajita Chicken	1	659
Fireside Jack	1	699
Garden	1	390
Giant Panda Wrap	1	556
Grilled Cheese	1	480
Ham & Swiss On Rye	1	394
Hoot Owl	1	641
Italian Asiago Focaccia	1	901
Low Carb Wrap	1	308
Low Fat Ham	1	309
Low Fat Turkey	1	280
Mountain Bird	1	691
Peanut Butter & Jelly	1	387
Reuben's Peak	1	540
Rising Sunflower	1	591
Roast Turkey & Bacon	1	522
Rockside Focaccia	1	958
Sasquash	1	408
The Early Bear Bagel + Bacon	1	530
The Early Bear English Muffin + Bacon	1	344
The Early Bear English Muffin + Sausage	1	514
The Moose	1	976
Turkey On Whole Wheat	1	602
SOUPS		
Aztec Black Bean	1 serv	162
Baked Potato Mountain Chowder	1 serv	352
Chicken & Dumpling	1 serv	249
Chicken Gumbo	1 serv	123
Chicken Noodle	1 serv	165
Chicken w/ Wild Rice	1 serv	313
Cream Of Broccoli w/ Cheddar	1 serv	264
French Onion	1 serv	121
Grande Chili	1 serv	351

FOOD	PORTION	CALS
In Bread Bowl Aztec Black Bean	1 serv	545
In Bread Bowl Baked Potato Mountain Chowder	1 serv	735
In Bread Bowl Chicken & Dumplings	1 serv	632
In Bread Bowl Chicken Gumbo	1 serv	506
In Bread Bowl Chicken Noodle	1 serv	548
In Bread Bowl Chicken w/ Wild Rice	1 serv	696
In Bread Bowl Cream Of Broccoli w/ Cheddar	1 serv	647
In Bread Bowl French Onion	1 serv	504
In Bread Bowl Grande Chili	1 serv	734
In Bread Bowl New England Clam Chowder	1 serv	653
In Bread Bowl Normandy Vegetable Cheddar	1 serv	728
In Bread Bowl Tomato Florentine	1 serv	533
New England Clam Chowder	1 serv	270
Normandy Vegetable Cheddar	1 serv	345
Tomato Florentine	1 serv	150

BEN & JERRY'S

Sugar Cone	1	48
FROZEN YOGURT		
Black Raspberry Low Fat	½ cup	140
Cherry Garcia	½ cup	170
Chocolate Fudge Brownie	½ cup	190
Half Baked	½ cup	210
Phish Food	½ cup	230
ICE CREAM		
Brownie Batter	½ cup	310
Butter Pecan	½ cup	290
Cherry Garcia	½ cup	250
Chocolate Chip Cookie Dough	½ cup	280
Chocolate Chocolate Cookie	½ cup	280
Chocolate For A Change	½ cup	270
Chocolate Fudge Brownie	½ cup	280
Chubby Hubby	½ cup	330
Chunky Monkey	½ cup	300
Coffee For A Change	½ cup	240
Coffee Heath Bar Crunch	½ cup	310
Everything But The	½ cup	320
Fudge Central	½ cup	300
Half Baked	½ cup	280
Karamel Sutra	½ cup	290

FOOD	PORTION	CALS
Makin' Whoopie Pie	½ cup	270
Mint Chocolate Cookie	½ cup	270
New York Super Fudge Chunk	½ cup	270
Oatmeal Cookie Chunk	½ cup	280
One Sweet Whirled	½ cup	280
Organic Chocolate Fudge Brownie	½ cup	260
Organic Strawberry	½ cup	200
Organic Sweet Cream & Cookies	½ cup	240
Organic Vanilla	½ cup	220
Peanut Butter Cup	½ cup	380
Peanut Butter Me Up	½ cup	330
Phish Food	½ cup	280
Pistachio Pistachio	½ cup	280
Uncanny Cashew	½ cup	290
Vanilla Almond	1 bar (3.7 oz)	340
Vanilla Heath Bar Crunch	½ cup	300
Vanilla For A Change	½ cup	240
SORBETS		
Berry Berry Extraordinary	½ cup	100
Mango Lime	½ cup	100
Strawberry Kiwi	½ cup	100

BIG APPLE BAGELS
BAGELS

Apple Cinnamon	1	332
Banana Nut	1	340
Blueberry	1	330
Cheddar Herb	1	352
Chocolate Chip	1	348
Cinnamon Raisin	1	336
Cinnamon Sugar	1	175
Cranberry Walnut	1	352
Egg	1	328
Everything	1	336
Garlic	1	330
Honey Oat	1	320
Jalapeno	1	350
Onion	1	336
Pizzah Bagel	1	481
Plain	1	334

FOOD	PORTION	CALS
Poppy	1	344
Pumpernickel	1	332
Salt	1	324
Sesame	1	358
Spinach	1	356
Strawberry	1	342
Tomato Basil	1	322
Vegetable	1	318
Wheat	1	330
SANDWICHES		
All American Duo	1	762
Big Apple Club	1	797
Breakfast BLT	1	704
Chicken Caesar	1	611
Classic Turkey	1	552
Enchilada Bagellata	1	522
Grilled Chicken	1	571
Hoely Guacamole	1	476
Kick-N Roast Beef	1	579
Lox & Cream Cheese	1	602
Mediterranean Veg-Out	1	506
Morning Classic	1	486
Northern Omelette	1	699
Roma Italian	1	764
Toasted Cafe Chicken Melt	1	815
Toasted Deli Style Turkey	1	732
Toasted Roast Beef Parmesan Grinder	1	583
Toasted Spicy Italian Sub	1	770
Toasted Tuna Melt	1	641
Turkey Club	1	782

BILLY'S BURGER HUT
BEVERAGES

Shake Chocolate	1 (20 oz)	420
Shake Vanilla	1 (20 oz)	320
MAIN MENU SELECTIONS		
Big Billy's Roast Beef Sub	1	843
Billyburger	1	426
Billyburger w/ Cheese	1	498
Billy's Best Red Potato Salad	1 serv	190

FOOD	PORTION	CALS
Billy's Biggest Burger ½ Pounder w/ Everything	1	852
Billy's Famous 7 Layer Salad	1 serv	558
Billy's Seafood Sandwich	1	399
Caesar Side Salad	1 serv	360
Chili w/ Cheese & Onion	1 serv	380
Cowboy Cobb Salad	1 serv	735
French Fries	1 reg	230
Onion Rings	1 serv	250
Super Billy Burger w/ Bacon	1	663

BLIMPIE
COOKIES

Chocolate Chunk	1	200
Macadamia White Chunk	1	210
Oatmeal Raisin	1	190
Peanut Butter	1	220
Sugar	1	330

SALAD DRESSINGS AND TOPPINGS

Caesar Dressing	1 serv (1.5 oz)	208
Cracked Peppercorn Dressing	1 serv (1.5 oz)	237
Frank's Red Hot Buffalo Sauce	1 serv (1 oz)	13
French's Honey Mustard	1 tbsp	5
GourMayo Chipotle Chili	1 tbsp	50
GourMayo Sun Dried Tomato	1 tbsp	50
GourMayo Wasabi Horseradish	1 tbsp	50
Guacamole	1 serv (1.5 oz)	194
Oil & Vinegar	1 serv	36
Pesto Dressing	1 serv (1 oz)	132

SALADS

Antipasto	1 reg serv	244
Chef	1 reg serv	212
Chili Ole	1 reg serv	480
Grilled Chicken w/ Caesar Dressing	1 reg serv	347
Grilled Chicken w/o Dressing	1 serv	139
Roast Beef 'N Blue	1 reg serv	390
Seafood	1 reg serv	122
Tuna	1 reg serv	261
Zesto Pesto Turkey	1 reg serv	370

SANDWICHES

6 Inch Hot Sub BLT	1	588

FOOD	PORTION	CALS
6 Inch Hot Sub Buffalo Chicken	1	400
6 Inch Hot Sub Buffalo Chicken w/o Cheese	1	320
6 Inch Hot Sub ChiliMax	1	511
6 Inch Hot Sub Grilled Chicken	1	373
6 Inch Hot Sub Meatball	1	572
6 Inch Hot Sub MexiMelt	1	425
6 Inch Hot Sub Pastrami	1	507
6 Inch Hot Sub Steak & Onion Melt	1	440
6 Inch Hot Sub VegiMax	1	395
6 Inch Sub Blimpie Best	1	476
6 Inch Sub Club	1	440
6 Inch Sub Ham & Cheese	1	436
6 Inch Sub Roast Beef	1	468
6 Inch Sub Roast Beef w/o Cheese	1	388
6 Inch Sub Seafood	1	355
6 Inch Sub Tuna	1	493
6 inch Sub Turkey	1	424
6 Inch Sub Turkey w/o Cheese	1	344
Cheddar	1 slice	52
Grilled Subs Beef Turkey & Cheddar	1	600
Grilled Subs Cuban	1	462
Grilled Subs Pastrami	1	462
Grilled Subs Reuben	1	630
Provolone	1 slice	80
Swiss	1 slice	80
Wraps Beef & Cheddar	1	714
Wraps Chicken Caesar	1	646
Wraps Southewestern	1	674
Wraps Steak & Onions	1	716
Wraps Ultimate BLT	1	831
Wraps Zesty Italian	1	638
SIDE ORDERS		
Cole Slaw	1 serv (5 oz)	180
Macaroni Salad	1 serv (5 oz)	360
Mustard Potato Salad	1 serv (5 oz)	160
Potato Chips Cheddar & Sour Cream	1 bag	210
Potato Chips Jalapeno	1 bag	210
Potato Chips Lea & Perrins Barbecue	1 bag	210
Potato Chips Regular	1 bag	210
Potato Chips Romano & Garlic	1 bag	210

FOOD	PORTION	CALS
Potato Chips Sour Cream & Onion	1 bag	210
Potato Salad	1 serv (5 oz)	270
SOUPS		
Chicken w/ White & Wild Rice	1 serv (8 oz)	230
Cream Of Broccoli & Cheese	1 serv (8 oz)	190
Cream Of Potato	1 serv (8 oz)	190
Garden Vegetable	1 serv (8 oz)	80
Grande Chili w/ Beans & Beef	1 serv (8 oz)	250
Homestyle Chicken Noodle	1 serv (8 oz)	120
Tomato Basil w/ Raviolini	1 serv (8 oz)	110
Vegetable Beef	1 serv (8 oz)	80

BOB EVANS
BAKED SELECTIONS

FOOD	PORTION	CALS
Biscuit	1	277
Bread Apple Walnut	1 slice	142
Bread Banana Nut	1 slice	186
Bread Garlic	1 slice	218
Bread Sourdough	1	130
Bun Kaiser	1	167
Bun Mini	1	105
English Muffin	1	139
Roll Cinnamon Swirl Frosted	1	607
Roll Cinnamon Swirl Unfrosted	1	510
Roll Dinner	1	201
Texas Toast	1 slice	120
BEVERAGES		
Cocoa Cola	12.5 oz	145
Coffee Decafe	7 oz	5
Coffee Regular	7 oz	2
Creamer Half & Half	0.5 oz	40
Creamer Non-Dairy	0.5 oz	19
Diet Coke	12.5 oz	4
Dr Pepper	12.5 oz	145
Hot Chocolate	1 serv (8.8 oz)	142
Hot Tea	7 oz	2
Iced Tea	9.4 oz	3
Iced Tea Blackberry	9.4 oz	92
Iced Tea Strawberry	9.4 oz	120
Kool Aid Ice Blue Raspberry Lemonade	1 kids cup (8 oz)	70

FOOD	PORTION	CALS
Lemonade	12 oz	136
Lemonade Blackberry	12 oz	214
Lemonade Strawberry	12 oz	242
Root Beer	12.5 oz	145
Sprite	12.5 oz	142
Strawberry Splash	12.5 oz	218
BREAKFAST SELECTIONS		
Bacon	1 piece	36
Belgian Waffle	1	351
Canadian Bacon	1 piece	21
Country Biscuit Breakfast	1 serv	841
Egg Hardboiled	1	60
Egg Over Easy	1	93
Eggs Scrambled	1 serv	170
Eggs Benedict	1 serv	514
French Toast	1 slice	135
Fruit Cup	1 serv	164
Grits	1 serv	187
Ham Smoked	1 slice	66
Home Fries	1 serv	193
Hotcake Blueberry	1	192
Hotcake Buttermilk	1	176
Hotcake Cinnamon	1	166
Hotcake Multigrain	1	208
Lite Sausage Breakfast	1 serv	479
Mush	1 serv	73
Oatmeal Plain	1 serv	185
Omelette Border	1	847
Omelette Cheese	1	457
Omelette Farmer's Market	1	634
Omelette Garden Harvest	1 serv	437
Omelette Ham & Cheese	1 serv	486
Omelette Sausage & Cheese	1 serv	729
Omelette Southwestern Chicken	1 serv	641
Omelette Western	1 serv	503
Pot Roast Hash Breakfast	1 serv	698
Sausage	1 link	117
Sausage Lite	1 link	100
Skillet Chicken Cordon Bleu	1 serv	880

FOOD	PORTION	CALS
Skillet Sunshine	1 serv	754
Strawberry Yogurt	1 serv	145
CHILDREN'S MENU SELECTIONS		
Colorful Cool Cakes	1 serv	542
Garden Salad	1 kid serv	41
Hot Diggety Dog Plain	1	446
L'il Homesteader	1 serv	414
Mac & Cheese	1 serv	330
Mini Cheeseburger	1 serv	252
Pizza Pizzazz	1 serv	520
Plenty O Pancakes	1 serv	515
Quesadilla Chicken	1 serv	542
Smiley Face Potatoes	1 serv	335
Spaghetti & Meatballs	1 serv	523
Sundae Fudge Blast	1 serv	254
Sundae Oreo Cookies 'n' Cream	1 serv	315
Sundae Rainbow	1 serv	320 ·
Sundae	1 serv	325
Reese's I'm Smiling		
DESSERTS		
A La Mode Vanilla Ice Cream	1 serv	159
Cake Hershey's Hot Fudge	1 slice	688
Cake Pineapple Upside Down	1 slice	500
Oreo Cheesecake	1 slice	625
Peach Cobbler	1 serv	499
Pie Apple Dumpling	1 slice	682
Pie Banana Cream	1 slice	456
Pie Coconut Cream	1 slice	461
Pie French Silk	1 slice	653
Pie Lemon Meringue	1 slice	536
Pie No Sugar Added Apple	1 slice	483
Pie Reese's Peanut Butter Cup	1 slice	1130
Pie Strawberry Supreme	1 slice	589
Sundae Fudge	1	501
Sundae Reese's	1 serv	769
MAIN MENU SELECTIONS		
Applesauce	1 serv	101
Baked Potato Loaded	1	427
Baked Potato Plain	1	207
Broccoli Florets	1 serv	156

FOOD	PORTION	CALS
Broccoli Florets Cheddar	1 serv	230
Carrots Glazed	1 serv	188
Catfish Grilled New Orleans	1 piece	255
Cheeseburger Bacon Plain	1	1005
Cheeseburger Plain	1	691
Chicken Quesadilla	1 serv	502
Chicken & Broccoli Alfredo	1 serv	826
Chicken Fried	1 piece	291
Chicken Grilled	1 piece	229
Chicken Pot Pie	1 serv	758
Chicken Tenders Grilled	1 piece	103
Chicken-N-Noodle	1 serv	407
Coleslaw	1 serv	198
Corn Buttered	1 serv	225
Cottage Cheese	1 serv	122
Country Fried Steak w/ Gravy	1 serv	535
Country Fried Steak w/o Gravy	1 serv	481
Dressing Bread & Celery	1 serv	362
Fish Market Halibut	1 piece	209
French Fries	1 serv	217
Green Beans w/ Ham	1 serv	83
Grilled Garden Vegetables	1 serv	290
Hamburger Patty	1	388
Hamburger Plain	1	585
Hamburger Shroomin' Onion Plain	1	695
Home Fries	1 serv	193
Mashed Potatoes	1 serv	171
Meat Loaf	1 serv	626
Mushrooms Grilled	1 serv	152
Onion Rings	1 serv	460
Open Faced Roast Beef Dinner	1 serv	633
Pork Chop Dinner	1 serv	466
Pork Chop Dinner w/ Garlic Herb Butter	1 serv	624
Pork Chop Dinner w/ Wildfire Barbecue Sauce	1 serv	645
Rice Pilaf	1 serv	163
Salmon	1 serv	334
Salmon w/ Garlic Herb Butter	1 serv	491
Salmon w/ Wildfire Barbecue Sauce	1 serv	512
Sandwich Bob's BLT	1	795
Sandwich Chicken Salad	1	694

FOOD	PORTION	CALS
Sandwich Fish Market Haddock	1	570
Sandwich Fried Chicken	1	508
Sandwich Fried Chicken Club	1	994
Sandwich Grilled Cheese	1	391
Sandwich Grilled Chicken	1	447
Sandwich Grilled Chicken Club	1	993
Sandwich Pot Roast	1	728
Sandwich Turkey Bacon Melt	1	872
Seniors Chicken & Broccoli Alfredo	1 serv	513
Seniors Chicken Pot Pie	1 serv	758
Seniors Spaghetti & Meatballs	1 serv	617
Seniors Steak Tips & Noodles	1 serv	550
Seniors Stir-Fry Grilled Chicken	1 serv	479
Spaghelli & Marinara Sauce	1 serv	619
Spaghetti w/ Meatballs	1 serv	1087
Steak Monterey	1 serv	584
Steak Tips & Noodles	1 serv	985
Stir-Fry Grilled Chicken	1 serv	728
Stir-Fry Grilled Shrimp	1 serv	713
Stir-Fry Vegetable	1 serv	497
T-Bone Steak Plain	1 serv	1335
T-Bone Steak w/ Garlic Herb Butter	1 serv	1492
Turkey & Dressing	1 serv	542
SALAD DRESSINGS AND TOPPINGS		
Dressing Bleu Cheese	1 serv (1.5 oz)	220
Dressing Colonial	1 serv (1.5 oz)	232
Dressing French	1 serv (1.5 oz)	219
Dressing Honey Mustard	1 serv (1.5 oz)	192
Dressing Hot Bacon	1 serv (1.5 oz)	106
Dressing Lite Italian	1 serv (1.5 oz)	82
Dressing Oriental	1 serv (1.5 oz)	194
Dressing Ranch	1 serv (1.5 oz)	156
Dressing Ranch Lite	1 serv (1.5 oz)	103
Dressing Raspberry Vinaigrette	1 serv (1.5 oz)	155
Dressing Thousand Island	1 serv (1.5 oz)	212
Dressing Wildfire Ranch	1 serv (1.5 oz)	212
Gravy Chicken	1 serv (3 oz)	60
Gravy Country	1 serv (3 oz)	54
Gravy Sausage	1 serv (7 oz)	244

FOOD	PORTION	CALS
Syrup	1 serv (3 oz)	213
Syrup Sugar Free	1 serv (3 oz)	47
Topping Oregon Berry	1 serv (3 oz)	49
Topping Strawberry	1 serv (3 oz)	50
Whipped Topping	1 serv	69
SALADS		
Chicken Salad Plate	1 serv	789
Cobb Salad w/ Grilled Chicken	1 serv	778
Country Spinach w/ Grilled Chicken	1 serv	532
Frisco Salad w/ Fried Chicken	1 serv	672
Frisco Salad w/ Grilled Chicken	1 serv	599
Fruit & Yogurt	1 serv	414
Raspberry Grilled Chicken	1 serv	637
Speciality Side	1 serv	174
Wildfire Fried Chicken Salad	1 serv	806
Wildfire Grilled Chicken Salad	1 serv	733
SOUPS		
Bean	1 cup	125
Cheddar Baked Potato	1 cup	307
Vegetable Beef	1 cup	198
BOJANGLES		
Biscuit	1	243
Biscuit + Bacon	1	290
Biscuit + Bacon Egg Cheese	1	550
Biscuit + Cajun Filet	1	454
Biscuit + Country Ham	1	270
Biscuit + Egg	1	400
Biscuit + Sausage	1	350
Biscuit + Smoked Sausage	1	380
Biscuit + Steak	1	649
Botato Rounds	1 serv	235
Buffalo Bites	1 serv	180
Cajun Pintos	1 serv	110
Cajun Spiced Breast	1 serv	278
Cajun Spiced Leg	1 serv	284
Cajun Spiced Thigh	1 serv	310
Cajun Spiced Wing	1 serv	355
Chicken Supremes	1 serv	337
Corn On The Cob	1 serv	140

FOOD	PORTION	CALS
Dirty Rice	1 serv	166
Green Beans	1 serv	25
Macaroni & Cheese	1 serv	198
Marinated Cole Slaw	1 serv	136
Potatoes w/o Gravy	1 serv	80
Sandwich Cajun Filet w/o Mayo	1	337
Sandwich Cajun Filet w/ Mayo	1	437
Sandwich Grilled Filet w/ Mayo	1	335
Sandwich Grilled Filet w/o Mayo	1 serv	235
Seasoned Fries	1 serv	344
Southern Style Breast	1 serv	261
Southern Style Leg	1 serv	254
Southern Style Thigh	1 serv	308
Southern Style Wing	1 serv	337
Sweet Biscuit Bo Berry	1	220
Sweet Biscuit Cinnamon	1	320

BOSTON MARKET
DESSERTS

FOOD	PORTION	CALS
Apple Pie	1 slice	550
Brownie Caramel Pecan	1	900
Brownie Chocolate	1	580
Chocolate Cake	1 serv	290
Chocolate Mania	1 serv	290
Cookie Chocolate Chip	1	390
Cookie Oatmeal Scotchie	1	390
Cornbread	1 piece	120
Strawberry Bliss	1 serv	100

MAIN MENU SELECTIONS

FOOD	PORTION	CALS
½ Spicy Tuscan Rotisserie Chicken	1 serv	630
½ Sweet Garlic Rotisserie Chicken w/ Skin	1 serv	590
¼ Dark Spicy Tuscan Rotisserie Chicken	1 serv	340
¼ Dark Sweet Rotisserie Chicken No Skin	1 serv	190
¼ Dark Sweet Rotisserie Chicken w/ Skin	1 serv	320
¼ White Spicy Tuscan Rotisserie Chicken	1 serv	200
¼ White Sweet Garlic Rotisserie Chicken No Skin Or Wing	1 serv	170
¼ White Sweet Rotisserie Chicken w/ Skin & Wing	1 serv	280
Butternut Squash	1 serv	150
Carver Meatloaf w/ Cheese	1	1070

FOOD	PORTION	CALS
Carver Chicken w/ Cheese & Sauce	1	670
Carver Turkey w/ Cheese & Sauce	1	690
Coleslaw	1 serv	310
Cranberry	1 serv	120
Creamed Spinach	1 serv	260
Crispy Baked Country Chicken w/ Gravy	1 serv	440
Double Sauced Angus Meatloaf	1 serv	510
Garlic Dill New Potatoes	1 serv	130
Green Bean Casserole	1 serv	80
Green Beans	1 serv	70
Homestyle Mashed Potatoes & Gravy	1 serv	230
Honey Glazed Ham	1 serv	210
Hot Cinnamon Apples	1 serv	250
Macaroni & Cheese	1 serv	280
Mashed Potatoes	1 serv	210
Meatloaf Double Sauce Angus & Chunky Tomato	1 serv	550
Meatloaf Double Sauced Angus & Beef Gravy	1 serv	580
Pot Pie Pastry Topped	1	750
Poultry Gravy	1 serv	15
Roasted Sirloin	5 oz	270
Rotisserie Turkey Hand Carved	1 serv	170
Savory Stuffing	1 serv	190
Seasonal Fruit Salad	1 serv	70
Squash Casserole	1 serv	330
Steamed Vegetable Medley	1 serv	30
Sweet Corn	1 serv	180
Sweet Potato Casserole	1 serv	280
SALADS		
Asian Rotisserie Chicken Salad No Dressing or Noodles	1 serv	270
Asian Rotisserie Chicken Salad w/ Dressing & Noodles	1 serv	540
Caesar	1 entree	470
Caesar Rotisserie Chicken	1 serv	640
Caesar Side Salad	1 serv	300
Southwest Chicken Salad	1 serv	750
SOUPS		
Chicken Tortilla + Toppings	1 serv	170
Hearty Chicken Noodle	1 cup	101
Tortilla Soup No Toppings	1 serv	80

FOOD	PORTION	CALS
BOSTON PIZZA		
CHILDREN'S MENU SELECTIONS		
Corkscrews n' Cheese	1 serv	870
Dino Fingers & Fries w/ Ketchup	1 serv	680
Grill Cheese Sandwich w/ Fries & Ketchup	1 serv	770
Mini Lasagna	1 serv	400
Pint Sized Ham Pizza	1 serv	430
Potato Smiles	1 serv	580
Stuffed Pizza w/ Fries & Ketchup	1 serv	850
Super Spaghetti	1 serv	340
MAIN MENU SELECTIONS		
Baked Onion Soup	1 serv	210
Bayou Chicken Strips w/ Dipping Sauce	1 serv	370
BBQ Ribs w/ Fries	1 serv	2220
BBQ Ribs w/ Garlic Mashed Potatoes	1 serv	1760
BBQ Ribs w/ Spaghetti	1 serv	1870
Boston's Extreme Double Order	1 serv	1660
Boston's Extreme Starter Order	1 serv	940
Bruschetta	1 serv	640
Buffalo Chicken Fingers w/ Caesar Salad	1 serv	650
Buffalo Chicken Fingers w/ Fries	1 serv	1430
Buffalo Chicken Fingers w/ Light Ranch	1 serv	600
Cactus Cuts & Dip	1 serv	1380
Carne Amore	1 full order	1250
Cheese Toast	1 serv	400
Cheese Toast	1 basket	800
Chicken & Rib Combo	1 serv	1470
Chicken & Rib Combo w/ Fries	1 serv	1920
Chicken & Rib Combo w/ Spaghetti	1 serv	1590
Chicken Fingers w/ Caesar Salad	1 serv	640
Chicken Fingers w/ Fries	1 serv	1420
Chicken Fingers w/ Light Ranch	1 serv	590
Chips & Salsa	1 serv	830
Deluxe Cheese Bread	1 basket	890
Deluxe Cheese Toast	1 serv	420
Dry Ribs	1 serv	1270
Fettuccini Cajun Shrimp	1 full order	1200
Fettuccini Four Cheese	1 full order	1370
Fettuccini Jambalaya	1 full order	1360
Fettuccini Spicy Chicken & Spinach	1 full order	1330

FOOD	PORTION	CALS
Fries	1 serv	700
Garlic Toast w/ Garlic Margarine	1 slice	170
Garlic Twist Bread	1 basket	1080
Garlic Twist Bread	1 serv	540
Homestyle Macaroni	1 full order	1490
Italian Pizza Bread w/ Dip	1 serv	1000
Ketchup	1 serv (2 oz)	20
Lasagna Boston's	1 full order	820
Lasagna Mediterranean	1 full order	870
Lasagna Seafood	1 full order	970
Linguini Chicken & Mushroom	1 full order	1320
Mashed Potatoes	1 serv	240
Mexican Beef w/ Sour Cream	1 serv	970
Mini Tortellini	1 serv	490
Nachos	1 full order	1540
Nachos Beef	1 full order	1760
Nachos Chicken	1 full order	1630
NY Steak Sandwich w/ Fries	1 serv	1580
Penne Baked 3 Cheese	1 full order	990
Penne Italiano	1 full order	1160
Penne Pisa Pesto	1 full order	1270
Penne Roast Veggie	1 full order	900
Pizza Bread w/o Meat Sauce	1 serv	520
Plain Pasta w/ Alfredo Sauce	1 full order	1200
Plain Pasta w/ Creamy Tomato Sauce	1 full order	1070
Plain Pasta w/ Marinara Sauce	1 full order	870
Plain Pasta w/ Meatsauce	1 full order	910
Plain Pasta w/ Seafood Sauce	1 full order	1050
Plain Pasta w/ Spicy Tomato Sauce	1 full order	880
Plain Pasta w/ Tex Mex Sauce	1 full order	940
Potato Skins	1 full order	860
Quesadilla Chicken w/ Sour Cream	1 serv	770
Quesadilla Garden Veggie w/ Sour Cream	1 serv	750
Quesadilla Sundried Tomato w/ Sour Cream	1 serv	890
Shrimp Dinner w/ Fries	1 serv	1510
Shrimp Dinner w/ Garlic Mashed Potatoes	1 serv	1050
Shrimp Dinner w/ Spaghetti	1 serv	1180
Side Tossed Salad w/ House Dressing	1 serv	170
Sirloin Steak Dinner w/ Fries	1 serv	1910
Sirloin Steak Dinner w/ Garlic Mashed Potatoes	1 serv	1450

FOOD	PORTION	CALS
Sirloin Steak Dinner w/ Spaghetti	1 serv	1580
Smokey Mountain Spaghetti	1 full order	1860
Spaghetti w/ Meatsauce	1 serv	370
Spinach & Artichoke Dip w/ Tortilla Chips	1 serv	890
Steak & Shrimp Dinner w/ Fries	1 serv	1760
Steak & Shrimp Dinner w/ Garlic Mashed Potatoes	1 serv	1310
Steak & Shrimp Dinner w/ Spaghetti	1 serv	1430
The Ribber w/ Fries	1 serv	1470
The Ribber w/ Garlic Mashed Potatoes	1 serv	1010
The Ribber w/ Spaghetti	1 serv	1140
Tortellini w/ Alfredo Sauce	1 full order	1220
Tortellini w/ Creamy Tomato Sauce	1 full order	1370
Tortellini w/ Marinara Sauce	1 full order	1180
Tortellini w/ Meatsauce	1 full order	1500
Tortellini w/ Seafood Sauce	1 full order	1360
Tortellini w/ Spicy Tomato Sauce	1 full order	1180
Tortellini w/ Tex Mex Sauce	1 full order	1240
Veal Parmigan w/ Fries	1 serv	1550
Veal Parmigan w/ Garlic Mashed Potatoes	1 serv	1090
Veal Parmigan w/ Spaghetti	1 serv	1220
Wings BBQ Double Order	1 serv	1700
Wings BBQ Starter Size	1 serv	960
Wings Cajun Double Order	1 serv	1610
Wings Cajun Starter Size	1 serv	910
Wings Honey Garlic Double Order	1 serv	1720
Wings Honey Garlic Starter Size	1 serv	970
Wings Screamin' Hot Double Order	1 serv	1630
Wings Screamin' Hot Starter Size	1 serv	920
Wings Teriyaki Double Order	1 serv	1690
Wings Teriyaki Starter Size	1 serv	950
Wings Thai Double Order	1 serv	1870
Wings Thai Starter Size	1 serv	1040
PIZZA		
Bacon Double Cheeseburger Individual	1 pie	1210
Bacon Double Cheeseburger Large	1 slice	350
Bacon Double Cheeseburger Medium	1 slice	300
Boston Royal Individual	1 pie	770
Boston Royal Large	1 slice	230
Boston Royal Medium	1 slice	200

FOOD	PORTION	CALS
Cajun Chicken Individual	1 pie	780
Cajun Chicken Large	1 slice	250
Cajun Chicken Medium	1 slice	200
Californian Individual	1 pie	580
Californian Large	1 slice	190
Californian Medium	1 slice	160
Four Cheese Individual	1 pie	800
Four Cheese Large	1 slice	260
Four Cheese Medium	1 slice	240
Great White Individual	1 pie	880
Great White Large	1 slice	260
Great White Medium	1 slice	220
Hawaiian Individual	1 pie	690
Hawaiian Large	1 slice	220
Hawaiian Medium	1 slice	180
Meat Lovers Individual	1 pie	1120
Meat Lovers Large	1 slice	330
Meat Lovers Medium	1 slice	280
Pepperoni Individual	1 pie	760
Pepperoni Large	1 slice	240
Pepperoni Medium	1 slice	200
Pepperoni & Mushroom Individual	1 pie	760
Pepperoni & Mushroom Large	1 slice	250
Pepperoni & Mushroom Medium	1 slice	200
Perogy Individual	1 pie	1010
Perogy Large	1 slice	330
Perogy Medium	1 slice	280
Popeye Individual	1 pie	730
Popeye Large	1 slice	240
Popeye Medium	1 slice	200
Rustic Italian Individual	1 pie	940
Rustic Italian Large	1 slice	310
Rustic Italian Medium	1 slice	250
Sante Fe Chicken Individual	1 pie	800
Sante Fe Chicken Large	1 slice	260
Sante Fe Chicken Medium	1 slice	220
Super Veggie Individual	1 pie	850
Super Veggie Large	1 slice	280
Super Veggie Medium	1 slice	230
Thai Chicken Individual	1 pie	870

FOOD	PORTION	CALS
Thai Chicken Large	1 slice	280
Thai Chicken Medium	1 slice	240
The Basic Individual	1 pie	620
The Basic Large	1 slice	200
The Basic Medium	1 slice	160
The Deluxe Individual	1 pie	780
The Deluxe Large	1 slice	240
The Deluxe Medium	1 slice	190
Tropical Chicken Individual	1 pie	1060
Tropical Chicken Large	1 slice	340
Tropical Chicken Medium	1 slice	280
Tuscan Individual	1 pie	900
Tuscan Large	1 slice	290
Tuscan Medium	1 slice	240
Vegetarian Individual	1 pie	670
Vegetarian Large	1 slice	220
Vegetarian Medium	1 slice	170
Zorba The Greek Individual	1 pie	810
Zorba The Greek Large	1 slice	270
Zorba The Greek Medium	1 slice	220
SALADS		
Boston's Cobb Salad	1 serv	1100
Caesar Salad	1 reg	260
Caesar Salad Meal Sized	1 serv	690
Greek Salad	1 serv	500
Greek Salad Meal Sized	1 serv	1110
House Dressing	1 serv (2 oz)	136
Spinach Salad	1 serv	190
Spinach Salad Meal Sized	1 serv	500
Taco Salad Beef w/ Sour Cream & Salsa	1 serv	640
Taco Salad Chicken w/ Sour Cream & Salsa	1 serv	520
Thai Chicken Salad	1 serv	730
Tossed Garden Greens w/ House Dressing	1 serv	170
Veggie Plate w/ Low Fat Ranch Dressing	1 serv	180
SANDWICHES		
BBQ Beef w/ Fries	1 serv	1580
Beef Dip w/ Fries & Au Jus	1 serv	1560
Boston Cheesesteak w/ Fries & Au Jus	1 serv	1790
Boston Brute w/ Fries	1 serv	1420
Buffalo Chicken w/ Fries	1 serv	1720

FOOD	PORTION	CALS
Chicken Foccacia w/ Fries	1 serv	1350
Spicy Italian Sausage w/ Caesar Salad	1 serv	1070
Stromboli Chicken w/ Caesar Salad	1 serv	1020
Stromboli Perogy w/ Caesar Salad	1 serv	1120
Stromboli Sante Fe w/ Caesar Salad	1 serv	1000
Super Ham & Cheese w/ Fries	1 serv	1370
Tango Chicken Wrap w/ Caesar Salad	1 serv	740

BREWSTER'S COFFEE

FOOD	PORTION	CALS
Americano	1 serv (16 oz)	12
Black Forest Coffee	1 serv (16 oz)	198
Cafe Caramello	1 serv (16 oz)	212
Cappuccino 2% Milk	1 serv (16 oz)	195
Cappuccino Fat Free Milk	1 serv (16 oz)	133
Italiano 2% Milk	1 serv (16 oz)	131
Italiano Fat Free Milk	1 serv (16 oz)	89
Jittery Monkey 2% Milk	1 serv (16 oz)	482
Jittery Monkey Fat Free Milk	1 serv (16 oz)	429
Latte 2% Milk	1 serv (16 oz)	212
Latte Cinnamon Toast 2% Milk	1 serv	299
Latte Cinnamon Toast Fat Free Milk	1 serv (16 oz)	240
Latte Creme Caramel 2% Milk	1 serv (16 oz)	303
Latte Creme Caramel Fat Free Milk	1 serv (16 oz)	244
Latte Fat Free Milk	1 serv (16 oz)	145
Latte Oregon Chai Tea 2% Milk	1 serv (16 oz)	274
Latte Oregon Chai Tea Fat Free Milk	1 serv (16 oz)	231
Latte Raspberry Cheesecake 2% Milk	1 serv (16 oz)	319
Latte Raspberry Cheesecake Fat Free Milk	1 serv (16 oz)	259
Mocha w/ Whipped Cream 2% Milk	1 serv (16 oz)	454
Mocha w/ Whipped Cream Fat Free Milk	1 serv (16 oz)	392

BRUEGGER'S BAGELS
BAGELS

FOOD	PORTION	CALS
Blueberry	1	330
Chocolate Chip	1	310
Cinnamon Raisin	1	320
Cinnamon Sugar	1	340
Everything	1	310
Garlic	1	310
Honey Grain	1	330
Jalapeno Bagel	1	310

FOOD	PORTION	CALS
Onion	1	310
Orange Cranberry	1	330
Plain	1	300
Poppy Seed	1	310
Pumpernickel	1	320
Rosemary Olive Oil	1	350
Salt	1	300
Sesame	1	320
Sun Dried Tomato	1	320
DESSERTS		
Blondies	1	370
Brownie Chocolate Chunk	1	330
Brownie Mint	1	300
Bruegger Bar	1	420
Cappuccino Bar	1	420
Luscious Lemon Bar	1	350
Oatmeal Cranberry Mountains	1	430
Raspberry Sammies	1	270
SANDWICH FILLINGS		
Atlantic Smoked Salmon	2 oz	90
Cream Cheese Bacon Scallion	2 tbsp	100
Cream Cheese Chive	2 tbsp	100
Cream Cheese Garden Veggie	2 tbsp	90
Cream Cheese Garden Veggie Light	2 tbsp	60
Cream Cheese Herb Garlic Light	2 tbsp	70
Cream Cheese Honey Walnut	2 tbsp	110
Cream Cheese Jalapeno	2 tbsp	100
Cream Cheese Light Strawberry	2 tbsp	70
Cream Cheese Olive Pimento	2 tbsp	100
Cream Cheese Plain	2 tbsp	90
Cream Cheese Plain Light	2 tbsp	70
Cream Cheese Smoked Salmon	2 tbsp	100
Cream Cheese Wildberry	2 tbsp	100
Hummus	2 tbsp	60
Tuna Salad	1 serv (2.5 oz)	180
SANDWICHES		
Atlantic Smoked Salmon	1	470
Chicken Breast	1	440
Chicken Fajita	1	500
Chicken Salad w/ Mayo	1	460

FOOD	PORTION	CALS
Deli-Style Ham w/ Honey Mustard	1	440
Egg Cheese	1	480
Egg Cheese Sausage	1	680
Egg Cheese Bacon	1	560
Egg Cheese Ham	1	520
Garden Veggie	1	390
Herby Turkey	1	530
Leonardo Da Veggie	1	460
Santa Fe Turkey	1	480
Turkey w/ Mayo	1	480

BURGER KING
BEVERAGES
Aquafina Water	1 bottle	0
Coffee Black	1 lg	10
Coffee Black	1 sm	0
Coke Classic	1 sm	160
Coke Classic	1 lg	330
Coke Classic frzn	1 sm	370
Diet Coke	1 sm	0
Dr Pepper	1 lg	410
Dr Pepper	1 sm	160
Milk 1%	1	100
Minute Maid Cherry frzn	1 sm	370
Minute Maid Orange Juice	1 serv	140
Shake Chocolate	1 sm	620
Shake Strawberry	1 sm	620
Shake Vanilla	1 sm	560
Sprite	1 lg	320
Sprite	1 sm	160

BREAKFAST SELECTIONS
Croissan'wich Bacon Egg & Cheese	1	360
Croissan'wich Egg & Cheese	1	320
Croissan'wich Ham Egg & Cheese	1	360
Croissan'wich Sausage Egg & Cheese	1	520
Croissan'wich w/ Sausage & Cheese	1	420
French Toast Sticks	5 pieces	390
Hash Browns	1 lg	390
Hash Browns	1 sm	230

FOOD	PORTION	CALS
Sourdough Breakfast Sandwich Bacon Egg & Cheese	1	380
Sourdough Breakfast Sandwich Ham Egg & Cheese	1	380
Sourdough Breakfast Sandwich Sausage Egg & Cheese	1	540
DESSERTS		
Chocolate Chip Cookies	2	440
Hershey Sundae Pie	1	300
MAIN MENU SELECTIONS		
Bacon Cheeseburger	1	400
Bacon Double Cheeseburger	1	580
Baguette Santa Fe Fire Grilled Chicken	1	350
Baguette Savory Mustard Fire Grilled Chicken	1	350
Baguette Smokey BBQ Fire Grilled Chicken	1	350
Baja BBQ Sauce	1 serv	14
BK Veggie Burger	1	340
Cheeseburger	1	360
Chicken Tenders	8 pieces	340
Chicken Tenders	5 pieces	210
Chili	1 serv	190
Dipping Sauce Sweet And Sour	1 serv	40
Double Cheeseburger	1	540
Double Hamburger	1	450
Double Whopper	1	980
Double Whopper w/ Cheese	1	1070
Dutch Apple Pie	1 serv	340
French Fries No Salt Added	1 lg	500
French Fries No Salt Added	1 sm	230
French Fries Salted	1 sm	230
French Fries Salted	1 lg	500
Hamburger	1	310
Onion Rings	1 sm	180
Onion Rings	1 lg	480
Sandwich BK Fish Filet	1	520
Sandwich Grilled Chicken Caesar Club	1	540
Sandwich Original Chicken	1	560
Sandwich Whopper	1	580
Whopper	1	710
Whopper Jr.	1	390
Whopper Jr. w/ Cheese	1	440

FOOD	PORTION	CALS
Whopper w/ Cheese	1	800
SALAD DRESSINGS AND TOPPINGS		
Breakfast Syrup	1 serv	80
Dipping Sauce Barbecue	1 serv	35
Dipping Sauce Honey	1 serv	90
Dipping Sauce Honey Mustard	1 serv	90
Dipping Sauce Ranch	1 serv	140
Dipping Sauce Zesty Onion Ring	1 serv	150
Dressing Kraft Catalina	1 serv	180
Dressing Kraft Fat Free Ranch	1 serv	60
Dressing Kraft Ranch	1 serv	220
Dressing Light Done Right Light Italian	1 serv	50
Dressing Signature Creamy Caesar	1 serv	140
Fire Roasted Sauce	1 serv	9
Grape Jam	1 serv	30
Peppers & Onions Flame Roasted	1 serv	18
Savory Mustard Sauce	1 serv	21
Strawberry Jam	1 serv	30
SALADS		
Chicken Caesar w/o Dressing And Croutons	1 serv	230
Side Salad w/o Dressing	1 serv	25

BURGERVILLE
BEVERAGES

FOOD	PORTION	CALS
Milkshake Black Forest	1 (16 oz)	600
Milkshake Blackberry	1 (16 oz)	610
Milkshake Caramel Apple	1 (16 oz)	540
Milkshake Chocolate	1 (16 oz)	520
Milkshake Fresh Strawberry	1 (16 oz)	560
Milkshake Mocha Perk	1 (16 oz)	590
Milkshake Pumpkin	1 (16 oz)	460
Milkshake Vanilla	1 (16 oz)	500
Smoothies Chocolate Monkey	1 (16 oz)	470
Smoothies Fresh Blackberry	1 (16 oz)	420
Smoothies Fresh Raspberry	1 (16 oz)	470
Smoothies Fresh Strawberry	1 (16 oz)	390
Smoothies Strawberry Splash	1 (16 oz)	310
Smoothies Triple Berry Blast	1 (16 oz)	360
BREAKFAST SELECTIONS		
American Cheese	2 slices	90

FOOD	PORTION	CALS
Bagel Bacon Egg	1	450
Bagel Cheese	1	290
Bagel Ham Egg	1	450
Bagel Plain	1	310
Bagel Sausage Egg	1	640
Biscuit Bacon Egg	1	400
Biscuit Ham Egg	1	400
Biscuit Sausage Egg	1	590
Tillamook Cheese	1 slice	120
MAIN MENU SELECTIONS		
Cheeseburger	1	370
Cheeseburger Double Beef	1	470
Cheeseburger Pepper Bacon	1	680
Cheeseburger Tillamook	1	630
Cheeseburger Walla Walla Onion	1	679
Chicken Strips	5 pieces	550
Colossal	1	530
French Fries	1 kid size	220
French Fries	1 reg	390
Gardenburger	1	460
Gardenburger Spicy Black Bean	1	550
Halibut	3 pieces	230
Hamburger	1	320
Onion Rings Walla Walla	3 pieces	485
Roasted Turkey Salad w/o Hazelnuts	1 serv	375
Rogue River Blue Cheese Bacon Burger	1	510
Sandwich Crispy Chicken	1	450
Sandwich Deluxe Crispy Chicken	1	610
Sandwich Grilled Chicken	1	350
Sandwich Halibut	1	490
Sandwich Turkey Club	1	490
Side Salad w/o Dressing	1 serv	70
Smoked Salmon Salad w/o Hazelnuts	1 serv	370
Sweet Potato Fries	1 serv	530
Turkey Burger	1	470
CAPTAIN D'S SEAFOOD		
Baked Chicken Dinner	1 serv	350
Baked Fish Dinner	1 serv	390
Baked Potato	1 serv	190

FOOD	PORTION	CALS
Baked Salmon Dinner	1 serv	470
Carb Counter Chicken Dinner	1 serv	320
Carb Counter Fish Dinner	1 serv	350
Cole Slaw	1 serv	150
Corn On The Cob	1 serv	150
Fresh Steamed Broccoli	1 serv	25
Green Beans	1 serv	90
Rice Pilaf	1 serv	160
Shrimp Scampi Dinner	1 serv	370
Side Salad w/o Dressing	1	30
Tuscan Style Vegetables	1 serv	30

CARIBOU COFFEE

FOOD	PORTION	CALS
Black Forest Mocha	1 med	553
Black Forest Wild Drink	1 med	553
Cappuccino	1 med (16 oz)	113
Cappuccino 2%	1 med (16 oz)	162
Caramel Hirise	1 med (16 oz)	414
Chai Latte 2%	1 med (16 oz)	286
Chai Skim	1 med (16 oz)	236
Cooler Caramel	1 med (12 oz)	450
Cooler Chocolate	1 med (12 oz)	257
Cooler Coffee	1 med (16 oz)	230
Cooler Espresso	1 med (16 oz)	193
Cooler Mint Oreo	1 med (12 oz)	614
Cooler Vanilla	1 med (16 oz)	257
Glacier Gum	2 pieces	5
Hot Apple Blast	1 med	379
Latte 2%	1 med (16 oz)	171
Latte Skim	1 med (16 oz)	121
Latte Skinny Bou Low Cal	1 med	120
Lite White Berry	1 med (16 oz)	311
Mint Condition	1 med (16 oz)	520
Mints All Flavors	3 pieces	5
Mocha 2%	1 med (16 oz)	347
Mocha Skim	1 med (16 oz)	302
Mocha Turtle	1 med (16 oz)	559
Smoothie Passion Green Tea	1 med (16 oz)	252
Smoothie Raspberry	1 med (12 oz)	293
Smoothie Strawberry Banana	1 med (16 oz)	253
Smoothie Wild Berry	1 med (16 oz)	235

FOOD	PORTION	CALS
CARL'S JR.		
BAKED SELECTIONS		
Cheese Danish	1	400
Cheesecake Strawberry Swirl	1 serv	290
Chocolate Cake	1 serv	300
Chocolate Chip Cookie	1	350
Muffin Blueberry	1	340
Muffin Bran Raisin	1	370
BEVERAGES		
Coca-Cola Classic	1 reg (21 oz)	220
Coffee	1 reg (12 oz)	2
Diet Coke	1 reg (21 oz)	tr
Dr. Pepper	1 reg (21 oz)	200
Hot Chocolate	1 serv (12 oz)	120
Iced Tea	1 reg (12 oz)	5
Lemonade Minute Maid Orange	1 reg (21 oz)	200
Milk 1%	1 (10 fl oz)	150
Minute Maid Orange Soda	1 reg (21 oz)	200
Nestea Raspberry	1 reg (21 oz)	160
Orange Juice	1 (10 oz)	150
Ramblin' Root Beer	1 reg (21 oz)	220
Shake Chocolate	1 reg (32 oz)	770
Shake Strawberry	1 reg (32 oz)	750
Shake Vanilla	1 reg (32 oz)	700
Sprite	1 reg (21 oz)	200
BREAKFAST SELECTIONS		
Bacon	2 strips	45
Breakfast Burrito	1	560
Breakfast Quesadilla	1	370
English Muffin w/ Margarine	1	210
French Toast Dips w/o Syrup	1 serv	370
Grape Jelly	1 serv (0.5 oz)	40
Hash Brown Nuggets	1 serv	330
Sausage	1 patty	190
Scrambed Eggs	1 serv	180
Sourdough Breakfast	1 serv	410
Strawberry Jam	1 serv (0.5 oz)	40
Sunrise Sandwich w/o Meat	1	360
Table Syrup	1 serv (1 oz)	90

FOOD	PORTION	CALS
MAIN MENU SELECTIONS		
American Cheese	1 sm	50
BBQ Sauce	1 serv (1.1 oz)	50
Breadstick	1 (0.3 oz)	35
Carl's Famous Star	1	590
Chicken Stars	6 pieces	260
CrissCut Fries	1 serv	410
Croutons	1 serv (0.5 oz)	30
Double Sourdough Bacon Cheeseburger	1	880
Double Western Bacon Cheeseburger	1	920
Famous Bacon Cheeseburger	1	700
French Fries	1 med	460
French Fries	1 kid size	250
Hamburger	1	280
Honey Sauce	1 serv (1 oz)	90
Mustard Sauce	1 serv (1 oz)	50
Onion Rings	1 serv	430
Potato Bacon & Cheese	1	640
Potato Broccoli & Cheese	1 serv	530
Potato Plain w/o Margarine	1	290
Potato Sour Cream & Chives	1	430
Salsa	1 serv (0.9 oz)	10
Sandwich Bacon Swiss Crispy Chicken	1	760
Sandwich Carl's Catch Fish	1	530
Sandwich Charbroiled Sirloin Steak	1	550
Sandwich Chargrilled Chicken Club	1	470
Sandwich Chargrilled Santa Fe Chicken	1	540
Sandwich Chargrilled BBQ Chicken	1	290
Sandwich Ranch Crispy Chicken	1	660
Sandwich Southwest Spicy Chicken	1	620
Sandwich Spicy Chicken	1	480
Sandwich Western Bacon Crispy Chicken	1	750
Sourdough Bacon Cheeseburger	1	640
Sourdough Ranch Bacon Cheeseburger	1	720
Super Star	1	790
Sweet N'Sour Sauce	1 serv (1 oz)	50
Swiss Cheese	1 serv	50
Western Bacon Cheeseburger	1	660
Zucchini	1 serv	320

FOOD	PORTION	CALS
SALAD DRESSINGS		
1000 Island	1 serv (2 oz)	230
Blue Cheese	1 serv (2 oz)	320
French Fat Free	1 serv (2 oz)	60
House	1 serv (2 oz)	220
Italian Fat Free	1 serv (2 oz)	15
SALADS		
Salad-To-Go Charbroiled Chicken	1 serv	200
Salad-To-Go Garden	1	50
CARVEL		
BEVERAGES		
Carvelanche w/ Topping	1 (16 oz)	600
Regular Fizzlers	1 (16 oz)	340
Thick Shake Chocolate	1 (16 oz)	720
Thick Shake Reduced Fat Chocolate	1 (16 oz)	520
Thick Shake Reduced Fat Vanilla	1 (16 oz)	460
ICE CREAM		
Cake Butterscotch Dream	1 slice (4 oz)	260
Cake Celebration	1 slice (4 oz)	200
Cake Cookies & Cream	1 serv (4 oz)	240
Cake Fudge Drizzle	1 slice (4 oz)	240
Cake Game Ball	1 slice (4 oz)	330
Cake Holiday	1 slice (4 oz)	200
Cake Lil'Love	1 piece (4 oz)	200
Cake Lil'Love All Vanilla	1 piece (4.4 oz)	330
Cake Sinfully Chocolate	1 slice (4 oz)	240
Cake Strawberries & Cream	1 slice (4 oz)	270
Chocolate	4 oz	190
Chocolate No Fat	4 oz	120
Flying Saucer 98% Fat Free Black Raspberry	1	170
Flying Saucer 98% Fat Free Chocolate	1	170
Flying Saucer 98% Fat Free Coffee	1	190
Flying Saucer 98% Fat Free Maple	1	190
Flying Saucer 98% Fat Free Mint	1	190
Flying Saucer 98% Fat Free Pistachio	1	190
Flying Saucer 98% Fat Free Strawberry	1	190
Flying Saucer 98% Fat Free Vanilla	1	190
Flying Saucer Chocolate	1	230
Flying Saucer Vanilla	1	240

FOOD	PORTION	CALS
Vanilla	4 oz	200
Vanilla No Fat	4 oz	120
Vanilla No Sugar Added	4 oz	130
ICES		
Italian Ice Blue Raspberry	4 oz	70
Italian Ice Bubble Gum	4 oz	70
Italian Ice Cherry	4 oz	100
Italian Ice Chocolate Ice Cream	4 oz	90
Italian Ice Cotton Candy	4 oz	70
Italian Ice Lemon	4 oz	70
Italian Ice Mango	4 oz	70
Italian Ice Orange	4 oz	70
Italian Ice Vanilla Ice Cream	4 oz	90
Italian Ice Watermelon	4 oz	70
Sherbet All Flavors	4 oz	140

CHICKEN OUT ROTISSERIE

MAIN MENU SELECTIONS

Apple Cornbread Stuffing	1 serv (6 oz)	215
Baked Potato Wedges	1 serv (6 oz)	110
Biscuit	1	150
Chicken Breast Skinless	1 serv (6 oz)	210
Chicken Burger w/o Cheese	1	285
Chunky Cinnamon Applesauce	1 serv (6 oz)	60
Creamed Spinach w/ Artichokes	1 serv (6 oz)	160
Farm Fresh Cole Slaw	1 serv (6 oz)	55
French Baguette	1	80
Fresh Fruit Salad	1 serv (6 oz)	77
Mandarin Walnut Cranberry Relish	1 serv (6 oz)	240
Mashed Sweet Potatoes	1 serv (6 oz)	120
Oriental Green Beans	1 serv (6 oz)	34
Pulled White Meat	1 serv (6 oz)	180
Real Cheese & Macaroni	1 serv (6 oz)	311
Red Skin Mashed Potatoes	1 serv (6 oz)	181
Rice Pilaf	1 serv (6 oz)	140
Roasted Peas Corn & Carrots	1 serv (6 oz)	120
Rotisserie Chicken Quarter Dark No Skin	1 serv	232
Rotisserie Chicken Quarter White No Skin	1 serv	196

FOOD	PORTION	CALS
Sandwich BBQ Pulled Chicken	1	406
Sandwich Grilled Chicken Breast	1	350
Sandwich Open Faced Pulled Chicken	1	682
Sandwich Pulled Chicken	1	320
Sandwich Signature Chicken Salad	1	370
Steamed Broccoli & Carrots	1 serv (6 oz)	30
Vegetarian Baked Beans	1 serv (6 oz)	150
Wrap Chinese Chicken Salad w/o Dressing	1	330
Wrap Fajita	1	360
Wrap Fresh Vegetable Salad w/o Dressing	1	170
Wrap Grilled Chicken Caesar	1	355
Wrap Pesto Chicken	1	405
Wrap Pulled Chicken	1	300
Wrap Skinless Grilled Chicken	1	330
SALAD DRESSINGS		
Balsamic Vinaigrette	1 oz	18
Caesar	1 oz	55
Chinese	1 oz	72
Low Fat Honey Mustard	1 oz	23
Ranch	1 oz	90
Southwestern	1 oz	85
SALADS		
Caesar w/ Grilled Chicken w/o Dressing	½ serv	235
Caesar w/o Dressing	½ serv	140
Chicken Salad Apricot	1 serv (6 oz)	300
Chicken Salad BBQ Pulled	1 serv (6 oz)	263
Chicken Salad Chinese w/o Dressing	½ serv	210
Chicken Salad Pesto	1 serv (6 oz)	285
Chicken Salad Pulled w/o Dressing	½ serv	204
Chicken Salad Santa Fe w/o Dressing	½ serv	240
Chicken Salad Signature	1 serv (6 oz)	230
Garden w/ Grilled Chicken w/o Dressing	½ serv	200
Garden w/o Dressing	½ serv	25
Young Spinach w/ Grilled Chicken w/o Dressing	½ serv	270
Young Spinach w/o Dressing	½ serv	180
SOUPS		
Chicken Noodle	1 serv (6 oz)	130
Vegetable Minestrone	1 serv (6 oz)	96

FOOD	PORTION	CALS
CHICK-FIL-A		
BEVERAGES		
Coca-Cola Classic	1 sm	110
Diet Coke	1 sm	0
Diet Lemonade	1 sm	25
Ice Tea Sweetened	1 sm	80
Ice Tea Unsweetened	1 sm	0
Lemonade	1 sm	170
BREAKFAST SELECTIONS		
Bagel Chicken Egg & Cheese	1	500
Bagel Wheat	1	220
Biscuit Bacon	1	300
Biscuit Bacon & Egg	1	390
Biscuit Bacon Egg Cheese	1	440
Biscuit Buttered	1	270
Biscuit Chicken	1	420
Biscuit Chicken w/ Cheese	1	470
Biscuit Egg	1	350
Biscuit Egg Cheese	1	400
Biscuit Sausage	1	410
Biscuit Sausage Egg	1	500
Biscuit Sausage Egg Cheese	1	550
Biscuit w/ Gravy	1	330
Burrito Chicken	1	420
Burrito Sausage	1	460
Chick-N-Minis	1 serv	270
Hashbrowns	1 serv	260
DESSERTS		
Cheesecake	1 slice	340
Fudge Nut Brownie	1	330
Icedream Cone	1 sm	160
Lemon Pie	1 slice	390
MAIN MENU SELECTIONS		
Carrot & Raisin Salad	1 sm	170
Chicken Filet	1	230
Chicken Filet Chargrilled	1	100
Chick-N-Strips	4	290
Cole Slaw	1 sm	260
Cool Wrap Chargrilled Chicken	1	390
Cool Wrap Chicken Caesar	1	460

FOOD	PORTION	CALS
Cool Wrap Spicy Chicken	1	380
Fruit Cup	1 serv	60
Hearty Breast of Chicken Soup	1 cup	140
Nuggets	8	260
Polynesian Sauce	1 pkg	110
Sandwich Chargrilled Chicken	1	270
Sandwich Chicken	1	410
Sandwich Chicken Deluxe	1	420
Sandwich Chicken Salad On Wheat Bread	1	350
Waffle Fries w/o Salt	1 sm	280
Waffle Potato Fries	1 sm	270
SALAD DRESSINGS AND SAUCES		
Barbecue Sauce	1 pkg	45
Blue Cheese	2 tbsp	150
Buffalo Sauce	1 pkg	15
Buttermilk Ranch	2 tbsp	160
Buttermilk Ranch Sauce	1 pkg	110
Caesar	2 tbsp	160
Fat Free Honey Mustard	2 tbsp	60
Honey Mustard	1 pkg	45
Honey Roasted BBQ Sauce	1 pkg	60
Light Italian	2 tbsp	15
Raspberry Vinaigrette Reduced Fat	2 tbsp	80
Spicy	2 tbsp	140
Thousand Island	2 tbsp	150
SALADS		
Chargrilled Chicken Garden Salad	1 serv	180
Chick-N-Strips Salad	1 serv	390
Croutons Garlic & Butter	1 pkg	50
Honey Roasted Sunflower Kernels	1 pkg	80
Side Salad	1 serv	60
Southwest Chargrilled Salad	1 serv	240
Tortilla Strips	1 pkg	70

CHILI'S
CHILDREN'S MENU SELECTIONS

Corn Dog	1	250
Grilled Chicken Platter	1 serv	140
Little Chicken Crispers	1 serv	590
Little Mouth Burger	1 serv	280

FOOD	PORTION	CALS
Little Mouth Cheeseburger	1 serv	350
Macaroni & Cheese	1 serv	510
Pepper Pal Pasta w/ Alfredo	1 serv	410
Pepper Pal Pasta w/ Marinara	1 serv	290
Pizza	1	570
Rib Basket	1 serv	370
Sandwich Grilled Cheese	1 serv	420
Sandwich Grilled Chicken	1 serv	140
DESSERTS		
Cheesecake	1 serv	760
Chocolate Chip Paradise Pie w/ Vanilla Ice Cream	1 serv	1600
Frosty Chocolate Shake w/ Chocolate Sprinkles	1 serv	850
Molten Chocolate Cake w/ Vanilla Ice Cream	1 serv	1270
MAIN MENU SELECTIONS		
Awesome Blossom	1 serv	2710
Baby Back Ribs & Chicken	1 serv	1460
Black Bean Burger	1 serv	650
Boneless Buffalo Wings	1 serv	1250
Boneless Shangai Wings	1 serv	1260
Bottomless Tostada Chips	1 basket	400
Burger Bacon	1 serv	1080
Burger BBQ Ranch	1 serv	1110
Burger Chipotle Bleu Cheese Bacon	1 serv	1090
Burger Ground Peppercorn	1 serv	1050
Burger Mushroom Swiss	1 serv	1100
Burger Oldtimer	1 serv	800
Chicken Crispers	1 serv	1870
Cinnamon Apples	1 serv	210
Citrus Fire Chicken & Shrimp	1 serv	760
Classic Nachos	1 serv	1570
Country Fried Steak	1 serv	1890
Fried Cheese w/ Marinara Sauce	1 serv	1210
Garlic Toast	1 piece	200
Grilled Baby Back Ribs	1 serv	1370
Grilled Salmon w/ Garlic & Herbs	1 serv	700
Guiltless Grill Chicken Pita	1 serv	550
Guiltless Grill Chicken Platter	1 serv	580
Guiltless Grill Chicken Sandwich	1 serv	490
Guiltless Grill Salmon	1 serv	480

FOOD	PORTION	CALS
Guiltless Grill Tomato Basil Pasta	1 serv	650
Homestyle Fries	1 serv	520
Kettle Black Beans	1 serv	140
Loaded Mashed Potatoes	1 serv	560
Margarita Grilled Chicken	1 serv	690
Monterey Chicken	1 serv	1170
Pasta Cajun Chicken	1 serv	1460
Pasta Grilled Shrimp Alfredo	1 serv	1340
Pasta Tomato Basil Chicken	1 serv	860
Pita Chicken Caesar	1 serv	650
Pita Chicken Fajita	1 serv	450
Pita Steak Fajita	1 serv	580
Quesadillas Fajita Chicken	1 serv	1720
Quesadillas Fajita Combo	1 serv	1840
Quesadillas Fajita Steak	1 serv	1970
Ribeye Cajun	1 serv	870
Ribeye Flame Grilled	1 serv	960
Rice	1 serv	210
Sandwich Cajun Chicken	1 serv	820
Sandwich Chicken Ranch	1 serv	1150
Sandwich Chili's Cheesesteak	1 serv	1010
Sandwich Grilled Chicken	1 serv	840
Sandwich Smoked Turkey	1 serv	930
Sauteed Mushrooms Onions & Bell Peppers	1 serv	120
Seasonal Grilled Veggies	1 serv	90
Seasonal Steamed Veggie w/ Parmesan Cheese	1 serv	60
Sirloin Chili's Classic	1 serv	530
Sirloin Honey BBQ	1 serv	800
Skillet Queso	1 serv	670
Southwestern Eggrolls	1 serv	810
Steamed Broccoli	1 serv	80
Sweet Corn On The Cob	1 serv	180
Triple Play	1 serv	2330
Wings Over Buffalo	1 serv	1140
SALAD DRESSINGS AND SAUCES		
Dressing Asian Sesame Ginger	1 serv (2 oz)	250
Dressing Avocado Ranch	1 serv (2 oz)	150
Dressing Bleu Cheese	1 serv (2 oz)	330
Dressing Caesar	1 serv (2 oz)	350

FOOD	PORTION	CALS
Dressing Chipotle Ranch	1 serv (2 oz)	170
Dressing Citrus Balsamic Vinaigrette	1 serv (2 oz)	350
Dressing Creamy Cilantro	1 serv (2 oz)	300
Dressing Honey Lime	1 serv (2 oz)	270
Dressing Honey Mustard	1 serv (2 oz)	260
Dressing Low Fat Ranch	1 serv (2 oz)	110
Dressing No Fat Balsamic Vinaigrette	1 serv (2 oz)	50
Dressing No Fat Honey Mustard	1 serv (2 oz)	90
Dressing Ranch	1 serv (2 oz)	240
Dressing Thousand Island	1 serv (2 oz)	270
Sauce Peanut Dipping	1 serv (2 oz)	190
Sauce Picante Salsa	1 serv (2 oz)	40
Sauce Sesame Dipping	1 serv (2 oz)	70
SALADS		
Boneless Buffalo Chicken	1 serv	870
Chicken Caesar w/ Dressing	1 serv	1010
Crispy Chicken	1 serv	810
Dinner Caesar w/ Dressing	1 serv	430
Dinner House	1 serv	140
Grilled Caribbean	1 serv	440
Lettuce Wraps	1 serv	330
Lime Grilled Shrimp Caesar w/ Dressing	1 serv	980
Quesadilla Explosion	1 serv	850
Southwestern Cobb	1 serv	650
SOUPS		
Broccoli Cheese	1 cup	160
Chicken Enchilada	1 cup	220
Chicken Noodle	1 cup	50
Chicken Tortilla	1 cup	140
Chili w/ Cheese	1 cup	500
New England Clam Chowder	1 cup	470
Potato	1 cup	220
Southwestern Vegetable	1 cup	110
CHIPOTLE		
Barbacoa	1 serv (5 oz)	285
Black Beans	1 serv (4 oz)	130
Carnitas	1 serv (4 oz)	227
Cheese	1 serv (1 oz)	110

FOOD	PORTION	CALS
Chicken	1 serv (4 oz)	219
Chips	1 serv (4 oz)	490
Crispy Taco Shells	4	240
Fajita Vegetables	1 serv (3 oz)	100
Flour Tortilla	1 (13 inch)	340
Flour Tortilla	1 (6 inch)	300
Guacamole	1 serv (4 oz)	170
Lettuce	1 serv (1 oz)	5
Pinto Beans	1 serv (4 oz)	138
Rice	1 serv (5 oz)	240
Salsa Corn	1 serv (4 oz)	100
Salsa Tomato	1 serv (4 oz)	25
Sour Cream	1 serv (2 oz)	120
Steak	1 serv (4 oz)	230
Tomatillo Green	1 serv (2 oz)	15
Tomatillo Red	1 serv (2 oz)	28

CHURCH'S CHICKEN
DESSERTS

Apple Pie	1 pie	280
Edward's Double Lemon Pie	1 pie	300
Edward's Strawberry Cream Cheese Pie	1 pie	280

MAIN MENU SELECTIONS

Breast	1 serv	200
Cajun Rice	1 reg	130
Chicken Fried Steak w/ White Gravy	1 serv	470
Cole Slaw	1 reg	92
Collard Greens	1 reg	25
Corn On The Cob	1 ear	139
French Fries	1 reg	210
Honey Butter Biscuit	1	250
Jalapeno Cheese Bombers	4 pieces	240
Krispy Tender Strips	1 piece	137
Leg	1 serv	140
Macaroni & Cheese	1 reg	210
Mashed Potatoes & Gravy	1 reg	90
Okra	1 reg	210
Sweet Corn Nuggets	1 reg	250
Tender Crunchers	6-8 pieces	411

FOOD	PORTION	CALS
Thigh	1 serv	230
Whole Jalapeno Peppers	2	10
Wing	1 serv	250
SAUCES		
BBQ	1 pkg	29
Creamy Jalapeno	1 pkg	102
Honey Mustard	1 pkg	111
Purple Pepper	1 pkg	21
Sweet & Sour	1 pkg	31

CINNABON

Caramel Pecanbon	1	890
Cinnabon	1 reg	670

COLD STONE CREAMERY

Waffle Cone Dipped	1	310
Waffle Cone Dipped w/ Candy	1	390
Waffle Cone Or Bowl	1	160
FROZEN YOGURT		
Cheesecake	1 serv (6 oz)	170
Low Fat Chocolate	1 serv (6 oz)	230
Nonfat Coffee	1 serv (6 oz)	220
Nonfat Sweet Cream	1 serv (6 oz)	220
ICE CREAM		
Amaretto	1 serv (6 oz)	390
Banana	1 serv (6 oz)	370
Black Cherry	1 serv (6 oz)	390
Butter Pecan	1 serv (6 oz)	390
Cake A Cheesecake Named Desire	1 slice (5 oz)	410
Cake Butterfinger Bonanza	1 slice (5 oz)	450
Cake Celebration Sensation	1 slice (4.5 oz)	350
Cake Chocolate Chipper	1 slice (4.6 oz)	450
Cake Coffeehouse Crunch	1 slice (5 oz)	530
Cake Cookie Dough Delirium	1 slice (4.8 oz)	420
Cake Cookies & Creamery	1 slice (4.5 oz)	390
Cake Midnight Delight	1 slice (5.3 oz)	510
Cake MMMMMM Chip	1 slice (4.5 oz)	380
Cake Peanut Butter Playground	1 slice (5 oz)	490
Cake Raspberry Truffle Temptation	1 slice (5 oz)	480
Cake Snicker's Supreme	1 slice (5 oz)	510
Cake Strawberry Passion	1 slice (5 oz)	380

FOOD	PORTION	CALS
Cake Zebra Stripes	1 slice (4.8 oz)	400
Cake Batter	1 serv (6 oz)	410
Candy Cane	1 serv (6 oz)	420
Caramel Latte	1 serv (6 oz)	400
Carrot Cake Batter	1 serv (6 oz)	450
Cheesecake	1 serv (6 oz)	390
Chocolate	1 serv (6 oz)	390
Cinnamon	1 serv (6 oz)	400
Coconut	1 serv (6 oz)	390
Coffee	1 serv (6 oz)	400
Cookie Batter	1 serv (6 oz)	450
Cotton Candy	1 serv (6 oz)	390
Dark Chocolate Peppermint	1 serv (6 oz)	410
Egg Nog	1 serv (6 oz)	400
Expresso	1 serv (6 oz)	350
French Vanilla	1 serv (6 oz)	400
Irish Cream	1 serv (6 oz)	390
Macadamia Nut	1 serv (6 oz)	390
Mango	1 serv (6 oz)	370
Mint	1 serv (6 oz)	400
Mocha	1 serv (6 oz)	390
Oatmeal Batter	1 serv (6 oz)	400
Orange Dreamsicle	1 serv (6 oz)	380
Peanut Butter	1 serv (6 oz)	440
Pecan Praline	1 serv (6 oz)	400
Pistachio	1 serv (6 oz)	390
Pumpkin	1 serv (6 oz)	390
Raspberry	1 serv	390
Sinless Sans Fat Sweet Cream	1 serv (6 oz)	160
Strawberry	1 serv (6 oz)	380
Sweet Cream	1 serv (6 oz)	390
Vanilla Bean	1 serv (6 oz)	400
White Chocolate	1 serv (6 oz)	390
MIX-INS AND TOPPINGS		
Almond Joy	1 piece	180
Apple Pie Filling	¾ oz	60
Banana	½	60
Black Cherries	¾ oz	80
Blackberries	¾ oz	10
Blueberries	¾ oz	10

FOOD	PORTION	CALS
Brownies	1 piece	180
Butterfinger	½ bar	140
Caramel Topping	1 oz	110
Cashews	1 oz	170
Chocolate Chips	1 oz	130
Cinnamon	⅛ tsp	15
Coconut	1 oz	80
Cookie Dough	1 piece	180
Fat Free Butterscotch	1 oz	80
Fat Free Caramel	1 oz	80
Fat Free Fudge	1 oz	80
Fudge Topping	1 oz	110
Granola	1 oz	120
Gumballs	1 oz	120
Gummi Bears	1 oz	120
Heath Candy	1 bar	110
Honey	1 oz	90
Kit Kat	½ bar	100
Krackel Candy	½ bar	130
M&M's	1 oz	170
M&M's Peanut	1 oz	150
Macadamia Nuts	1 oz	180
Maraschino Cherry	1	5
Marshmallow Creme	1 oz	100
Marshmallows	1 oz	100
Nestle Crunch	½ bar	130
Nilla Wafers	3	70
Oreo Cookies	2	120
Peach Pie Filling	1 oz	60
Peanut Butter	¾ oz	150
Peanuts	1 oz	200
Pecan Pralines	1 oz	210
Pecans	1 oz	140
Pie Crust Graham Cracker	1 oz	110
Pie Crust Oreo	1 oz	180
Pistachio Nuts	1 oz	210
Raisins	1 oz	80
Raspberries	¾ oz	15
Red Hot Candy	1 oz	130
Reese's Peanut Butter Cup	1 piece	190

FOOD	PORTION	CALS
Reese's Pieces	1 oz	170
Roasted Almonds	1 oz	190
Sliced Almonds	1 oz	210
Snickers	½ bar	170
Sprinkles Chocolate	1 oz	25
Sprinkles Rainbow	1 oz	25
Strawberries	¾ oz	20
Toasted Coconut	1 oz	180
Walnuts	1 oz	130
Whip Topping	1 serv	50
White Chocolate Chips	1 oz	160
Whoppers	1 oz	100
Yellow Sponge Cake	1 piece	70
York Peppermint Patties	2 pieces	120
SORBET		
Sinless Lemon	1 serv	180
Sinless Raspberry	1 serv (6 oz)	200
Sinless Tangerine	1 serv (6 oz)	200

COLOMBO FROZEN YOGURT
Strawberry Lowfat	½ cup	110
Strawberry Nonfat	½ cup	100

DAIRY QUEEN
FOOD SELECTIONS
Chicken Breast Fillet Sandwich	1 (6.7 oz)	430
Chicken Strip Basket	1 serv (14.5 oz)	1000
Chili 'n' Cheese Dog	1 (5 oz)	330
DQ Homestyle Bacon Double Cheeseburger	1 (8.9 oz)	610
DQ Homestyle Cheeseburger	1 (5.3 oz)	340
DQ Homestyle Double Cheeseburger	1 (7.7 oz)	540
DQ Homestyle Hamburger	1 (4.8 oz)	290
DQ Ultimate Burger	1 (9.4 oz)	670
French Fries	1 med (3.9 oz)	440
French Fries	1 sm (4 oz)	350
Grilled Chicken Sandwich	1 (6.5 oz)	310
Hot Dog	1 (3.5 oz)	240
Onion Rings	1 serv (4 oz)	320
The Great Steakmelt Basket	1 serv (13.2 oz)	770

FOOD	PORTION	CALS
ICE CREAM		
Banana Split	1 (12.9 oz)	510
Blizzard Chocolate Sandwich Cookie	1 med (11.4 oz)	640
Blizzard Chocolate Sandwich Cookie	1 sm (12 oz)	520
Blizzard Chocolate Chip Cookie Dough	1 med (15.4 oz)	950
Blizzard Chocolate Chip Cookie Dough	1 sm (12 oz)	660
Breeze Heath	1 med (14.2 oz)	710
Breeze Heath	1 sm (10.2 oz)	470
Breeze Strawberry	1 med (13.4 oz)	460
Breeze Strawberry	1 sm (12 oz)	320
Buster Bar	1 (5.2 oz)	450
Chocolate Malt	1 med (19.9 oz)	880
Chocolate Malt	1 sm (14.7 oz)	650
Cone Chocolate	1 med (6.9 oz)	340
Cone Chocolate	1 sm (5 oz)	240
Cone Vanilla	1 med (6.9 oz)	330
Cone Vanilla	1 lg (8.9 oz)	410
Cone Vanilla	1 sm (5 oz)	230
Cone Yogurt	1 med (6.9 oz)	260
Cone Dipped	1 med (7.7 oz)	490
Cone Dipped	1 sm (5.5 oz)	340
Cup Of Yogurt	1 med (6.7 oz)	230
Dilly Bar Chocolate	1 (3 oz)	210
DQ 8 Inch Round Cake Undecorated	⅛ of cake (6.2 oz)	340
DQ Fudge Bar No Sugar Added	1 (2.3 oz)	50
DQ Lemon Freez'r	½ cup (3.2 oz)	80
DQ Nonfat Frozen Yogurt	½ cup (3 oz)	100
DQ Sandwich	1 (2.1 oz)	200
DQ Soft Serve Chocolate	½ cup (3.3 oz)	150
DQ Soft Serve Vanilla	½ cup (3.3 oz)	140
DQ Treatzza Pizza Heath	⅛ of pie (2.3 oz)	180
DQ Treatzza Pizza M&M	⅛ of pie (2.4 oz)	190
DQ Vanilla Orange Bar No Sugar Added	1 (2.3 oz)	60
Frozen Hot Chocolate	1 (20.9 oz)	860
Misty Slush	1 sm (15.9 oz)	220
Misty Slush	1 med (20.9 oz)	290
Peanut Buster Parfait	1 (10.7 oz)	730
Pecan Mudslide Treat	1 (4.6 oz)	650
Shake Chocolate	1 med (18.9 oz)	770
Shake Chocolate	1 sm (13.9 oz)	560

FOOD	PORTION	CALS
S'more Galore Parfait	1 (10.7 oz)	730
Starkiss	1 (3 oz)	80
Strawberry Shortcake	1 (8.5 oz)	430
Sundae Chocolate	1 med (8.2 oz)	400
Sundae Chocolate	1 sm (5.7 oz)	280
Yogurt Sundae Strawberry	1 med (8.2 oz)	280

D'ANGELO'S SANDWICH SHOP
CHILDREN'S MENU SELECTIONS

FOOD	PORTION	CALS
D'Lite Turkey	1 kidz	217
Sub Cheeseburger	1 kidz	294
Sub Ham & Cheese	1 kidz	214
Sub Meatball	1 kidz	330
Sub Tuna	1 kidz	450

SALAD DRESSINGS AND TOPPINGS

FOOD	PORTION	CALS
Bacon	1 serv	64
Bleu Cheese	1 serv (1 oz)	152
Buffalo Sauce	1 serv (1 oz)	10
Caesar	1 serv (1 oz)	140
Caesar Fat Free	1 serv (1 oz)	20
Creamy Italian	1 serv (1 oz)	122
Cucumbers	3 slices	2
Greek Dressing w/ Feta	1 serv (3 oz)	227
Honey Mustard Dressing	1 serv (1 oz)	150
Hot Peppers	1 serv	0
Mayonnaise	2 tbsp	236
Mayonnaise Fat Free	1 pkg	10
Mustard Honey Dijon	2 tbsp	60
Mustard Yellow	2 tbsp	20
Olive Oil Vinaigrette	1 serv (3 oz)	170
Olive Oil Blend	2 tbsp	239
Ranch Lite	1 serv (3 oz)	240
Sesame Ginger	1 serv (1 oz)	170

SALADS

FOOD	PORTION	CALS
Antipasto Salad w/o Dressing	1 serv	275
Asian Chicken w/o Dressing	1 serv	224
Caesar w/ Dressing	1 serv	474
Chef w/o Dressing	1 serv	273

FOOD	PORTION	CALS
Chicken Caesar w/ Dressing	1 serv	532
Chicken Stir Fry w/o Dressing	1 serv	166
Cobb w/o Dressing	1 serv	289
Greek w/o Dressing	1 serv	298
Lobster w/o Dressing	1 serv	385
Roast Beef w/o Dressing	1 serv	146
Tossed Garden w/o Dressing	1 serv	47
Turkey w/o Dressing	1 serv	157
SANDWICHES		
D'Lite Chicken Stir Fry	1 sm	426
D'Lite Fresh Veggie	1	348
D'Lite Grilled Chicken Breast	1 sm	387
D'Lite Ham & Cheese	1 sm	351
D'Lite Roast Beef	1 sm	353
D'Lite Turkey	1 sm	364
D'Lite Turkey Cranberry	1 sm	460
Pokket BLT & Cheese	1 sm	421
Pokket Caesar Salad	1 sm	643
Pokket Capacola & Cheese	1 sm	426
Pokket Cheeseburger	1 sm	481
Pokket Chicken Caesar Salad	1 sm	701
Pokket Chicken Club	1 sm	559
Pokket Chicken Honey Dijon	1 sm	527
Pokket Chicken Salad	1 sm	705
Pokket Chicken Stir Fry	1 sm	425
Pokket Classic Veggie No Cheese	1 sm	238
Pokket Greek	1 sm	812
Pokket Grilled Chicken	1 sm	328
Pokket Ham & Cheese	1 sm	349
Pokket Ham & Salami	1 sm	412
Pokket Hamburger	1 sm	422
Pokket Italian	1 sm	574
Pokket Lobster	1 sm	568
Pokket Meatball	1 sm	600
Pokket Mortadella & Cheese	1 sm	505
Pokket Seafood Salad	1 sm	532
Pokket Steak	1 sm	335
Pokket Steak & Cheese	1 sm	407
Pokket Tuna	1 sm	791
Sub Cheeseburger	1 sm	542

FOOD	PORTION	CALS
Sub Chicken Club	1 sm	619
Sub Chicken Honey Dijon	1 sm	587
Sub Chicken Salad	1 sm	769
Sub Chicken Stir Fry	1 sm	487
Sub Classic Veggie	1 sm	465
Sub Grilled Chicken	1 sm	387
Sub Ham & Cheese	1 sm	412
Sub Ham & Salami	1 sm	474
Sub Hamburger	1 sm	482
Sub Italian	1 sm	637
Sub Lobster	1 sm	628
Sub Meatball	1 sm	663
Sub Mortadella & Cheese	1 sm	568
Sub Number 9	1 sm	475
Sub Pastrami	1 sm	526
Sub Pepperoni	1 sm	614
Sub Roast Beef	1 sm	350
Sub Salad	1 sm	298
Sub Salami & Cheese	1 sm	597
Sub Seafood Salad	1	595
Sub Steak	1 sm	383
Sub Steak & Cheese	1 sm	455
Sub Steak Tip	1 sm	486
Sub Stuffed Turkey	1 sm	1036
Sub Tuna	1 sm	853
Sub Turkey	1 sm	361
Sub Turkey Club	1 sm	360
Wrap Asian Chicken Salad	1	914
Wrap BLT & Cheese	1	500
Wrap Buffalo Chicken Salad	1	778
Wrap Caesar Salad	1	669
Wrap Capacola & Cheese	1	451
Wrap Cheese	1	631
Wrap Cheeseburger	1	569
Wrap Chef	1	832
Wrap Chicken Caesar Salad	1	788
Wrap Chicken Cobb	1	855
Wrap Chicken Filet & Bacon	1	643
Wrap Chicken Honey Dijon	1	619
Wrap Chicken Salad	1	780

FOOD	PORTION	CALS
Wrap Chicken Stir Fry	1	511
Wrap Classic Veggie	1	490
Wrap Greek	1	761
Wrap Grilled Chicken	1	420
Wrap Ham & Cheese	1	436
Wrap Ham & Salami	1	499
Wrap Hamburger	1	509
Wrap Italian	1	654
Wrap Lobster	1	766
Wrap Meatball	1	687
Wrap Mortadella & Cheese	1	592
Wrap Number 9	1	494
Wrap Pastrami	1	550
Wrap Pepperoni	1	638
Wrap Roast Beef	1	374
Wrap Salad	1	322
Wrap Salami & Cheese	1	605
Wrap Seafood Salad	1	619
Wrap Steak	1	402
Wrap Steak & Cheese	1	474
Wrap Steak Tip	1	374
Wrap Tuna	1	881
Wrap Turkey	1	385
Wrap Turkey Club	1	435
SOUPS		
#9 Steak & Cheese	1 sm	280
Chicken Noodle	1 sm	130
Hearty Vegetable	1 sm	40
Lobster Bisque	1 sm	360
New England Clam Chowder	1 sm	270
Santa Fe Chipotle Vegetable	1 sm	130
Shrimp & Roasted Corn	1 sm	250
Thanksgiving Everyday	1 sm	250

DELTACO
BEVERAGES

FOOD	PORTION	CALS
Coffee	1 serv (8 oz)	0
Coke Classic	1 lg (20 oz)	230
Coke Classic	1 med (12 oz)	150
Coke Classic	1 sm (10 oz)	120
Coke Classic Best Value	1 serv (27 oz)	320

FOOD	PORTION	CALS
Diet Coke	1 lg (20 oz)	5
Diet Coke	1 med (12 oz)	0
Diet Coke	1 sm (10 oz)	0
Diet Coke Best Value	1 serv (27 oz)	10
Iced Tea	1 lg (20 oz)	5
Iced Tea	1 med (12 oz)	0
Iced Tea	1 sm (10 oz)	0
Iced Tea Best Value	1 serv (27 oz)	10
Milk 1% Lowfat	1 serv (11 oz)	130
Mr Pibb	1 lg (20 oz)	230
Mr Pibb	1 med (12 oz)	150
Mr Pibb	1 sm (10 oz)	120
Mr Pibb Best Value	1 serv (27 oz)	320
Orange Juice	1 serv (11 oz)	140
Shake Chocolate	1 lg (15 oz)	680
Shake Chocolate	1 sm (11.4 oz)	520
Shake Strawberry	1 lg (15 oz)	540
Shake Strawberry	1 sm (11.4 oz)	410
Shake Vanilla	1 lg (15 oz)	550
Shake Vanilla	1 sm (11.4 oz)	420
Sprite	1 lg (20 oz)	230
Sprite	1 med (12 oz)	140
Sprite	1 sm (10 oz)	110
Sprite Best Value	1 serv (27 oz)	310
BREAKFAST SELECTIONS		
Burrito Breakfast	1 (3.8 oz)	250
Burrito Egg & Cheese	1 (7.5 oz)	450
Burrito Macho Bacon & Egg	1 (15.9 oz)	1030
Burrito Steak & Egg	1 (9 oz)	580
Quesadilla Bacon & Egg	1 (6.1 oz)	450
Side of Bacon	2 strips (0.3 oz)	50
MAIN MENU SELECTIONS		
Beans 'n Cheese Cup	1 serv (7.7 oz)	260
Burrito Combo	1 (8.2 oz)	490
Burrito Del Beef	1 (8 oz)	550
Burrito Del Classic Chicken	1 (8.5 oz)	580
Burrito Deluxe Combo	1 (10.7 oz)	530
Burrito Deluxe Del Beef	1 (10.5 oz)	590
Burrito Green	1 (5 oz)	280
Burrito Macho Beef	1 (18.9 oz)	1170

FOOD	PORTION	CALS
Burrito Macho Combo	1 (19.4 oz)	1050
Burrito Red	1 (5 oz)	270
Burrito Red Regular	1 (7.5 oz)	390
Burrito Regular Green	1 (7.5 oz)	400
Burrito Spicy Chicken	1 (8.7 oz)	480
Burrito The Works	1 (10.2 oz)	480
Cheeseburger	1 (4.6 oz)	330
Del Cheeseburger	1 (5.6 oz)	430
Double Del Cheeseburger	1 (7.1 oz)	560
Fries	1 reg (5 oz)	350
Fries	1 sm (3 oz)	210
Fries Best Value	1 serv (7 oz)	490
Fries Chili Cheese	1 serv (10.5 oz)	670
Fries Deluxe Chili Cheese	1 serv (11.9 oz)	710
Get A Lot Meals #1 Combo Burrito Fries Drink	1 meal	980
Get A Lot Meals #2 Del Classic Chicken Burrito Fries Drink	1 meal	1080
Get A Lot Meals #3 Regular Red Burrito Fries Drink	1 meal	890
Get A Lot Meals #4 Two Chicken Soft Tacos Fries Drink	1 meal	910
Get A Lot Meals #5 Taco Combo Burrito Drink	1 meal	790
Get A Lot Meals #6 Two Tacos Quesadilla Drink	1 meal	960
Get A Lot Meals #7 Macho Combo Burrito Fries Drink	1 meal	1530
Get A Lot Meals #8 Two Big Fat Tacos Fries Drink	1 meal	802
Get A Lot Meals #9 Double Del Cheeseburger Fries Drink	1 meal	1050
Nachos	1 serv (4 oz)	380
Nachos Macho	1 serv (17 oz)	1200
Quesadilla Chicken	1 (6.8 oz)	580
Quesadilla Regular	1 (5.3 oz)	500
Quesadilla Spicy Jack Chicken	1 (6.8 oz)	570
Quesadilla Spicy Jack Regular	1 (5.3 oz)	490
Rice Cup	1 serv (4 oz)	150
Soft Taco	1 (2.8 oz)	160
Soft Taco Chicken	1 (3.3 oz)	210
Taco	1 (2.2 oz)	160
Taco Big Fat	1 (5.4 oz)	320

FOOD	PORTION	CALS
Taco Big Fat Chicken	1 (5.4 oz)	340
Taco Big Fat Steak	1 (5.4 oz)	390
Taco Salad Deluxe	1 (18.8 oz)	760
Tostada Salad	1 (4.5 oz)	210

DENNY'S
BEVERAGES

FOOD	PORTION	CALS
2% Milk	10 oz	151
Apple Juice	1 reg	126
Cappuccino French Vanilla	8 oz	100
Cappuccino Original	8 oz	100
Chocolate Milk	10 oz	235
Grapefruit	1 serv (10 oz)	162
Hot Chocolate	8 oz	100
Lemonade	16 oz	150
Malted Milk Shake Chocolate Or Vanilla	12 oz	583
Orange Juice	10 oz	126
Raspberry Ice Tea	16 oz	78
Tomato Juice	1 serv (10 oz)	56

BREAKFAST SELECTIONS

FOOD	PORTION	CALS
All American Slam	1 serv	816
Applesauce	1 serv	60
Bacon	4 strips	162
Bagel Dry	1	235
Banana	1	110
Belgian Waffle	1	619
Breakfast Dagwood	1 serv	1446
Buttermilk Hotcakes	3	466
Cantaloupe	¼	32
Chicken Fajita Skillet	1 serv	855
Corned Beef Hash Slam	1 serv	668
Country Fish Potatoes	1 serv	394
Egg	1	120
English Muffin Dry	1	125
Fabulous French Toast	1 serv	1146
Farmer's Slam	1 serv	1200
French Slam	1 serv	1119
Fruit Mix	1 serv	36
Grand Slam Slugger	1 serv	927
Grapefruit	½	60

FOOD	PORTION	CALS
Grapes	1 serv	55
Grits	1 serv	80
Ham & Cheddar Omelette	1 serv	595
Ham & Cheese Omelette w/ Eggbeaters	1 serv	468
Ham Slice	1	94
Hashed Browns	1 serv	197
Hashed Browns Covered	1 serv	280
Hashed Browns Covered & Smothered	1 serv	493
Honeydew	¼	31
Lumberjack Slam w/ Hash Browns	1 serv	1035
Meat Lover's Skillet	1 serv	1031
Moon Over My Hammy	1 serv	841
Oatmeal	1 serv	100
Oatmeal Deluxe	1 serv	460
Original Grand Slam	1 serv	665
Ready To Eat Cereal	1 serv	100
Sausage	4 links	354
Scram Slam	1 serv	827
Senior Belgian Waffle Slam	1 serv	399
Senior Omelette	1 serv	429
Sirloin Steak & Eggs	1 serv	675
Slim Slam	1 serv	438
T-Bone Steak & Eggs	1 serv	991
Toast Dry	1 slice	92
Two Egg Breakfast w/ Hash Browns	1 serv	825
Ultimate Omelette	1 serv	611
Vegggie Cheese Omelette	1 serv	494
CHILDREN'S MENU SELECTIONS		
Burgerlicious	1 serv	296
Burgerlicious w/ Cheese	1 serv	341
Dennysaur Chicken Nuggets	1 serv	190
Frenchtastic Slam	1 serv	452
Junior Fish & Chips	1 serv	698
Junior Grand Slam	1 serv	397
Junior Shrimps Ahoy!	1 serv	411
Oreo Blender Blaster	1 serv	580
Pizza Party	1 serv	400
Smiley-Face Hotcakes w/ Meat	1 serv	463
Smiley-Face Hotcakes w/o Meat	1 serv	344
The Big Cheese	1 serv	334

FOOD	PORTION	CALS
DESSERTS		
Apple Pie	1 serv	470
Banana Split	1	894
Carrot Cake	1 serv	799
Cheesecake	1 serv	580
Chocolate Topping	1 serv	317
Chocolate Peanut Butter Pie	1 serv	653
Double Scoop Sundae	1 serv	375
Float Rootbeer or Coke	12 oz	280
Hot Fudge Brownie A La Mode	1 serv	997
Milkshake Vanilla Or Chocolate	12 oz	560
Oreo Blender Blaster	1 serv	895
Single Scoop Sundae	1 serv	188
MAIN MENU SELECTIONS		
Albacore Tuna Melt	1 serv	640
Applesauce	1 serv	60
Bacon Lettuce & Tomato	1	610
Baked Potato Plain	1	220
BBQ Chicken Sandwich	1 serv	1089
Bread Stuffing Plain	1 serv	100
Buffalo Chicken Sandwich	1 serv	708
Buffalo Chicken Strips	5 pieces	734
Buffalo Wings	12 pieces	856
Burger Bacon Cheddar	1	875
Burger BBQ	1 serv	953
Burger Boca	1 serv	601
Burger Classic	1	694
Burger Classic w/ Cheese	1	852
Burger Mushroom Swiss	1 serv	880
Carrots In Honey Glaze	1 serv	80
Chicken Strips	5 pieces	720
Chicken Ranch Melt	1 serv	758
Chicken Strips	1 serv	635
Club Sandwich	1	718
Coleslaw	1 serv	274
Corn In Butter Sauce	1 serv	120
Cottage Cheese	1 serv	72
Country Fried Steak	1 serv	644
Fish & Chips Dinner	1 serv	955
French Fries Unsalted	1 serv	423

FOOD	PORTION	CALS
Fried Shrimp Dinner	1 serv	219
Fried Shrimp & Shrimp Scampi	1 serv	346
Green Beans w/ Bacon	1 serv	60
Grilled Cheese Sandwich	1	510
Grilled Chicken Dinner	1 serv	130
Grilled Chicken Sandwich	1	469
Ham & Swiss On Rye	1	417
Herb Toast	1 serv	170
Hoagie Chicken Melt	1	751
Hoagie Philly Melt	1 serv	874
Mashed Potatoes Plain	1 serv	168
Mozzarella Sticks	8 pieces	710
Onion Rings	1 serv	381
Patty Melt	1	798
Pot Roast Dinner w/ Gravy	1 serv	292
Roast Turkey & Stuffing w/ Gravy	1 serv	388
Sampler	1 serv	1405
Seasoned Fries	1 serv	261
Senior Chicken Strip Dinner	1 serv	285
Senior Club	1 serv	540
Senior Country Fried Steak	1 serv	341
Senior Fish & Chips	1 serv	756
Senior French Slam	1 serv	820
Senior Fried Shrimp Dinner	1 serv	129
Senior Grilled Chicken Breast	1 serv	200
Senior Pot Roast	1 serv	160
Senior Starter	1 serv	544
Senior Turkey & Stuffing	1 serv	220
Shrimp Scampi Skillet Dinner	1 serv	289
Sirloin Steak Dinner	1 serv	337
Sliced Tomatoes	3 slices	13
Smothered Cheese Fries	1 serv	767
Steak & Shrimp Dinner	1 serv	645
T-Bone Steak Dinner	1 serv	860
The Super Bird Sandwich	1	620
Turkey Breast On Multigrain w/o Mayo	1	277
SALAD DRESSINGS AND TOPPINGS		
BBQ Sauce	1.5 oz	47
Bleu Cheese	1 oz	163
Blueberry Topping	1 serv	71

FOOD	PORTION	CALS
Caesar	1 oz	133
Cherry Topping	1 serv	57
Cream Cheese	1 oz	100
French	1 oz	106
Fudge Topping	1 serv	201
Gravy Brown	1 serv	13
Gravy Chicken	1 serv	14
Gravy Country	1 serv	17
Honey Mustard	1 serv	160
Low Calorie Italian	1 oz	15
Marinara Sauce	1 serv	48
Ranch	1 oz	129
Ranch Fat Free	1 serv	25
Sour Cream	1.5 oz	91
Strawberry Topping	1 serv	77
Syrup	3 tbsp	143
Syrup Sugar Free	1 serv	23
Tartar Sauce	1 serv	225
Thousand Island	2 tbsp	170
Thousand Island	1 oz	118
Whipped Margarine	1 serv	87
Whipped Cream	2 tbsp	23
SALADS		
Garden Salad w/ Albacore Tuna	1 serv	444
Garden Salad w/ Fried Chicken Strips	1 serv	438
Garden Salad w/ Grilled Chicken Breast	1 serv	264
Grilled Chicken Caesar Salad w/ Dressing	1 serv	600
Side Caesar w/ Dressing	1 serv	362
Side Garden Salad w/o Dressing	1 serv	113
SOUPS		
Chicken Noodle	1 serv	60
Clam Chowder	1 serv	624
Cream Of Broccoli	1 serv	574
Vegetable Beef	1 serv	79

DESERT MOON CAFE
CHILDREN'S MENU SELECTIONS

Burrito Bean & Cheese	1 serv	650
Kids Nachos	1 serv	500
Kids Taco w/ Chicken	1	280

FOOD	PORTION	CALS
Kids Taco w/ Steak	1	290
Kidsadilla	1 serv	630
MAIN MENU SELECTIONS		
Alamo Burger	1	810
Burrito Adobe Moon w/ Chicken	1	730
Burrito Adobe Moon w/ Steak	1	750
Burrito Black Bean w/ Chicken	1	770
Burrito Black Bean w/ Steak	1	790
Burrito Full Moon w/ Chicken	1	620
Burrito Full Moon w/ Steak	1	640
Burrito Get It Smothered	1	120
Burrito Harvest Wrap w/ Chicken	1	620
Burrito Harvest Wrap w/ Steak	1	300
Enchilada Mesa	1	710
Enchilada Queso	1	730
Enchilada Shrimp	1	830
Fajita Platter w/ Chicken	1 serv	1160
Fajita Platter w/ Shrimp	1 serv	1060
Fajita Platter w/ Steak	1	1190
Hell Canyon Chili	1 serv	260
Mucho Nachos	1 serv	800
Mucho Nachos w/ Chicken	1 serv	900
Mucho Nachos w/ Steak	1 serv	920
Pizza Texas BBQ	1	330
Quesadilla Baja Chicken	1	650
Quesadilla Coyote w/ Chicken	1	660
Quesadilla Coyote w/ Steak	1	680
Quesadilla Sonoran	1	660
Rice Bowl Black Bean w/ Chicken	1 serv	790
Rice Bowl Black Bean w/ Steak	1 serv	820
Rice Bowl Chili w/ Chicken	1 serv	760
Rice Bowl Chili w/ Steak	1 serv	790
Rice Bowl Shrimp Creole	1 serv	910
Shrimp Dippers	1 serv	430
Soup Black Bean	1 serv	360
Soup Tortilla	1 serv	330
Taco Acapulco Shrimp	1	230
Taco Classic w/ Chicken	1	190
Taco Classic w/ Steak	1	200

FOOD	PORTION	CALS
Taco Fajita w/ Chicken	1	200
Taco Fajita w/ Steak	1	210
SALAD DRESSINGS AND SAUCES		
BBQ Sauce	1 serv (1 oz)	50
Buffalo Wing Sauce	1 serv (1 oz)	45
Dressing Bleu Cheese	1 serv (2 oz)	300
Dressing Creamy Caesar	1 serv (2 oz)	320
Dressing Honey Dijon Fat Free	1 serv (2 oz)	80
Dressing Lite Ranch	1 serv (2 oz)	150
Dressing Lite Raspberry Vinaigrette	1 serv (2 oz)	150
Dressing Poblano	1 serv (1 oz)	150
Guacamole	1 serv (2 oz)	100
Pepper Cream Sauce	1 serv (2 oz)	100
Pico De Gallo	1 serv (2 oz)	15
Salsa Black Bean	1 serv (2 oz)	20
Salsa Fruit	1 serv (2 oz)	60
Salsa Mild Tomato	1 serv (2 oz)	15
Salsa Rattlesnake	1 serv (2 oz)	15
SALADS W/O TORTILLA BOWL		
Caesar	1 serv	530
Caesar w/ Chicken	1 serv	640
Caesar w/ Shrimp	1 serv	570
Chopped Chicken	1 serv	520
Taco w/ Chicken	1 serv	310
Taco w/ Steak	1 serv	340

DOMINO'S PIZZA
12 INCH MEDIUM PIZZAS

FOOD	PORTION	CALS
Deep Dish Cheese Only	2 slices	482
Hand Tossed America's Favorite Feast	1 serv	508
Hand Tossed Bacon Cheeseburger Feast	2 slices	549
Hand Tossed Barbeque Feast	2 slices	506
Hand Tossed Cheese Only	2 slices	375
Hand Tossed Deluxe Feast	2 slices	465
Hand Tossed ExtravaganZZa Feast	2 slices	576
Hand Tossed Hawaiian Feast	2 slices	450
Hand Tossed MeatZZa Feast	2 slices	560
Hand Tossed Pepperoni Feast	2 slices	534
Hand Tossed Vegi Feast	2 slices	439
Thin Crust Cheese	¼ pie	273

FOOD	PORTION	CALS
Toppings Pineapple	1 serv	12
DESSERTS		
Cinna Stix	1 serv	111
Sweet Icing	1 serv	283
MAIN MENU SELECTIONS		
Breadstick	1	116
Buffalo Chicken Kickers	1 piece	47
Buffalo Wings Barbeque	1 piece	50
Buffalo Wings Hot	1 piece	45
Cheesy Bread	1 piece	142
TOPPINGS		
Blue Cheese	1 serv	223
Hot Sauce	1 serv	14
Medium Pizza Anchovies	1 serv	34
Medium Pizza Bacon	1 serv	102
Medium Pizza Banana Peppers	1 serv	5
Medium Pizza Beef	1 serv	78
Medium Pizza Cheddar Cheese	1 serv	57
Medium Pizza Extra Cheese	1 serv	49
Medium Pizza Green Olives	1 serv	19
Medium Pizza Green Peppers	1 serv	4
Medium Pizza Ham	1 serv	23
Medium Pizza Italian Sausage	1 serv	77
Medium Pizza Mushrooms	1 serv	6
Medium Pizza Onion	1 serv	5
Medium Pizza Pepperoni	1 serv	74
Medium Pizza Ripe Olives	1 serv	21
Ranch	1 serv	197

DONATOS PIZZA
PIZZA

FOOD	PORTION	CALS
Dessert Apple	¼ pie	722
Dessert Cherry	¼ pie	818
Original	¼ pie	660
Original Chicken Vegy Medley	¼ pie	500
Original Chicken Vegy Medley No Cheese	¼ pie	392
Original Founders	¼ pie	737
Original Hawaiian	¼ pie	620
Original Hawaiian No Cheese	¼ pie	411
Original Mariachi Beef	¼ pie	613

FOOD	PORTION	CALS
Original Mariachi Chicken	¼ pie	580
Original Serious Cheese	¼ pie	640
Original Serious Meat	¼ pie	817
Original Vegy	¼ pie	564
Original Vegy No Cheese	¼ pie	370
Original Works	¼ pie	729
Traditional Chicken Vegy Medley	¼ pie	647
Traditional Founders	¼ pie	900
Traditional Hawaiian	¼ pie	794
Traditional Mariachi Beef	¼ pie	797
Traditional Mariachi Chicken	¼ pie	770
Tradtional Original	¼ pie	928
Tradtional Serious Cheese	¼ pie	830
Traditional Serious Meat	¼ pie	977
Traditional Vegy	¼ pie	752
Traditional Works	¼ pie	892
SALAD DRESSINGS		
Italian	1 serv (1.5 oz)	230
Italian Lite	1 serv (1.5 oz)	20
SALADS		
Grilled Chicken w/o Dressing	1 serv	314
Italian Chef w/o Dressing	1 serv	338
Side w/o Dressing	1 serv	106
SIDE ORDERS		
Breadsticks	2	220
Chicken Wings Hot	5	449
Chicken Wings Mild	5	451
Three Cheese Garlic Bread	1 bun	605
SUBS		
Big Don Italian	1 serv	705
Big Don Lite Italian	1 serv	631
Grilled Chicken	1 serv	786
Ham & Cheese Italian	1 serv	609
Ham & Cheese Lite Italian	1 serv	534
Southwest Turkey	1 serv	710
Steak & Cheese	1 serv	929
Vegy Italian	1 serv	730
Vegy Lite Italian	1 serv	661

FOOD	PORTION	CALS
DUNKIN' DONUTS		
BAGELS AND CREAM CHEESE		
Bagel Blueberry	1	330
Bagel Cinnamon Raisin	1	330
Bagel Everything	1	370
Bagel Harvest	1	350
Bagel Onion	1	320
Bagel Plain	1	320
Bagel Poppyseed	1	370
Bagel Reduced Carb w/ Cheese	1	380
Bagel Salsa	1	310
Bagel Salt	1	370
Bagel Sesame	1	380
Bagel Wheat	1	330
Cream Cheese Chive	2 oz	170
Cream Cheese Garden Vegetable	2 oz	170
Cream Cheese Lite	2 oz	110
Cream Cheese Plain	2 oz	190
Cream Cheese Salmon	2 oz	170
Cream Cheese Strawberry	2 oz	190
BAKED SELECTIONS		
Apple Fritter	1	300
Biscuit	1	250
Bismark Chocolate Iced	1	340
Coffee Roll	1	270
Coffee Roll Chocolate Frosted	1	290
Coffee Roll Maple Frosted	1	290
Coffee Roll Vanilla Frosted	1	290
Cookie Chocolate Chunk	2	220
Cookie Chocolate Chunk w/ Walnuts	2	230
Cookie Oatmeal Raisin Pecan	2	220
Cookie White Chocolate Chunk	2	230
Croissant Plain	1	330
Danish Apple	1	330
Danish Cheese	1	340
Danish Strawberry Cheese	1	320
Donut Apple Crumb	1	230
Donut Apple Crumb Cake	1	290
Donut Apple N' Spice	1	200
Donut Bavarian Kreme	1	210

FOOD	PORTION	CALS
Donut Black Raspberry	1	210
Donut Blueberry	1	290
Donut Blueberry Crumb	1	240
Donut Boston Kreme	1	240
Donut Bow Tie	1	300
Donut Chocolate Coconut	1	300
Donut Chocolate Frosted	1	360
Donut Chocolate Glazed	1	290
Donut Chocolate Kreme Filled	1	270
Donut Cinnamon	1	330
Donut Double Chocolate	1	310
Donut Frosted Lemon	1	240
Donut Glazed	1	350
Donut Glazed Ginerbread	1	260
Donut Glazed Lemon	1	240
Donut Jelly Filled	1	210
Donut Lemon Burst	1	300
Donut Maple Frosted	1	210
Donut Marble Frosted	1	200
Donut Old Fashioned	1	300
Donut Powdered	1	330
Donut Strawberry	1	210
Donut Strawberry Frosted	1	210
Donut Sugar Raised	1	170
Donut Vanilla Kreme Filled	1	270
Donut Whole Wheat Glazed	1	310
Eclair	1	270
English Muffin	1	160
French Cruller	1	150
Fritter Glazed	1	260
Muffin Banana Walnut	1	540
Muffin Blueberry	1	470
Muffin Chocolate Chip	1	630
Muffin Coffee Cake	1	580
Muffin Corn	1	510
Muffin Cranberry Orange	1	440
Muffin Honey Bran Raisin	1	480
Muffin Reduced Fat Blueberry	1	400
Munchkins Chocolate Glazed	3	200

FOOD	PORTION	CALS
Munchkins Cinnamon	4	270
Munchkins Glazed	3	280
Munchkins Jelly Filled	5	210
Munchkins Lemon Filled	4	170
Munchkins Plain	4	270
Munchkins Powdered	4	270
Munchkins Sugar Raised	7	220
Stick Cinnamon	1	450
Stick Glazed	1	490
Stick Glazed Chocolate	1	470
Stick Jelly	1	530
Stick Plain	1	420
Stick Powdered	1	450
BEVERAGES		
Cappuccino	1 (10 oz)	60
Cappuccino w/ Soy Milk	1 (10 oz)	70
Cappuccino w/ Soy Milk Sugar	1 (10 oz)	120
Cappuccino w/ Sugar	1 (10 oz)	130
Coffee Blueberry	1 (10 oz)	20
Coffee Caramel	1 (10 oz)	20
Coffee Chocolate	1 (10 oz)	20
Coffee Cinnamon	1 (10 oz)	20
Coffee Coconut	1 (10 oz)	20
Coffee French Vanilla	1 (10 oz)	20
Coffee Hazelnut	1 (10 oz)	20
Coffee Marshmallow	1 (10 oz)	20
Coffee Regular	1 (10 oz)	15
Coffee Toasted Almond	1 (10 oz)	20
Coffee w/ Cream	1 (10 oz)	70
Coffee w/ Cream Sugar	1 (10 oz)	120
Coffee w/ Milk	1 (10 oz)	35
Coffee w/ Milk Sugar	1 (10 oz)	80
Coffee w/ Skim Milk	1 (10 oz)	25
Coffee w/ Skim Milk Sugar	1 (10 oz)	70
Coffee w/ Sugar	1 (10 oz)	60
Coolatta Lemonade	1 (16 oz)	240
Coolatta Strawberry Fruit	1 (16 oz)	290
Coolatta Tropicana Orange	1	370
Coolatta Vanilla Bean	1 (16 oz)	440
Coolatta Coffee w/ 2% Milk	1 (16 oz)	190

FOOD	PORTION	CALS
Coolatta Coffee w/ Cream	1 (16 oz)	350
Coolatta Coffee w/ Milk	1 (16 oz)	210
Coolatta Coffee w/ Skin Milk	1 (16 oz)	170
Dunkaccino	1 (10 oz)	230
Expresso	1 (2 oz)	0
Expresso w/ Sugar	1 (2 oz)	30
Hot Chocolate	1 (10 oz)	220
Iced Coffee	1 (16 oz)	15
Iced Coffee w/ Cream	1 (16 oz)	70
Iced Coffee w/ Cream Sugar	1 (16 oz)	120
Iced Coffee w/ Milk	1 (16 oz)	35
Iced Coffee w/ Milk Sugar	1 (16 oz)	80
Iced Coffee w/ Skim Milk	1 (16 oz)	25
Iced Coffee w/ Skim Milk Sugar	1 (16 oz)	70
Iced Coffee w/ Sugar	1 (16 oz)	60
Iced Latte	1 (16 oz)	120
Iced Latte Caramel Creme	1 (16 oz)	260
Iced Latte Caramel Swirl	1 (16 oz)	240
Iced Latte Caramel Swirl w/ Skim Milk	1 (16 oz)	180
Iced Latte Lite	1 (16 oz)	80
Iced Latte Mocha Almond	1 (16 oz)	290
Iced Latte Mocha Swirl	1 (16 oz)	240
Iced Latte Mocha Swirl w/ Skim Milk	1 (16 oz)	180
Iced Latte w/ Skim Milk	1 (16 oz)	70
Iced Latte w/ Skim Milk Sugar	1 (16 oz)	120
Iced Latte w/ Sugar	1 (16 oz)	170
Latte	1 (10 oz)	120
Latte Caramel Creme	1 (10 oz)	260
Latte Caramel Swirl	1 (10 oz)	230
Latte Caramel Swirl w/ Soy Milk	1 (10 oz)	210
Latte Lite	1 (10 oz)	70
Latte Mocha Almond	1 (10 oz)	290
Latte Mocha Swirl	1 (10 oz)	230
Latte Mocha Swirl w/ Soy Milk	1 (10 oz)	210
Latte w/ Soy Milk	1 (10 oz)	90
Latte w/ Soy Milk Sugar	1 (10 oz)	150
Latte w/ Sugar	1 (10 oz)	160
Tea Regular Or Decaffeinated	1 (10 oz)	0
Tea w/ Milk	1 (10 oz)	25
Tea w/ Milk Sugar	1 (10 oz)	70

FOOD	PORTION	CALS
Tea w/ Skim Milk	1 (10 oz)	25
Tea w/ Skim Milk Sugar	1 (10 oz)	60
Tea w/ Sugar	1 (10 oz)	50
Turbo Ice	1 (16 oz)	120
Vanilla Chai	1 (10 oz)	230
SANDWICHES		
Bagel Bacon Egg Cheese	1	540
Bagel Egg Cheese	1	470
Bagel Ham Egg Cheese	1	510
Bagel Sausage Egg Cheese	1	660
Biscuit Egg Cheese	1	410
Biscuit Sausage Egg Cheese	1	610
Croissant Bacon Egg Cheese	1	520
Croissant Egg Cheese	1	550
Croissant Ham Egg Cheese	1	520
Croissant Sausage Egg Cheese	1	490
English Muffin Bacon Egg Cheese	1	360
English Muffin Egg Cheese	1	280
English Muffin Ham Egg Cheese	1	310
English Muffin Sausage Egg Cheese	1	530
Panini Meatball	1	480
Panini Southwestern Chicken	1	420
Panini Steak	1	450

EINSTEIN BROS BAGELS
BAGELS AND BREADS

FOOD	PORTION	CALS
Bagel Asiago Cheese	1	360
Bagel Cranberry Special	1	350
Bagel Egg	1	340
Bagel Honey Whole Wheat	1	320
Bagel Jalapeno	1	330
Bagel Lucky Green	1	320
Bagel Mango	1	360
Bagel Marble Rye	1	340
Bagel Potato	1	350
Bagel Power	1	410
Bagel Power w/ Peanut Butter	1	750
Bagel Pumpkin	1	330
Bagel Roasted Red Pepper & Pesto	1	410
Bagel Six Cheese	1	390

FOOD	PORTION	CALS
Bagel Spicy Nacho	1	450
Bagel Spinach Florentine	1	410
Bagel Croutons	¼ cup	25
Bagel Twist	1	220
Bread Ciabatta	1 serv	320
Chocolate Chip	1	370
Chopped Garlic	1	380
Chopped Onion	1	330
Cinnamon Raisin Swirl	1	350
Cinnamon Sugar	1	330
Dark Pumpernickel	1	320
Everything	1	340
Focaccia Cheese Pizza	1 serv	500
Focaccia Margherita	1 serv	400
Focaccia Pepperoni Pizza	1 serv	590
Nutty Banana	1	360
Plain	1	320
Poppy Dip'd	1	350
Roll Challah	1	300
Salt	1	330
Sesame Dip'd	1	380
Sun Dried Tomato	1	320
Wild Blueberry	1	350
BEVERAGES		
Americano	1 reg	1
Cafe Latte	1 reg	140
Cafe Latte Nonfat	1 reg	100
Cappuccino	1 reg	90
Cappuccino Nonfat	1 reg	60
Chai 2% Milk	1 reg	210
Chai Skim Milk	1 reg	190
Coffee	1 reg	0
Espresso	1 reg	1
Half & Half	2 tbsp	40
Hot Chocolate	1 reg	290
Hot Chocolate Lower Fat	1 reg	260
Hot Tea All Flavors	1 cup	0
Iced Americano	1 serv	1
Iced Coffee	1 serv	0
Iced Latte	1 serv	120

FOOD	PORTION	CALS
Iced Latte Nonfat	1 serv	90
Iced Mocha	1 serv	210
Iced Mocha Low Fat	1 serv	180
Mocha	1 reg	230
Mocha Low Fat	1 reg	190
DESSERTS		
Brownie Iced	1	550
Brownie Iced w/ Walnuts	1	600
Cherry Figure 8	1	400
Cinnamon Roll	1	810
Cookie Chocolate Chunk	1	640
Cookie Oatmeal Raisin	1	600
Cookie Peanut Butter	1	640
Muffin Banana Nut	1	640
Muffin Blueberry	1	540
Muffin Chocolate Chip	1	620
Pound Cake Lemon Iced	1 slice	540
Pound Cake Marble	1 slice	460
Rice Krispy Bar	1	420
Scone Blueberry w/ Icing	1	450
Scone Lemon Currant	1	430
Strudel Cinnamon Walnut	1 piece	550
Sweetie Pie	1	620
SALAD DRESSINGS		
Asian Sesame	2 tbsp	80
Caesar	2 tbsp	150
Chipotle Vinaigrette	2 tbsp	110
Horseradish Sauce	2 tbsp	170
Raspberry Vinaigrette	2 tbsp	160
Thousand Island	2 tbsp	110
SALADS		
Asian Chicken Salad	1 serv (14.5 oz)	550
Bros Bistro	1 serv (9.5 oz)	520
Chicken Caesar	1 serv (12.5 oz)	750
Chicken Chipotle Salad	1 serv	710
Chicken Salad On Greens	1 serv (10.5 oz)	210
Egg Salad	1 serv (4 oz)	200
Fresh Fruit Cup	1 serv (8 oz)	110
Mixed Greens	1 serv (3.5 oz)	228
Potato	½ cup	290
Tuna Salad On Greens	1 serv (10.5 oz)	170

FOOD	PORTION	CALS
SANDWICHES		
12 Grain Bread Deli Chicken Salad	1	440
12 Grain Bread Deli Egg Salad	1	490
12 Grain Bread Deli Ham	1	560
12 Grain Bread Deli Roast Beef	1	560
12 Grain Bread Deli Smoked Turkey	1	530
12 Grain Bread Deli Tuna Salad	1	440
12 Grain Bread Deli Turkey Pastrami	1	540
12 Grain Bread Ultimate Toasted Cheese w/ Tomato	1	870
Bagel Chicken Salad	1	500
Bagel Egg Bacon	1	580
Bagel Egg Ham	1	530
Bagel Egg Salad	1	560
Bagel Egg Sausage	1	550
Bagel Ham	1	450
Bagel Holey Cow	1	900
Bagel Hummus & Feta	1	540
Bagel New York Lox	1	660
Bagel Original	1	480
Bagel Roast Beef	1	460
Bagel Rueben Deli	1	660
Bagel Salmon & Shmear	1	650
Bagel Sante Fe	1	650
Bagel Smoked Turkey	1	420
Bagel Tasty Turkey	1	570
Bagel The Veg Out	1	490
Bagel Tuna Salad	1	470
Bagel Turkey Pastrami	1	440
Challah Club Mex	1	750
Challah Cobbie	1	630
Challah Deli Chicken Salad	1	480
Challah Deli Egg Salad	1	430
Challah Deli Pastrami	1	480
Challah Deli Roast Beef	1	500
Challah Deli Smoked Turkey	1	470
Challah Deli Tuna Salad	1	370
Challah Deli Turkey Ham	1	500
Challah EBBQ Chicken	1	380

FOOD	PORTION	CALS
Challah Roasted Chicken & Smoked Gouda	1	440
Chicago Bagel Dog Asiago	1	740
Chicago Bagel Dog Chili Cheese	1	810
Chicago Bagel Dog Everything	1	730
Chicago Bagel Dog Onion w/o Cheese	1	680
Country White Deli Chicken Salad	1	540
Country White Deli Egg Salad	1	590
Country White Deli Ham	1	660
Country White Deli Roast Beef	1	660
Country White Deli Smoked Turkey	1	630
Country White Deli Tuna Salad	1	510
Country White Deli Turkey Pastrami	1	640
Country White Ultimate Toasted Cheese w/ Tomato	1	870
Panini Cali Club	1	730
Panini Cuban Ham	1	700
Panini Denver Omelet Breakfast	1	740
Panini Italian Chicken	1	770
Panini Taos Turkey	1	740
Panini Ultimate Toasted Cheese	1	900
Roll Ups Albuquerque Turkey	1	790
Roll Ups Thai Vegetable w/ Chicken	1	670
Roll Ups Thai Vegetables	1	630
SOUPS		
Broccoli Sharp Cheddar	1 cup	230
Chicken & Wild Rice	1 cup	190
Chicken Noodle	1 cup	220
Clam Chowda	1 cup	160
Minestroni Low Fat	1 cup	180
Tomato Bisque	1 cup	190
Tortilla	1 cup	90
Turkey Chili	1 cup	140
SPREADS		
Butter	1 tbsp	100
Butter & Margarine Blend	1 tbsp	60
Cream Cheese Blueberry	1 tbsp	70
Cream Cheese Cappuccino	2 tbsp	70
Cream Cheese Garden Vegetable	2 tbsp	60
Cream Cheese Honey Almond Reduced Fat	2 tbsp	70
Cream Cheese Jalapeno Salsa	1 tbsp	60

FOOD	PORTION	CALS
Cream Cheese Maple Walnut Raisin	2 tbsp	60
Cream Cheese Onion & Chive	2 tbsp	70
Cream Cheese Plain	2 tbsp	60
Cream Cheese Plain Reduced Fat	2 tbsp	60
Cream Cheese Pumpkin	2 tbsp	100
Cream Cheese Smoked Salmon	2 tbsp	60
Cream Cheese Strawberry	2 tbsp	70
Cream Cheese Sun Dried Tomato & Basil	2 tbsp	60
Fruit Spread Apricot	1 serv	75
Fruit Spread Grape	1 serv (1 oz)	75
Fruit Spread Strawberry	1 serv (1 oz)	75
Honey Butter	1 tbsp	90
Hummus	1 serv	110
Mayo Ancho Lime	1 tbsp	50
Mustard French Dijon	1 tsp	10
Mustard Grain Dijon	1 tsp	5
Mustard Honey	1 tsp	15
Mustard Raspberry	2 tbsp	50
Mustard Yellow	1 tbsp	5
Peanut Butter	2 tbsp	190
Salsa Ancho Lime	¼ cup	20

EL POLLO LOCO
DESSERTS

FOOD	PORTION	CALS
Churro	1	179
Fosters Freeze Soft Serve	1 cup	180

MAIN MENU SELECTIONS

FOOD	PORTION	CALS
Bowl Chicken Caesar	1 serv	535
Bowl Pollo	1 serv	545
Bowl Veggie	1 serv	570
Bowl Veggie w/o Cheese	1 serv	529
Burrito BRC	1 serv	530
Burrito Caesar	1 serv	895
Burrito Chicken Lover's	1 serv	525
Burrito Classic Chicken	1	580
Burrito Spicy	1 serv	555
Burrito Twice Grilled	1 serv	835
Burrito Ultimate Chicken	1 serv	685
Chicken Breast	1 piece	153
Chicken Leg	1 piece	86

FOOD	PORTION	CALS
Chicken Thigh	1 piece	120
Chicken Wing	1	83
Cole Slaw	1 serv	206
Corn Cobbette	1 serv	80
French Fries	1 serv	444
Fresh Vegetables	1 serv	70
Gravy	1 serv (1 oz)	107
Mashed Potatoes	1 serv	97
Nachos Chicken	1 serv	1420
Pinto Beans	1 serv	165
Popcorn Chicken	1 serv	226
Potato Salad	1 serv	256
Quesadilla Cheese	1 serv	495
Quesadilla Chicken	1 serv	593
Smokey Black Beans	1 serv	306
Spanish Rice	1 serv	165
Taco Al Carbon Chicken	1 serv	135
Taco Soft Chicken	1	237
Taquitos Chicken	2	370
Tortilla Chips	1 serv	426
Tortilla Corn	1 (4.5 inch)	40
Tortilla Corn	1 (6 inches)	70
Tortilla Flour	1 (6.5 inch)	110
Tortilla Flour	1 (12 inches)	325
Tortilla Spicy Tomato	1 (12 inches)	270
Tostada Salad	1 serv	700
SALAD DRESSINGS AND TOPPINGS		
Bleu Cheese	1 serv (1.5 oz)	230
Buttermilk Ranch	1 serv (1.5 oz)	220
Creamy Chipotle	1 (0.5 oz)	75
Creamy Cilantro	1 serv (0.5 oz)	80
Guacamole	1 serv (1 oz)	30
Hot Sauce Jalapeno	1 pkg (0.5 oz)	5
Light Italian	1 serv (1.5 oz)	20
Salsa Avocado	1 serv (1 oz)	20
Salsa House	1 serv (1 oz)	6
Salsa Pico De Gallo	1 serv (1 oz)	10
Salsa Spicy Chipotle	1 serv (1 oz)	7
Sour Cream	1 serv (1 oz)	60
Thousand Island	1 serv (1.5 oz)	220

FOOD	PORTION	CALS
SALADS		
Caesar	1 serv	565
Ceasar w/o Dressing	1 serv	250
Fiesta Salad	1 serv	755
Fiesta Salad w/o Dressing	1 serv	450
Garden Salad	1 serv	110
Macaroni & Cheese	1 serv	381
Tostada Salad w/o Shell	1 serv	360
FAZOLI'S		
DESSERTS		
Cheesecake	1 slice	290
Cheesecake Turtle	1 slice	420
Cookie Milk Chocolate Chunk	1	360
Lemon Ice	1 serv	190
Specialty Cheesecake	1 serv	300
Strawberry Topping	1 serv	35
MAIN MENU SELECTIONS		
Baked Chicken Parmesan	1 serv	740
Baked Spaghetti Parmesan	1 serv	700
Baked Ziti	1 reg	750
Baked Ziti	1 sm	490
Breadstick	1	140
Breadstick Dry	1	90
Broccoli Fettuccine Alfredo	1 reg	830
Broccoli Fettuccine Alfredo	1 sm	560
Cheese Ravioli w/ Marinara Sauce	1 serv	480
Cheese Ravioli w/ Meat Sauce	1 serv	510
Classic Sampler	1 serv	710
Fettuccine Alfredo	1 reg	800
Fettuccine Alfredo	1 sm	530
Fettuccine w/ Shrimp & Scallop	1 serv	590
Homestyle Lasagna	1 serv	440
Homestyle Lasagna w/ Broccoli	1 serv	420
Minestrone Soup	1 serv	120
Peppery Chicken Alfredo	1 serv	610
Pizza Cheese	1 serv	460
Pizza Combination Double Slice	1 serv	570
Pizza Pepperoni	1 serv	530
Pizza Baked Spaghetti	1 serv	750

FOOD	PORTION	CALS
Spaghetti w/ Marinara Sauce	1 reg	620
Spaghetti w/ Marinara Sauce	1 sm	420
Spaghetti w/ Meat Sauce	1 reg	670
Spaghetti w/ Meat Sauce	1 sm	450
Spaghetti w/ Meatballs	1 reg	1020
Spaghetti w/ Meatballs	1 sm	730
SALAD DRESSINGS		
Honey French	1 serv	150
House Italian	1 serv	110
Ranch	1 serv	150
Reduced Calorie Italian	1 serv	50
Thousand Island	1 serv	130
SALADS		
Caesar Side Salad	1	220
Chicken & Pasta Caesar Salad	1	500
Chicken Caesar Salad	1	420
Chicken Finger Salad	1	190
Chicken Finger Salad w/ Bacon & Honey Mustard	1	400
Garden Salad	1	25
Garden Salad w/ Balsamic Vinaigrette	1	120
Italian Chef Salad	1	260
Pasta Salad	1 serv	590
SANDWICHES		
Panini Chicken Caesar Club	1	660
Panini Chicken Pesto	1	510
Panini Four Cheese & Tomato	1	720
Panini Ham & Swiss	1	600
Panini Italian Club	1	670
Panini Italian Deli	1	660
Panini Smoked Turkey	1	710
Submarinos Club	half	1100
Submarinos Ham & Swiss	1	1000
Submarinos Meatball	half	1260
Submarinos Original	half	1160
Submarinos Pepperoni Pizza	half	1060
Submarinos Turkey	half	990

FOOD	PORTION	CALS
FRESHENS		
PRETZELS		
Bites	1 serv (3 oz)	255
Gourmet	1 (6 oz)	510
SMOOTHIES		
Berry Berry	1 serv (21 oz)	280
Blueberry Breeze	1 serv (21 oz)	396
Caribbean Craze	1 serv (21 oz)	315
Cayman Cooler	1 serv (21 oz)	320
Club Trim	1 serv (21 oz)	291
Fitness Fuel	1 serv (21 oz)	521
Immune Support	1 serv (21 oz)	377
Jamaican Jammer	1 serv (21 oz)	378
Maui Mango	1 serv (21 oz)	354
Mocha Coffee	1 serv (21 oz)	385
Mystic Mango	1 serv (21 oz)	407
Orange Shooter	1 serv (21 oz)	330
Orange Sunrise	1 serv (21 oz)	367
Peach Sunset	1 serv (21 oz)	388
Peachy Pineapple	1 serv (21 oz)	415
Peanut Butter Chocolate	1 serv (21 oz)	312
Pina Colada	1 serv (21 oz)	451
Pineapple Passion	1 serv (21 oz)	389
Raspberry Royale	1 serv (21 oz)	346
Rockin' Raspberry	1 serv (21 oz)	332
Strawberry Shooter	1 serv (21 oz)	251
Strawberry Squeeze	1 serv (21 oz)	313
Vanilla Coffee	1 serv (21 oz)	438
Vanilla Fudge	1 serv (21 oz)	275
GREAT STEAK & POTATO COMPANY		
Baked Potato w/ Broccoli & Cheese	1 serv (12 oz)	340
Chicken Philadelphia	1 serv (10 oz)	640
Chicken Teriyaki	1 serv (11 oz)	580
Fresh Cut Fries	1 reg	540
Fresh Cut Fries	1 serv	920
Fresh Cut Fries	1 sm	460
Great Potato w/ Steak	1 serv (14 oz)	600
Great Potato w/ Turkey	1 serv (14 oz)	610

FOOD	PORTION	CALS
Great Salad Experience w/ Chicken w/o Dressing	1 serv (15oz)	260
Great Steak	1 lg (18 oz)	1070
Great Steak	1 serv (11 oz)	660
Ham Delight	1 serv (11 oz)	710
Turkey Philadelphia	1 serv (10 oz)	690
Veggi Delight	1 serv (7 oz)	570

HAAGEN-DAZS
FROZEN YOGURT

FOOD	PORTION	CALS
Pinapple Coconut	½ cup	230
Soft Serve Nonfat Chocolate	½ cup	110
Soft Serve Nonfat Chocolate Mousse	½ cup	80
Soft Serve Nonfat Coffee	½ cup	110
Soft Serve Nonfat Strawberry	½ cup	110
Soft Serve Nonfat Vanilla	½ cup	110
Soft Serve Nonfat Vanilla Mousse	½ cup	70
Soft Serve Nonfat White Chocolate	½ cup	110
Vanilla Fudge	½ cup	160
Vanilla Raspberry Swirl	½ cup	130

ICE CREAM

FOOD	PORTION	CALS
Bailey's Irish Cream	½ cup	270
Bar Chocolate	1 (2.7 oz)	200
Bar Chocolate & Dark Chocolate	1 (3.6 oz)	350
Bar Coffee	1 (2.7 oz)	190
Bar Coffee & Almond Crunch	1 (3.7 oz)	370
Bar Vanilla	1 (2.7 oz)	190
Bar Vanilla & Almonds	1 (3.7 oz)	380
Bar Vanilla & Milk Chocolate	1 (3.5 oz)	340
Belgian Chocolate Chocolate	½ cup	330
Brownies A La Mode	½ cup	280
Butter Pecan	½ cup	300
Cappuccino Commotion	½ cup	310
Chocolate	½ cup	269
Chocolate Chocolate Chip	½ cup	300
Chocolate Chocolate Mint	½ cup	300
Chocolate Swiss Almond	½ cup	300
Coffee	½ cup	250
Coffee Mocha Chip	½ cup	270
Cookie Dough Dynamo	½ cup	310

FOOD	PORTION	CALS
Cookies & Cream	½ cup	270
Cookies & Fudge	½ cup	180
Deep Chocolate Peanut Butter	½ cup	350
Dulce De Leche Caramel	½ cup	270
Lowfat Coffee Fudge	½ cup	170
Macadamia Brittle	½ cup	280
Macadamia Nut	½ cup	320
Mint Chip	½ cup	280
Pistachio	½ cup	280
Pralines & Cream	½ cup	280
Rum Raisin	½ cup	260
Strawberry	½ cup	250
Vanilla	½ cup	250
Vanilla Chocolate Chip	½ cup	290
Vanilla Swiss Almond	½ cup	290
SORBET		
Bar Raspberry & Vanilla	1 (2.5 oz)	90
Mango	½ cup	120
Orange	½ cup	120
Raspberry	½ cup	120
Soft Serve Raspberry	½ cup	110
Strawberry	½ cup	120
Zesty Lemon	½ cup	120

HARDEE'S
MAIN MENU SELECTIONS

Monster Thickburger	1	1400
SALAD DRESSINGS		
French Fat Free	1 serv (2 oz)	70

HUNGRY HOWIE'S
MAIN MENU SELECTIONS

Howie Wings	6 (3 oz)	180
Three Cheeser Bread	1 serv	370
PIZZA		
Large Cheese	1 slice	175
Large Cheese + Bacon	1 slice	208
Large Cheese + Beef	1 slice	197
Large Cheese + Black Olives	1 slice	181
Large Cheese + Green Olives	1 slice	181
Large Cheese + Green Peppers	1 slice	175

FOOD	PORTION	CALS
Large Cheese + Ham	1 slice	179
Large Cheese + Mushrooms	1 slice	175
Large Cheese + Onions	1 slice	175
Large Cheese + Pepperoni	1 slice	191
Large Cheese + Pineapple	1 slice	388
Large Cheese + Sausage	1 slice	195
Medium Cheese	1 slice	153
Medium Cheese + Bacon	1 slice	179
Medium Cheese + Beef	1 slice	177
Medium Cheese + Black Olives	1 slice	159
Medium Cheese + Green Olives	1 slice	159
Medium Cheese + Green Peppers	1 slice	155
Medium Cheese + Ham	1 slice	159
Medium Cheese + Mushrooms	1 slice	155
Medium Cheese + Onions	1 slice	155
Medium Cheese + Pepperoni	1 slice	171
Medium Cheese + Pineapple	1 slice	158
Medium Cheese + Sausage	1 slice	175
Small Cheese	1 slice	121
Small Cheese + Bacon	1 slice	138
Small Cheese + Beef	1 slice	137
Small Cheese + Black Olives	1 slice	125
Small Cheese + Green Olives	1 slice	125
Small Cheese + Green Peppers	1 slice	122
Small Cheese + Ham	1 slice	126
Small Cheese + Mushrooms	1 slice	123
Small Cheese + Onions	1 slice	122
Small Cheese + Pepperoni	1 slice	136
Small Cheese + Pineapple	1 slice	124
Small Cheese + Sausage	1 slice	136
SALADS		
Antipasto Salad w/o Dressing	1 lg	101
Chef Salad w/o Dressing	1 lg	99
Garden Salad w/o Dressing	1 lg	17
Greek Salad w/o Dressing	1 lg	109
SANDWICHES		
Sub Deluxe Italian	½ sub	506
Sub Ham & Cheese	½ sub	475
Sub Pizza	½ sub	689
Sub Pizza Special	½ sub	606

FOOD	PORTION	CALS
Sub Steak Cheese Mushroom	½ sub	491
Sub Turkey	½ sub	466
Sub Turkey Club	½ sub	556
Sub Vegetarian	½ sub	530

IHOP

Pancake Buckwheat	1 (1.7 oz)	110
Pancake Buttermilk	1 (1.7 oz)	110
Pancake Country Griddle	1 (2 oz)	120
Pancake Harvest Grain 'N Nut	1 (2.25 oz)	180

JACK IN THE BOX
BEVERAGES

Barq's Root Beer	1 serv (20 oz)	180
Coca-Cola Classic	1 serv (20 oz)	170
Coffee	1 serv (12 oz)	5
Diet Coke	1 serv (20 oz)	0
Dr Pepper	1 serv (20 oz)	190
Ice Cream Shake Caramel	1 serv (16 oz)	660
Ice Cream Shake Chocolate	1 (16 oz)	660
Ice Cream Shake Oreo	1 serv (16 oz)	670
Ice Cream Shake Strawberry	1 serv (16 oz)	640
Ice Cream Shake Strawberry Banana	1 serv (16 oz)	700
Ice Cream Shake Vanilla	1 (16 oz)	570
Iced Tea	1 serv (20 oz)	0
Lowfat Milk 2%	1 serv (8 oz)	140
Orange Juice	1 serv (10 oz)	140
Sprite	1 serv (20 oz)	160

BREAKFAST SELECTIONS

Breakfast Sandwich Sourdough	1	440
Breakfast Sandwich Ultimate	1	730
Breakfast Jack	1	310
Croissant Sausage	1	680
Croissant Supreme	1	570
French Toast Sticks	4 pieces	430
Hash Brown	1 serv	150
Sandwich Extreme Sausage	1	720

DESSERTS

Cheesecake	1 serv	310
Double Fudge Cake	1 serv	310

FOOD	PORTION	CALS
MAIN MENU SELECTIONS		
American Cheese	1 slice	45
Bacon Cheddar Potato Wedges	1 serv	770
Cheeseburger Bacon Bacon	1	910
Cheeseburger Bacon Ultimate	1	1120
Cheeseburger Junior Bacon	1	540
Cheeseburger Ultimate	1	990
Chicken Breast Pieces	4	360
Chicken Breast Strips	1 serv	500
Chicken Fajita Pita	1	330
Chicken Sandwich	1	410
Dipping Sauce Barbeque	1 serv (1.6 oz)	45
Egg Rolls	1	130
Fish & Chips	1 serv	610
French Fries	1 lg	580
French Fries	1 med	410
French Fries	1 sm	330
Hamburger	1	310
Hamburger w/ Cheese	1	360
Jumbo Jack	1	600
Jumbo Jack w/ Cheese	1	690
Onion Rings	1 serv	500
Philly Cheesesteak	1	580
Salsa	1 serv (1 oz)	10
Sandwich Roasted Turkey	1	580
Sandwich Ultimate Club	1	640
Seasoned Curly Fries	1 serv	400
Sour Cream	1 serv (1 oz)	60
Sourdough Grilled Chicken Club	1	520
Sourdough Jack	1	700
Spicy Crispy Chicken	1	730
Stuffed Jalapeno	3 pieces	230
Swiss Style Cheese	1 slice	40
Taco	1	170
Taco Monster	1	260
Turkey Jack	1	700
SALAD DRESSINGS AND TOPPINGS		
Almonds Roasted Slivered	1 serv (0.7 oz)	130
Asian Sesame	1 serv (2.5 oz)	230
Bacon Ranch	1 serv (2.5 oz)	320

FOOD	PORTION	CALS
Balsamic Vinaigrette Low Fat	1 serv (2.5 oz)	40
Country Crock Spread	1 pkg	25
Creamy Southwest Dressing	1 serv (2.5 oz)	270
Croutons	1 serv (0.5 oz)	60
Dipping Sauce Buttermilk House	1 serv (0.9 oz)	130
Dipping Sauce Frank's Red Hot Buffalo	1 serv (1 oz)	10
Dipping Sauce Sweet & Sour	1 serv (1 oz)	45
Grape Jelly	1 serv (0.5 oz)	35
Herb Mayo Sauce Low Fat	1 serv (1.5 oz)	45
Ketchup	1 pkg (0.3 oz)	10
Marinara Sauce	1 serv (0.9 oz)	15
Mustard	1 pkg	0
Ranch	1 serv (2.5 oz)	390
Ranch Lite	1 serv (2.5 oz)	190
Soy Sauce	1 serv (0.3 oz)	5
Syrup	1 serv (1.5 oz)	130
Taco Sauce	1 serv (0.3 oz)	0
Tartar Sauce	1 serv (1.5 oz)	210
Thousand Island	1 serv (2 oz)	160
Vinegar	1 serv	0
Wonton Strips	1 serv (0.7 oz)	110
SALADS		
Asian Salad	1 serv	140
Chicken Club Salad	1 serv	290
Side Salad	1 serv	50
Southwest Chicken	1 serv	320
JAMBA JUICE		
Jambolas Honey Nut Energy	1 serv	192
Jambolas Mighty Multi Grain	1 serv	208
Jambolas Mind Over Blueberry	1 serv	170
Jambolas Pizza Protein	1 serv	199
Mango-A-Go-Go	1 reg (24 oz)	460
Orchard Oasis	1 reg (24 oz)	440
Protein Berry Pizazz	1 reg (24 oz)	470
Razzmatazz	1 reg (24 oz)	440
JERSEY MIKE'S		
Ham On Wheat	1	240
Ham On White	1	240
Ham/Turkey Wheat	1	230

FOOD	PORTION	CALS
Ham/Turkey White	1	240
Roast Beef Wheat	1	290
Roast Beef White	1	280
Turkey On Wheat	1	230
Turkey On White	1	230
Veggie On Wheat	1	170
Veggie On White	1	170

KENTUCKY FRIED CHICKEN
BEVERAGES

FOOD	PORTION	CALS
Diet Pepsi	1 sm	0
Mt. Dew	1 sm	150
Pepsi	1 sm (11 oz)	140

DESSERTS

FOOD	PORTION	CALS
Cake Double Chocolate Chip	1 slice	400
Cherry Cheesecake Parfait	1 serv	300
Lil' Bucket Chocolate Creme	1 serv	270
Lil' Bucket Fudge Brownie	1	270
Lil' Bucket Lemon Creme	1 serv	400
Lil' Bucket Strawberry Shortcake	1 serv	200
Pie Apple	1 slice	270
Pie Lemon Meringue	1 slice	310
Pie Pecan	1 slice	370
Pie Strawberry Creme	1 slice	270

MAIN MENU SELECTIONS

FOOD	PORTION	CALS
BBQ Beans	1 serv	230
Biscuit	1	190
Boneless Wings HBBQ Sauced	7 pieces	600
Chicken Pot Pie	1 serv	770
Cole Slaw	1 serv	190
Corn On The Cob	1 ear (3 inch)	70
Crispy Strips	3	400
Extra Crispy Breast	1 serv	490
Extra Crispy Drumstick	1	160
Extra Crispy Thigh	1	370
Extra Crispy Whole Wing	1	190
Green Beans	1 serv	50
Hot & Spicy Breast	1 serv	460
Hot & Spicy Drumstick	1	150
Hot & Spicy Thigh	1	400

FOOD	PORTION	CALS
Hot & Spicy Whole Wing	1	180
Hot Wings	6 pieces	450
Mac & Cheese	1 serv	130
Mashed Potatoes w/o Gravy	1 serv	110
Mashed Potatoes With Gravy	1 serv	120
Original Recipe Breast	1 serv	380
Original Recipe Breast w/o Skin Or Breading	1 serv	140
Original Recipe Drumstick	1	140
Original Recipe Thigh	1	360
Original Recipe Whole Wing	1	150
Popcorn Chicken	1 reg serv	450
Potato Salad	1 serv	180
Potato Wedges	1 sm	240
Sandwich HBBQ	1	300
Sandwich Original Recipe w/ Sauce	1	450
Sandwich Tender Roast w/ Sauce	1	390
Sandwich Tender Roast w/o Sauce	1	260
Sandwich Twister	1	670
Sandwich Zinger w/ Sauce	1	680
Sandwich Zinger w/o Sauce	1	540
Sandwiches Original Recipe w/o Sauce	1	320
Wings HBBQ Sauced	6 pieces	540

KOO-KOO-ROO

FOOD	PORTION	CALS
Original Breast	1 piece	187
Original Chicken Dark	3 pieces	320
Rotisserie Chicken Breast & Wing	1 serv	355
Rotisserie Chicken Leg & Thigh	1 serv	300
Rotisserie Half Chicken	1 serv	655
Sandwich BBQ Chicken	1	562
Sandwich Chicken Caesar	1	781
Sandwich Original Chicken	1	661
Traditional Turkey Dinner	1 serv	692
Turkey Pot Pie	1 serv	883
Turkey Sandwich Hand Carved	1	599
Wrap Caesar Chicken	1	757
Wrap Chipotle Chicken	1	924

KRISPY KREME

FOOD	PORTION	CALS
Apple Fritter	1	380
Caramel Kreme Crunch	1	350

FOOD	PORTION	CALS
Chocolate Iced Glazed w/ Sprinkles	1	260
Chocolate Malted Kreme	1	390
Chocolate Iced	1	250
Chocolate Iced Cake	1	270
Chocolate Iced Creme Filled	1	350
Chocolate Iced Cruller	1	290
Chocolate Iced Custard Filled	1	300
Chocolated Iced w/ Sprinkles	1	290
Cinnamon Apple Filled	1	290
Cinnamon Bun	1	260
Cinnamon Sugar Cake	1	280
Cinnamon Twist	1	230
Coffee & Kreme	1	360
Dulce De Leche	1	290
Glazed Blueberry	1	340
Glazed Creme Filled	1	340
Glazed Devil's Food	1	340
Glazed Lemon Filled	1	290
Glazed Raspberry Filled	1	300
Glazed Sour Cream	1	340
Glazed Strawberry Filled	1	290
Glazed Cinnamon	1	210
Glazed Cruller	1	240
Glazed Custard Filled	1	290
Glazed Filled Blueberry	1	290
Glazed Twist	1	210
Honey & Oat	1	340
Key Lime Pie	1	330
Maple Iced	1	240
Maple Iced Cake	1	270
New York Cheesecake	1	330
Original Glazed	1	200
Powdered Blueberry Filled	1	290
Powdered Cake	1	280
Powdered Creme Filled	1	340
Powdered Raspberry	1	300
Powdered Strawberry Filled	1	260
Pumpkin Spice Cake	1	340
Sugar Coated	1	200
Traditional Cake	1	230

FOOD	PORTION	CALS
Vanilla Iced Creme Fill	1	340
Vanilla Iced Glazed	1	240
Vanilla Iced Cake w/ Sprinkles	1	270
Vanilla Iced Custard Filled	1	290
Vanilla Iced Raspberry Filled	1	350
Vanilla Iced Raspberry Glazed	1	350

KRYSTAL
BEVERAGES
FOOD	PORTION	CALS
Coco Cola Classic frzn	1 (16 oz)	130
Cocoa Cola Classic	1 sm (16 oz)	129
Diet Coke	1 sm (16 oz)	tr
Sprite	1 sm (16 oz)	126

BREAKFAST SELECTIONS
FOOD	PORTION	CALS
Biscuit	1	270
Biscuit And Gravy	1	280
Biscuit Bacon Egg & Cheese	1	390
Biscuit Chik	1	360
Biscuit Sausage	1	480
Country Breakfast	1 serv	660
Kryspers	1 serv	190
Krystal Sunriser	1	240
Scrambler	1 serv	440

DESSERTS
FOOD	PORTION	CALS
Fried Apple Turnover	1	220
Lemon Icebox Pie	1 serv	260

MAIN MENU SELECTIONS
FOOD	PORTION	CALS
Chik'n Bites	1 sm	310
Chik'n Bites Salad	1 serv	290
Fries	1 med	470
Fries Chili Cheese	1 serv	540
Krystal	1	160
Krystal Bacon Cheese	1	190
Krystal Cheese	1	180
Krystal Chik	1	240
Krystal Chili	1 serv	200
Krystal Double	1	260
Krystal Double Cheese	1	310
Pup	1	170

FOOD	PORTION	CALS
Pup Chili Cheese	1	210
Pup Corn	1	260

LITTLE CAESARS
MAIN MENU SELECTIONS

FOOD	PORTION	CALS
Baby Pan! Pan!	1 piece	360
Crazy Bread	1 piece	90
Crazy Bread Cinnamon	2 pieces	100
Crazy Sauce	1 serv (4 oz)	45
Deli Sandwich Ham & Cheese	1	640
Deli Sandwich Italian	1	800
Deli Sandwich Veggie	1	600
Italian Cheese Bread	1 piece	130

PIZZA

FOOD	PORTION	CALS
14 Inch Round Meatsa	1/10 pie	280
14 Inch Round Supreme	1/10 pie	270
14 Inch Round Veggie	1/10 pie	240
14 Inch Thin Crust Cheese	1/10 pie	160
16 Inch Round Cheese	1/12 pie	220
18 Inch Round Cheese	1/14 pie	230
Deep Dish Large	1/8 pie	320
Deep Dish Medium	1/8 pie	230

SALAD DRESSINGS

FOOD	PORTION	CALS
Caesar	1 serv (1.5 oz)	230
Greek	1 serv (1.5 oz)	270
Italian	1 serv (1.5 oz)	220
Italian Fat Free	1 serv (1.5 oz)	25
Ranch	1 serv (1.5 oz)	230

SALADS

FOOD	PORTION	CALS
Antipasto	1 serv	140
Caesar	1 serv	90
Greek	1 serv	128
Tossed Salad	1 serv	100

TOPPINGS PER SLICE

FOOD	PORTION	CALS
Bacon	1 serv	41
Beef	1 serv	20
Black Olives	1 serv	12
Extra Cheese	1 serv	26
Green Peppers	1 serv	2
Ham	1 serv	5

FOOD	PORTION	CALS
Italian Sausage	1 serv	22
Mushrooms	1 serv	2
Onion	1 serv	3
Pepperoni	1 serv	26
Pineapple	1 serv	7
Tomato	1 serv	2

LONG JOHN SILVER'S
BEVERAGES

Coca Cola	1 sm	150
Diet Coke	1 sm	0
Sprite	1 sm	140

DESSERTS

Pie Chocolate Cream	1 pie	310
Pie Pecan	1 pie	370
Pie Pineapple Cream	1 pie	290

MAIN MENU SELECTIONS

Baked Cod	1 piece	120
Battered Chicken	1 piece	140
Battered Fish	1 piece	230
Battered Shrimp	1 piece	45
Breaded Clams	1 serv	240
Cheesesticks	3 pieces	140
Clam Chowder	1 bowl	220
Corn Cobbette	1 piece	90
Crumblies	1 serv	170
Crunchy Shrimp	21 pieces	330
Fries	1 reg	230
Hushpuppy	1 piece	60
Rice	1 serv	180
Sandwich Chicken	1	360
Sandwich Fish	1	440
Sandwich Ultimate Fish	1	500
Slaw	1 serv	200

MAGGIE MOO'S

Ice Cream Fat Free	½ cup	80
Ice Cream Low Carb Sugar Added	½ cup	100
Ice Cream Udderly Cream	½ cup	180
Sorbet	½ cup	90

FOOD	PORTION	CALS
MANHATTAN BAGEL		
Blueberry	1	260
Cheddar Cheese	1	270
Chocolate Chip	1	290
Cinnamon Raisin	1	280
Cranberry Orange	1	270
Egg	1	270
Everything	1	290
Garlic	1	270
Jalapeno Cheddar	1	260
Marble	1	260
Oat Bran	1	260
Oat Bran Raisin Walnut	1	270
Onion	1	270
Plain	1	260
Poppy	1	300
Pumpernickel	1	250
Rye	1	260
Salt	1	260
Sesame	1	310
Spinach	1	270
Sun-Dried Tomato	1	260
Whole Wheat	1	260
MARBLE SLAB CREAMERY		
Cone Honey Wheat	1	130
Cone Sugar	1	130
Cone Vanilla Cinnamon	1	130
Frozen Yogurt Nonfat	½ cup	100
Frozen Yogurt Nonfat No Sugar Added	½ cup	90
Ice Cream Reduced Fat	1 serv (6.75 oz)	390
Ice Cream Superpremium	1 serv (6.75 oz)	450
Sorbet	½ cup	90
MAUI WOWI		
Smoothie Rip Sticks All Flavors	1	88
MAX & ERMA'S		
Black Bean Roll Up	1 serv	401
Black Bean Salsa	½ cup	215
Fruit Smoothie	1 serv	124

FOOD	PORTION	CALS
Garden Grill Sandwich w/ Tex Mex Dressing	1	569
Garlic Breadstick	1	156
Hula Bowl w/ Fat Free Honey Mustard Dressing w/o Breadsticks	1 serv	583
Salad Dressing Fat Free French	2 tbsp	126
Salad Dressing Fat Free Honey Mustard	2 tbsp	60
Salad Dressing Tex Mex	2 tbsp	33
Sugar Snap Peas w/ Lemon Pepper Butter	1 serv (4 oz)	106

MCDONALD'S
BAKED SELECTIONS
Cinnamon Roll Warm	1	420

BEVERAGES
Apple Juice	1 box (6.75 oz)	90
Chocolate Milk 1% Low Fat	8 oz	170
Coca-Cola Classic	1 sm (16 oz)	150
Coffee	1 (12 oz)	0
Diet Coke	1 sm (16 oz)	0
Half & Half Creamer	1 pkg	15
Hi-C Orange	1 sm (16 oz)	160
Iced Tea Unsweetened	1 (16 oz)	0
Milk Lowfat 1%	1 serv (8 oz)	100
Orange Juice	1 sm (12 oz)	140
Powerade Mountain Blast	1 sm (16 oz)	100
Sprite	1 sm (16 oz)	150
Triple Shake Chocolate	1 (16 oz)	580
Triple Shake Strawberry	1 (16 oz)	560
Triple Shake Vanilla	1 (16 oz)	550

BREAKFAST SELECTIONS
Big Breakfast	1 serv	730
Biscuit	1	240
Biscuit Bacon Egg Cheese	1	440
Biscuit Sausage	1	410
Biscuit Sausage w/ Egg	1	500
Deluxe Breakfast	1 serv	1220
English Muffin Buttered	1	150
Hash Browns	1 serv	140
Hotcakes Margarine & Syrup	1 serv	600
Hotcakes & Sausage	1 serv	770
Hotcakes Plain	1 serv	340

FOOD	PORTION	CALS
McGriddles Sausage	1	420
McGriddles Sausage Egg Cheese	1	560
McMuffin Egg	1	450
McMuffin Sausage	1	370
Sausage	1 patty	170
Sausage Burrito	1	300
Scrambled Eggs	2	180
DESSERTS		
Apple Dippers	1 pkg	35
Apple Pie Baked	1	250
Carmel Dip Low Fat	1 pkg	70
Cinnamon Roll Deluxe Warm	1	590
Cookie Chocolate Chip	1 (1.1 oz)	160
Cookie Chocolate Chip	1 pkg	270
Cookie Oatmeal	1 (1.1 oz)	140
Cookie Sugar	1 (1.1 oz)	150
Fruit 'n Yogurt Parfait	1 serv	160
Ice Cream Cone Reduced Fat Vanilla	1	150
McDonaldland Cookies	1 pkg	250
McFlurry M&M	1 (12 oz)	620
McFlurry Oreo	1 (12 oz)	560
Peanuts For Sundae	1 serv	45
Sundae Hot Caramel	1	340
Sundae Hot Fudge	1	340
Sundae Strawberry	1	280
MAIN MENU SELECTIONS		
Big Mac	1	560
Big N' Tasty	1	470
Big N' Tasty w/ Cheese	1	520
Cheeseburger	1	310
Cheeseburger Double	1	460
Chicken McNuggets	4 pieces	170
Chicken Selects	3 pieces	380
Crispy Chicken Classic	1	500
Crispy Chicken Club	1	680
Crispy Chicken Ranch BLT	1	580
Filet-O-Fish	1	400
French Fries	1 sm (2.6 oz)	230
Grilled Chicken Classic	1	420

FOOD	PORTION	CALS
Grilled Chicken Club	1	590
Grilled Chicken Ranch BLT	1	490
Hamburger	1	260
McChicken	1	370
McChicken Hot 'n Spicy	1	380
Quarter Pounder	1	420
Quarter Pounder Double w/ Cheese	1	730
Quarter Pounder w/ Cheese	1	510
SALAD DRESSINGS AND SAUCES		
Honey	1 pkg (0.5 oz)	50
Newman's Own Cobb	1 pkg (2 oz)	120
Newman's Own Creamy Caesar	1 pkg (2 oz)	190
Newman's Own Low Fat Balsamic Vinaigrette	1 pkg (1.5 oz)	40
Newman's Own Low Fat Family Recipe Italian	1 pkg (1.6 oz)	50
Newman's Own Ranch	1 pkg (2 oz)	170
Sauce Barbecue	1 pkg (1 oz)	45
Sauce Chipotle Barbecue	1 pkg	70
Sauce Creamy Ranch	1 pkg (1.5 oz)	200
Sauce Hot Mustard	1 pkg (1 oz)	50
Sauce Spicy Buffalo	1 pkg (1.5 oz)	60
Sauce Sweet 'N Sour	1 pkg (1 oz)	50
Sauce Tangy Honey	1 pkg (1.5 oz)	70
Mustard		
SALADS		
Bacon Ranch w/ Crispy Chicken	1 serv	340
Bacon Ranch w/ Grilled Chicken	1 serv	260
Bacon Ranch w/o Chicken	1 serv	140
Caesar w/ Crispy Chicken	1 serv	300
Caesar w/ Grilled Chicken	1 serv	220
Caesar w/o Chicken	1 serv	90
California Cobb w/ Crispy Chicken	1 serv	360
California Cobb w/ Grilled Chicken	1 serv	280
California Cobb w/o Chicken	1 serv	160
Croutons Butter Garlic	1 pkg	60
Fruit & Walnut	1 serv	310
Side Salad	1 serv	20

MIAMI SUBS

FOOD	PORTION	CALS
Burger Deluxe	1	784
Cheeseburger Deluxe	1	859

FOOD	PORTION	CALS
Cheeseburger Deluxe Bacon	1	919
Cheesesteak Classic	1 (6 inch)	420
Cheesesteak Original	1 (6 inch)	409
Cheesesteak Works	1 (6 inch)	532
Chicken Philly Classic	1 (6 inch)	551
Mozzarella Sticks	1 serv	757
Onion Rings	1 serv	869
Pita Chicken	1	392
Pita Gyros	1	662
Platter Chicken Breast	1 serv	743
Platter Gyros	1 serv	1420
Salad Caesar w/ Dressing	1 serv	459
Salad Chicken Caesar w/ Dressing	1 serv	609
Salad Chicken Club	1 serv	490
Salad Garden	1 serv	310
Salad Greek	1 serv	284
Salad Greek Side w/ Dressing	1 serv	78
Spicy Fries	1 reg	532
Subs 6 Inch Ham And Cheese	1	452
Subs 6 Inch Italian Deli	1	516
Subs 6 Inch Meatball	1	491
Subs 6 Inch Tuna	1	468
Subs 6 Inch Turkey	1	484
Wings w/ Fries Celery & Blue Cheese	1 serv	1020

MR. HERO
DESSERTS

Cheesecake	1 serv	350
Cheesecake w/ Cherries	1 serv	385

MAIN MENU SELECTIONS

Breadstick w/ Sauce	1 serv	291
Cheddar Cheese Sauce	1 serv	60
Onion Rings	1 serv	564
Potato Waffers	1 serv	334
Spaghetti Dinner	1 serv	606
Spaghetti w/ Meatballs	1 serv	846

SALAD DRESSINGS

Buttermilk	1 serv (2 oz)	290
Creamy Italian	1 serv (2 oz)	190
Fat Free French	1 serv (2 oz)	70

FOOD	PORTION	CALS
Fat Free Ranch	1 serv (2 oz)	70
SALADS		
Croutons	1 serv	59
Garden Salad	1 serv	36
Grilled Chicken	1 serv	225
Seafood Crab	1 serv	452
Side Salad	1 serv	27
Tuna	1 serv	745
SANDWICHES		
Cheesesteaks Grilled Steak	7 inch	450
Cheesesteaks Hot Buttered Deluxe	7 inch	566
Cold Subs Classic Italian	7 inch	586
Cold Subs Tuna & Cheese	7 inch	666
Cold Subs Turkey & Cheese	7 inch	453
Cold Subs Ultimate Italian	7 inch	608
Hot Subs Grilled Chicken Philly	7 inch	438
Hot Subs Meatball	7 inch	620
Hot Subs Romanburger	7 inch	717
Round Bacon Cheeseburger	1	352
Round Chicken	1	420
Round Fish	1	412
Round Tuna	1	302
MR. PITA		
Cranberry Turkey	1 reg	424
Grilled Raspberry Chicken	1 reg	342
Grilled Chicken & Broccoli	1 reg	373
Grilled Chicken Caesar	1 reg	353
Grilled Hawaiian Chicken	1 reg	375
Ultra Combo	1 reg	354
Ultra Grilled Chicken	1 reg	367
Ultra Supreme	1 reg	350
Ultra Turkey	1 reg	343
MRS. FIELDS		
Brownie Double Fudge	1 (2.7 oz)	360
Brownie Frosted Fudge	1 (3.7 oz)	440
Brownie Pecan Fudge	1 (2.7 oz)	340
Brownie Pecan Pie	1 (2.7 oz)	340
Brownie Walnut Fudge	1 (2.7 oz)	380
Bundt Cake Banana Walnut	1 piece (2.9 oz)	350

FOOD	PORTION	CALS
Bundt Cake Banana Walnut w/ Chocolate Chips	1 piece (2.9oz)	370
Bundt Cake Blueberry	1 piece (2.9 oz)	270
Bundt Cake Raspberry	1 piece (2.9 oz)	270
Bundt Cake White w/ Chocolate Chips	1 piece (2.9 oz)	350
Cookie Butter Toffee	1 (2.3 oz)	290
Cookie Cinnamon Sugar	1 (2.3 oz)	300
Cookie Coconut Macadamia	1 (2.3 oz)	280
Cookie Debra's Special	1 (2.3 oz)	280
Cookie Milk Chocolate	1 (2.3 oz)	280
Cookie Milk Chocolate & Walnuts	1 (2.3 oz)	320
Cookie Milk Chocolate Macadamia	1 (2.3 oz)	320
Cookie Oatmeal Chocolate Chip	1 (2.3 oz)	280
Cookie Oatmeal Raisin & Walnuts	1 (2.3 oz)	280
Cookie Peanut Butter	1 (2.3 oz)	310
Cookie Peanut Butter w/ Milk Chocolate Chips	1 (2.3 oz)	300
Cookie Semi-Sweet Chocolate	1 (2.3 oz)	280
Cookie Semi-Sweet Chocolate & Walnuts	1 (2.3 oz)	310
Cookie White Chunk Macadamia	1 (2.3 oz)	310
Jumbo Cookie Snickerdoodle	1 (5 oz)	640
Nibbler Cookies	2 (0.9 oz)	110
Nibbler Cookies Chewy Chocolate Fudge	2 (0.9 oz)	110
Nibbler Cookies Cinnamon Sugar	2 (0.9 oz)	120
Nibbler Cookies Debra's Special	2 (0.9 oz)	100
Nibbler Cookies M&M	2 (0.9 oz)	110
Nibbler Cookies Milk Chocolate	2 (0.9 oz)	110
Nibbler Cookies Milk Chocolate w/ Walnuts	2 (0.9 oz)	120
Nibbler Cookies Peanut Butter	2 (0.9 oz)	110
Nibbler Cookies Semi-Sweet Chocolate	2 (0.9 oz)	110
Nibbler Cookies Triple Chocolate	2 (0.9 oz)	110
Nibbler Cookies White Chunk Macadamia	2 (0.9 oz)	120

MY FAVORITE MUFFIN
BAGELS

Blueberry	1	320
Cinnamon Raisin	1	310
Honey Grain	1	310
Plain	1	310
Russian Black Bread	1	320
Sour Dough	1	310
Whole Wheat	1	310

FOOD	PORTION	CALS
MUFFINS		
Banana Nut	⅓ jumbo	195
Blueberry	⅓ jumbo	168
Blueberry Cheesecake	⅓ jumbo	199
Boston Cream Pie	⅓ jumbo	176
Cherry Cheesecake	⅓ jumbo	170
Chocolate Cheesecake	⅓ jumbo	202
Chocolate Chip	⅓ jumbo	211
Cinnamon Crumb Cake	⅓ jumbo	212
Cinnamon Swirl Cheesecake	⅓ jumbo	214
Deep Dish Apple Pie	⅓ jumbo	177
Double Chocolate	⅓ jumbo	201
Fat Free Blueberry	⅓ jumbo	108
Fat Free Cherry Pie	⅓ jumbo	109
Fat Free Chocolate Eclair	⅓ jumbo	120
Fat Free Chocolate Marble	⅓ jumbo	125
Fat Free Cinnamon Bun	⅓ jumbo	168
Fat Free Raspberry Amaretto	⅓ jumbo	127
Golden Corn Bread	⅓ jumbo	197
Lemon Poppyseed	⅓ jumbo	201
Pumpkin Spice	⅓ jumbo	181
NATHAN'S		
¼ Pound Burger	1	537
¼ Pound Burger w/ Cheese	1	850
Bacon Cheeseburger	1	707
Cheesesteak Chicken	1 serv	565
Cheesesteak Original	1	741
Cheesesteak Supreme	1 serv	786
Chicken Tender Pita	1	610
Chicken Tenders	3 pieces	512
Cole Slaw	1 serv	213
Corn Muffin	1	163
Famous Hot Dog	1	309
Fish N Chips	1 serv	1538
French Fries	1 reg	547
Hot Dog Nuggets	6 pieces	351
Hush Puppy	2 pieces	277
Onion Rings	1 sm	559
Platter Chicken Breast	1 serv	943

FOOD	PORTION	CALS
Platter Chicken Tender	1 serv	1301
Sandwich Chicken Tender	1	725
Sandwich Fish	1	469
Sandwich Grilled Chicken	1	524
Seafood Sampler	1 serv	3379
Shrimp N Chips	1 serv	2051
Super Burger	1	864

OLD SPAGHETTI FACTORY
CHILDREN'S MENU SELECTIONS

Grilled Cheese Sandwich	1 serv	360
Macaroni & Cheese	1 serv	350
Spaghetti w/ Tomato Sauce	1 serv	300
Spaghetti w/ Tomato Sauce & Meatballs	1 serv	440

DESSERTS

Caramel Turtle Pie	1 serv	660
Mud Pie	1 serv	680
New York Cheese Cake w/ Strawberry Topping	1 serv	690

MAIN MENU SELECTIONS

Baked Chicken	1 dinner serv	880
Caesar Salad	1 sm	330
Caesar Salad Dinner Chicken	1 serv	1280
Chicken Marsala	1 dinner serv	960
Fettuccine Alfredo	1 dinner serv	1130
Fettuccine Chicken	1 dinner serv	960
Lasagne	1 dinner serv	630
Parmigiana Chicken	1 dinner serv	840
Parmigiana Eggplant	1 dinner serv	670
Pot Pourri	1 dinner serv	710
Ravioli Spinach & Cheese	1 dinner serv	480
Salmon Tuscany	1 dinner serv	680
Sandwich Meatball	1	860
Sandwich Sausage	1	730
Sandwich Tuscan Chicken	1	1060
Seafood Cheddar Melt	1 serv	790
Spaghetti w/ Clam Sauce	1 dinner serv	690
Spaghetti w/ Clam Sauce & Mizithra	1 dinner serv	960
Spaghetti w/ Meat & Clam Sauces	1 dinner serv	980
Spaghetti w/ Meat Sauce	1 dinner serv	470
Spaghetti w/ Meat Sauce & Mizithra	1 dinner serv	850

FOOD	PORTION	CALS
Spaghetti w/ Meat Sauce & Sausage	1 dinner serv	830
Spaghetti w/ Meatballs	1 dinner serv	840
Spaghetti w/ Mizithra	1 dinner serv	1010
Spaghetti w/ Mushroom & Clam Sauces	1 dinner serv	830
Spaghetti w/ Mushroom & Meat Sauces	1 dinner serv	460
Spaghetti w/ Mushroom Sauce	1 dinner serv	460
Spaghetti w/ Mushroom Sauce & Mizithra	1 dinner serv	850
Spaghetti w/ Tomato & Mizithra	1 dinner serv	840
Spaghetti w/ Tomato & Meat Sauces	1 dinner serv	460
Spaghetti w/ Tomato Sauce	1 dinner serv	440
Spaghetti w/ Tomato Sauce & Clam Sauce	1 dinner serv	560
Starter Garlic Cheese Bread	1 serv	1220
Starter Meatballs	1 serv	910
Starter Sausage	1 serv	690
Starter Tortellini	1 serv	930
Tortellini Mortadella & Chicken	1 dinner serv	930
SOUPS		
Chicken Mulligatawny	1 serv	250
Chicken Orzo	1 serv	90
Clam Chowder	1 serv	380
Cream Of Broccoli	1 serv	220
Mediterranean White Bean	1 serv	150
Minestrone	1 serv	120

ON THE BORDER
CHILDREN'S MENU SELECTIONS

FOOD	PORTION	CALS
Border Chicken Strips	1 serv	570
Corn Dog	1	320
Crispy Taco Mexican Dinner Beef	1 serv	740
Crispy Taco Mexican Dinner Chicken	1 serv	740
Hamburger	1	390
Nachos Bean & Cheese	1 serv	980
Nachos Cheese	1 serv	670
Quesadillas Chicken	1 serv	720
Sandwich Grilled Chicken	1	630
Soft Taco Mexican Dinner Beef	1 serv	840
Soft Taco Mexican Dinner Chicken	1 serv	750
Sundae w/ Chocolate Syrup	1 serv	300
Sundae w/ Strawberry Puree	1 serv	340

FOOD	PORTION	CALS
DESSERTS		
Border Brownie Sundae	1	440
Chocolate Turtle Empanadas	1 serv	1280
Dulce De Leche Cheesecake	1 serv	1160
Kahlua Ice Cream Pie	1 serv	850
Sizzling Apple Crisp	1 serv	960
Sopapillas	1 serv	1230
Vanilla Ice Cream	1 scoop	180
MAIN MENU SELECTIONS		
Bacon Wrapped Shrimp	1 serv	730
Baja Chicken	1 serv	610
Bandera Sirloin	1 serv	640
Beans Black	1 serv	180
Beans Refried	1 serv	290
Black Bean & Corn Relish	1 serv	80
Border Chimichanga Fajita Chicken w/ Onions & Mushrooms	1 serv	1230
Border Chimichanga Ground Beef	1 serv	1310
Border Chimichanga Spicy Chicken	1 serv	1160
Border Sampler	1 serv	1940
Bordurrito Big Beef w/ Side Salad	1 serv	1600
Bordurrito Big Chicken w/ Side Salad	1 serv	1420
Burrito Beef	1 serv	1080
Burrito Chicken	1 serv	880
Burrito Three Sauce Fajita Chicken	1 serv	870
Burrito Three Sauce Fajita Steak	1 serv	1050
Carne Asada & Shrimp	1 serv	1040
Cheese Chile Rellano	1	880
Cheesy Pepper Jack Mashed Potatoes	1 serv	380
Chicken Flautas Appetizer	1 serv	970
Chile Con Queso	1 bowl	390
Chile Con Queso	1 cup	250
Corona Extra Dinner	1 serv	2040
Crispy Taco Beef	1	330
Crispy Taco Chicken	1	240
Crispy Taco Veggie	1	250
Dos XX Fish Tacos	1 serv	1590
Empanadas Beef	1	440
Empanadas Chicken	1	390
Empanadas Chicken	1 serv	1090

FOOD	PORTION	CALS
Empanadas Ground Beef	1 serv	1150
Enchilada Beef	1	340
Enchilada Cheese & Onion	1	410
Enchilada Chicken	1	350
Fajita Chicken Con Queso	1 skillet	1130
Fajitas 7 Pepper Steak	1 serv	910
Fajitas Blackened Chicken w/ Portobello Mushrooms	1 serv	640
Fajitas Carnitas	1 serv	830
Fajitas Grilled Vegetables w/ Portobello Mushrooms	1 serv	390
Fajitas Jalapeno BBQ Chicken	1 serv	760
Fajitas Mesquite Grilled Chicken	1 serv	440
Fajitas Mesquite Grilled Steak	1 serv	620
Fajitas Monterey Ranch Chicken	1 serv	840
Fajitas Shrimp	1 serv	750
Fajitas Ultimate	1 serv	1230
Firecracker Stuffed Jalapenos	1 serv	980
French Fries	1 serv	390
Grande Fajita Nachos Beef	1 serv	1970
Grande Fajita Nachos Chicken	1 serv	1890
Grande Fajita Nachos Combo	1 serv	1940
Guacamole	1 serv	130
Guacamole Live	1 serv	570
Margarita Chicken	1 serv	290
Mexican Rice	1 serv	220
Mexican Shrimp Scampi	1 serv	740
Pico Chicken & Shrimp	1 serv	730
Quesadillas Combo Fajita	1 serv	1450
Quesadillas Double Stacked Club	1 serv	1860
Quesadillas Fajita Chicken	1 serv	1430
Quesadillas Fajita Steak	1 serv	1530
Quesadillas Spinach & Mushroom	1 serv	1420
Ranchiladas	1 serv	1360
Red Chili Ribeye	1 serv	900
Salmon Mexican	1 serv	650
Sandwich Chicken Blackened w/ French Fries	1 serv	1510
Sandwich Chicken Grilled w/ French Fries	1 serv	1430
Sauteed Shrimp	4	170
Shaken Margarita Shrimp Cocktail	1 serv	280

FOOD	PORTION	CALS
Shaken Margarita Shrimp Cocktail w/ Tortilla Chips	1 serv	780
Soft Taco Beef	1	340
Soft Taco Chicken	1	250
Soft Taco Veggie	1	210
Superior Dinner	1 serv	1350
Tamale	1	310
Tortilla Corn	3	230
Tortilla Soup	1 bowl	350
Tortillas Flour	3	300
Tres Enchilada Dinner Beef	1 serv	1010
Tres Enchilada Dinner Cheese	1 serv	1210
Tres Enchilada Dinner Chicken	1 serv	1040
Ultimate Loaded Queso	1 serv	900
Vegetables Grilled	1 serv	50
Vegetables Sauteed	1 serv	70
SALAD DRESSINGS AND SAUCES		
Chili Con Carne Sauce	1 serv (2 oz)	70
Chipotle Mayonnaise	1 serv (1 oz)	190
Dressing Chipotle Honey Mustard	1 serv (2 oz)	310
Dressing Ranch	1 serv (2 oz)	220
Dressing Smoked Jalapeno Vinaigrette	1 serv (2 oz)	230
Dressing Sweet Pepper Vinaigrette	1 serv (2 oz)	270
Dressing Fat Free Balsamic Vinaigrette	1 serv (2 oz)	50
Dressing Lo Fat Ranch	1 serv (2 oz)	110
Parrila Butter	1 serv (1 oz)	120
Pico De Gallo	1 scoop	20
Ranchero Sauce	1 serv (2 oz)	18
Salsa	1 serv (2 oz)	25
Sour Cream	1 serv (2 oz)	140
SALADS		
Chopped Chicken w/ Dressing	1 serv	1330
Fiesta Blackened Chicken w/ Dressing	1 serv	1150
Fiesta Chicken w/ Dressing	1 serv	1140
Grande Taco Beef	1 serv	1450
Grande Taco Chicken	1 serv	1280
House	1 serv	170
Sizzling Fajita Chicken	1 serv	760
Sizzling Fajita Steak	1 serv	910

FOOD	PORTION	CALS
PANDA EXPRESS		
MAIN MENU SELECTIONS		
BBQ Pork	1 serv	350
Beef & Broccoli	1 serv	150
Beef w/ String Beans	1 serv	170
Black Pepper Chicken	1 serv	180
Chicken w/ Mushrooms	1 serv	130
Chicken w/ Potato	1 serv	220
Chicken w/ String Beans	1 serv	170
Egg Roll Chicken	1 (3 oz)	190
Fried Shrimp	6 pieces	260
Mandarin Chicken	1 serv	250
Mixed Vegetables	1 serv	70
Orange Chicken	1 serv	480
Spicy Chicken w/ Peanuts	1 serv	200
Spring Roll Veggie	1 (1.7 oz)	80
Steamed Rice	1 serv	330
String Beans w/ Fried Tofu	1 serv	180
Sweet & Sour Chicken	1 serv	310
Sweet & Sour Pork	1 serv	410
Vegetable Chow Mein	1 serv	330
Vegetable Fried Rice	1 serv	390
SAUCES		
Hot	2 tsp	10
Hot Mustard	1 serv	18
Mandarin	1 serv	70
Soy	1 tbsp	16
Sweet & Sour	1 serv	60
PANERA BREAD		
BAGELS AND SPREADS		
Bagel Asiago Cheese	1	330
Bagel Blueberry	1	320
Bagel Cinnamon Crunch	1	490
Bagel Dutch Apple & Raisin	1	340
Bagel Everything	1	290
Bagel French Toast	1	340
Bagel Mochachip Swirl	1	340
Bagel Nine Grain	1	290
Bagel Peanut Butter Crunch	1	400

FOOD	PORTION	CALS
Bagel Plain	1	280
Bagel Sesame	1	310
Cream Cheese Hazelnut Reduced Fat	1 serv (2 oz)	150
Cream Cheese Honey Walnut Reduced Fat	1 serv (2 oz)	150
Cream Cheese Mocha Reduced Fat	1 serv (2 oz)	160
Cream Cheese Plain	1 serv (2 oz)	190
Cream Cheese Plain Reduced Fat	1 serv (2 oz)	130
Cream Cheese Raspberry Reduced Fat	1 serv (2 oz)	120
Cream Cheese Smoked Salmon Reduced Fat	1 serv (2 oz)	120
Cream Cheese Sun Dried Tomato Reduced Fat	1 serv (2 oz)	140
Cream Cheese Veggie Reduced Fat	1 serv (2 oz)	130
Hummus Roasted Garlic	1 serv (2 oz)	100
BEVERAGES		
Caffe Mocha	1 serv (11.5 oz)	360
Homestyle Lemonade	1 serv (16 oz)	80
Hot Chocolate	1 serv (11 oz)	350
IC Cappuccino Chip	1 serv (16 oz)	590
IC Caramel	1 serv (16 oz)	550
IC Honeydew Green Tea	1 serv (16 oz)	270
IC Mocha	1 serv (16 oz)	520
IC Spice	1 serv (16 oz)	470
Iced Green Tea	1 serv (16 oz)	60
Latte Caffe	1 serv (8.5 oz)	120
Latte Caramel	1 serv (11 oz)	400
Latte Chai Tea	1 serv (10 oz)	210
Latte House	1 serv (10.8 oz)	320
BREADS		
Artisan Country	1 slice	120
Artisan French	1 slice (2 oz)	110
Artisan Kalamata Olive	1 slice (2 oz)	140
Artisan Multigrain	1 slice (2 oz)	120
Artisan Raisin Pecan	1 slice (2 oz)	140
Artisan Sesame Semolina	1 slice (2 oz)	120
Artisan Stone Milled Rye	1 slice (2 oz)	110
Artisan Three Cheese	1 slice (2 oz)	120
Artisan Three Seed	1 slice	130
Ciabatta	1 (6 oz)	430
Cinnamon Raisin	1 slice (2 oz)	160
Focaccia Asiago Cheese	1 slice (2 oz)	150
Focaccia Basil Pesto	1 slice (2 oz)	150

FOOD	PORTION	CALS
Focaccia Rosemary & Onion	1 slice (2 oz)	140
French	1 slice (2 oz)	130
French Roll	1 (2.25 oz)	140
Holiday	1 slice (2 oz)	150
Honey Wheat	1 slice (2 oz)	140
Nine Grain	1 slice (2 oz)	150
Rye	1 slice (2 oz)	140
Sourdough	1 slice (2 oz)	120
Sourdough Roll	1 (2.5 oz)	160
Sourdough Soup Bowl	1 serv (8 oz)	500
Sunflower	1 slice (2 oz)	160
Tomato Basil	1 slice (2 oz)	130
DESSERTS		
Bear Claw	1	380
Brownie Caramel Pecan	1	470
Brownie Chocolate Raspberry	1	370
Brownie Very Chocolate	1	460
Cinnamon Roll	1	560
Cobblestone	1	560
Coffee Cake Cherry Cheese	1	190
Cookie Chocolate Chipper	1	420
Cookie Chocolate Duet w/ Walnuts	1	410
Cookie Nutty Chocolate Chipper	1	440
Cookie Nutty Oatmeal Raisin	1	350
Cookie Shortbread	1	340
Croissant Apple	1	260
Croissant Cheese	1	300
Croissant Chocolate	1	440
Croissant French	1	265
Croissant Raspberry Cheese	1	280
Danish Apple	1	510
Danish Cheese	1	590
Danish Cherry	1	520
Danish Georgia Peach	1	580
Danish German Chocolate	1	770
Macaroon Chocolate Hazelnut	1	270
Mini Bundt Cake Carrot Walnut	1	430
Mini Bundt Cake Lemon Poppyseed	1	460
Mini Bundt Cake Pineapple Upside Down	1	450
Muffie Banana Nut	1	260

FOOD	PORTION	CALS
Muffie Chocolate Chip	1	240
Muffie Pumpkin	1	270
Muffin Banana Nut	1	470
Muffin Blueberry	1	450
Muffin Chocolate Chip	1	540
Muffin Pumpkin	1	510
Muffin Low Fat Tripleberry	1	300
Pecan Roll	1	520
Scone Cinnamon Chip	1	560
Scone Orange	1	530
Strudel Apple Raisin	1	390
Strudel Cherry	1	400
SALADS		
Asian Sesame Chicken	1 serv	370
Caesar	1 serv	350
Caesar Grilled Chicken	1 serv	470
Classic Cafe	1 serv	380
Fandango	1 serv	400
Greek	1 serv	520
SANDWICHES		
Asiago Roast Beef	1	730
Bacon Turkey Bravo	1	770
Chicken Salad On Artisan Sesame Semolina	1	730
Chicken Salad On Nine Grain	1	640
Garden Veggie	1	570
Italian Combo	1	1050
Panini Coronado Carnitas	1	810
Panini Frontega Chicken	1	860
Panini Portobello & Mozzarella	1	650
Panini Turkey Artichoke	1	810
Peanut Butter & Jelly On French	1	450
Sierra Turkey	1	950
Smoked Ham On Artisan Stone Milled Rye	1	930
Smoked Ham On Rye	1	650
Smoked Turkey Breast On Artisan Country	1	590
Smoked Turkey On Sourdough	1	440
Tuna Salad On Artisan Multigrain	1	830
Tuna Salad On Honey Wheat	1	720
Turkey Fresco	1	580
Tuscan Chicken	1	950

FOOD	PORTION	CALS
SOUPS		
Baked Potato	1 serv	260
Boston Clam Chowder	1 serv	210
Broccoli Cheddar	1 serv	230
Cream Of Chicken & Wild Rice	1 serv	200
Forest Mushroom	1 serv	140
French Onion	1 serv	220
Low Fat Chicken Noodle	1 serv	100
Low Fat Vegetarian Garden Vegetable	1 serv	90
Low Fat Vegetarian Black Bean	1 serv	100
Vegetarian Santa Fe Roasted Corn	1 serv	130
PAPA JOHNS		
OTHER MENU SELECTIONS		
Bread Sticks	1 serv	140
Cheese Sticks	1 serv	180
Chickenstrips	1	83
Cinnapie	1 serv	114
PIZZA 14 INCH		
Original All The Meats	⅛ pie	405
Original BBQ Chicken & Bacon	⅛ pie	369
Original Cheese	⅛ pie	290
Original Chicken Alfredo	⅛ pie	310
Original Garden Fresh	⅛ pie	287
Original Hawaiian BBQ Chicken	⅛ pie	376
Original Pepperoni	⅛ pie	343
Original Sausage	⅛ pie	336
Original Spinach Alfredo	⅛ pie	303
Original The Works	⅛ pie	370
Thin Crust All The Meat	⅛ pie	371
Thin Crust BBQ Chicken & Bacon	⅛ pie	336
Thin Crust Cheese	⅛ pie	238
Thin Crust Chicken Alfredo	⅛ pie	276
Thin Crust Garden Fresh	⅛ pie	228
Thin Crust Hawaiian BBQ Chicken	⅛ pie	324
Thin Crust Pepperoni	⅛ pie	294
Thin Crust Sausage	⅛ pie	303
Thin Crust Spinach Alfredo	⅛ pie	251
Thin Crust The Works	⅛ pie	315

FOOD	PORTION	CALS
SALAD DRESSINGS AND SAUCES		
BBQ Sauce	1 serv	48
Buffalo Sauce	1 serv	25
Cheese Sauce	1 serv	60
Garlic Sauce	1 serv	235
Honey Mustard Dressing	1 serv	170
Pizza Sauce	1 serv	25
Ranch Dressing	1 serv	140
PAPA MURPHY'S		
PIZZA		
Deeper Dish Traditional	⅛ pie	440
Delite Large Cheese	⅒ pie	130
Delite Large Hawaiian	⅒ pie	140
Delite Large Meat	⅒ pie	190
Delite Large Pepperoni	⅒ pie	160
Delite Large Veggie	⅒ pie	150
Family Size Cheese	1⁄12 pie	270
Gourmet Family Size Chicken Garlic	1⁄12 pie	320
Gourmet Family Size Classic Italian	1⁄12 pie	360
Gourmet Family Size Veggie	1⁄12 pie	300
Papa's Family Size All Meat	1⁄12 pie	370
Papa's Family Size Cheese	1⁄12 pie	270
Papa's Family Size Cowboy	1⁄12 pie	370
Papa's Family Size Favorite	1⁄12 pie	380
Papa's Family Size Hawaiian	1⁄12 pie	290
Papa's Family Size Murphy's Combo	1⁄12 pie	480
Papa's Family Size Pepperoni	1⁄12 pie	310
Papa's Family Size Perfect	1⁄12 pie	300
Papa's Family Size Rancher	1⁄12 pie	330
Papa's Family Size Specialty	1⁄12 pie	340
Papa's Family Size Veggie Combo	1⁄12 pie	300
Stuffed Big Murphy	⅛ pie	380
Stuffed Chicago Style	⅛ pie	370
SALADS		
Club	1 serv	190
Garden	1 serv	160
Italian	1 serv	220

FOOD	PORTION	CALS
PICCADILLY CAFETERIA		
DESSERTS		
Gelatin Sugar Free	1 serv	0
Sugar Free Blueberry Pie	1 serv	314
Sugar Free Cherry Pie	1 serv	334
Sugar Free Chocolate Almond Pie	1 serv	611
MAIN MENU SELECTIONS		
Bass Blackened	1 serv	408
Bass Cajun Baked	1 serv	260
Bass Stuffed	1 serv	447
Beef Chopped Steak	1 serv	382
Beef Chopped Steak Fried	1 serv	225
Beef Roast Leg	1 sm serv	353
Broccoli Florets	1 serv	90
Broccoli w/ Cheese Sauce	1 serv	55
Brussels Sprouts	1 serv	92
Cabbage Steamed Bacon Seasoned	1 serv	108
Cabbage Steamed Buttered	1 serv	68
Catfish Filet Blackened	1 serv	523
Catfish Filet Cajun Baked	1 serv	401
Catfish Filet Stuffed	1 serv	561
Cauliflower Buttered	1 serv	73
Chicken Baked Cajun Boneless Breast	1 serv	428
Chicken Baked Quarters	1 serv	828
Chicken Barbecued Quarters	1 serv	472
Chicken Breast Italian Boneless Breast	1 serv	371
Chicken Breast Mesquite Smoke	1 serv	212
Chicken Breast Mesquite w/ BBQ Sauce	1 serv	240
Chicken Breast Southwestern	1 serv	315
Chicken Grilled Breast	1 serv	345
Chicken Half Rotisserie Herb	1 serv	833
Chicken Rotisserie Herb Dark Meat	1 serv	823
Chicken Rotisserie Herb White Meat	1 serv	602
Corn	1 serv	125
Cottage Cheese	1 serv	117
Filet Mignon	1 (6 oz)	184
Green Beans	1 serv	136
Green Collard Mustard Turnip	1 serv	135
Greens Turnip w/ Diced Turnips	1 serv	150
Grouper Filet Baked	1 piece (6 oz)	305

FOOD	PORTION	CALS
New York Strip	1 (10 oz)	871
Okra Creole	1 serv	77
Okra Fried	1 serv	240
Peas & Sugar Snapped Mixed	1 serv	102
Pork Loin Marinated Boneless	1 serv	365
Pork Loin Roast Bone In	1 serv	373
Ribeye	1 (10 oz)	1038
Roast Beef	1 serv	481
Roll Parker House	1	147
Roll Whole Wheat	1	231
Shrimp Fried	1 serv	499
Tilapia Baked	1 serv	210
Tilapia Cajun Baked	1 serv	263
Trout Almondine Baked	1 lg serv	457
Trout Cajun Baked	1 lg serv	517
Trout Filet Baked	1 lg serv	464
Turkey Breast Carved	1 serv	302
Vegetables Mixed	1 serv	95
SALAD DRESSINGS AND TOPPINGS		
Au Jus	1 serv	6
Blue Cheese	2 tbsp	160
Cheese Sauce	2 oz	35
French	2 tbsp	130
Italian	2 tbsp	140
Ranch	2 tbsp	150
Ranch Fat Free	2 tbsp	36
SALADS		
Asparagus & Tomato	1 serv	86
Caesar	1 serv	141
Cauilflower	1 serv	118
Chef	1 sm serv	146
Cole Slaw Kosher Style	1 serv	140
Coleslaw Italian	1 serv	163
Combination	1 serv	63
Cucumber & Celery	1 serv	74
Cucumber & Tomato	1 serv	41
Cucumber Mix	1 serv	61
Cucumbers & Sour Cream	1 serv	90
Louisianne Bowl	1 serv	42
Mexican	1 serv	58

FOOD	PORTION	CALS
Piccadilly Bowl	1 serv	27
Piccadilly Fruit	1 serv	76
Shrimp Ramoulade	1 serv	521
Spring Bowl	1 reg serv	24
Tomato Cucumber & Onion	1 serv	44
Vegetable Combo w/ Cherry Tomatoes	1 serv	66
SOUPS		
Gumbo Chicken & Sausage No Rice	1 serv	224
Gumbo Chicken No Rice	1 serv	89
PIZZA HUT		
APPETIZERS		
Breadstick	1	150
Breadstick Cheese	1	200
Hot Wings	2 pieces	110
Mild Wings	2 pieces	110
BEVERAGES		
Diet Pepsi	1 med (14 oz)	0
Mt. Dew	1 med (14 oz)	190
Pepsi	1 med (14 oz)	180
DESSERTS		
Apple Pizza	1 slice	260
Cherry Pizza	1 slice	240
Cinnamon Sticks	2	170
PIZZA		
Fit 'N Delicious Diced Chicken Mushroom Jalapeno	1 med slice	170
Fit 'N Delicious Diced Chicken Red Onion Green Pepper	1 med slice	170
Fit 'N Delicious Diced Red Tomato Mushroom Jalapeno	1 med slice	150
Fit 'N Delicious Green Pepper Red Onion Diced Red Tomato	1 med slice	150
Fit 'N Delicious Ham Pineapple Diced Red Tomato	1 med slice	160
Fit 'N Delicious Ham Red Onion Mushroom	1 med slice	160
Hand Tossed Cheese	1 med slice	240
Hand Tossed Chicken Supreme	1 med slice	230
Hand Tossed Ham	1 med slice	220
Hand Tossed Meat Lover's	1 med slice	300

FOOD	PORTION	CALS
Hand Tossed Pepperoni	1 med slice	250
Hand Tossed Pepperoni Lover's	1 med slice	300
Hand Tossed Super Supreme	1 med slice	300
Hand Tossed Supreme	1 med slice	270
Hand Tossed Veggie Lover's	1 med slice	220
Pan Cheese	1 med slice	280
Pan Chicken Supreme	1 med slice	280
Pan Ham	1 med slice	260
Pan Meat Lover's	1 med slice	340
Pan Pepperoni	1 med slice	290
Pan Pepperoni Lover's	1 med slice	340
Pan Super Supreme	1 med slice	340
Pan Supreme	1 med slice	320
Pan Veggie Lover's	1 med slice	260
Personal Pan Cheese	1 pie	630
Personal Pan Chicken Supreme	1 pie	620
Personal Pan Meat Lover's	1 pie	800
Personal Pan Pepperoni	1 pie	660
Personal Pan Pepperoni Lover's	1 pie	800
Personal Pan Super Supreme	1 pie	790
Personal Pan Supreme	1 pie	750
Personal Pan Veggie Lover's	1 pie	580
Stuffed Crust Cheese	1 lg slice	360
Stuffed Crust Chicken Supreme	1 lg slice	380
Stuffed Crust Ham	1 lg slice	340
Stuffed Crust Meat Lover's	1 lg slice	450
Stuffed Crust Pepperoni	1 lg slice	370
Stuffed Crust Pepperoni Lover's	1 lg slice	420
Stuffed Crust Super Supreme	1 lg slice	440
Stuffed Crust Supreme	1 lg slice	400
Stuffed Crust Veggie Lover's	1 lg slice	360
Thin'N Crispy Cheese	1 med slice	200
Thin'N Crispy Chicken Supreme	1 med slice	200
Thin'N Crispy Ham	1 med slice	180
Thin'N Crispy Meat Lover's	1 med slice	270
Thin'N Crispy Pepperoni	1 med slice	210
Thin'N Crispy Pepperoni Lover's	1 med slice	260
Thin'N Crispy Super Supreme	1 med slice	260
Thin'N Crispy Supreme	1 med slice	240
Thin'N Crispy Veggie Lover's	1 med slice	180

FOOD	PORTION	CALS
XL Full House Cheese	1 slice	280
XL Full House Chicken Supreme	1 slice	270
XL Full House Ham	1 slice	260
XL Full House Meat Lover's	1 slice	380
XL Full House Pepperoni	1 slice	290
XL Full House Pepperoni Lover's	1 slice	310
XL Full House Super Supreme	1 slice	330
XL Full House Supreme	1 slice	310
XL Full House Veggie Lover's	1 slice	280
SALAD DRESSINGS AND SAUCES		
Dipping Cup White Icing	1 serv	170
Dipping Sauce Breadstick	1 serv	45
Dipping Sauce Wing Blue Cheese	1 serv	230
Dipping Sauce Wing Ranch	1 serv	210
Dressing Caesar	2 tbsp	150
Dressing French	2 tbsp	140
Dressing Italian	2 tbsp	140
Dressing Ranch	2 tbsp	100
Dressing Thousand Island	2 tbsp	110
Dressing Lite Italian	2 tbsp	60
Dressing Lite Ranch	1 tbsp	70

P.J. CHANG'S CHINA BISTRO

Cantonese Scallops	1 serv	305
Chicken w/ Black Bean Sauce	1 serv	426
Pin Rice Noodles	1 serv	270
Vegetable Chow Fun	1 serv	677

QUIZNO'S

Cookie Oatmeal Chocolate Chip	1	360
Cookie w/ Reese's Pieces	1	360
Sub Honey Burbon Chicken	1 sm	329
Sub Sierra Turkey w/ Raspberry Chipotle Sauce	1 sm	350
Sub Turkey Lite	1 sm	334
Sub Tuscan Chicken Salad	1 sm	326

RANCH 1
MAIN MENU SELECTIONS

Baked Potato w/ Broccoli	1 serv	510
Baked Potato w/ Cheese	1 serv	790
Baked Potato w/ Chicken	1 serv	610

FOOD	PORTION	CALS
Chicken Tenders	1 serv	370
Fajita Grilled Chicken	1	330
Fruit Cup	1 serv	90
Hot Pasta Grilled Chicken	1 serv	590
Platter Grilled Chicken & Vegetables	1 serv	790
Ranch Fries	1 lg	420
Ranch Fries	1 reg	350
Sandwich American Rancher	1	390
Sandwich Grilled Chicken Philly	1	450
Sandwich Ranch Classic	1	370
Sandwich Spicy Grilled Chicken	1	420
Sandwich Club	1	470
SALADS		
Gourmet Greens	1 serv	220
Gourmet Greens w/ Chicken	1 serv	350
Zesty Caesar	1 serv	180
Zesty Chicken Caesar	1 serv	290

RAX
MAIN MENU SELECTIONS

FOOD	PORTION	CALS
Baked Potato	1	207
Baked Potato w/ Butter	1	306
Baked Potato w/ Cheese	1 serv	270
Baked Potato w/ Cheese Bacon	1 serv	336
Baked Potato w/ Cheese Broccoli	1 serv	281
Baked Potato w/ Sour Cream Topping	1 serv	257
BBC Sandwich	1	716
BBQ Beef Sandwich	1	399
Cheddar Melt	1	346
Deluxe Sandwich	1	521
Grilled Chicken Sandwich	1	526
Jr. Deluxe Sandwich	1	367
Mushroom Melt	1	599
Philly Melt	1	537
Regular Rax	1	388
Turkey Bacon Club	1	680
Turkey Sandwich	1	484
SALAD DRESSINGS		
1000 Island	1 serv	130
Blue Cheese	1 serv	145

FOOD	PORTION	CALS
Buttermilk Ranch	1 serv	175
Catalina Fat Free	1 serv	32
Creamy Caesar	1 serv	140
Honey French	1 serv	140
Italian Fat Free	1 serv	12
Ranch Fat Free	1 serv	30
Vinaigrette	1 serv	30
SALADS		
Garden	1 serv	220
Grilled Chicken	1 serv	160
Side Salad	1 serv (19 oz)	40
SOUPS		
Chicken Noodle	1 serv	113
Chili	1 serv	158
Cream Of Broccoli	1 serv	95

RED LOBSTER
BEVERAGES

Coffee	1 cup	0
Dannon Spring Water	1 glass	0
Diet Coke	1 serv	0
Hot Tea	1 cup	0
Iced Tea Unsweetened	1 glass	0
Lemonade Light	1 glass	5
Michelob Ultra	1 glass	95
Perrier Water	1 glass	0
Sutter Home Cabernet Sauvignon	1 glass	138
Sutter Home Chardonnay	1 glass	147
MAIN MENU SELECTIONS		
Baked Potato Plain	1	170
Baked Potato w/ Pico De Gallo Topping	1 serv	185
Cheddar Bay Biscuit	1	160
Fresh Buttered Vegetables	1 serv	143
Garden Salad	1 serv	52
Light House Broiled Flounder	1 serv	240
Light House Grilled Chicken	1 serv	527
Light House Jumbo Shrimp Cocktail Dinner	1 serv	243
Light House King Crab Legs	1 serv	490
Light House Live Maine Lobster	1 serv	145
Light House Main Lobster Tail	1 serv	104

FOOD	PORTION	CALS
Light House Rainbow Trout	1 lunch serv	273
Light House Rock Lobster Tail	1 serv	256
Light House Salmon	1 serv	578
Light House Salmon	1 lunch serv	258
Light House Snow Crab Legs	1 serv	262
Light House Tilapia	1 serv	346
Light House Tilapia	1 lunch serv	186
Seasoned Fresh Broccoli	1 serv	60
Shrimp Cocktail	1 jumbo	146
Wild Rice Pilaf	1 serv	208
SALAD DRESSINGS AND TOPPINGS		
Large Cocktail Sauce	1 serv	68
Lemon Wedge	1 serv	8
Melted Butter	1 serv	183
Red Wine Vinaigrette	1 serv	49
Topping Petite Shrimp	1 serv	30

RUBIO'S
MAIN MENU SELECTIONS

FOOD	PORTION	CALS
Black Beans	1 serv	220
Burritos Baja Carne Asada	1	710
Burritos Baja Carnitas	1	660
Burritos Baja Chicken	1	640
Burritos Carne Asada Especial w/ Black Beans	1	970
Burritos Carne Asada Especial w/ Pinto	1	950
Burritos Chicken Especial w/ Black Beans	1	920
Burritos Chicken Especial w/ Pinto	1	900
Burritos Fish	1	780
Burritos HealthMex Chicken	1	520
Burritos HealthMex Veggie	1	470
Burritos Lobster	1	660
Burritos Mahi Mahi	1	630
Burritos Shrimp	1	650
Carne Asada	1 serv	1430
Chips	1 serv	430
Grilled Grande Bowl Asada Black Beans	1 serv	770
Grilled Grande Bowl Asada Pinto	1 serv	760
Grilled Grande Bowl Chicken Black Beans	1 serv	710
Grilled Grande Bowl Chicken Pinto	1 serv	700
Guacamole	1 sm	170

FOOD	PORTION	CALS
Nachos Grande	1 serv	1270
Nachos Grande w/ Chicken	1 serv	1380
Pinto Beans	1 serv	190
Quesadillas Carne Asada	1	1010
Quesadillas Cheese	1	860
Quesadillas Grilled Chicken	1	860
Quesadillas Lobster	1	820
Quesadillas Shrimp	1	810
Roasted Chipotle	1 serv (1.5 oz)	10
Salsa Picante	1 serv (1.5 oz)	30
Salsa Regular	1 serv (1.5 oz)	15
Salsa Verde	1 serv (1.5 oz)	5
Tacos Carne Asada	1	220
Tacos Fish	1	310
Tacos Fish Especial	1	370
Tacos Grilled Chicken	1	300
Tacos Grilled Fish	1	310
Tacos HealthMex w/ Chicken	1	170
Taquitos	3	310
SALADS AND SALAD DRESSINGS		
Grilled Chicken Chopped Salad	1 serv	540
HealthMex Chicken	1 serv	220
Low Carb Chicken	1 serv	480
Serrano Grape Dressing	1 serv (1.3 oz)	10
RUBY TUESDAY'S		
Cajun Chicken Salad w/ Ranch Dressing	1 serv	636
Peppercorn Mushroom Sirloin	1 serv	947
SBARRO		
Baked Ziti	1 serv (14 oz)	830
Meat Lasagna	1 serv (17 oz)	730
Pizza Cheese	1 serv (6 oz)	450
Pizza Pepperoni	1 serv (6 oz)	510
Pizza Sausage	1 serv (10 oz)	640
Pizza Sausage & Pepperoni Stuffed	1 serv (11 oz)	880
Pizza Spinach & Broccoli Stuffed	1 serv (11 oz)	710
Pizza Supreme	1 serv (10 oz)	600
Pizza Veggie Slice	1 serv (10 oz)	490
Spaghetti w/ Sauce	1 serv (18 oz)	630

FOOD	PORTION	CALS
SCHLOTZSKY'S DELI		
SANDWICHES		
Light & Flavorful Albacore Tuna	1 (13 oz)	530
Light & Flavorful Chicken Breast	1 (15 oz)	540
Light & Flavorful Dijon Chicken	1 sm (10 oz)	330
Light & Flavorful Dijon Chicken	1 (15 oz)	500
Light & Flavorful Pesto Chicken	1 (14 oz)	510
Light & Flavorful Santa Fe Chicken	1 (17 oz)	640
Light & Flavorful Smoked Turkey Breast	1 (13 oz)	500
Light & Flavorful The Vegetarian	1 (12 oz)	520
Original Cheese	1 (14 oz)	850
Original Ham & Cheese	1 (17 oz)	790
Original Turkey	1 (17 oz)	1020
Specialty Deli Albacore Tuna Melt	1 (16 oz)	820
Specialty Deli BLT	1 (10 oz)	580
Specialty Deli Chicken Club	1 (16 oz)	690
Specialty Deli Corned Beef	1 (12 oz)	590
Specialty Deli Corned Beef Reuben	1 (15 oz)	830
Specialty Deli Pastrami & Swiss	1 (15 oz)	860
Specialty Deli Pastrami Reuben	1 (16 oz)	920
Specialty Deli Roast Beef	1 (14 oz)	620
Specialty Deli Roast Beef & Cheese	1 (17 oz)	850
Specialty Deli Texas Schlotzsky	1 (16 oz)	820
Specialty Deli The Philly	1 (16 oz)	820
Specialty Deli Turkey & Bacon Club	1 (17 oz)	870
Specialty Deli Turkey Guacamole	1 (16 oz)	680
Specialty Deli Turkey Reuben	1 (16 oz)	860
Specialty Deli Vegetable Club	1 (13 oz)	580
Specialty Deli Western Vegetarian	1 (12 oz)	650
The Original	1 (14 oz)	940
SKIPPERS		
CHILDREN'S MENU SELECTIONS		
Kids Catch Chicken Tenderloin + Chips & Kids Side	1 serv	560
Kids Catch Fish Bites + Chips & Kids Side	1 serv	490
Kids Catch Sandwich Grilled Cheese + Chips & Kids Side	1 serv	620
Kids Catch Shrimp + Chips & Kids Side	1 serv	520

FOOD	PORTION	CALS
MAIN MENU SELECTIONS		
Baked Potato Plain	1	210
Basket Chicken & Fish + Chips & Slaw	1 serv	620
Basket Chicken & Shrimp + Chips & Slaw	1 serv	760
Basket Chicken + Chips & Slaw	1 pieces	730
Basket Clam Strips + Chips & Slaw	1 serv	890
Basket Clams & Fish + Chips & Slaw	1 serv	740
Basket Original Recipe Shrimp + Chips & Slaw	1 serv	800
Basket Popcorn Shrimp + Chips & Slaw	1 serv	750
Basket Prawn & Fish + Chips & Slaw	1 serv	730
Basket Prawn Seafood + Chips & Slaw	1 serv	720
Basket Shrimp & Fish + Chips & Slaw	1 serv	650
Basket Shrimp Trio + Chips & Slaw	1 serv	1040
Clam Chowder	1 cup	120
Clam Strips	1 serv	270
Fish Bites + Chips & Slaw	6 pieces	490
French Fries	1 reg	180
Grilled Veggies	1 serv	35
Halibut + Chips & Slaw	1 serv	580
Homestyle Chicken Tenderloin	1 piece	190
Hush Puppies	3 pieces	240
Original Fish Fillet	1 piece	80
Original Fish + Chips & Slaw	2 pieces	510
Original Shrimp	9 pieces	220
Sandwich Fish + Chips & Slaw	1 serv	800
Sandwich Fried Chicken + Chips & Slaw	1	1260
Sandwich Grilled Chicken + Chips & Slaw	1	1070
Skipper's Platter + Chips & Slaw	1 serv	930
SALADS		
Caesar	1 sm	150
Caesar w/ Chicken	1 sm	340
Caesar w/ Salmon	1 sm	350
Green Salad w/o Dressing	1 sm	25
SMOOTHIE KING		
Activator Chocolate	1 (20 oz)	429
Activator Strawberry	1 (20 oz)	559
Activator Vanilla	1 (20 oz)	429
Banana Boat	1 (20 oz)	520
Coconut Surprise	1 (20 oz)	457

FOOD	PORTION	CALS
Coffee Smoothie Hazelnut	1 (20 oz)	118
Coffee Smoothies Amaretto	1 (20 oz)	118
Coffee Smoothies French Roast	1 (20 oz)	164
Coffee Smoothies French Vanilla	1 (20 oz)	118
Coffee Smoothies Irish Creme	1 (20 oz)	118
Coffee Smoothies Mocha	1 (20 oz)	206
HeaterZ Banana Nut	1	400
HeaterZ Blueberry Muffin	1	370
HeaterZ Chocolate Peanut Butter Cup	1	380
HeaterZ Cinnamon Oatmeal Raisin	1	420
HeaterZ Coconut	1	440
HeaterZ Coffee Amaretto	1 (12 oz)	177
HeaterZ Coffee French Roast	1 (12 oz)	172
HeaterZ Coffee French Vanilla	1 (12 oz)	177
HeaterZ Coffee Hazelnut	1 (12 oz)	177
HeaterZ Coffee Irish Creme	1 (12 oz)	177
HeaterZ Coffee Mocha	1 (12 oz)	266
High Protein Almond Mocha	1 (20 oz)	402
High Protein Banana	1 (20 oz)	412
High Protein Chocolate	1 (20 oz)	401
High Protein Lemon	1 (20 oz)	390
High Protein Pineapple	1 (20 oz)	380
Hot Coffee Amaretto	1 (12 oz)	168
Hot Coffee French Roast	1 (12 oz)	164
Hot Coffee French Vanilla	1 (12 oz)	168
Hot Coffee Hazelnut	1 (12 oz)	168
Hot Coffee Irish Creme	1 (12 oz)	168
Hot Coffee Mocha	1 (12 oz)	209
Iced Coffee Amaretto	1 (20 oz)	168
Iced Coffee French Roast	1 (20 oz)	164
Iced Coffee French Vanilla	1 (20 oz)	168
Iced Coffee Hazelnut	1 (20 oz)	168
Iced Coffee Irish Creme	1 (20 oz)	168
Iced Coffee Mocha	1 (20 oz)	209
Kid Cup Berry Interesting	1	150
Kid Cup Choc-A-Laka	1	210
Kid Cup Gimmi-Grape	1	170
Kid Cup Smarti Tarti	1	150
Low Carb All Flavors	1 (20 oz)	225
Low Fat Angel Food	1 (20 oz)	330

FOOD	PORTION	CALS
Low Fat Blackberry Dream	1 (20 oz)	343
Low Fat Caribbean Way	1 (20 oz)	392
Low Fat Celestial Cherry High	1 (20 oz)	285
Low Fat Cherry Picker	1 (20 oz)	360
Low Fat Cranberry Supreme	1 (20 oz)	577
Low Fat Cranberry Cooler	1 (20 oz)	538
Low Fat Grape Expectations	1 (20 oz)	399
Low Fat Grape Expectations II	1 (20 oz)	529
Low Fat Healthy Apple	1 (20 oz)	380
Low Fat Immune Builder	1 (20 oz)	333
Low Fat Instant Vigor	1 (20 oz)	359
Low Fat Island Treat	1 (20 oz)	334
Low Fat Lemon Twist Banana	1 (20 oz)	339
Low Fat Lemon Twist Strawberry	1 (20 oz)	399
Low Fat Light & Fluffy	1 (20 oz)	389
Low Fat Mangofest	1 (20 oz)	320
Low Fat Muscle Punch	1 (20 oz)	339
Low Fat Muscle Punch Plus	1 (20 oz)	340
Low Fat Orange Ka-BAM	1 (20 oz)	320
Low Fat Peach Slice	1 (20 oz)	341
Low Fat Peach Slice Plus	1 (20 oz)	471
Low Fat Pep Upper	1 (20 oz)	334
Low Fat Pineapple Pleasure	1 (20 oz)	331
Low Fat Pineapple Surf	1 (20 oz)	440
Low Fat Raspberry Sunrise	1 (20 oz)	335
Low Fat Strawberry X-Treme	1 (20 oz)	370
Low Fat Strawberry Kiwi Breeze	1 (20 oz)	300
Low Fat Youth Fountain	1 (20 oz)	267
Malts	1 (20 oz)	887
Mo'cuccino	1 (20 oz)	420
Peanut Power	1 (20 oz)	502
Peanut Power Plus Grape	1 (20 oz)	703
Peanut Power Plus Strawberry	1 (20 oz)	632
Pina Colada Island	1 (20 oz)	550
Power Punch	1 (20 oz)	430
Power Punch Plus	1 (20 oz)	499
Shakes	1 (20 oz)	875
Slim-N-Trim Chocolate	1 (20 oz)	270
Slim-N-Trim Orange Vanilla	1 (20 oz)	199
Slim-N-Trim Strawberry	1 (20 oz)	357

FOOD	PORTION	CALS
Slim-N-Trim Vanilla	1 (20 oz)	227
Super Punch	1 (20 oz)	425
Super Punch Plus	1 (20 oz)	516
The Hulk Chocolate	1 (20 oz)	846
The Hulk Strawberry	1 (20 oz)	953
The Hulk Vanilla	1 (20 oz)	846
Yogurt D-Lite	1 (20 oz)	335

SONIC DRIVE-IN
ADD-ONS

FOOD	PORTION	CALS
Bacon	1 serv (0.5 oz)	80
Cheddar Cheese Shredded	1 serv (1 oz)	104
Cheese	1 serv (0.7 oz)	70
Chili	1 serv (1 oz)	52
Cone Coat Chocolate	1 serv (1 oz)	143
Green Chilies	1 serv (1 oz)	10
Hickory Barbecue Sauce	1 serv (1 oz)	41
Honey Mustard Dressing	1 serv (1.1 oz)	110
Jalapenos Nachos Sliced	1 serv (1 oz)	5
Malt	1 serv (1 oz)	104
Maraschino Cherry	1 serv (8 g)	10
Marinara Sauce	1 serv (1 oz)	15
Ranch Dressing	1 serv (1 oz)	147
Slaw	1 serv (0.9 oz)	45
Sweet Pickle Relish	1 serv (1.1 oz)	40
Syrup Blue Coconut	1 serv (1 oz)	65
Syrup Cherry	1 serv (1 oz)	64
Syrup Chocolate	1 serv (1 oz)	74
Syrup Grape	1 serv (1 oz)	63
Syrup Vanilla	1 serv (1 oz)	61
Syrup Watermelon	1 serv (1 oz)	71
Thousand Island Dressing	1 serv (1 oz)	150
Topping Pineapple	1 serv (1.5 oz)	108
Topping Strawberry	1 serv (1 oz)	101
Topping Strawberry	1 serv (1.2 oz)	38

BEVERAGES

FOOD	PORTION	CALS
Barqs Root Beer	1 lg	333
Barqs Root Beer	1 sm	160
Coca-Cola	1 lg	291
Coca-Cola	1 sm	139

FOOD	PORTION	CALS
Diet Coca-Cola	1 lg	3
Diet Coca-Cola	1 sm	1
Diet Sprite	1 lg	8
Diet Sprite	1 sm	4
Dr Pepper	1 lg	300
Dr Pepper	1 sm	144
Float or Flurry Blue Coconut Slush	1 reg	424
Limeade	1 lg	303
Limeade	1 sm	143
Limeade Cherry	1 lg	361
Limeade Cherry	1 sm	169
Limeade Strawberry	1 lg	341
Limeade Strawberry	1 sm	172
Slush Blue Coconut	1 lg	521
Slush Watermelon	1 lg	526
Sprite	1 lg	288
Sprite	1 sm	138
BREAKFAST SELECTIONS		
Breakfast Burrito	1	731
Fruit Taquitos	1 serv	302
Sunrise	1 reg	224
Sunrise	1 lg	368
Toaster Bacon Egg & Cheese	1	500
Toaster Ham Egg & Cheese	1	436
Toaster Sausage Egg & Cheese	1	570
DESSERTS		
Banana Split	1 serv	467
Chocolate Covered Shake Banana	1 reg	625
Chocolate Covered Shake Cherry	1 reg	587
Chocolate Covered Shake Peanut Butter	1 reg	678
Chocolate Covered Shake Strawberry	1 reg	608
Cream Pie Shake Banana	1 reg	775
Cream Pie Shake Chocolate	1 reg	795
Cream Pie Shake Coconut	1 reg	721
Dish Of Vanilla	1 serv	265
Float or Flurry Cherry Slush	1 reg	421
Float or Flurry Coca-Cola	1 reg	379
Float or Flurry Dr Pepper	1 reg	377
Float or Flurry Grape Slush	1 reg	423
Float or Flurry Orange Slush	1 reg	422

FOOD	PORTION	CALS
Float or Flurry Rootbeer	1 reg	386
Float or Flurry Watermelon Slush	1 reg	427
Ice Cream Cone	1	285
Shake Banana	1 reg	508
Shake Chocolate	1 reg	564
Shake Pineapple	1 reg	615
Shake Strawberry	1 reg	510
Shake Vanilla	1 reg	454
Sonic Blast Butterfinger	1 reg	636
Sonic Blast M&M	1 reg	641
Sonic Blast Oreo	1 reg	638
Sonic Blast Reese's	1 reg	658
Sundae Chocolate	1 serv	362
Sundae Hot Fudge	1 serv	392
Sundae Pineapple	1 serv	399
Sundae Strawberry	1 serv	322
MAIN MENU SELECTIONS		
Ched'R'Peppers	1 serv	256
Cheese Fries	1 lg	322
Cheese Fries	1 reg	265
Cheese Tater Tots	1 reg	329
Cheese Tots	1 lg	435
Chicken Strip Dinner	1 serv	749
Chicken Strip Snack	1 serv	272
Chicken Strips	2	184
Chili Cheese Fries	1 lg	357
Chili Cheese Fries	1 reg	299
Chili Cheese Tater Tots	1 reg	363
Chili Cheese Tots	1 lg	547
Corn Dog	1	262
Extra Long Coney Cheese	1	666
Extra Long Coney Plain	1	483
French Fries	1 lg	252
French Fries	1 reg	195
Fritos Chili Pie	1 serv	611
Hot Dog Plain	1	262
Jr. Burger	1	353
Mozzarella Sticks	1 serv	382
No.1 Hamburger	1	577
No.1 Sonic Cheeseburger	1	647

FOOD	PORTION	CALS
No.2 Hamburger	1	481
No.2 Sonic Cheeseburger	1	551
Onion Rings	1 lg	507
Onion Rings	1 reg	331
Regular Coney Cheese	1	366
Regular Coney Plain	1	262
Sandwich Breaded Chicken	1	582
Sandwich Country Fried Steak	1	748
Sandwich Grilled Chicken	1	343
Super Sonic No.1	1	929
Super Sonic No.2	1	839
SuperSonic Onion Rings	1 serv	706
SuperSonic Tots	1 serv	485
SuperSonic Fries	1 serv	358
Tater Tots	1 lg	365
Tater Tots	1 reg	259
Toaster Sandwich Bacon Cheddar Burger	1	675
Toaster Sandwich BLT	1	581
Toaster Sandwich Chicken Club	1	675
Toaster Sandwich Country Fried Steak	1	708
Toaster Sandwich Grilled Cheese	1	282
Wrap Chicken Strip	1	574
Wrap Grilled Chicken	1	539
Wrap w/o Ranch Chicken Strip	1	428
Wrap w/o Ranch Grilled Chicken	1	393

SOUPLANTATION
BREADS AND MUFFINS

FOOD	PORTION	CALS
Bread Low Fat Sourdough	1 slice	150
Breads Indian Grain Low Fat	1 slice	200
Cornbread Buttermilk Low Fat	1 piece	140
Focaccia Big Hearth Pizza	1	140
Focaccia Bruschetta	1 piece	130
Focaccia Pepperoni	1 piece	160
Focaccia Roasted Potato	1 piece	150
Focaccia Sauteed Vegetables	1 piece	150
Focaccia Tomatillo	1 piece	140
Focaccia Low Fat Garlic Parmesan	1 piece	100
Muffin Apple Cinnamon Bran 96% Fat Free	1	80
Muffin Apple Raisin	1	150

FOOD	PORTION	CALS
Muffin Banana Nut	1	150
Muffin Big Blue Blueberry	1	310
Muffin Black Forest	1	230
Muffin Cappuccino Chip	1	160
Muffin Caribbean Key Lime	1	170
Muffin Cherry Nut	1	150
Muffin Chocolate Brownie	1	170
Muffin Chocolate Chip	1	170
Muffin Country Blackberry	1	170
Muffin French Quarter Praline	1	290
Muffin Georgia Peach Poppyseed	1	150
Muffin Lemon	1	140
Muffin Low Fat Chile Corn	1	140
Muffin Macadamia Nut Spice	1	220
Muffin Maple Walnut	1	230
Muffin Nutty Peanut Butter	1	170
Muffin Pumpkin Raisin	1 piece	150
Muffin Strawberry Buttermilk	1	140
Muffin Sweet Orange & Cranberry	1	200
Muffin Taffy Apple	1	160
Muffin Tropical Papaya Coconut	1	180
Muffin Zucchini Nut	1	150
Muffin 96% Fat Free Cranberry Orange Bran	1	80
Muffin 96% Fat Free Fruit Medley Bran	1	80
DESSERTS		
Cobbler Apple	½ cup	350
Cobbler Blissful Blueberry	½ cup	380
Cobbler Cherry	½ cup	340
Cobbler Cranberry Apple	½ cup	370
Cobbler Peach	½ cup	360
Cookie Chocolate Chip	1 sm	70
Fat Free Apple Medley	½ cup	70
Fat Free Banana Royale	½ cup	80
Fat Free Frozen Yogurt Chocolate	½ cup	95
Jello Fat Free All Flavors	½ cup	80
Jello Fat Free Sugar Free All Flavors	½ cup	10
Pudding Banana	½ cup	160
Pudding Low Fat Butterscotch	½ cup	140
Pudding Low Fat Chocolate	½ cup	140
Pudding Low Fat Rice	½ cup	110

FOOD	PORTION	CALS
Pudding Vanilla	½ cup	140
Soft Serve Reduced Fat Vanilla	½ cup	140
Tapioca Low Fat	½ cup	140
MAIN MENU SELECTIONS		
Alfredo Broccoli w/ Basil	1 cup	380
Alfredo Fettuccine	1 cup	390
Alfredo Four Cheese	1 cup	390
Alfredo Roasted Garlic & Asiago	1 cup	330
Alfredo Roasted Mushroom w/ Rosemary	1 cup	380
Alfredo Southwestern	1 cup	350
Beef Stroganoff	1 cup	340
Carbonara Pasta	1 cup	280
Chili Arizona	1 cup	220
Chili Cheatin' Heart	1 cup	300
Chili Deep Kettle House Low Fat	1 cup	230
Chili Longhorn Beef	1 cup	190
Chili Rock N' Mole	1 cup	240
Chili Santa Fe Black Bean Low Fat	1 cup	190
Chili Texas Red	1 cup	240
Chili Three Bean Turkey Low Fat	1 cup	140
Chili Vegetarian	1 cup	150
Creamy Herb Chicken	1 cup	310
Creamy Pepper Jack	1 cup	290
Garden Vegetable w/ Italian Sausage	1 cup	300
Garden Vegetable w/ Meatballs	1 cup	270
Greek Mediterranean	1 cup	290
Italian Vegetable Beef	1 cup	270
Italian Sausage w/ Red Pepper Puree	1 cup	250
Lemon Cream & Asparagus	1 cup	230
Linguini w/ Clam Sauce	1 cup	380
Low Fat Oriental Green Bean & Noodle	1 cup	240
Macaroni & Cheese	1 cup	260
Nutty Mushroom	1 cup	390
Pasta Florentine	1 cup	360
Penne Arrabbiatta	1 cup	340
Pesto Cilantro Lime	1 cup	370
Roasted Eggplant Marinara	1 cup	340
Smoked Salmon & Dill	1 cup	360
Tuscany Sausage w/ Capers & Olives	1 cup	240
Vegetable Ragu	1 cup	250

FOOD	PORTION	CALS
Vegetarian Marinara w/ Basil	1 cup	260
Walnut Pesto	1 cup	310
SALAD DRESSINGS		
Bacon	2 tbsp	120
Balsamic Vinaigrette	1 tbsp	180
Basil Vinaigrette	2 tbsp	160
Blue Cheese	1 tbsp	140
Creamy Italian	2 tbsp	120
Fat Free Honey Mustard	2 tbsp	45
Honey Mustard	2 tbsp	150
Italian Fat Free	2 tbsp	20
Kahlena French	2 tbsp	120
Parmesan Pepper Cream	2 tbsp	160
Ranch	2 tbsp	130
Ranch Fat Free	2 tbsp	50
Reduced Calorie Cucumber	2 tbsp	80
Roasted Garlic	2 tbsp	140
Thousand Island	2 tbsp	110
SALADS		
Ambrosia w/ Cocount	½ cup	170
Antipasto w/ Peppered Salami	1 cup	140
Artichoke Rice	½ cup	160
Aunt Doris' Red Pepper Slaw Fat Free	½ cup	70
Baja Bean & Cilantro Low Fat	½ cup	180
Bartlett Pear & Walnut	1 cup	180
BBQ Julienne Chopped	1 cup	190
BBQ Smokehouse w/ Bacon & Peanuts	1 cup	190
Caesar Asiago	1 cup	190
California Cobb	1 cup	180
Cape Cod Spinach w/ Walnuts	1 cup	170
Carrot Ginger w/ Herb Vinaigrette	½ cup	150
Carrot Raisin Low Fat	½ cup	90
Chicken Tortilla	1 cup	180
Chinese Krab	½ cup	160
Citrus Noodle w/ Snow Peas	½ cup	140
Country French w/ Bacon	1 cup	210
Ensalada Azteca	1 cup	130
Field Corn & Very Wild Rice	½ cup	170
Greek	1 cup	120
Greek Couscous w/ Feta	½ cup	170

FOOD	PORTION	CALS
Italian Garden Vegetable	½ cup	110
Italian Sub Salad w/ Turkey & Salami	1 cup	260
Italian White Bean	½ cup	140
Joan's Blue BLT	1 cup	250
Joan's Broccoli Madness	½ cup	180
Lemon Rice w/ Cashews	½ cup	160
Mandarin Noodles w/ Broccoli Low Fat	½ cup	120
Mandarin Shells w/ Almonds	½ cup	120
Mandarin Spinach w/ Carmelized Walnuts	1 cup	170
Marinated Summer Vegetables Fat Free	½ cup	80
Mediterranean	1 cup	150
Monterey Blue w/ Peanuts	1 cup	200
Moroccan Marinated Vegetables Low Fat	½ cup	90
Old Fashioned Macaroni Salad w/ Ham	½ cup	180
Oriental Ginger Slaw w/ Krab Low Fat	½ cup	70
Penne w/ Chicken In Citrus Vinaigrette Low Fat	½ cup	130
Pesto Orzo w/ Pinenuts	1 cup	220
Pesto Pasta	½ cup	160
Pineapple Coconut Slaw	½ cup	150
Poppyseed Coleslaw	½ cup	120
Potato BBQ	½ cup	160
Potato Dijon w/ Garlic Dill Vinaigrette	½ cup	150
Potato German	½ cup	120
Potato Jalapeno	½ cup	140
Potato Picnic	½ cup	150
Potato Southern Dill Low Fat	½ cup	120
Ragin' Cajun	1 cup	200
Ranch House BLT Salad w/ Turkey	1 cup	180
Red Potato & Tomato	½ cup	120
Roasted Vegetables w/ Feta & Olives	1 cup	140
Roasted Potato Salad w/ Chipotle Chili Vinaigrette	½ cup	140
Roma Tomatoes Mozzarella & Basil	1 cup	120
San Francisco Herb Rice	½ cup	170
Shrimp & Seafood	½ cup	200
Smoked Turkey & Spinach w/ Almonds	1 cup	190
Sonoma Spinach w/ Honey Dijon Vinaigrette	1 cup	210
Southern Black Eyed Pea	½ cup	130
Southwestern Rice & Beans	½ cup	90
Spiced Pecans & Roasted Vegetables	1 cup	180
Spicy Southwestern Pasta Low Fat	½ cup	130

FOOD	PORTION	CALS
Spinach Gorgonzola w/ Spiced Pecans	1 cup	210
Strawberry Fields w/ Carmelized Walnuts	1 cup	130
Summer Barley w/ Black Beans Low Fat	½ cup	110
Summer Lemon w/ Spiced Pecans	1 cup	220
Thai Noodle w/ Peanut Sauce	½ cup	170
Three Bean Marinade	½ cup	170
Tomato Cucumber Marinade	½ cup	80
Traditional Spinach w/ Bacon	1 cup	160
Tuna Tarragon	½ cup	240
Turkey Chutney Pasta	½ cup	230
Watercress & Orange	1 cup	90
Wild Rice & Chicken	½ cup	300
Won Ton Chicken Happiness	1 cup	150
Zesty Tortellini	½ cup	190
SOUPS		
Albino Bean Chicken	1 cup	190
Albondigas Locas	1 cup	210
Autumn Root Vegetable w/ Wild Rice	1 cup	80
Baked Potato & Cheese w/ Bacon	1 cup	290
Be Wild With Mushroom	1 cup	220
Big Chunk Chicken Noodle Low Fat	1 cup	160
Black Bean Sausage Fling	1 cup	350
Black Bean & Chorizo	1 cup	230
Bombay Lentil Low Fat	1 cup	160
Broc On	1 cup	220
Broccoli Cheese	1 cup	280
Butternut Squash	1 cup	140
Cheese Stuffed Cappelletti	1 cup	130
Chesapeake Corn Chowder	1 cup	280
Chicken Got Smoked	1 cup	350
Chicken Tortilla w/ Jalapeno Chiles & Tomatoes Low Fat	1 cup	100
Chunky Potato Cheese w/ Thyme	1 cup	210
Classical French Onion	1 cup	130
Classical Minestrone Low Fat	1 cup	120
Classical Shrimp Bisque	1 cup	240
Country Corn & Red Potato Chowder	1 cup	160
Cream Of Broccoli	1 cup	210
Cream of Mushroom	1 cup	290
Cream Of Rosemary Potato	1 cup	270

FOOD	PORTION	CALS
Cream Of Chicken	1 cup	260
Creamy Vegetable Chowder	1 cup	200
Devotion To The Ocean	1 cup	220
El Paso Lime & Chicken	1 cup	160
Field Of Creams Cauliflower w/ Cheese	1 cup	260
Field Of Creams Celery	1 cup	210
Field Of Creams Spinach	1 cup	280
Field Of Creams Tomato Basil	1 cup	220
Fire Roasted Green Chili & Corn Chowder	1 cup	230
Garden Fresh Vegetable Low Fat	1 cup	110
Garlic Kickin Roasted Chicken	1 cup	140
Hungarian Vegetable Low Fat	1 cup	120
Irish Potato Leek	1 cup	250
Living On The Veg	1 cup	90
Manhattan Clam Chowder	1 cup	130
Mulligatawny	1 cup	210
Navy Bean w/ Ham	1 cup	340
Neighbor Joe's Gumbo	1 cup	280
Posole	1 cup	150
Ratatouille Provencale Fat Free	1 cup	110
Roasted Mushroom w/ Sage	1 cup	320
Spicy Sausage & Pasta	1 cup	310
Split Pea w/ Ham	1 cup	350
Tomato Chipotle Bisque	1 cup	240
Tomato Parmesan & Vegetables Low Fat	1 cup	120
Toot Your Horn For Crab & Corn	1 cup	290
Vegetarian Lentils & Brown Rice Low Fat	1 cup	130
Yankee Clipper Clam Chowder w/ Bacon	1 cup	330

STARBUCKS
BAKED SELECTIONS

Baby Bundt Cake Chocolate	1	330
Bagel	1	430
Bagel Cinnamon Raisin	1	440
Bagel Sesame	1	440
Bar Caramel Apple	1	310
Bar Carrot Cake	1	420
Bar Lemon	1	310
Bar Oreo Dream	1	420
Bar Toffee Crunch	1	430

FOOD	PORTION	CALS
Biscotti Chocolate Hazelnut	1	110
Biscotti Vanilla Almond	1	110
Brownie Caramel	1	580
Brownie Enrobed Espresso	1	430
Brownie Espresso	1	370
Brownie Milk Chocolate Peanut Butter	1	460
Bundt Cake Lemon Yogurt	1 serv	350
Caramel Pecan Sticky Roll	1	730
Cinnamon Roll	1	620
Cinnamon Twist	1	320
Coffee Cake	1 serv	570
Coffee Cake Apple Walnut	1 serv	320
Coffee Cake Blueberry Walnut	1 serv	340
Coffee Cake Cinnamon Walnut	1 serv	360
Coffee Cake Crumble Berry	1 serv	520
Coffee Cake Hazelnut	1 serv	630
Coffee Cake Sour Cream	1 serv	420
Cookie Black And White	1	430
Cookie Double Chocolate Chunk	1 serv	430
Cookie Oatmeal Raisin	1	390
Cookie White Chocolate Macadamia Nut	1	470
Crisp Cinnamon Twist	1	60
Croissant Almond	1	330
Croissant Butter w/ Apricot Glaze	1	320
Croissant Chocolate	1	350
Croissant Raspberry & Cream Cheese	1	260
Crumb Cake	1 serv	670
Crumb Cake Key Lime	1 serv	550
Danish Apple w/ Mocha Swirls	1	370
Danish Cheese w/ Mocha Swirls	1	460
Danish Raspberry w/ Mocha Swirls	1	370
Graham Dark Chocolate	1	140
Graham Milk Chocolate	1	140
Madeline	1	80
Muffin Blueberry	1	380
Muffin Chocolate Cream Cheese	1	450
Muffin Cranberry Orange	1	410
Muffin Morning Sunrise	1	330
Pound Cake Banana	1 serv	360
Pound Cake Cranberry Walnut	1 serv	390

FOOD	PORTION	CALS
Pound Cake Iced Carrot	1 serv	540
Pound Cake Iced Lemon	1 serv	500
Pound Cake Marble	1 serv	400
Pound Cake Orange Poppy	1 serv	490
Pound Cake Pumpkin	1 serv	310
Pound Cake Zucchini	1 serv	370
Pullman Banana	1 serv	400
Pullman Chocolate	1	380
Pullman Cranberry Walnut	1	360
Pullman Lemon Glazed	1	370
Pullman Marble Chocolate Chip	1	440
Pullman Orange Poppy Cheese	1	450
Pullman Pumpkin	1	370
Scone Blueberry	1	460
Scone Butterscotch Pecan	1	520
Scone Cinnamon Chip w/ Icing	1	510
Scone Maple Oat w/ Icing	1	490
Scone Apricot Currant	1	450
Scone Raspberry	1	440
Shortbread	1	100
BEVERAGES		
Apple Juice	1 grande	230
Blended Coffee Of The Week	1 grande	10
Cafe Americano	1 grande	150
Cafe Au Lait Nonfat Milk	1 grande	90
Cafe Au Lait Soy Milk	1 grande	110
Cafe Latte Whole Milk	1 grande	260
Cafe Misto Cafe Au Lait Whole Milk	1 grande	140
Cafe Mocha Whip Whole Milk	1 grande	400
Caffe Latte Nonfat Milk	1 grande	160
Caffe Latte Soy Milk	1 grande	210
Caffe Mocha No Whip Whole Milk	1 grande	300
Caffe Mocha No Whip Nonfat Milk	1 grande	230
Caffe Mocha No Whip Soy Milk	1 grande	260
Caffe Mocha Whip Nonfat Milk	1 grande	330
Caffe Mocha Whip Soy Milk	1 grande	360
Cappuccino Nonfat Milk	1 grande	100
Cappucino Soy Milk	1 grande	120
Caramel Apple Cider No Whip	1 grande	300
Caramel Apple Cider Whip	1 grande	410

FOOD	PORTION	CALS
Caramel Macchiato Nonfat Milk	1 grande	230
Caramel Macchiato Soy Milk	1 grande	300
Caramel Macchiato Whole Milk	1 grande	320
Caramel Mocha Whip Soy Milk	1 grande	440
Caramel Mocha No Whip Soy Milk	1 grande	340
Caramel Mocha No Whip Whole Milk	1 grande	370
Caramel Mocha Whip Nonfat Milk	1 grande	410
Caramel Mocha Whip Whole Milk	1 grande	470
Caramel Mocha No Whip Nonfat Milk	1 grande	300
Chocolate Nonfat Milk	1 grande	240
Chocolate Whole Milk	1 grande	340
Cinnamon Spice Mocha No Whip Nonfat Milk	1 grande	250
Cinnamon Spice Mocha No Whip Whole Milk	1 grande	330
Cinnamon Spice Mocha Whip Nonfat Milk	1 grande	350
Cinnamon Spice Mocha Whip Whole Milk	1 grande	430
Cinnamon Spice No Whip Soy Milk	1 grande	290
Cinnamon Spice Whip Soy Milk	1 grande	390
Espresso Decaf Coffee Of The Week	1 grande	10
Frappuccino Blended Coffee	1 grande	230
Frappuccino Blended Coffee Mocha Coconut No Whip Whole Milk	1 grande	400
Frappuccino Caramel Blended Coffee No Whip	1 grande	280
Frappuccino Caramel Blended Coffee Whip	1 grande	430
Frappuccino Chocolate Blended Creme Whip	1 grande	530
Frappuccino Chocolate Blended Creme No Whip	1 grande	400
Frappuccino Chocolate Brownie Blended Coffee No Whip	1 grande	370
Frappuccino Chocolate Brownie Blended Coffee Whip	1 grande	510
Frappuccino Chocolate Malt Blended Creme No Whip	1 grande	470
Frappuccino Chocolate Malt Blended Creme Whip	1 grande	610
Frappuccino Mocha Blended Coffee No Whip	1 grande	290
Frappuccino Mocha Blended Coffee Whip	1 grande	420
Frappuccino Mocha Blended Coffee Whip	1 grande	550
Frappuccino Mocha Malt Blended Coffee No Whip	1 grande	430
Frappuccino Mocha Malt Blended Coffee Whip	1 grande	570

FOOD	PORTION	CALS
Frappuccino Tazo Chai Creme Blended Tea No Whip	1 grande	370
Frappuccino Tazo Chai Creme Blended Tea Whip	1 grande	500
Frappuccino Tazoberry Blended Tea	1 grande	190
Frappuccino Tazoberry Creme Blended Tea No Whip	1 grande	330
Frappuccino Tazoberry Creme Blended Tea Whip	1 grande	460
Frappuccino Vanilla Blended Creme No Whip	1 grande	350
Frappuccino Vanilla Blended Creme Whip	1 grande	480
Frappuccino White Chocolate Mocha Blended Coffee No Whip	1 grande	320
Frappuccino White Chocolate Mocha Blended Coffee Whip	1 grande	450
Hot Chocolate No Whip Whole Milk	1 grande	340
Hot Chocolate No Whip Nonfat Milk	1 grande	240
Hot Chocolate Whip Nonfat Milk	1 grande	340
Hot Chocolate Whip Whole Milk	1 grande	440
Iced Cafe Latte Whole Milk	1 grande	160
Iced Cafe Mocha Whip Nonfat Milk	1 grande	310
Iced Cafe Mocha Whip Soy Milk	1 grande	330
Iced Caffe Americano	1 grande	20
Iced Caffe Mocha No Whip Whole Milk	1 grande	220
Iced Caffe Mocha Whip Whole Milk	1 grande	350
Iced Caffe Latte Nonfat Milk	1 grande	100
Iced Caffe Latte Soy Milk	1 grande	120
Iced Caffe Mocha No Whip Nonfat Milk	1 grande	180
Iced Caffe Mocha No Whip Soy Milk	1 grande	200
Iced Caramel Macchiato Nonfat Milk	1 grande	100
Iced Caramel Macchiato Soy Milk	1 grande	230
Iced Caramel Macchiato Whole Milk	1 grande	270
Iced Shaken Coffee	1 grande	80
Iced Tazo Chai Nonfat Milk	1 grande	230
Iced Tazo Chai Whole Milk	1 grande	270
Iced White Chocolate Mocha No Whip Soy Milk	1 grande	340
Iced White Chocolate Mocha No Whip Whole Milk	1 grande	360
Iced White Chocolate Mocha Whip Nonfat Milk	1 grande	450
Iced White Chocolate Mocha Whip Soy Milk	1 grande	470

FOOD	PORTION	CALS
Iced White Chocolate Mocha Whip Whole Milk	1 grande	490
Iced White Chocolate No Whip Nonfat Milk	1 grande	320
Milk Nonfat	1 grande	160
Steamed Apple Cider	1 grande	230
Steamed Nonfat Milk	1 grande	160
Steamed Whole Milk	1 grande	270
Tazo Chai Whole Milk	1 grande	290
Tazo Chai Nonfat Milk	1 grande	230
Tazo Iced Tea	1 grande	80
Tazo Tea Lemonade	1 grande	120
Vanilla Creme Whip Nonfat Milk	1 grande	340
Vanilla Creme Whip Whole Milk	1 grande	440
Vanilla Creme No Whip Nonfat Milk	1 grande	240
Vanille Creme No Whip Whole Milk	1 grande	340
White Chocolate Mocha No Whip Nonfat Milk	1 grande	340
White Chocolate Mocha No Whip Whole Milk	1 grande	410
White Chocolate Mocha Whip Nonfat Milk	1 grande	440
White Chocolate Mocha Whip Whole Milk	1 grande	510
White Chocolate No Whip Soy Milk	1 grande	370
White Chocolate Whip Soy Milk	1 grande	440
White Hot Chocolate No Whip Nonfat Milk	1 grande	390
White Hot Chocolate No Whip Whole Milk	1 grande	480
White Hot Chocolate Whip Nonfat Milk	1 grande	490
White Hot Chocolate Whip Whole Milk	1 grande	580
Whole Milk	1 grande	270
TOPPINGS		
Caramel	1 tbsp	15
Chocolate	1 tsp	5
Flavored Sugar Free Syrup	1 pump	0
Flavored Syrup	1 pump	20
Mocha Syrup	1 pump	25
Sprinkles	1 serv	0

STEAK ESCAPE
BEVERAGES

FOOD	PORTION	CALS
Coca Cola	12 oz	110
Coca Cola	44 oz	430
Diet Coke	12 oz	0
Diet Coke	44 oz	0
Hi-C Fruit Punch	12 oz	116

FOOD	PORTION	CALS
Hi-C Fruit Punch	44 oz	452
Lemonade	12 oz	126
Lemonade	44 oz	488
Sprite	44 oz	430
Sprite	12 oz	110
CHILDREN'S MENU SELECTIONS		
Kids Fries	1 serv	249
Kids Tenders	2 pieces	240
Sandwich Chicken	1	205
Sandwich Ham	1	183
Sandwich Steak	1	210
Sandwich Turkey	1	183
MAIN MENU SELECTIONS		
12 Inch Sandwich Grand Cobbler	1	680
12 Inch Sandwich Grand Escape	1	776
12 Inch Sandwich Grandest Chicken	1	770
12 Inch Sandwich Great Escape	1	776
12 Inch Sandwich Hambrosia	1	684
12 Inch Sandwich Ragin' Cajun	1	756
12 Inch Sandwich Turkey Club	1	675
12 Inch Sandwich Vegetarian	1	524
12 Inch Sandwich Wild West BBQ	1	841
7 Inch Sandwich Grand Cobbler	1	380
7 Inch Sandwich Grand Escape	1	435
7 Inch Sandwich Grandest Chicken	1	425
7 Inch Sandwich Great Escape	1	428
7 Inch Sandwich Hambrosia	1	382
7 Inch Sandwich Ragin' Cajun	1	418
7 Inch Sandwich Turkey Club	1	390
7 Inch Sandwich Vegetarian	1	302
7 Inch Sandwich Wild West BBQ	1	469
Fries	1 serv (32 oz)	996
Fries	1 serv (12 oz)	498
Fries Loaded Bacon & Cheddar	1 serv	905
Fries Loaded Ranch & Bacon	1 serv	1044
Smashed Potatoes Loaded Bacon & Cheddar	1 serv	636
Smashed Potatoes Loaded Ranch & Bacon	1 serv	692
Smashed Potatoes Plain	1 serv	246
Smashed Potatoes w/ Chicken	1 serv	318
Smashed Potatoes w/ Ham	1 serv	336

FOOD	PORTION	CALS
Smashed Potatoes w/ Steak	1 serv	391
Smashed Potatoes w/ Turkey	1 serv	336
SALAD DRESSINGS AND TOPPINGS		
American Cheese	1 slice	101
Bacon	1 serv (1 oz)	80
BBQ Sauce	1 serv (1 oz)	40
Black Olives	1 serv (1 oz)	32
Brown Mustard	1 serv (1 oz)	0
Cheddar Cheese	1 slice	116
Dressing Italian	1 serv (0.5 oz)	51
Dressing Ranch	1 serv (0.5 oz)	83
Lettuce	1 serv (1 oz)	2
Margarine	1 serv (1 oz)	203
Mayonnaise	1 serv (1 oz)	101
Peppers Jalapeno	1 serv (1.5 oz)	11
Peppers Mild	1 serv (1.5 oz)	11
Provolone Cheese	1 slice	80
Sour Cream	1 serv (1 oz)	61
Swiss Cheese	1 slice	100
Tomatoes	1 serv (2 oz)	24
SALADS		
Grilled Salad w/ Chicken	1 serv	175
Grilled Salad w/ Ham	1 serv	130
Grilled Salad w/ Steak	1 serv	185
Grilled Salad w/ Turkey	1 serv	130
Side	1 serv	40

SUBWAY
BEVERAGES

FOOD	PORTION	CALS
Fruizle Smoothie Berry Lishus	1 sm (13 oz)	113
Fruizle Smoothie Berry Lishus w/ Banana	1 sm (17 oz)	221
Fruizle Smoothie Peach Pizazz	1 sm (12 oz)	103
Fruizle Smoothie Pineapple Delight w/ Banana	1 sm (17 oz)	241
Fruizle Smoothie Pineapple Delite	1 sm (13 oz)	133
Fruizle Smoothie Sunrise Refresher	1 sm (12 oz)	119
COOKIES		
Chocolate Chip	1	215
Chocolate Chunk	1	217
Double Chocolate	1	209

FOOD	PORTION	CALS
M&M	1	215
Oatmeal Raisin	1	210
Peanut Butter	1	221
Sugar	1	227
White Macadamia Nut	1	221
SALAD DRESSINGS		
Fat Free French	1 serv (2 oz)	70
Fat Free Italian	1 serv (2 oz)	20
Fat Free Ranch	1 serv (2 oz)	60
SALADS		
BMT	1 serv	275
Cold Cut Trio	1 serv	234
Ham	1 serv	112
Meatball	1 serv	320
Roast Beef	1 serv	117
Roasted Chicken Breast	1 serv	130
Seafood & Crab	1 serv	197
Steak & Cheese	1 serv	181
Subway Club	1 serv	146
Subway Melt	1 serv	203
Tuna	1 serv	238
Turkey Breast	1 serv	105
Turkey Breast & Ham	1 serv	117
Veggie Delight	1 serv	50
SANDWICHES		
6 Inch Steak & Cheese	1	362
6 Inch Sub BMT	1	456
6 Inch Sub Cold Cut Trio	1	415
6 Inch Sub Ham	1	261
6 Inch Sub Meatball	1	501
6 Inch Sub Roast Beef	1	267
6 Inch Sub Roasted Chicken Breast	1	291
6 Inch Sub Seafood & Crab	1	378
6 Inch Sub Subway Club	1	296
6 Inch Sub Tuna	1	419
6 Inch Sub Turkey Breast	1	254
6 Inch Sub Turkey Breast & Ham	1	267
6 Inch Sub Veggie Delight	1	200
6 Inch Subway Melt	1	384

FOOD	PORTION	CALS
American Cheese Triangles	2	41
Asiago Caesar Sauce	1.5 tbsp	110
Bacon Strips	2	45
Breakfast Bacon & Egg	1	321
Breakfast Cheese & Egg	1	317
Breakfast Ham & Egg	1	338
Breakfast Western Egg	1	300
Cheddar Triangles	2	59
Cucumber Slices	3	2
Deli Ham	1	210
Deli Roast Beef	1	223
Deli Tuna	1	325
Deli Turkey Breast	1	215
Deli Style Roll	1	165
Dijon Horseradish	1.5 tbsp	91
Dijon Horseradish Melt	6 inch	465
Fat Free Red Wine Vinaigrette	1.5 tbsp	29
Fat Free Sweet Onion	1.5 tbsp	38
Green Pepper Strips	3 (0.2 oz)	2
Hearty Italian Bread	6 inch	207
Honey Mustard	1.5 tbsp	28
Honey Mustard Ham	6 inch	311
Honey Oat Bread	6 inch	249
Italian Bread	6 inch	178
Lettuce	1 serv (0.7 oz)	3
Mayonnaise	1 tbsp	111
Mayonnaise Light	1 tbsp	46
Moneterey Cheddar Bread	6 inch	235
Mustard	2 tsp	7
Olive Oil Blend	1 tsp	45
Olive Rings	3 (3 g)	3
Onions	1 serv (0.5 oz)	5
Parmesan Oregano Bread	6 inch	211
Pepperjack Cheese Triangles	2	40
Pickle Chips	3 pieces (0.3 oz)	1
Provolone Circles	2 halves	51
Red Wine Vinaigrette Club	6 inch	350
Roasted Garlic Bread	6 inch	225
Sourdough Bread	6 inch	208
Southwest Sauce	1.5 tbsp	86

FOOD	PORTION	CALS
Southwest Turkey Bacon	6 inch	407
Sweet Onion Chicken Teriyaki	6 inch	374
Swiss Triangles	2	53
Tomato Slices	3 (1.2 oz)	7
Vinegar	1 tsp	1
Wheat Sub	6 inch	186
Wrap Chicken Bacon Ranch w/ Swiss	1	480
Wrap Turkey Bacon Melt	1	430
SOUPS		
Black Bean	1 cup	180
Brown & Wild Rice w/ Chicken	1 cup	190
Cheese w/ Ham & Bacon	1 cup	230
Chicken & Dumplings	1 cup	130
Cream Of Broccoli	1 cup	130
Cream Of Potato w/ Bacon	1 cup	210
Golden Broccoli Cheese	1 cup	180
Hearty Chili Beef	1 cup	250
Minestrone	1 cup	70
New England Clam Chowder	1 cup	140
Potato Cheese Chowder	1 cup	210
Roasted Chicken Noodle	1 cup	90
Tomato Bisque	1 cup	90
Vegetable Beef	1 cup	90
TACO BELL		
Bean Burrito	1	370
Border Bowl Zesty Chicken	1 serv	730
Border Bowl Zesty Chicken w/o Dressing	1 serv	500
Burrito 7 Layer	1	530
Burrito Chili Cheese	1	390
Burrito Grilled Chicken	1	680
Burrito Spicy Chicken	1	430
Burrito Supreme Beef	1	440
Burrito ¼ Lb Bean Especial	1	600
Burrito ½ Lb Beef & Potato	1	530
Burrito ½ Lb Combo Beef	1	470
Burrito Fiesta Chicken	1	370
Burrito Fiesta Steak	1	370
Burrito Supreme Chicken	1	410
Burrito Supreme Steak	1	420

FOOD	PORTION	CALS
Chalupa Baja Beef	1	430
Chalupa Baja Chicken	1	400
Chalupa Baja Steak	1	400
Chalupa Nacho Cheese Beef	1	380
Chalupa Nacho Cheese Chicken	1	350
Chalupa Nacho Cheese Steak	1	350
Chalupa Supreme Beef	1	390
Chalupa Supreme Chicken	1	370
Chalupa Supreme Steak	1	370
Cheesy Fiesta Potatoes	1 serv	280
Cinnamon Twists	1 serv	160
Empanada Caramel Apple	1	290
Enchirito Beef	1	380
Enchirito Chicken	1	350
Enchirito Steak	1	360
Express Taco Salad	1 serv	630
Express Taco Salad w/o Chips	1 serv	410
Fiesta Taco Salad	1 serv	870
Fiesta Taco Salad w/o Shell	1 serv	500
Gordita Baja Beef	1	350
Gordita Baja Chicken	1	320
Gordita Baja Steak	1	320
Gordita Nacho Cheese Beef	1	300
Gordita Nacho Cheese Chicken	1	270
Gordita Nacho Cheese Steak	1	270
Gordita Supreme Beef	1	310
Gordita Supreme Chicken	1	290
Gordita Supreme Steak	1	280
Mexican Pizza	1 serv	550
Mexican Rice	1 serv	210
MexiMelt	1 serv	290
Nacho Supreme	1 serv	450
Nachos	1 serv	320
Nachos Bellgrande	1 serv	780
Pintos 'n Cheese	1 serv	180
Quesadilla Cheese	1 serv	490
Quesadilla Chicken	1	540
Quesadilla Steak	1	540
Soft Taco Beef	1	210
Soft Taco Grande	1	450

FOOD	PORTION	CALS
Soft Taco Grilled Steak	1	280
Soft Taco Ranchero Chicken	1	270
Soft Taco Supreme Beef	1	260
Southwest Steak Bowl	1 serv	700
Taco	1	170
Taco Double Decker	1	340
Taco Spicy Chicken	1	180
Taco Supreme	1	220
Taco Supreme Double Decker	1	380
Tostada	1	250

TACO CABANA

FOOD	PORTION	CALS
Black Beans	1 serv (4 oz)	111
Borracho Beans	1 serv (4 oz)	108
Breakfast Taco Bacon & Egg	1	246
Breakfast Taco Barbacoa	1	307
Breakfast Taco Chorizo & Egg	1	248
Breakfast Taco Potato & Egg	1	234
Burrito Bean & Cheese	1	710
Burrito Beef	1	653
Burrito Black Bean	1	559
Burrito Chicken	1	665
Calabacita	1 serv (4 oz)	78
Chips	1 serv (2 oz)	285
Elotes	1	220
Fajitas Beef	1 serv (4 oz)	245
Fajitas Chicken Dark	1 serv (4 oz)	236
Fajitas Chicken White	1 serv (4 oz)	191
Grilled Chicken Dark	1 serv (4.5 oz)	298
Grilled Chicken Dark No Skin	1 serv (3.4 oz)	170
Grilled Chicken White	1 serv (5 oz)	295
Grilled Chicken White No Skin	1 serv (3.8 oz)	167
Guacamole	1 serv (1 oz)	48
Queso	1 serv (3 oz)	184
Refried Beans	1 serv (4 oz)	171
Sour Cream	1 serv (1 oz)	57
Spanish Rice	1 serv (4 oz)	181
Taco Bean & Cheese	1	292
Taco Black Bean	1	216
Taco Carne Guisada	1	202

FOOD	PORTION	CALS
Taco Crispy Beef	1	148
Taco Soft Chicken	1	217
Tortilla Corn	1 6-inch	70
Tortilla Flour	1 6-inch	129
Tortilla Soup	1 lg	371
Tortilla Soup	1 sm	249

TACO JOHN'S
DESSERTS

FOOD	PORTION	CALS
Apple Grande	1 serv	240
Choco Taco	1 serv	300
Churro	1 serv	230
Cinnamon Mini Swirl	1 piece	10

MAIN MENU SELECTIONS

FOOD	PORTION	CALS
Burrito Bean	1	380
Burrito Beefy	1	430
Burrito Chicken & Potato	1	460
Burrito Combination	1	400
Burrito Meat & Potato	1	490
Burrito Super	1	450
Crispy Taco	1 serv	180
Mexican Rice	1 serv	250
Nachos	1 serv	380
Potato Oles	1 sm	440
Potato Oles	1 sm	440
Potato Oles	1 lg	790
Potato Oles Bravo	1 serv	580
Potato Oles Super	1 serv	980
Potato Oles w/ Nacho Cheese	1 serv	550
Quesadilla Cheese	1	480
Quesadilla Chicken	1	540
Refried Beans	1 serv	400
Sierra Taco Beef	1	430
Sierra Taco Chicken	1	390
Softshell Taco	1	220
Softshell Taco Chicken	1	190
Super Nachos	1 serv	830
Super Nachos Chicken	1 serv	780
Taco Bravo	1 serv	340

FOOD	PORTION	CALS
Taco Burger	1	280
Texas Chili	1 serv	270
SALAD DRESSINGS AND TOPPINGS		
Bacon Ranch Dressing	1 serv (3 oz)	250
Barbecue Sauce	1 serv (2 oz)	70
Chipotle Cream Sauce	1 serv (3 oz)	450
Creamy Italian Dressing	1 serv (3 oz)	260
Guacamole	1 serv (2 oz)	90
Hot Sauce	1 serv (1 oz)	5
House Dressing	1 serv (3 oz)	140
Jalapenos	1 serv (2 oz)	15
Mild Sauce	1 serv (1 oz)	5
Nacho Cheese	1 serv (3 oz)	120
Pico De Gallo	1 serv (2 oz)	15
Ranch Dressing	1 serv (3 oz)	280
Salsa	1 serv (2 oz)	20
Sour Cream	1 serv (2 oz)	120
Super Hot Sauce	1 serv (1 oz)	10
SALADS		
Chicken Festiva w/o Dressing	1 serv	400
Chicken Taco w/o Dressing	1	530
Side w/o Dressing	1 serv	80
Taco w/o Dressing	1 serv	580
TACOTIME		
DESSERTS		
Cinnamon Crustos	1 serv	373
Fruit Filled Empanada	1 serv	250
MAIN MENU SELECTIONS		
Burrito Beef Bean & Cheese	1 serv	617
Burrito Casita	1 serv	647
Burrito Chicken & Black Bean	1 serv	400
Burrito Chicken BLT	1 serv	580
Burrito Crisp Bean	1 serv	427
Burrito Crisp Chicken	1	422
Burrito Crisp Meat	1 serv	552
Burrito Soft Bean	1	380
Burrito Soft Meat	1 serv	491
Burrito Veggie	1 serv	491
Burrito Big Juan Beef	1 serv	640

FOOD	PORTION	CALS
Burrito Big Juan Chicken	1 serv	620
Cheddar Fries	1 lg	704
Cheddar Fries	1 sm	352
Cheddar Melt	1 serv	205
Mexi-Fries	1 lg	532
Mexi-Fries	1 sm	266
Mexi-Rice	1 serv	159
Nachos	1 serv	680
Nachos Deluxe	1 serv	1048
Refritos Cheese Sauce Chips	1 serv	326
Stuffed Fries	1 lg	990
Stuffed Fries	1 sm	490
Taco Cheeseburger	1	633
Taco Crisp	1	295
Taco Soft	1 serv	316
Taco Soft ½ lb	1 serv	512
Taco Soft ½ lb Chicken	1 serv	387
Taco Super Soft	1 serv	510
SALAD DRESSINGS AND TOPPINGS		
1000 Island Dressing	1 serv (1 oz)	120
Green Sauce	1 serv (1 oz)	5
Original Hot Sauce	1 serv (1 oz)	10
Salsa Fresca	1 serv (1 oz)	65
SALADS		
Chicken Fiesta	1 serv	390
Taco	1 reg	479
Taco Salad Chicken	1 serv	370
Tostada	1 serv	628

TASTI D-LITE

Vanilla	1 sm (4 oz)	40

TGI FRIDAY'S

Sizzling Chicken & Broccoli	1 serv	700
Sizzling NY Strip Steak w/ Blue Cheese & Broccoli	1 serv	684

TIM HORTONS
BAGELS AND CREAM CHEESE

Blueberry	1	200
Cinnamon Raisin	1	300
Cream Cheese Light	1.5 oz	90

FOOD	PORTION	CALS
Cream Cheese Plain	1.5 oz	140
Everything	1	300
Multigrain	1	300
Onion	1	295
Plain	1	290
Poppy Seed	1	300
Sesame Seed	1	300
Whole Wheat & Honey	1	300
BAKED SELECTIONS		
Biscuit Southern Country Cranberry	1	470
Biscuit Southern Country Raspberry	1	470
Cake Black Forest	1 serv	500
Cake Celebration	1 serv	500
Cake Chocolot Fantasy	1 serv	420
Cake Shadow	1 serv	430
Cookie Chocolate Chip	1	150
Cookie Macaroon	1	140
Cookie Oatcakes	1	190
Cookie Oatmeal Raisin	1	150
Cookie Peanut Butter	1	170
Cookie Peanut Butter Chocolate Chunk	1	170
Croissant Butter	1	210
Croissant Cheese	1	240
Danish Cherry Cheese	1	380
Donut Apple Fritter	1	300
Donut Chocolate Dip	1	230
Donut Chocolate Glazed	1	360
Donut Dutchie	1	280
Donut Honey Dip	1	230
Donut Maple Dip	1	250
Donut Old Fashion Glazed	1	270
Donut Old Fashion Plain	1	220
Donut Sour Cream Plain	1	280
Donut Sugar Twist	1	230
Donut Walnut Crunch	1	320
Donut Filled Angel Cream	1	280
Donut Filled Blueberry	1	220
Donut Filled Boston Cream	1	230
Donut Filled Canadian Maple	1	230
Donut Filled Strawberry	1	220

OOD	PORTION	CALS
Donuts Honey Stick	1	280
Muffin Blueberry Bran	1	300
Muffin Carrot Whole Wheat	1	410
Muffin Chocolate Chip	1	390
Muffin Low Fat Carrot	1	260
Muffin Low Fat Cranberry	1	260
Muffin Low Fat Honey	1	290
Muffin Oatbran Carrot 'n Raisin	1	340
Muffin Oatbran 'n Apple	1	350
Muffin Oatmeal Raisin	1	430
Muffin Raisin Bran	1	380
Muffin Wild Blueberry	1	330
Pie Apple	1 serv	540
Pie Banana Cream	1 serv	440
Pie Cherry	1 serv	570
Pie Chocolate Cream	1 serv	490
Tart Fresh Strawberry	1 serv	220
Tart Raisin Butter	1 serv	330
Tea Biscuit Plain	1	220
Tea Biscuit Raisin	1	250
Timbits Chocolate Glazed	1	70
Timbits Dutchie	1	60
Timbits Filled Banana Cream	1	45
Timbits Filled Lemon	1	50
Timbits Filled Spiced Apple	1	80
Timbits Filled Strawberry	1	50
Timbits Honey Dip	1	50
Timbits Old Fashion Plain	1	45
BEVERAGES		
Apple Juice	1 (9 oz)	140
Cafe Mocha	1 (10 oz)	250
Cappuccino English Toffee	1 (10 oz)	130
Cappuccino French Vanilla	1 (10 oz)	130
Cappuccino Iced	1 (16 oz)	430
Chocolate Milk	1 (14 oz)	280
Coffee Decaffeinated + Sugar & Cream	1 (10 oz)	80
Coffee + Sugar & Cream	1 (10 oz)	80
Coke	1 (14 oz)	170
Diet Coke	1 (14 oz)	1
Fruit Punch	1 (10 oz)	150

FOOD	PORTION	CALS
Hot Chocolate	1 (10 oz)	200
Iced Tea	1 (14 oz)	130
Milk 2%	1 (14 oz)	210
Orange Juice	1 (10 oz)	140
Sprite	1 (14 oz)	160
Tea + Sugar & Milk	1 (10 oz)	45
SANDWICHES		
Albacore Tuna Salad	1 serv	350
Black Forest Ham & Swiss	1 serv	640
Chunky Chicken Salad	1 serv	380
Fireside Roast Beef	1 serv	470
Garden Vegetable	1 serv	460
Harvest Turkey Breast	1 serv	470
SOUPS		
Barley & Wild Rice	1 serv	120
Chicken Noodle	1 serv	100
Chili	1 serv	320
Cream Of Broccoli	1 serv	190
Cream of Mushroom	1 serv	195
Hearty Vegetable	1 serv	130
Minestrone	1 serv	125
Potato Bacon	1 serv	195
Vegetable Beef Barley	1 serv	110

TJ CINNAMONS

Cinnachips	1 bag (10 oz)	1130
Cinnamon Twist	1	260
Coffee Black	1 (12 oz)	0
Mocha Chill w/ Whipped Cream	1 (12.5 oz)	310
Mocha Chill w/o Whipped Cream	1 (12.5 oz)	260
Original Roll w/o Icing	1	500
Original Roll w/ Cream Cheese Icing	1	651
Pecan Sticky Roll	1	690

TOGO'S
SALAD DRESSINGS

1000 Island	1 serv (2.3 oz)	231
Caesar	1 serv (2.3 oz)	241
Oriental	1 serv (2.3 oz)	221
Ranch	1 serv (2.3 oz)	321
Reduced Calorie Italian	1 serv (2.3 oz)	60

FOOD	PORTION	CALS
Reduced Calorie Ranch	1 serv (2.3 oz)	191
SALADS		
Caesar Salad	1 serv	471
Garden Salad	1 serv	256
Oriental Salad	1 serv	499
Potato Salad	1 serv (4 oz)	215
Taco Salad	1 serv	943
SANDWICHES		
Albacore Tuna	1 sm	701
Avocado & Turkey	1 sm	675
Avocado & Alfalfa Sprouts	1 sm	637
Bar-B-Q Beef	1 sm	724
California Roasted Chicken	1 sm	510
Cheese Swiss American Provolone	1 sm	859
Chunky Chicken Salad	1 sm	636
Egg Salad w/ Cheese	1 sm	728
Ham & Cheese	1 sm	661
Hot Pastrami	1 sm	705
Hummus	1 sm	668
Italian Salami & Cheese	1 sm	770
Italian Salami Capicolla Mortadella Cotto & Provolone	1 sm	736
Meatballs w/ Pizza Sauce & Parmesan	1 sm	707
Pastrami Reuben	1 sm	875
Roast Beef Hot & Cold	1 sm	552
Turkey & Cranberry	1 sm	623
Turkey & Bacon Club	1 sm	667
Turkey & Cheese	1 sm	638
Turkey & Ham w/ Cheese	1 sm	670
WENDY'S		
BEVERAGES		
Cola	11 oz	130
Diet Cola	11 oz	0
Frosty Junior	6 oz	170
Frosty Medium	16 oz	440
Frosty Small	12 oz	330
Lemon-Lime Soda	11 oz	130
CHILDREN'S MENU SELECTIONS		
French Fries Kid's Meal	1 serv (3.2 oz)	270

FOOD	PORTION	CALS
Kid's Meal Cheeseburger	1 (4.2 oz)	310
Kid's Meal Hamburger	1 (3.9 oz)	270
Kids'Meal Chicken Nuggets	4 pieces (2.1 oz)	190
MAIN MENU SELECTIONS		
¼ lb Hamburger Patty	1 (2.6 oz)	200
2 oz Hamburger Patty	1 (1.3 oz)	100
American Cheese	1 slice (0.6 oz)	70
American Cheese Jr.	1 slice (0.4 oz)	45
Bacon	1 strip (4 g)	20
Big Bacon Classic	1 (9.9 oz)	580
Breaded Chicken Fillet	1 (3.5 oz)	230
Cheddar Shredded	2 tbsp (0.6 oz)	70
Chicken Breast Fillet Sandwich	1 (7.3 oz)	430
Chicken Club Sandwich	1 (7.6 oz)	470
Chicken Nuggets	5 pieces (2.6 oz)	230
Chili	1 lg (12 oz)	310
Chili	1 sm (8 oz)	210
Classic Single w/ Everything	1 (7.6 oz)	410
French Fries	1 Biggie (5.6 oz)	470
French Fries	1 Great Biggie (6.7 oz)	570
French Fries	1 med (5 oz)	420
Grilled Chicken Fillet	1 (2.9 oz)	110
Grilled Chicken Sandwich	1 (6.6 oz)	300
Honey Mustard Reduced Calorie	1 tsp (7 g)	25
Hot Stuffed Baked Potato Bacon & Cheese	1 (12.6 oz)	530
Hot Stuffed Baked Potato Broccoli & Cheese	1 (14.4 oz)	470
Hot Stuffed Baked Potato Plain	1 (10 oz)	310
Jr. Bacon Cheeseburger	1 (5.8 oz)	380
Jr. Cheeseburger	1 (4.5 oz)	310
Jr. Cheeseburger Deluxe	1 (6.3 oz)	360
Kaiser Bun	1 (2.5 oz)	200
Ketchup	1 tsp (7 g)	10
Lettuce	1 leaf (0.5 oz)	0
Mayonnaise	1 ½ tsp (9 g)	30
Mustard	½ tsp (5 g)	5
Nuggets Sauce Barbeque	1 pkg (1 oz)	45
Nuggets Sauce Honey Mustard	1 pkg (1 oz)	130
Nuggets Sauce Sweet & Sour	1 pkg (1 oz)	50
Onion	4 rings (0.5 oz)	5
Pickles	4 slices (0.4 oz)	0

FOOD	PORTION	CALS
Saltines	2 (0.2 oz)	25
Sandwich Bun	1 (2 oz)	160
Spicy Chicken Fillet	1 (3.6 oz)	210
Spicy Chicken Sandwich	1 (7.5 oz)	410
Tomatoes	1 slice (0.9 oz)	5
Whipped Margarine	1 pkg (0.5 oz)	70
SALAD DRESSINGS		
Blue Cheese	1 pkg (2 oz)	360
French	1 pkg (2 oz)	250
Hidden Valley Ranch	1 pkg (2 oz)	200
Hidden Valley Ranch Reduced Fat Reduced Calorie	1 pkg (2 oz)	120
Italian Reduced Fat Reduced Calorie	1 pkg (2 oz)	80
Italian Caesar	1 pkg (1.5 oz)	230
Thousand Island	1 pkg (2 oz)	260
SALADS		
Ceasar Side Salad w/o Dressing	1 (3.2 oz)	110
Deluxe Garden Salad w/o Dressing	1 (9.5 oz)	110
Grilled Chicken Salad w/o Dressing	1 (11.9 oz)	200
Side Salad w/o Dressing	1 (5.4 oz)	60
Soft Breadstick	1 (1.5 oz)	130
Taco Chips	15 (1.5 oz)	210
Taco Salad w/o Dressing	1 (16.4 oz)	380
WETZEL'S PRETZELS		
Original w/ Butter	1	320
Original w/o Butter	1	280
WHATABURGER		
BAKED SELECTIONS		
Cinnamon Roll	1	860
BEVERAGES		
Cherry Coke	1 lg (44 oz)	343
Cherry Coke	1 sm (20 oz)	169
Coca Cola Classic	1 lg (44 oz)	327
Coca Cola Classic	1 sm (20 oz)	161
Coffee	1 sm (8 oz)	30
Creamer Nondairy	1 pkg	15
Diet Coke	1 lg (44 oz)	0
Diet Coke	1 sm (20 oz)	0
Diet Dr Pepper	1 sm (20 oz)	0

FOOD	PORTION	CALS
Dr Pepper	1 sm (20 oz)	147
Fanta Strawberry	1 sm (20 oz)	177
Fanta Strawberry	1 lg (44 oz)	360
Fruit Drink	1 lg (44 oz)	244
Fruit Drink	1 sm (20 oz)	121
Lemonade	1 lg (44 oz)	320
Lemonade	1 sm (20 oz)	158
Lipton Iced Tea	1 med	0
Milk 2%	8 oz	120
Orange Juice	1 serv	140
Orange Soda	1 sm (20 oz)	173
Orange Soda	1 lg (44 oz)	350
Shake Chocolate	1 sm (20 oz)	616
Shake Strawberry	1 sm (20 oz)	620
Shake Vanilla	1 sm (20 oz)	559
Sprite	1 lg (44 oz)	320
Sprite	1 sm	158
CHILDREN'S MENU SELECTIONS		
Kid's Justaburger	1	306
Kid's Chicken Strips	1 serv	382
MAIN MENU SELECTIONS		
Biscuit Buttermilk	1	300
Biscuit w/ Bacon	1	375
Biscuit w/ Bacon Egg & Cheese	1	476
Biscuit w/ Egg & Cheese	1	446
Biscuit w/ Sausage	1	517
Biscuit w/ Sausage Egg & Cheese	1	663
Biscuit w/ Sausage Gravy	1	491
Breakfast Platter w/ Bacon	1 serv	698
Breakfast Platter w/ Sausage	1 serv	840
Breakfast On A Bun Ranchero w/ Bacon	1	404
Breakfast On A Bun Ranchero w/ Sausage	1	546
Breakfast On A Bun w/ Bacon	1	398
Breakfast On A Bun w/ Sausage	1	540
Chicken Strips	2	382
Croutons Njoy Seasoned	1 pkg	35
French Fries	1 lg	514
French Fries	1 sm	257
Grape Jelly	1 pkg	35
Gravy White Peppered	1 serv	53

FOOD	PORTION	CALS
Hashbrown Sticks	1 serv	140
Honey	1 pkg	25
Hot Apple Pie	1	240
Justaburger	1	309
Ketchup	1 pkg	40
Margarine	1 pkg	23
Onion Rings	1 med	201
Pancake Syrup	1 pkg	120
Pancakes	1 serv	614
Pancakes w/ Bacon	1 serv	689
Pancakes w/ Sausage	1 serv	831
Picante Sauce	1 serv	5
Sandwich Egg	1	323
Sandwich Grilled Chicken	1	473
Sandwich Grilled Chicken Not Bun	1	190
Sandwich Whatacatch	1	473
Sandwich Whatachick'n	1	523
Strawberry Jam	1 pkg	40
Taquito Bacon & Egg	1	387
Taquito Potato & Egg	1	382
Taquito Sausage & Egg	1	389
Taquito w/ Bacon Egg & Cheese	1	432
Taquito w/ Potato Egg & Cheese	1	427
Taquito w/ Sausage Egg & Cheese	1	434
Texas Toast	1 serv	328
Whataburger	1	607
Whataburger Double Meat	1	857
Whataburger Double Meat No Bun	1	520
Whataburger Jr.	1	315
Whataburger No Bun	1	270
Whataburger Triple Meat	1	1107
Whataburger w/ Bacon & Cheese	1	810
Whatacatch	2 pieces	814
SALAD DRESSINGS		
Low Fat Ranch	1 pkg	66
Low Fat Vinaigrette	1 pkg	35
Ranch	1 pkg	310
Thousand Island	1 pkg	150
SALADS		
Chicken Strips	1 serv	419

FOOD	PORTION	CALS
Chicken Strips w/ Cheddar Cheese	1 serv	600
Chicken Strips w/ Cheddar Cheese & Bacon	1 serv	675
Garden Salad	1	49
Garden w/ Cheddar Cheese	1 serv	218
Garden w/ Cheddar Cheese & Bacon	1 serv	293
Grilled Chicken	1 serv	229
Grilled Chicken w/ Cheddar Cheese	1 serv	398
Grilled Chicken w/ Cheddar Cheese & Bacon	1 serv	473

WHITE CASTLE
BEVERAGES

FOOD	PORTION	CALS
Coca Cola	16 oz	200
Coffee Black	1 sm	6
Diet Coke	16 oz	0
Iced Tea	16 oz	90
Shake Chocolate	16 oz	250
Shake Vanilla	16 oz	260

MAIN MENU SELECTIONS

FOOD	PORTION	CALS
Bacon Cheeseburger	1	200
Cheese Sticks	3	250
Cheeseburger	1	160
Chicken Rings	6	210
Double Cheeseburger	1	290
Double Hamburger	1	240
French Fries	1 sm	115
Hamburger	1	140
Onion Rings	6	260
Sandwich Breakfast	1	340
Sandwich Chicken	1	190
Sandwich Chicken Ring	1	180
Sandwich Fish	1	180

WINCHELL'S DONUTS

FOOD	PORTION	CALS
Chocolate Bar	1	240
Chocolate Round	1	240
Chocolate Twist	1	240
Croissant	1	260
Glazed Round	1	230
Glazed Twist	1	230
Iced Chocolate	1	230
Traditional	1	215

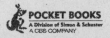
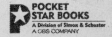